# Hearing Disorders: Clinical Research

# Hearing Disorders: Clinical Research

Editor: Sophie Silva

FOSTER ACADEMICS
www.fosteracademics.com

www.fosteracademics.com

FOSTER ACADEMICS

**Cataloging-in-Publication Data**

Hearing disorders : clinical research / edited by Sophie Silva.
p. cm.
Includes bibliographical references and index.
ISBN 978-1-63242-773-1
1. Hearing disorders. 2. Hearing disorders--Treatment. 3. Ear--Diseases--Treatment.
4. Deafness--Prevention. I. Silva, Sophie.
RF290 .H43 2019
617.8--dc23



Foster Academics,
118-35 Queens Blvd., Suite 400,
Forest Hills, NY 11375, USA

ISBN 978-1-63242-773-1 (Hardback)



Printed and bound in China.

# Contents

# Preface

Every book is initially just a concept; it takes months of research and hard work to give it the final shape in which the readers receive it. In its early stages, this book also went through rigorous reviewing. The notable contributions made by experts from across the globe were first molded into patterned chapters and then arranged in a sensibly sequential manner to bring out the best results.

Hearing disorders refer to the impairment in perceiving or processing auditory information. Hearing loss can be partial or complete, and may occur in one or both ears. Auditory processing disorder, hearing loss, tinnitus, endaural phenomena, hyperacusis and presbycusis are common hearing disorders. They may be acquired, inherited or caused due to perinatal problems and aging. Chronic ear infections can be a common cause of hearing loss. Syphilis and rubella infections during pregnancy can lead to hearing loss in children. Some cases of hearing loss can be addressed medically, while others are irreversible and therefore, permanent. When hearing loss occurs at a young age, it interferes with spoken language acquisition and development. Use of hearing aids, cochlear implants, sign language and subtitles can help individuals deal with this condition. Research aimed at the use of stem cell transplant and gene therapy for the regrowth of cochlear cells and nerve cells, and recovery of hearing loss is being actively explored. This book contains some path-breaking studies in the field of hearing disorders. It discusses the fundamentals as well as modern approaches in the management of hearing disorders and the recent researches in this domain. Researchers and students in this field will be assisted by this book.

It has been my immense pleasure to be a part of this project and to contribute my years of learning in such a meaningful form. I would like to take this opportunity to thank all the people who have been associated with the completion of this book at any step.

**Editor**

# Noise-Induced Hearing Loss in Korean Workers: Co-Exposure to Organic Solvents and Heavy Metals in Nationwide Industries

**Yoon-Hyeong Choi**[1], **KyooSang Kim**[2*¤]

**1** Department of Preventive Medicine, Gachon University Graduate School of Medicine, Incheon, Korea, **2** Occupational Safety and Health Research Institute, Korea Occupational Safety and Health Agency, Incheon, Korea

## Abstract

***Background:*** Noise exposure is a well-known contributor to work-related hearing loss. Recent biological evidence suggests that exposure to ototoxic chemicals such as organic solvents and heavy metals may be additional contributors to hearing loss. However, in industrial settings, it is difficult to determine the risks of hearing loss due to these chemicals in workplaces accompanied by excessive noise exposure. A few studies suggest that the effect of noise may be enhanced by ototoxic chemicals. Therefore, this study investigated whether co-exposure to organic solvents and/or heavy metals in the workplace modifies the risk of noise exposure on hearing loss in a background of excessive noise.

***Methods:*** We examined 30,072 workers nationwide in a wide range of industries from the Korea National Occupational Health Surveillance 2009. Data on industry-based exposure (e.g., occupational noise, heavy metals, and organic solvents) and subject-specific health outcomes (e.g., audiometric examination) were collected. Noise was measured as the daily 8-h time-weighted average level. Air conduction hearing thresholds were measured from 0.5 to 6 kHz, and pure-tone averages (PTA) (i.e., means of 2, 3, and 4 kHz) were computed.

***Results:*** In the multivariate linear model, PTA increment with occupational noise were 1.64-fold and 2.15-fold higher in individuals exposed to heavy metals and organic solvents than in unexposed individuals, respectively.

***Conclusion:*** This study provides nationwide evidence that co-exposure to heavy metals and/or organic solvents may exacerbate the effect of noise exposure on hearing loss in workplaces. These findings suggest that workers in industries dealing with heavy metals or organic solvents are susceptible to such risks.

**Editor:** Jonathan I. Matsui, Harvard University, United States of America

**Funding:** These authors have no support or funding to report.

**Competing Interests:** The authors have declared that no competing interests exist.

* E-mail: kyoosang@daum.net

¤ Current address: Department of Occupational Environmental Medicine, Seoul Medical Center, Seoul, Korea

## Introduction

Work-related hearing loss is a critical issue in workplace safety and health. The U.S. National Institute for Occupational Safety and Health (NIOSH) and the occupational safety and health community designated hearing loss as one of the 21 priority research areas in the 21st century [1]. Loud noise is a major risk factor for work-related hearing loss, and audiologists are well aware of the need for monitoring and protecting against noise in the workplace [2–4]. In fact, many countries have conducted surveillance and/or compensation programs to monitor workplace noise and identify occupational noise-induced hearing loss [5–8].

Evidence accumulated over recent decades suggests that exposure to neurotoxic chemicals is an additional contributor to occupational hearing loss. Some organic solvents, heavy metals, asphyxiants, and pesticides fall within this category and are widely used in many industries and occupations [9–11]. Organic solvents such as toluene ($C_7H_8$), styrene ($C_8H_8$), xylene ($C_8H_{10}$), isopropyl alcohol ($C_3H_8O$), and ethyl benzene ($C_8H_{10}$) have been widely studied for their ototoxicity. Indeed, animal experiments demonstrate sensorineural hearing loss with cochlear damage as a result of exposure to these chemicals [12–16]. Furthermore, several workplace studies suggest that such solvents are associated with an increased risk of hearing loss [17–22]. Heavy metals such as cadmium, lead, mercury, and manganese are reported to impair inner ear cells, leading to auditory function disorders in animal studies [23–27]. There is further evidence for their ototoxicity in human studies as well [28–30].

However, the effects of organic solvents and/or heavy metals on hearing loss in industrial settings are difficult to distinguish from the effect of noise [31]. In fact, many studies in workplaces involving exposure to both solvents and noise commonly assume noise to be the sole contributor to hearing loss; but, they could not observe the effects of solvents despite scientific plausibility that both noise and solvents have biological effects. A possible reason for the null findings of the ototoxic effects of solvents include diluted observation due to the dominant effect of noise; this is because workplaces using these chemicals are likely to be accompanied by excessive noise as well [32,33]. A few recent studies suggest that the effect of noise can be enhanced by ototoxic chemical exposure [34–38].

The Korea National Occupational Health Surveillance (KNOHS), also known as Korean Occupational Medical Examination Program [39], is a nationwide annual surveillance program designed to monitor problematic industries and their workers, including work-related hearing loss. The program includes audiometric testing, industrial-based noise measurement, and assessment of exposure to ototoxic chemicals (e.g., organic solvents and heavy metals).

Thus, the present study estimated the national burdens of occupational noise exposure on work-related hearing loss using nationwide data from various industries from the KNOHS 2009 and evaluated the hypothesis that co-exposure to heavy metals and/or organic solvents in the workplace modifies the risk of occupational noise exposure on hearing loss in a background of excessive noise.

## Methods

### Study population

The final study sample consisted of 30,072 employees aged 18 to 77 years registered in 1,935 industries from the KNOHS 2009; this program was established by the Ministry of Labor of Korea as part of a government program aimed at preventing and compensating for work-related hearing loss.

Data on industry-based exposure and subject-specific health outcomes were collected. The Occupational Safety and Health Research Institute (OSHRI) of the Korea Occupational Safety and Health Agency (KOSHA) compiled a list of all available industries registered with the Korea Ministry of Labor and administered the industries particularly in which the noise exposure level was ≥80 decibels of ambient noise (dBA). These industries were assigned to the KNOHS, which assessed noise exposure levels. All employees who have worked in these industries underwent audiometric examinations and interviews to obtain demographic and physical information. The initial sample included 300,741 participants for primary audiometric examination at limited frequencies (necessarily including 1 kHz) from the KNOHS 2009. From the initial sample, all employees who worked in the industries where the noise level was ≥85 dBA underwent an advanced audiometric examination at various frequencies.

For the present study, we selected participants who had measures in all available frequencies (i.e., 0.5, 1, 2, 3, 4, and 6 kHz); therefore, 64,974 subjects were eligible for inclusion in data analyses. We further excluded participants with missing information for covariate variables ($n = 33,782$), and additional participants were excluded for non-Korean ($n = 1,120$) (see Figure S1). The final analysis included 30,072 participants in the analysis.

### Ethics Statement

The KNOHS is a national dataset collected by the OSHRI that followed the Korean Occupational Safety and Health (OSH) Act [8]. The study protocol was approved by the Occupational Safety and Health Research Institute institutional review board, and written informed consent was provided by study participants.

### Occupational Noise Measures

For each industry, occupational noise exposure assessment was conducted at various onsite spots (1 to 2,109 spots depending on each industry's scale). Exposure was measured as a daily eight-hour time-weighted average (8HR TWA) using a sound level meter (SLM) and was based upon 5 dB exchange rate for calculating noise dose as a function of exposure time and level [40]. The mean noise value from these spot measurements for each industry was computed. All individuals who have worked in the industries with 8HR TWA ≥85 dBA (i.e., noisy industries) were selected to participate in an advanced audiometric examination component.

### Hearing Threshold Examination

An advanced audiometric examination was conducted at various frequencies in a silent room by health technicians trained by a KOSHA-certified audiologist. For standardized measurements, audiometric components, including an audiometer and headphones, and measurement environment followed the guidelines of the Korean Audiometric Quality Control Program [41]. Pure tone air conduction hearing thresholds were obtained for both ears at each frequency over intensity range of −10 to 120 dB and computed as a pure-tone average (PTA) of 2, 3, and 4 kHz following the definition of standard threshold shift of the Occupational Safety and Health Administration. Hearing loss was defined as PTA >25 dB in one or both ears. The details of audiometric examination have been described elsewhere [42]. Hearing thresholds at1 kHz were obtained only in a primary audiometric examination from an initial sampling stage and were not attained in advanced examination in a silent room by trained technicians.

### Ototoxic Chemical Exposures

Non-noise source exposures to organic chemicals and heavy metals were classified based on industries-database compiled by the OSHRI. The OSHRI administered a list of problematic industries exposed to occupational agents (i.e., organic chemicals and heavy metals) among all available industries registered with the Korea Ministry of Labor, similar to a list of problematic noisy industries. Each industry was classed as exposure or not to organic solvents and heavy metals, respectively. Organic solvent exposure was considered for toluene, isopropyl alcohol, and/or xylene (a mixture and individual elements); heavy metal exposure was considered for lead, cadmium, mercury, chrome, and/or manganese (a mixture). Exposure to a mixture was defined as exposure to one or more of the individual elements.

We modeled organic solvent exposure or heavy metal exposure as an exposure to a mixture, because workplaces are not solely exposed to any individual chemical but commonly exposed to a mixture. Instead, sensitivity analyses were examined in all individual organic solvents including toluene, isopropyl alcohol, and xylene. No data regarding individual types of heavy metals were available. Further details are available elsewhere (see File S1).

### Demographic and Potential Risk Variables

Data on demographic and potential risk variables were obtained through physical examinations and extensive interviews. Body mass index (BMI) was computed as weight in kilograms/height in meters squared. Hypertension was classified based on either systolic blood pressure ≥140 mmHg or diastolic blood pressure ≥ 90 mm Hg at the time of the examination.

### Statistical Analysis

All regression analyses began with univariate analyses to identify outliers and influential points. The statistically significant level was set as $P$ values less than 0.05. Linear regression was fit for the association of hearing thresholds in PTA and individual frequencies with occupational noise measures. To identify the influence of potential confounders, we developed a sequence of models — initially crude model; adjusted for age, age-squared, and sex; and further adjusted for BMI and hypertension. We also fit multivariate-adjusted linear regressions in subgroups stratified by age, sex, BMI, and hypertension as well as occupational exposures to organic solvents and heavy metals, in order to evaluate whether these factors modify the association of PTA with occupational noise exposure. Logistic regression was used to estimate odds ratio (ORs) for the hearing loss. All statistical analyses were performed using SAS (version 9.1) and R (2.13.1).

## Results

The KNOHS estimated that 64,974 Korean workers in 7,394 industries were exposed to a daily occupational noise ≥80 dB and that 77% of them had hearing loss (PTA > 25 dB in one or both ears) in 2009 (see Figure S1). Table 1 shows the characteristics of the 30,072 study participants, eligible for the analyses. Their mean ± standard deviation (SD) age was 44.4±9.3 years. Because hearing ability is strongly correlated with age, we computed age-adjusted means for hearing thresholds and other continuous variables. The age-adjusted mean PTA was 28.1±14.7 decibels hearing level (dBHL). The age-adjusted mean of occupational noise exposure was high at 88.6±5.3 dBA, which is unsurprising considering that participants were originally collected from the industries with problematic noise levels. Table 2 shows the occupational noise exposure levels by subject characteristics. Occupational noise exposure was higher for women, older workers, those more exposed to organic chemicals, those less exposed to heavy metals, and those with hypertension and a BMI <25 kg/m$^2$ (Table 2).

Table 3 presents the associations between occupational noise exposure and hearing thresholds on PTAs and at each frequency in covariate-adjusted models. In the crude model, occupational noise was significantly associated with elevated hearing thresholds at all frequencies and PTAs (Model A). After adjusting for age and sex, although the associations were attenuated over all frequencies and PTAs, their significance remained, except at 0.5 kHz (Model B). After further adjustment for BMI and hypertension, similar associations between occupational noise and increased hearing thresholds were observed (Model C). In the multivariate-adjusted Model C, the average increase in hearing thresholds in PTAs was 2.35 dBHL (95% confidence interval [CI], 2.05–2.64 dBHL) for an interquartile range (IQR) increase in occupational noise exposure. Further adjustment for occupational exposure to organic solvents and heavy metals did not alter the results (Model D). In all models, the largest rate increase in hearing thresholds with occupational noise exposure was observed at 3 kHz.

Table 4 shows the multivariate-adjusted associations of PTAs with occupational noise exposure in groups stratified according to participant status listed in Table 1. There was a significant increase in the associations of PTAs with occupational noise exposure with increasing age ($p_{interaction}$ = 0.004) and a marginally stronger association in women than in men ($p_{interaction}$ = 0.055).

We also evaluated whether the association between occupational noise exposure and hearing outcome is modified by co-exposure to ototoxic chemicals. Table 5 shows the multivariate-adjusted associations of PTA with occupational noise levels in groups stratified according to occupational organic solvent or heavy metal exposure. The PTA increment with the IQR increase in occupational noise was significantly higher in subjects exposed to organic solvents (versus non-exposed subjects, 4.43 dBHL [CI, 3.43–5.42] vs. 2.06 dBHL [CI, 1.75–2.37]) as well as in subjects exposed to heavy metals (vs. non-exposed subjects, 3.25 dBHL [CI, 2.58–3.92] vs. 1.98 dBHL [CI, 1.65–2.31]). When individual frequencies were examined, similar higher increments were observed in the organic solvent-exposed group at 3, 4, and 6 kHz as well as in the heavy metal-exposed group at 2 and 3 kHz compared to the respective non-exposed reference groups (see Table S1).

Logistic regression models revealed significantly greater odds of hearing loss with occupational noise levels in groups exposed to heavy metals and organic solvents than in the respective non-exposure reference groups (Table S2).

**Table 1.** General characteristics of study participants (N = 30,072[a]).

| Characteristic | Mean[b] ± SD |
|---|---|
| Occupational noise[c] | 88.6±5.3 |
| Age *(y)* | 44.4±9.3 |
| BMI *(kg/m$^2$)* | 23.6±3.0 |
| Sex [male; *n (%)*] | 27,857 (92.6) |
| Hypertension [*n (%)*] | 4,873 (16.2) |
| Hearing Thresholds *(dBHL)* | |
| *PTA at 2, 3, 4 Khz*[d] | 28.1±14.7 |
| *0.5 kHz* | 15.6±11.1 |
| *1 kHz*[e] | 15.8±12.2 |
| *2 kHz* | 18.8±14.3 |
| *3 kHz* | 28.4±17.4 |
| *4 kHz* | 37.3±18.3 |
| *6 kHz* | 41.6±20.3 |
| Hearing Loss[f] *(PTA>25dBHL, %)* | 20461, 68% |

[a]Participants (N = 33,072) are the individuals having all interest variables in this study: advanced audiometric measurements, age, occupational noise, sex, BMI, and hypertension.
[b]Age-adjusted means were presented.
[c]Occupational noise (a daily 8-hour time weighted average level in each industry).
[d]PTA (pure tone average) of standard threshold at 2, 3, 4 kHz frequencies.
[e]Hearing thresholds at 1 kHz were obtained from primary audiometric tests.
[f]Hearing Loss (PTA at 2, 3, 4 KHz frequencies > 25 dBHL).
SD, standard deviation.

## Discussion

The present study of a nationwide working population demonstrates association of occupational noise exposure with poorer hearing outcomes, and that individuals working in industries that particularly involve exposure to organic solvents and/or heavy metals are susceptible to an increased risk of hearing loss due to occupational noise, suggesting noise–organic solvent interaction and noise–heavy metal interaction.

Work-related hearing loss is one of the most common occupational hazards [1]. Noise is a well-known contributing factor. Thus, many researchers suggest the need to control noise exposure in order to reduce the burden of work-related hearing loss. Although many countries have implemented national programs to monitor and control noise levels in various industries, it is difficult to reduce noise exposure in many industries. Therefore, identifying susceptibility-related factors in conjunction

**Table 2.** Means and 95% confidence intervals of occupational noise exposure by participants characteristics.

| Characteristic | No. | Occupational noise (dBA), mean (95% C.I.) | *p-value*[a] |
|---|---|---|---|
| Age *(year)* | | | <0.001 |
| *10–29* | 2356 | 85.8 (85.6–86.0) | |
| *30–39* | 6995 | 87.9 (87.8–88.1) | |
| *40–49* | 10062 | 89.2 (89.1–89.3) | |
| *≥50* | 10659 | 90.7 (90.6–90.8) | |
| Sex | | | <0.001 |
| *Male* | 27857 | 89.0 (89.0–89.1) | |
| *Female* | 2215 | 90.8 (90.5–91.0) | |
| Body mass index *(kg/m²)* | | | <0.001 |
| *<25* | 20991 | 89.3 (89.3–89.4) | |
| *≥25* | 9081 | 88.7 (88.6–88.8) | |
| Hypertension | | | <0.001 |
| *No* | 25199 | 89.1 (89.0–89.1) | |
| *Yes* | 4873 | 89.6 (89.5–89.8) | |
| *Occupational exposure to heavy metals* | | | <0.001 |
| *Non exposure* | 27382 | 89.4 (89.4–89.5) | |
| *Exposure* | 2690 | 86.1 (85.9–86.3) | |
| *Occupational exposure to organic solvents* | | | <0.001 |
| *Non exposure* | 22164 | 89.0 (88.9–89.0) | |
| *Exposure* | 7908 | 89.7 (89.6–89.8) | |

CI, confidence interval
[a]*t*-test for binominal groups and *trend-P* for ordinal categorical groups were used.

with the avoidance of noise (the major risk factor) is important for effectively preventing occupational noise-induced hearing loss.

Despite biological evidence of the ototoxicity of industrial chemicals, previous studies in occupational settings assume noise to be the sole contributor to hearing loss and observed little effects of ototoxic chemicals. The dominant effect of loud noise in workplaces may explain why such previous studies did not find effects of ototoxic chemicals. Interestingly, 2 recent studies in a general population [43,44] report adverse effects of lead and cadmium exposure on hearing outcomes not in the group exposed to higher noise levels, but only in those exposed to lower or mid-noise levels; these findings support the notion that the observed risk due to heavy metals may be diluted by the greater risk due to noise. In fact, consistent with previous studies, the present sensitivity analysis stratified according to noise levels revealed that organic solvent exposure adversely affected hearing thresholds in a group exposed to mid-noise levels but found no effect of organic solvent exposure in a group exposed to more noise (Table S3). This suggests that noise exposure is basically the greatest contributing factor to hearing loss while ototoxic chemicals may have additive effects in low-noise environments (that is, when there remains room for additional damage) and should be approached as a modifiable factor in workplaces involving regular high noise levels.

The current study provides evidence of effect modification by the exposure to heavy metals and organic solvents. Individuals exposed to heavy metals and organic solvents had a higher risk of hearing loss in relation to noise than unexposed individuals. The effect sizes of PTA increment with occupational noise were 1.64-fold and 2.15-fold higher in individuals exposed to heavy metals and organic solvents than in unexposed individuals, respectively (3.25 vs. 1.98 dBHL and 4.43 vs. 2.06 dBHL, respectively; see Table 5). Such effect modifications were roughly comparable to estimated effect modification by sex (1.36-fold higher in women [3.19 dBHL] than in men [2.23 dBHL]) and age over 20 years (1.36-fold higher in subjects aged ≥50 years [2.79 dBHL] than in subjects in their 30s [2.05 dBHL]; see Table 4).

Few studies have evaluated the effect modification (i.e., interaction) by organic solvents or heavy metals on the risk of occupational noise towards hearing outcomes. Several small-scale workplace studies compared noise-only exposure cases and noise- and solvent-exposure cases with a control group (i.e., non-exposure). One such study examining 1,117 employees in the yacht, shipping, paint and lacquer, plastics, and footwear industries found an increased risk of hearing loss by co-exposure to solvents; the odds ratios (ORs) of hearing loss were 3.8 and 6.7–21.5 in the cases of noise only, and noise and solvents (i.e., mixtures, styrene, *n*-hexane plus toluene, or styrene plus toluene) compared to a control group, respectively [36]. Another study analyzing the responses of 701 dockyard workers to a questionnaire on exposure revealed that the OR of hearing loss increased approximately 3-fold in the group exposed to only noise but almost 5-fold in the group exposed to both noise and solvent [35]. Although these studies do not provide evidence of multiplicative interaction by solvents on the risk of noise towards hearing loss, they are broadly compatible with the present findings. A previous study of case-control design supported a potential interaction between noise and toluene; the risk of hearing loss was 11 times greater for noise- and toluene-exposure group compared with unexposed group. The estimated effects were larger than the sums of the individual effects [noise-only (4 times) and solvent-only (5 times)] [45]. To our knowledge, this is the first epidemiologic study

**Table 3.** Effect estimates (95% CI) of hearing thresholds (dBHL) with IQR increment in occupational noise exposure (dBA).

| Frequency | Model A[a] | | Model B[b] | | Model C[c] | | Model D[d] | |
|---|---|---|---|---|---|---|---|---|
| | Per noise IQR[e] | | Per noise IQR[e] | | Per noise IQR[e] | | Per noise IQR[e] | |
| | Estimate | (95% CI) | Estimate | (95% CI) | Estimate | (95% CI) | Estimate | (95% CI) |
| PTA[f] | 6.06 | (5.73, 6.39)* | 2.33 | (2.03, 2.62)* | 2.35 | (2.05, 2.64)* | 2.24 | (1.94, 2.54)* |
| 0.5 kHz | 0.54 | (0.32, 0.76)* | −0.10 | (−0.33, 0.12) | −0.12 | (−0.35, 0.11) | −0.14 | (−0.37, 0.09) |
| 1 kHz | 1.97 | (1.73, 2.22)* | 0.62 | (0.37, 0.87)* | 0.64 | (0.39, 0.89)* | 0.64 | (0.39, 0.89)* |
| 2 kHz | 4.22 | (3.92, 4.52)* | 1.72 | (1.43, 2.01)* | 1.71 | (1.43, 2.00)* | 1.65 | (1.36, 1.95)* |
| 3 kHz | 7.21 | (6.82, 7.59)* | 2.97 | (2.63, 3.32)* | 3.01 | (2.66, 3.36)* | 2.88 | (2.52, 3.23)* |
| 4 kHz | 6.75 | (6.34, 7.16)* | 2.29 | (1.93, 2.65)* | 2.32 | (1.96, 2.69)* | 2.19 | (1.82, 2.56)* |
| 6 kHz | 6.90 | (6.45, 7.34)* | 2.67 | (2.26, 3.07)* | 2.70 | (2.29, 3.11)* | 2.54 | (2.13, 2.95)* |

CI, confidence interval.
[a]Model A was a crude model.
[b]Model B was adjusted for age, $age^2$, sex.
[c]Model C: Model B + further adjusted for BMI, hypertension.
[d]Model D: Model C + further adjusted for occupational exposures to organic solvents and heavy metals.
[e]Hearing Thresholds (dBHL) change per interquartile range (IQR) of occupational noise, 94.26 dBA - 84.74 dBA: 9.52 dBA.
[f]PTA (pure tone average at 2, 3, 4 kHz).
*$p<0.05$.

**Table 4.** Multivariate-adjusted effect estimates (95% CI) of hearing thresholds (dBHL) with IQR increment in occupational noise exposure (dBA), stratified according to participant status.

| | | Per noise IQR[a] | p-value for |
|---|---|---|---|
| **Stratification variable** | **No.** | **Estimate (95% CI)** | **interaction** |
| Overall | 30072 | 2.35 (2.05, 2.64)* | |
| Age *(year)* | | | *0.004* |
| *≤29* | 2356 | 0.93 (0.17, 1.68)* | |
| *30–39* | 6995 | 2.05 (1.51, 2.58)* | |
| *40–49* | 10062 | 2.10 (1.58, 2.62)* | |
| *≥50* | 10659 | 2.79 (2.23, 3.35)* | |
| Sex | | | *0.055* |
| *Male* | 27857 | 2.23 (1.92, 2.54)* | |
| *Female* | 2215 | 3.19 (2.28, 4.09)* | |
| BMI *(kg/m)* | | | *0.573* |
| *<25* | 20991 | 2.35 (1.99, 2.70)* | |
| *≥25* | 9081 | 2.31 (1.78, 2.84)* | |
| Hypertension | | | *0.375* |
| *No* | 25199 | 2.26 (1.93, 2.58)* | |
| *Yes* | 4873 | 2.61 (1.91, 3.31)* | |

Models were adjusted for age, age$^2$, sex, BMI, and hypertension, defined in Model C, Table 3.
CI, confidence interval.
[a]PTA (dBHL) change per interquartile range (IQR) of occupational noise, 94.26 dBA - 84.74 dBA: 9.52 dBA.
*$p<0.05$.

to evaluate effect modifications by heavy metals on the association between noise and hearing outcomes in the workplace, although there is existing evidence for a main effect of heavy metals on hearing outcomes [4,28,46]. Nevertheless, the precise mechanisms underlying the observed effect modifications by heavy metals and organic solvents remain unclear. Previous animal experiments show that solvents such as toluene, styrene, xylene, isopropyl alcohol, and ethyl benzene damage the cochlea (predominantly the supporting and outer hair cells) and provoke irreversible sensorineural hearing loss [12–16]. Furthermore, heavy metals such as cadmium, lead, mercury, and manganese induce the impairment (i.e., apoptosis and/or degeneration) of inner ear receptor cells, leading to auditory neuronal function disorders [23–27]. These findings provide a possible explanation that heavy metals and/or organic solvents condition the cochlea for damage triggered by oxidative stress produced by noise exposure. In addition, heavy metals and organic solvents are associated with the regulation of intracellular calcium homeostasis [47,48], and thus, they may play an additional role in auditory hair cell death.

In the present study, the associations between occupational noise and poorer hearing outcomes were stronger, particularly at middle-to-high frequencies. In addition, effect modifications by heavy metals and organic solvents on the associations between noise and hearing outcomes were strong at middle-to-high

**Table 5.** Multivariate-adjusted effect estimates (95% CI) of hearing thresholds (dBHL) with IQR increment in occupational noise exposure (dBA), stratified according to occupational exposure to ototoxic chemicals.

| **Stratification variable** | | Per noise IQR[a] | *p-value* for interaction |
|---|---|---|---|
| | **No.** | **Estimate (95% CI)** | |
| Overall | 30072 | 2.35 (2.05, 2.64)* | |
| Heavy metals | | | *<.001* |
| *Non exposure* | 22164 | 1.98 (1.65, 2.31)* | |
| *Exposure* | 7908 | 3.25 (2.58, 3.92)* | |
| Organic solvents | | | *<.001* |
| *Non exposure* | 27382 | 2.06 (1.75, 2.37)* | |
| *Exposure* | 2690 | 4.43 (3.43, 5.42)* | |

Models were adjusted for age, age$^2$, sex, BMI, and hypertension, defined in Model C, Table 3.
CI, confidence interval.
[a]PTA (dBHL) change per interquartile range (IQR) of occupational noise, 94.26 dBA - 84.74 dBA: 9.52 dBA.
*$p<0.05$.

frequencies. These frequencies are known to be sensitive to noise [49,50]; therefore, the present observations suggests that heavy metals and organic solvents act as effect modifiers regulating "noise"-induced hearing loss.

This study investigated the effect caused by mixtures of organic solvent(s) or heavy metal(s) on the association between noise and hearing. Indeed, models including an individual organic solvent (e.g., toluene, isopropyl alcohol, and xylene) confirmed similar effect modifications to findings from models including a mixture of organic solvents (data not shown). However, there are no data for different types of heavy metals. Occupational environments do not expose workers solely to any given chemical; instead, workers are commonly exposed to a mixture of chemicals. Furthermore, molecular mechanisms involved in toxicity due to individual solvents (also, metals) are similar. Therefore, this study did not consider individual effects separately.

This study used a hearing outcome with a PTAs of 2, 3, and 4 kHz on a "standard threshold shift" as defined by the Occupational Safety and Health Administration rather than the most commonly used method of PTA definition at speech frequencies (i.e., 0.5, 1, 2, and 4 kHz) as defined by the World Health Organization (WHO). This is because hearing data at 1 kHz were collected only through a primary audiometric test and subsequently without an advanced examination by trained technicians in a silent room. Instead, sensitivity analyses were examined at all individual frequencies including 0.5 and 1 kHz.

The main strength of this study is its large sample population, which included over 30,000 available subjects in industries with problematic noise selected from an initial sample drawn from all industries registered with the Korean Department of Labor. In addition, the present data support the on-site measurement of noise exposure in all industries. Therefore, the present results extend the partial observations of previous epidemiological studies on work-related hearing loss, which are limited to certain occupations and particularly by the difficulty in assessing exposure, to a nationwide scale including a wide range of occupations/industries. In turn, this enabled us to observe co-exposure to noise and ototoxic chemicals in the workplace.

This study has several limitations that should be considered. First, occupational organic solvent and heavy metal exposure are classed as exposure or not, but no data regarding instrumental measured levels were available; thus, the present study may not account for variability in exposure levels of organic solvents and heavy metals. Moreover, noise and other ototoxic exposure were assigned only at the industrial level; exposure variation among different jobs/tasks within the same industry was not accounted for. Second, the present data do not provide information on various potential confounding factors such as smoking or exposure to non-occupational noise (e.g., residential and recreational). Therefore, the true associations of occupational noise and other ototoxic factors with hearing thresholds may be weaker than those reported in the present study. Third, it can be argued that the present findings regarding the effect modification by ototoxic chemicals on the association between noise and hearing loss are due to the correlation between ototoxic chemical exposure and high-level noise. However, the present results demonstrate the risk of hearing loss due to noise is higher in individuals exposed to heavy metals (see Table 5) even if they are exposed to less noise (see Table 2). Finally, although a nationwide representative sample of noise-exposed workers in Korea increased power to our findings, the observed effect modification may not apply to the general population. Because the present data were collected only from industries that have considerable noise levels, and therefore a majority of subjects may have work-related hearing loss and were male, our observations could be different from general populations exposed to low-level noise and who reflect half male and half female. We suggest more research is needed to confirm our evidence using a large sample of general adults.

The present study based on the Korea National Occupational Health Surveillance program estimates that more than 7,000 Korean industries involve occupational daily exposure to levels exceeding 85 dB. These industries include over 60,000 workers, 77% of whom have hearing loss attributable to their work. Indeed, it is difficult to control noise levels for all potentially problematic industries in a country. In addition, noise exposure is common in certain industries and occupations. Therefore, with the need for cost-effective control of noise, the present study provides data for establishing criteria for priority industries to implement monitoring and reduce occupational noise and chemicals to effectively lessen the national burden of work-related hearing loss.

## Conclusion

In conclusion, the present study supports the hypothesis that co-exposure to organic solvents and heavy metals may increase the risk of hearing loss due to noise exposure. The present findings suggest that the risk of noise-induced hearing loss may vary by industry. Furthermore, employees in industries dealing with heavy metals and/or organic solvents are susceptible to such risks, and these industries should prioritize noise and chemicals reduction to prevent work-related hearing loss.

## Supporting Information

**Figure S1 Study participants profile.**

**Table S1** Multivariate-adjusted effect estimates (95% CI) of hearing thresholds (dBHL) at individual frequencies with IQR increment in occupational noise exposure (dBA), stratified according to occupational exposure to ototoxic chemicals.

**Table S2** Multivariate-adjusted ORs (95% CIs) of hearing loss[a] with IQR increment in occupational noise exposure (dBA), stratified according to occupational exposure to ototoxic chemicals.

**Table S3** Multivariate-adjusted effect estimates (95% CIs) of hearing thresholds (dBHL) attributable to occupational exposure to ototoxic chemicals, stratified according to noise exposure levels (dBA).

**File S1 Methods: Ototoxic Chemical Exposures, References.**

## Author Contributions

Conceived and designed the experiments: YC KK. Performed the experiments: YC. Analyzed the data: YC. Contributed reagents/materials/analysis tools: YC KK. Wrote the paper: YC.

## References


1. CDC (2001) Work Related Hearing Loss. Atlanta, GA: Centers for Disease Control and Prevention.
2. Palmer KT, Griffin MJ, Syddall HE, Davis A, Pannett B, et al. (2002) Occupational exposure to noise and the attributable burden of hearing difficulties in Great Britain. Occupational and Environmental Medicine 59: 634–639.
3. Stanbury M, Rafferty AP, Rosenman K (2008) Prevalence of Hearing Loss and Work-Related Noise-Induced Hearing Loss in Michigan. Journal of Occupational and Environmental Medicine 50: 72–79.
4. Choi Y-H, Hu H, Tak S, Mukherjee B, Park SK (2012) Occupational Noise Exposure Assessment using O*NET and Its Application to a Study of Hearing Loss in the US General Population. Occupational and Environmental Medicine 69: 176–183.
5. CDC (2013) Occupational Hearing Loss Surveillance. Atlanta, GA: Centers for Disease Control and Prevention.
6. Meyer JD, Chen Y, McDonald JC, Cherry NM (2002) Surveillance for work-related hearing loss in the UK: OSSA and OPRA 1997-2000. Occup Med 52: 75–79.
7. Wu TN, Liou SH, Shen CY, Hsu CC, Chao SL, et al. (1998) Surveillance of noise-induced hearing loss in Taiwan, ROC: a report of the PRESS-NHL results. Prev Med 27: 65–69.
8. OSHRI (2010) Research on Occupational Exposures-Related Disease (I): the Korea National Occupational Health Surveillance 2009 on occupational audiological disorders. Incheon, Republich of Korea: The Occupational Safety and Health Research Institute, The Korea Occupational Safety and Health Agency.
9. Wallhagen MI, Strawbridge WJ, Cohen RD, Kaplan GA (1997) An increasing prevalence of hearing impairment and associated risk factors over three decades of the Alameda County Study. Am J Public Health 87: 440–442.
10. Fuente A, McPherson B (2006) Organic solvents and hearing loss: The challenge for audiology. International Journal of Audiology 45: 367–381.
11. Morata TC (2003) Chemical Exposure as a Risk Factor for Hearing Loss. Journal of Occupational and Environmental Medicine 45: 676–682.
12. Sliwinska-Kowalska M, Prasher D, Rodrigues C, Zamysłowska-Szmytke E, Campo P, et al. (2007) Ototoxicity of Organic Solvents - From Scientific Evidence to Health Policy. International Journal of Occupational Medicine and Environmental Health 20: 215–222.
13. Crofton K, Lassiter T, Rebert C (1994) Solvent-induced ototoxicity in rats: An atypical selective mid-frequency hearing deficit Hearing Research 80: 25–30.
14. Campo P, Lataye R, Loquet G, Bonnet P (2001) Styrene-induced hearing loss: a membrane insult. Hearing Research 154: 170–180.
15. Spandow O, Anniko M, Møller AR (1988) The round window as access route for agents injurious to the inner ear. American Journal of Otolaryngology 9: 327–335.
16. Cappaert NLM, Klis SFL, Muijser H, Kulig BM, Smoorenburg GF (2001) Simultaneous exposure to ethyl benzene and noise: synergistic effects on outer hair cells. Hearing Research 162: 67–79.
17. Sliwinska-Kowalska M, Zamyslowska-Szmytke E, Szymczak W, Kotylo P, Fiszer M, et al. (2001) Hearing loss among workers exposed to moderate concentrations of solvents. Scand J Work Environ Health 27: 335–342.
18. Sliwinska-Kowalska M, Zamyslowska-Szmytke E, Szymczak W, Kotylo P, Fiszer M, et al. (2003) Ototoxic Effects of Occupational Exposure to Styrene and Co-Exposure to Styrene and Noise. Journal of Occupational and Environmental Medicine 45: 15–24.
19. Abbate C, Giorgianni C, Munaò F, Brecciaroli R (1993) Neurotoxicity induced by exposure to toluene. International Archives of Occupational and Environmental Health 64: 389–392.
20. Varney NR, Kubu CS, Morrow LA (1998) Dichotic Listening Performances of Patients with Chronic Exposure to Organic Solvents. The Clinical Neuropsychologist 12: 107–112.
21. Morata TC, Fiorini AC, Fischer FM, Colacioppo S, Wallingford KM, et al. (1997) Toluene-induced hearing loss among rotogravure printing workers. Scandinavian Journal of Work, Environment and Health 23: 289–298.
22. Fuente A, Slade MD, Taylor T, Morata TC, Keith RW, et al. (2009) Peripheral and central auditory dysfunction induced by occupational exposure to organic solvents. J Occup Environ Med 51: 1202–1211.
23. Yamamura K, Terayama K, Yamamoto N, Kohyama A, Kishi R (1989) Effects of acute lead acetate exposure on adult guinea pigs: Electrophysiological study of the inner ear. Fundamental and Applied Toxicology 13: 509–515.
24. Lasky RE, Maier MM, Snodgrass EB, Hecox KE, Laughlin NK (1995) The effects of lead on otoacoustic emissions and auditory evoked potentials in monkeys. Neurotoxicology and Teratology 17: 633–644.
25. Jones LG, Prins J, Park S, Walton JP, Luebke AE, et al. (2008) Lead exposure during development results in increased neurofilament phosphorylation, neuritic beading, and temporal processing deficits within the murine auditory brainstem. The Journal of Comparative Neurology 506: 1003–1017.
26. Kim S-J, Jeong H-J, Myung N-Y, Kim M-C, Lee J-H, et al. (2008) The Protective Mechanism of Antioxidants in Cadmium-Induced Ototoxicity *in Vitro* and *in Vivo*. Environ Health Perspect 116: 854–862.
27. Ozcaglar H, Agirdir B, Dinc O, Turhan M, Kilinçarslan S, et al. (2001) Effects of cadmium on the hearing system. Acta Otolaryngol 121: 393–397.
28. Chuang H-Y, Kuo C-H, Chiu Y-W, Ho C-K, Chen C-J, et al. (2007) A case-control study on the relationship of hearing function and blood concentrations of lead, manganese, arsenic, and selenium. Science of The Total Environment 387: 79–85.
29. Choi YH, Hu H, Mukherjee B, Miller J, Park SK (2012) Environmental cadmium and lead exposures and hearing loss in u.s. Adults: the national health and nutrition examination survey, 1999 to 2004. Environ Health Perspect 120: 1544–1550.
30. Shargorodsky J, Curhan SG, Henderson E, Eavey R, Curhan GC (2011) Heavy metals exposure and hearing loss in US adolescents. Arch Otolaryngol Head Neck Surg 137: 1183–1189.
31. Sliwinska-Kowalska M (2008) Organic solvent exposure and hearing loss. Occupational and Environmental Medicine 65: 222–223.
32. Jacobsen P, Hein HO, Suadicani P, Parving A, Gyntelberg F (1993) Mixed solvent exposure and hearing impairment: an epidemiological study of 3284 men. The Copenhagen male study. Occup Med 43: 180–184.
33. Sass-Kortsak AM, Corey PN, Robertson JM (1995) An investigation of the association between exposure to styrene and hearing loss. Annals of Epidemiology 5: 15–24.
34. Vyskocil A, Truchon G, Leroux T, Lemay F, Gendron M, et al. (2011) A weight of evidence approach for the assessment of the ototoxic potential of industrial chemicals. Toxicology and Industrial Health 28:796–819.
35. Sliwinska-Kowalska M, Zamyslowska-Szmytke E, Szymczak W, Kotylo P, Fiszer M, et al. (2004) Effects of Coexposure to Noise and Mixture of Organic Solvents on Hearing in Dockyard Workers. Journal of Occupational and Environmental Medicine 46: 30–38.
36. Sliwinska-Kowalska M, Zamyslowska-Szmytke E, Szymczak W, Kotylo P, Fiszer M, et al. (2005) Exacerbation of noise-induced hearing loss by co-exposure to workplace chemicals. Environmental Toxicology and Pharmacology 19: 547–553.
37. Johnson A-C, Morata TC (2010) 142. Occupational exposure to chemicals and hearing impairment. The Nordic Expert Group for Criteria Documentation of Health Risks from Chemicals. Nordic Expert Group. Arbete och Hälsa; 44(4): 177 pp.
38. EU-OSHA (2009) Combined exposure to noise and ototoxic substances. Luxembourg: European Agency for Safety and Health at Work
39. Park J, Kim Y, Kim KS (1999) Remodeling of the occupational medical examination program in South Korea. Int Arch Occup Environ Health 72: 411–417.
40. OSHRI (2009) Occupational Health Surveillance Standard Methods: Noise. Incheon, Republic of Korea: The Occupational Safety and Health Research Institute, The Korea Occupational Safety and Health Agency.
41. Kim K-S (2007) Development of Korean Audiometric Quality Control Program for the Special Health Examination. Audiology 3: 9–16.
42. OSHRI (2009) Standard Methods for Manual Pure Tone Threshold Audiometry. Incheon, Republich of Korea: The Occupational Safety and Health Research Institute, The Korea Occupational Safety and Health Agency.
43. Park SK, Elmarsafawy S, Mukherjee B, Spiro Iii A, Vokonas PS, et al. (2010) Cumulative lead exposure and age-related hearing loss: The VA Normative Aging Study. Hearing Research 269: 48–55.
44. Choi Y-H, Hu H, Mukherjee B, Miller J, Park SK (2012) Environmental Cadmium and Lead Exposures and Hearing Loss in US Adults: the National Health and Nutrition Examination Survey, 1999 to 2004. Environ Health Perspectives Under review.
45. Morata TC, Dunn DE, Kretschmer LW, Lemasters GK, Keith RW (1993) Effects of occupational exposure to organic solvents and noise on hearing. Scand J Work Environ Health 19: 245–254.
46. Discalzi G, Fabbro D, Meliga F, Mocellini A, Capellaro F (1993) Effects of occupational exposure to mercury and lead on brainstem auditory evoked potentials. International Journal of Psychophysiology 14: 21–25.
47. Maguin K, Campo P, Parietti-Winkler C (2009) Toluene can perturb the neuronal voltage-dependent Ca2+ channels involved in the middle-ear reflex. Toxicol Sci 107: 473–481.
48. Sabolić I (2006) Common Mechanisms in Nephropathy Induced by Toxic Metals. Nephron Physiology 104: 107–114.
49. Rabinowitz PM, Galusha D, Slade MD, Dixon-Ernst C, Sircar KD, et al. (2006) Audiogram Notches in Noise-Exposed Workers. Ear and Hearing 27: 742–750.
50. Beckett WS (2003) Noise Induced Hearing Loss-Evidence Based Statement. Journal of Occupational and Environmental Medicine 45: 1029.

2

# Genetic Spectrum of Autosomal Recessive Non-Syndromic Hearing Loss in Pakistani Families

**Sobia Shafique[1,❡], Saima Siddiqi[2,❡], Margit Schraders[3,4,5], Jaap Oostrik[3,4,5], Humaira Ayub[1], Ammad Bilal[6], Muhammad Ajmal[1], Celia Zazo Seco[3,4,5], Tim M. Strom[7], Atika Mansoor[2], Kehkashan Mazhar[2], Syed Tahir A. Shah[1], Alamdar Hussain[1], Maleeha Azam[1], Hannie Kremer[3,4,5,8,*,¶], Raheel Qamar[1,9,*,¶]**

**1** COMSATS Institute of Information Technology, Park Road, Islamabad, Pakistan, **2** Institute of Biomedical and Genetic Engineering (IBGE), Islamabad, Pakistan, **3** Department of Otorhinolaryngology, Hearing and Genes, Radboud University Medical Center, Nijmegen, The Netherlands, **4** Nijmegen Centre for Molecular Life Sciences, Radboud University Medical Center, Nijmegen, The Netherlands, **5** Donders Institute for Brain, Cognition and Behaviour, Radboud University Medical Center, Nijmegen, The Netherlands, **6** Simon Fraser University, Vancouver, British Colombia, Canada, **7** Institute of Human Genetics, Helmholtz Zentrum München, German Research Center for Environmental Health, Neuherberg, Germany, **8** Department of Human Genetics, Radboud university medical center, Nijmegen, The Netherlands, **9** Al-Nafees Medical College & Hospital, Isra University, Islamabad, Pakistan

## Abstract

The frequency of inherited bilateral autosomal recessive non-syndromic hearing loss (ARNSHL) in Pakistan is 1.6/1000 individuals. More than 50% of the families carry mutations in *GJB2* while mutations in *MYO15A* account for about 5% of recessive deafness. In the present study a cohort of 30 ARNSHL families was initially screened for mutations in *GJB2* and *MYO15A*. Homozygosity mapping was performed by employing whole genome single nucleotide polymorphism (SNP) genotyping in the families that did not carry mutations in *GJB2* or *MYO15A*. Mutation analysis was performed for the known ARNSHL genes present in the homozygous regions to determine the causative mutations. This allowed the identification of a causative mutation in all the 30 families including 9 novel mutations, which were identified in 9 different families (*GJB2* (c.598G>A, p.Gly200Arg); *MYO15A* (c.9948G>A, p.Gln3316Gln; c.3866+1G>A; c.8767C>T, p.Arg2923* and c.8222T>C, p.Phe2741Ser), *TMC1* (c.362+18A>G), *BSND* (c.97G>C, p.Val33Leu), *TMPRSS3* (c.726C>G, p.Cys242Trp) and *MSRB3* (c.20T>G, p.Leu7Arg)). Furthermore, 12 recurrent mutations were detected in 21 other families. The 21 identified mutations included 10 (48%) missense changes, 4 (19%) nonsense mutations, 3 (14%) intronic mutations, 2 (9%) splice site mutations and 2 (9%) frameshift mutations. *GJB2* accounted for 53% of the families, while mutations in *MYO15A* were the second most frequent (13%) cause of ARNSHL in these 30 families. The identification of novel as well as recurrent mutations in the present study increases the spectrum of mutations in known deafness genes which could lead to the identification of novel founder mutations and population specific mutated deafness genes causative of ARNSHL. These results provide detailed genetic information that has potential diagnostic implication in the establishment of cost-efficient allele-specific analysis of frequently occurring variants in combination with other reported mutations in Pakistani populations.

**Editor:** Francesc Palau, Instituto de Ciencia de Materiales de Madrid - Instituto de Biomedicina de Valencia, Spain

**Funding:** This work was supported by Higher Education Commission (HEC) grant no 2155 to RQ under the National Research Program for Universities, by The Oticon Foundation (grant 09-3742 to HK), and by ZorgOnderzoek Nederland/Medische Wetenschappen (grant 40-00812-98-09047 to HK). The authors also acknowledge the Higher Education Commission of Pakistan for providing funds to S. Shafique and S. Siddiqi to work in The Netherlands. The funders had no role in study design, data collection and anlaysis, decision to publish, or preparation of the manuscript.

**Competing Interests:** The authors have declared that no competing interests exist.

* Email: Hannie.Kremer@radboudumc.nl (HK); raheelqamar@hotmail.com (RQ)

❡ These authors contributed equally to this work.

¶ These authors also contributed equally to this work.

## Introduction

Deafness or hearing loss is the most common congenital sensorineural disorder affecting about 1 in 1000 children. Genetic factors contribute to approximately half of the cases of hearing loss [1], which can be either syndromic or non-syndromic. The former is responsible for about 30% of prelingual deafness in combination with abnormalities of other organs. Non-syndromic deafness is usually due to abnormalities of the middle and/or the inner ear and is found in 70% of the hereditary cases [2]. The disease is genetically heterogeneous and currently 134 loci have been determined and 80 genes identified for the non-syndromic type (Hereditary Hearing Loss Homepage, URL: http://hereditaryhearingloss.org/). More than 400 syndromes are known with deafness as one of the symptoms and for many of these the causative genes have been identified (Online Mendelian Inheritance in Man: http://www.ncbi.nlm.nih.gov/omim).

Syndromic and non-syndromic hearing loss display an autosomal recessive, autosomal dominant, X-linked, Y-linked or mitochondrial pattern of inheritance [3]. Eighty percent of the early onset non-syndromic cases have an autosomal recessive inheritance pattern (ARNSHL), while autosomal dominant,

X-linked and mitochondrial non-syndromic deafness contribute to 18%, 1–3% and <1% of the cases, respectively [4]. In Pakistan, hearing impairment is severe and congenital in 70% of the cases and the increased occurrence of these conditions is due to a high rate of consanguineous marriages (60%); profound bilateral deafness occurs at 1.6 per 1000 individuals [5].

The genes most frequently involved in ARNSHL are those encoding gap junction protein beta 2 (*GJB2*, MIM# 121011), myosin XVA (*MYO15A*, MIM# 602666), transmembrane channel-like 1 (*TMC1*, MIM# 606706), solute carrier family 26 (anion exchanger) member 4 (*SLC26A4*, MIM# 605646), otoferlin (*OTOF*, MIM# 603681) and cadherin-related 23 (*CDH23*, MIM# 605516), each of which has been found to contain more than 20 different mutations, most of which have been reported in consanguineous families [6]. Mutations in *GJB2* are the most common cause of ARNSHL and explain up to 50% cases in the Mediterranean regions [7,8,9] while mutations in multiple genes have been shown to cause deafness in the remaining cases. In the Pakistani population mutations in *MYO15A* account for 5% of the recessive deafness [10].

In the present study a panel of 30 unrelated consanguineous Pakistani families was initially tested for involvement of *GJB2* and *MYO15A* followed by whole genome homozygosity mapping and candidate gene sequencing. This approach resulted in defining the mutation spectrum of the disease in the current panel.

## Materials and Methods

### Ethics statement

The current study conformed to the tenets of the Helsinki declaration and was approved by the Department of Biosciences Ethics Review Board of the COMSATS Institute of Information Technology, Islamabad, Pakistan. All patients, their normal hearing family members and 89 ethnically matched control individuals were informed about the purpose of the study and written consent was taken before recruitment and sampling. Informed written consent of minors was obtained from their guardians.

### Genotyping

A total of 30 consanguineous families with ARNSHL were ascertained from different regions of Punjab, Pakistan. Audiometery was performed on a few members from each family to determine the level of hearing loss.

Blood samples were collected in EDTA containing vacutainers. DNA extraction from these samples was carried out using a standard phenol-chloroform/organic method [11]. Microsatellite markers were analyzed as described previously [12] and Sanger sequencing was performed according to Schraders et al. [13]. Primers were designed using Primer3 software (URL: http://www.bioinformatics.nl/cgi-bin/primer3plus/primer3plus.cgi/; [14]). Primer sequences are available upon request. PCR was performed using standard conditions.

Prior to whole genome single nucleotide polymorphism (SNP) mapping all families were pre-screened for mutations in *GJB2* by Sanger sequence analysis. For the *MYO15A* locus, microsatellite markers (D17S1843, D17S2196, D17S783 and D17S1824) were genotyped and in families in which haplotype analysis showed compatibility with genetic linkage, Sanger sequence analysis was performed for *MYO15A*. For family 11DF, microsatellite markers (D9S166, D9S1806 and D9S1876) were used for exclusion of the *TMC1* region.

Families with no identified mutation in *GJB2* and *MYO15A* were further genotyped using the Illumina HumanOmniExpress whole genome single nucleotide polymorphism (SNP) microarray (>700 K SNPs) or the Illumina Human Linkage-12 panel according to the manufacturer's protocols. Homozygosity mapping was performed using an online tool Homozygosity Mapper (URL: http://www.homozygositymapper.org; [15]). The logarithm of odds (LOD) score for the homozygous regions identified in family DFR18 was calculated using the Gene Hunter v2.1r5 program in the easyLINKAGE plus v5.08 software package [16]. The exons and exon-intron boundaries of the known candidate genes (*BSND* (NM_057176.2), *GJB2* (NM_004004.5), *HGF* (NM_000601), *MYO15A* (NM_016239.3), *MSRB3* (NM_001031679.2), *SLC26A4* (NM_000441.1), *TMC1* (NM_138691.2), *TMPRSS3* (NM_024022.2) and *TMIE* (NM_147196)) present in the homozygous regions were sequenced in the proband of the families. Segregation analyses for identified mutations in the corresponding families were performed by Sanger sequencing except for family DFR24 and DFR18. In these families, the segregation of *TMPRSS3* and *MSRB3* mutations was analyzed with restriction digestion with the enzymes *AciI* and *TseI*, respectively (New England Biolabs Inc. UK).

Eighty nine ethnically matched controls were sequenced for the novel mutations identified in the current study. Control panel screening of *GJB2* (c.598G>A); *MYO15A* (c.9948G>A), (c.3866+1G>A), (c.8767C>T), (c.8222 T>C); *TMC1* (c.362+18A>G) and *BSND* (c.97G>C), variants was done by sanger sequencing. While for *TMPRSS3* (c.726C>G) and *MSRB3* (c.20T>G) variants *AciI* and *TseI* PCR-RFLP were performed, respectively.

### *In silico* prediction of the identified variants

*In silico* prediction of the identified variants was performed using online prediction tools. Sorting intolerant from tolerant (SIFT: http://sift.jcvi.org; [17]) and Polymorphism Phenotyping v2 (PolyPhen-2: http://genetics.bwh.harvard.edu/pph2; [18]) were used for analyses of missense changes. Effects on splicing were evaluated with NetGene2 (http://www.cbs.dtu.dk/services/NetGene2/; [19]). SignalP 4.0 (http://www.cbs.dtu.dk/services/SignalP-4.0/) was employed to predict the presence and location of the signal peptide/non-signal peptide cleavage sites [20]. In addition, the online tool, Have your Protein Explained (HOPE) (http://www.cmbi.ru.nl/hope/input) was used to predict the three dimensional structural changes at the protein level [21]. The exome variant server (EVS) and an in-house exome database (Human Genetics, Radboud University Medical Centre) were also searched for the presence of putative pathogenic variants.

### Minigene Construction and Splicing Assay (for c.362+18A>G mutation in *TMC1* and c.9948G>A mutation in *MYO15A*)

A plasmid containing the genomic region encompassing exons 3–5 of *RHO* inserted at the EcoRI/SalI sites in the pCI-NEO vector was used for *in vivo* splicing assays [22]. The plasmid was adapted from the Gateway cloning technology (Life technologies) according to the manufacturer's protocol. PCR amplified fragments of wild-type and mutant *TMC1* exon 8, along with flanking intronic sequences were generated with the following primers, 5′-GGGGACAAGTTTGTACAAAAAAGCAGGCTT-Ctgggtcctaatgttgactgc-3′ and 5′-GGGGACCACTTTGTACAA-GAAAGCTGGGTCggatttagaaaatcaatatcaggg-3′, that contain the attB1 and attB2 sites necessary for Gateway cloning. Similarly, amplified fragments of wild-type and mutant *MYO15A* exon 61 were generated using primers, 5′- GGGGACAAGTTTGTA-CAAAAAAGCAGGCTTCttccccaggagaaatggag-3′ and 5′- GGG-GACCACTTTGTACAAGAAAGCTGGGTCcagcttgctgggaag-

**Table 1.** Spectrum of recurrent *GJB2* mutations in Pakistani families with autosomal recessive non-syndromic hearing loss (ARNSHL).

| Mutation identified (Protein change) | Type of mutation | No. of families | No. of affected members | Frequency in EVS |
|---|---|---|---|---|
| c.71G>A (p.Trp24*) | Nonsense (homozygous) | 5 | 26 | Absent |
| c.231G>A (p.Trp77*) | Nonsense (homozygous) | 4 | 14 | AA = 0/AG = 1/GG = 4299 |
| c.35delG (p.Gly12Valfs*2) | Frameshift (homozygous) | 2 | 8 | Absent |
| c.35delG (p.Gly12Valfs*2) c.439G>A (p.Glu147Lys) | Missense (compound heterozygous) | 1 | 3 | Absent |
| c.380G>A (p.Arg127His)[#] | Missense (homozygous) | 2 | 4 | AA = 0/AG = 26/GG = 4274 |
| c.377_378insATGCGGA (p.Arg127Cysfs*85) | Frameshift (homozygous) | 1 | 2 | Absent |

As reference sequence NM_004004.5 was employed. EVS, exome variant server;
[#]The pathogenicity of this mutation is controversial.

gac-3′. Recombinant vectors were employed for transfection of HEK293T cells that were incubated at 37°C for 24 hours. RNA was then isolated from the transfected cells and reverse transcribed into cDNA and sequenced. Forward primer 5′-cggaggtcaacaacgagtct-3′ and reverse primer 5′-aggtgtaggggatgg-gagac-3′ were used to amplify and sequence the amplified cDNA fragments along with flanking *RHO* sequences as present in the vector.

## Results

All families in this study were consanguineous (Table S1) and all patients in these families were diagnosed with severe to profound congenital hearing loss. Causal mutations were identified in all 30 families and the 9 novel mutations identified in the current study were not present in any of the 89 ethnically matched control individuals.

Sequence analysis of *GJB2* in the current cohort identified 16 families with mutations in this gene (Table 1; Table 2) segregating with hearing loss. A recurrent nonsense mutation c.71G>A (p.Trp24*) was the most common and was found in 5 families (31%), followed by another nonsense variant, c.231G>A (p.Trp77*) that was identified in 4 families (25%; Table 1). In addition to the 6 recurrent *GJB2* mutations, a novel homozygous change c.598G>A (p.Gly200Arg) was found in one consanguineous family DFR10 (Table 2); as predicted by the HOPE server the larger side chain of the mutant residue arginine might well affect the proper folding of the cysteine rich domain. In addition, the residue resides in the conserved region of the protein (Figure 1; Figure S1A).

Out of the 9 novel mutations (Table 2) identified in the current study, 4 were present in *MYO15A*, of which 2 were splice site mutations (c.9948G>A and c.3866+1G>A), one was a nonsense (c.8767C>T) and one a missense mutation (c.8222 T>C). The c.9948G>A variant changes the last nucleotide of exon 61 and is predicted to affect the splice donor site. The splice donor site in the reference sequence has a highly confident score of 94%, which is reduced to a score of 24% in the mutant. To determine the effect of the c.9948G>A mutation on splicing, a minigene approach was used. This showed correct splicing of the wildtype *MYO15A* exon 61, while the c.9948G>A mutation almost completely abolished the normal splicing (Figure 2). NetGene2 predicted the abolition of the splice donor site of exon 5 as a result of the c.3866+1G>A mutation in intron 5 of *MYO15A*. The nonsense mutation c.8767C>T (p.Arg2923*) was novel and predicted to lead to the synthesis of a truncated protein, while the missense mutation c.8222 T>C, leads to the substitution of serine for phenylalanine (p.Phe2741Ser) at amino acid position 2741 that resides in the conserved region of the protein (Figure 1; Figure S1B). This missense change was predicted to be deleterious by SIFT and Polyphen2 (Table 2).

Haplotype analysis of STR-markers flanking *TMC1* showed compatibility with genetic linkage for family 11DF. Since sequence analysis of *TMC1* revealed a novel intronic mutation, c.362+18A>G, this family was not further analyzed by SNP-array genotyping. The variant segregated with the hearing loss in the family (Figure 1) and was predicted to create a novel splice donor site with a similar confidence score as the original splice donor site. To determine the effect of the c.362+18A>G mutation on splicing, a minigene approach was used. This revealed correct splicing of the wild-type *TMC1* exon 8, while the c.362+18A>G mutation resulted in a 17 bp extension of exon 8 (Figure 3). This leads to a frameshift and a premature stop codon (p.Glu122Tyrfs*10).

A novel homozygous missense mutation was identified in *TMPRSS3* (MIM_605511), c.726C>G (p.Cys242Trp) that co-segregated with hearing impairment in family DFR24 (Figure 1) and was predicted to be probably damaging by Polyphen2 and deleterious by SIFT (Table 2). This mutation is located in the peptidase S1 domain and the HOPE server predicted the abolition of the catalytic activity of TMPRSS3. In addition the amino acid substitution is present in a region of the protein that is conserved across different species (Figure S1D) and therefore probably affects the core structure of the peptidase domain (Figure 4).

In family DFR18 SNP microarray data analysis revealed a 17.6 Mb homozygous region on chromosome 12 flanked by SNPs rs7978381 and rs7976686, a LOD score of 2.7 was calculated for this region. The known deafness gene, *MSRB3* (MIM_613719), in the region was subsequently sequenced, revealing a novel homozygous nucleotide substitution c.20T>G (p.Leu7Arg) in exon 4 (Figure 1; Table 2). The leucine at position 7 is located in the signal peptide of the MSRB3 protein and as a result of the substitution by arginine this signal peptide loses its function as predicted by SignalP 4.0. Furthermore, the Leu7 residue is conserved across species (Figure S1E). The mutation abolishes a *TseI* restriction site, which allowed the segregation of this variant in the family to be checked by restriction digestion. By using the same analysis, this variant was also found heterozygously in 3 out of 178 ethnically matched control alleles.

The novel *BSND* (MIM_606412) missense mutation c.97G>C (p.Val33Leu) in family 7DF (Figure 1) was predicted to be deleterious by SIFT and Polyphen2 (Table 2) and Val33 is conserved across species (Figure S1C).

**Table 2.** Novel mutations identified in known genes for autosomal recessive non-syndromic hearing loss (ARNSHL) in the current study.

| Family ID | Size of homozygous regions (Mb) | Chr. | Flanking SNPs | Chr. position (in hg19) | Candidate gene (Acc. No.) | Mutation (Predicted protein change) | PhyloP; SIFT; Polyphen | NetGene2 | Frequency in EVS |
|---|---|---|---|---|---|---|---|---|---|
| DFR10 | ND | 13 | ND | ND | *GJB2* (NM_004004.5) | Ex-2: c.598G>A (p.Gly200Arg) | 3.43; Deleterious; Damaging | NA | Absent |
| DFR23 | ND | 17 | ND | ND | *MYO15A* (NM_016239.3) | Ex-61: c.9948G>A (p.Gln3316Gln) | NA | Abolition of splice site | Absent |
| 13DF | ND | 17 | ND | ND | *MYO15A* (NM_016239.3) | In-5: c.3866+1G>A (p.?) | NA | Abolition of splice site | AA = 0, AG = 1, GG = 6051 |
| DFR28 | ND | 17 | ND | ND | *MYO15A* (NM_016239.3) | Ex-50: c.8767C>T (p.Arg2923*) | NA | NA | TT = 0, TC = 1, CC = 6266 |
| DFR3 | ND | 17 | ND | ND | *MYO15A* (NM_016239.3) | Ex-45: c.8222T>C (p.Phe2741Ser) | 4.97; Deleterious; Damaging | NA | Absent |
| 11DF | ND | 9 | ND | ND | *TMC1* (NM_138691.2) | In-8: c.362+18A>G (p.Glu122Tyrfs*10) | NA | NA | Absent |
| 7DF | 8.40 | 1 | rs1242330; rs7521242 | 53,396,842–61,803,889 | *BSND* (NM_057176.2) | Ex-1: c.97G>C (p.Val33Leu) | 1.09 Deleterious; Damaging | NA | Absent |
| DFR24 | 3.49 | 21 | rs2838063; rs881969 | 42,929,129–46,421,694 | *TMPRSS3* (NM_024022.2) | Ex-8: c.726C>G (p.Cys242Trp) | −0.28 Deleterious; Damaging | NA | Absent |
| DFR18 | 2.92 | 12 | rs6581511; rs11176432 | 64,278,102–67,207,064 | *MSRB3* (NM_001031679.2) | Ex-4: c.20T>G (p.Leu7Arg) | 3.76; Tolerated; Possibly Damaging | NA | Absent |

Acc. No., accession number of reference sequence; Chr, chromosome; Ex, exon; EVS, exome variant server; hg19, human genome assembly 19; In, intron; NA, not applicable; ND, not determined; SNPs, single nucleotide polymorphisms; PhyloP, phylogenetic P-values; Polyphen, polymorphism phenotyping; SIFT, sorting intolerance from tolerance.

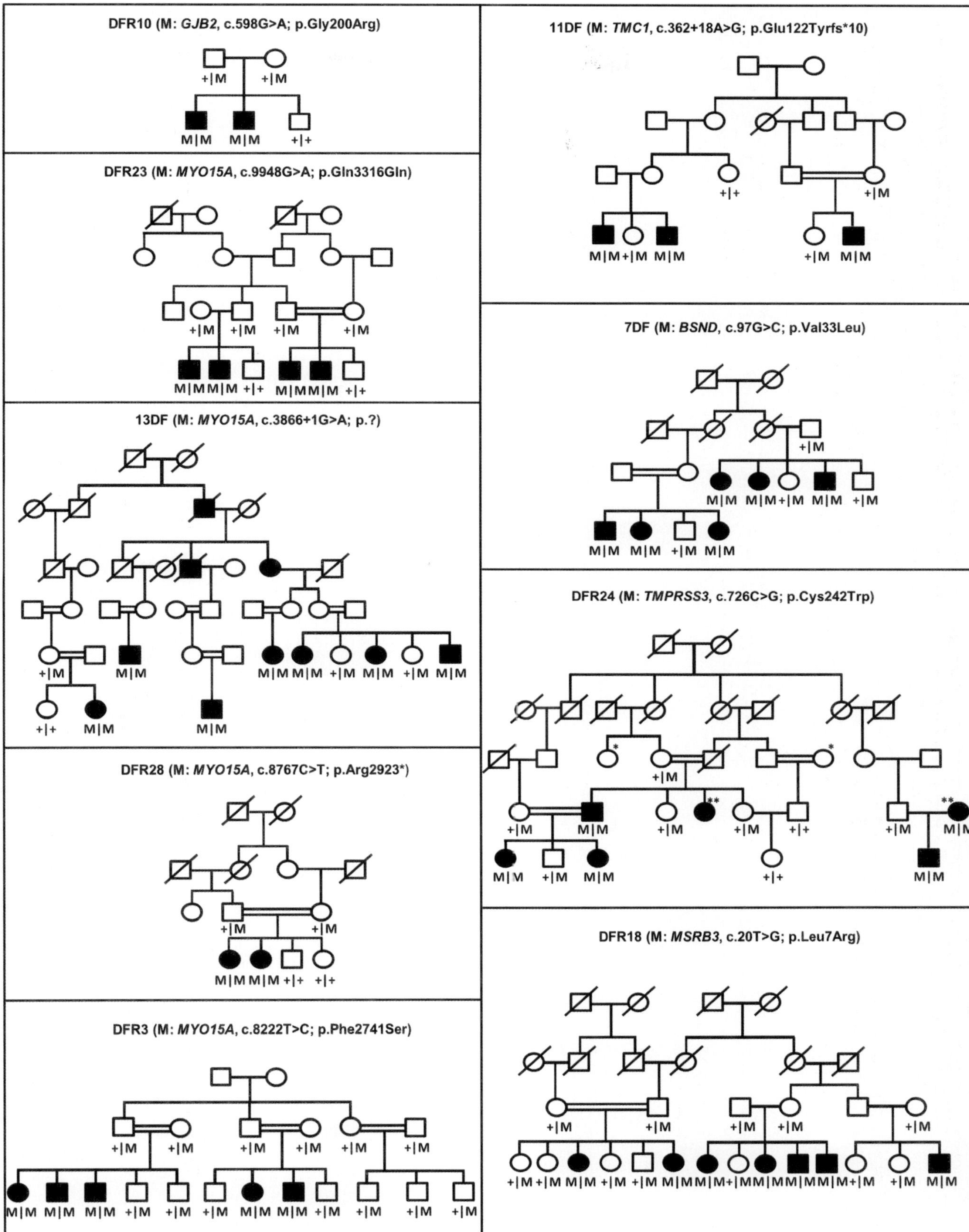


**Figure 1. Pedigrees and the segregation of novel mutations in known deafness genes.** Unfilled circles indicate unaffected females, unfilled squares indicate unaffected males, filled circles indicate affected females, filled squares indicate affected males, double lines represent consanguineous marriages, slashed line across the symbols indicate deceased individual, + indicates wild type allele, M indicates mutant allele.

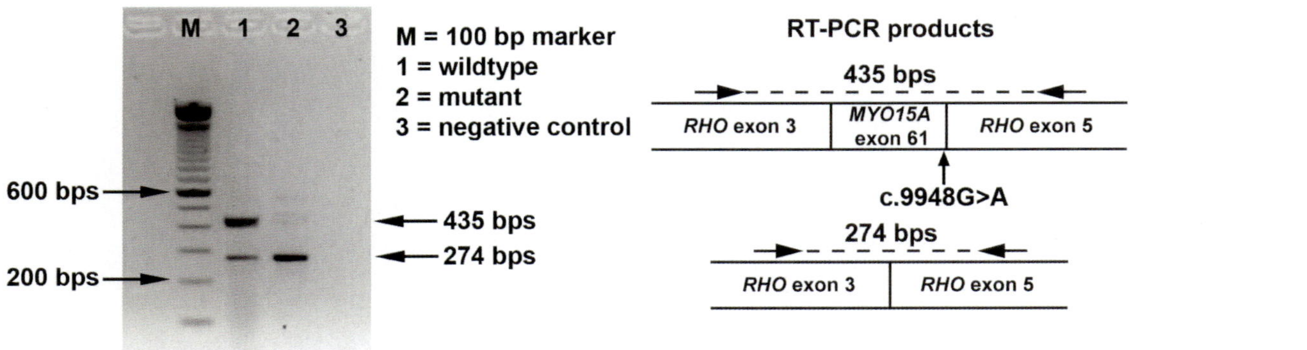


**Figure 2. Effect of MYO15A c. 9948G>A using a minigene approach.** An agarose gel containing RT-PCR products detected from HEK293T cells transfected with the wildtype and mutant minigene construct and a schematic representation of the identified splicing products. The RT-PCR products were verified by sequence analysis. The c.9948G>A mutation leads to skipping of exon 61.

Recurrent mutations in *TMC1* (c.1114G>A; p.Val372Met [23] and c.100C>T; p.Arg34* [24]), *HGF* (c.482+1991_2000delGATGATGAAA and c.482+1986_1988delTGA [25]), *SLC26A4* (c.1337A>G; p.Gln446Arg [26]) and *TMIE* (c.241C>T; p.Arg81Cys [27]) also segregated in the respective families and most likely are the disease causing mutations (Table 3).

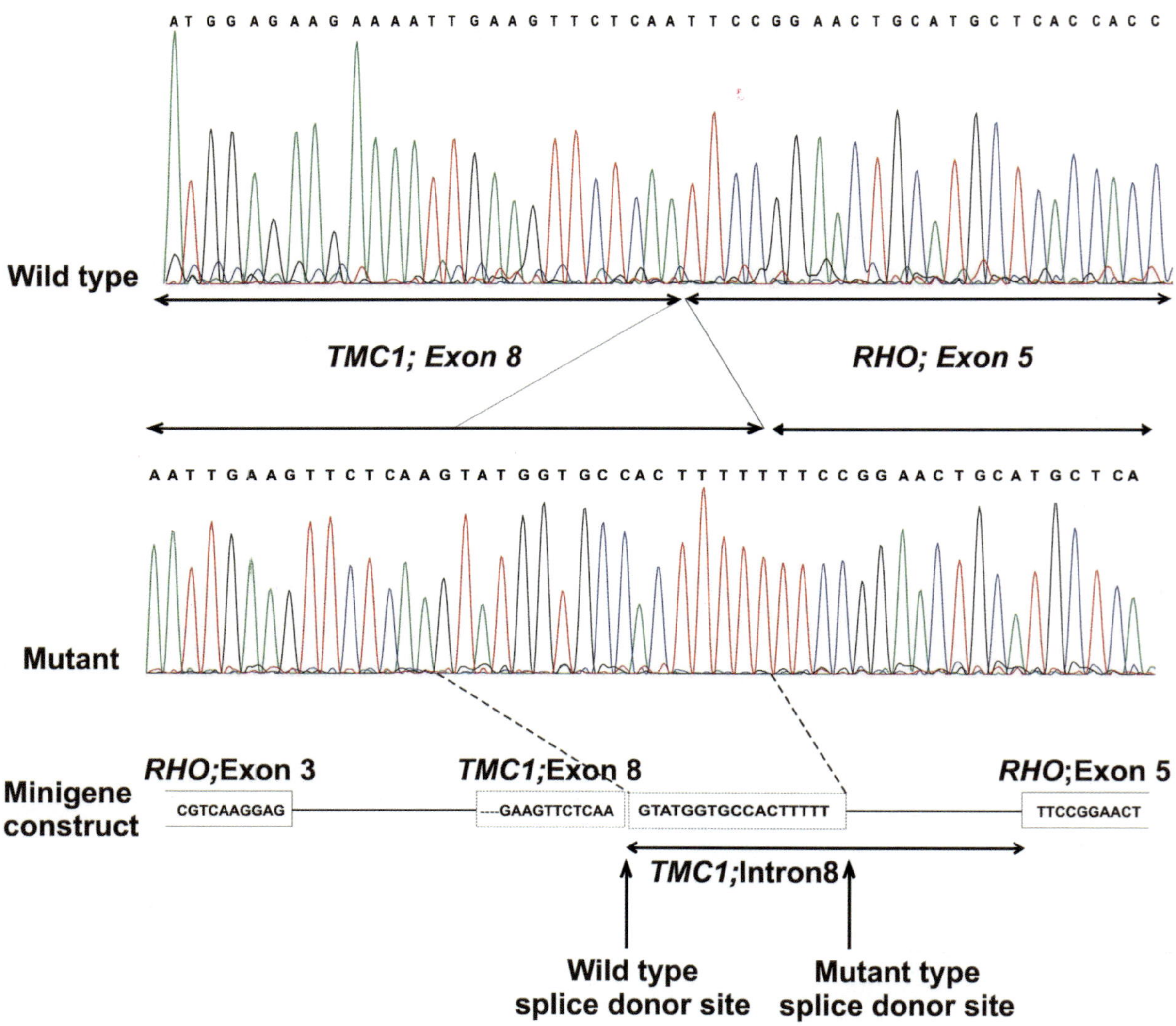


**Figure 3. Effect of *TMC1* intronic mutation c.362+18A>G using a minigene approach.** Electropherogram of the partial cDNA sequence of RNA derived from cells transfected with the pCI-NEO with either the mutant or wildtype *TMC1* exon 8. The mutation leads to the insertion of 17bp at the 3′end of exon 8, which can be predicted to result in a premature stop codon in exon 9 (p.Glu122Tyrfs*10).

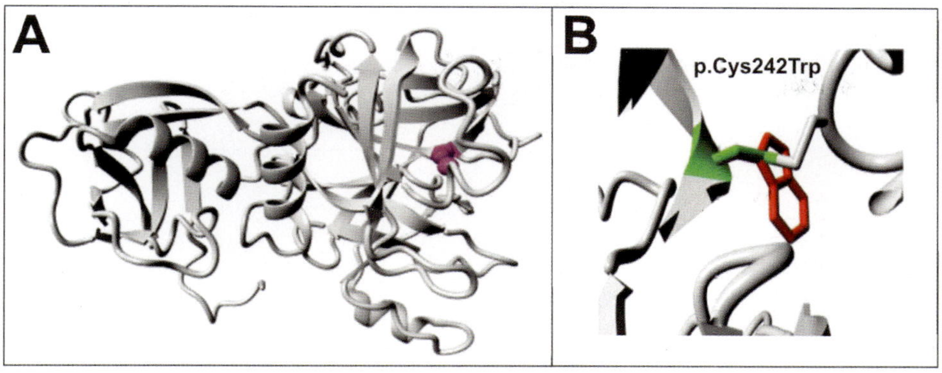


**Figure 4. Predicted effect of mutation c.726C>G (p.Cys242Trp) on the three dimensional structure of TMPRSS3.** A) Wild type protein structure with an intact disulphide bridge showing position of the mutated residue (magenta). B) Close-up view of the structure showing the wild type residue cysteine (green) and the mutant residue tryptophan (red). In case of the mutant residue there will be no disulphide bridge at this position.

## Discussion

In a cohort of 30 ARNSHL families the genetic defects were identified in 9 known deafness genes; *GJB2*, *MYO15A*, *TMC1*, *BSND*, *TMPRSS3*, *MSRB3*, *HGF*, *SLC26A4* and *TMIE*. In the current panel recurrent as well as novel mutations were detected, the novel mutations were identified in *GJB2*, *MYO15A*, *TMC1*, *BSND*, *TMPRSS3* and *MSRB3*.

*GJB2* was the most frequently mutated gene in these families. In this gene the novel mutation c.598G>A (p.Gly200Arg) affects a residue in the cysteine-rich domain that is involved in the formation of intramolecular disulphide bonds [28,29]. Although the effect of glycine on the intramolecular disulphide bond formation cannot be predicted, the mutant residue arginine may affect the proper folding of the cysteine-rich domain because of the larger size of the arginine side chain.

In two families the *GJB2* variant c.380G>A (p.Arg127His) was found to segregate with the hearing loss, being present homozygously in 4 affected members. Other studies have also reported deafness patients carrying this mutation homozygously [29,30,31]. Based upon the higher carrier frequency in patients as well as controls, Padma et al. [30] suggested that it is unlikely that this variant plays a pathogenic role in deafness. However, Matos et al. [32] have proposed that this mutation is likely to be pathogenic when influenced by other unknown genetic or environmental factors [32]. In the EVS, however, no homozygous occurrence of the mutated allele has been reported to date (Table S1). Identification of 4 p.Arg127His homozygous patients out of 125 deafness patients in the current study and the previously reported cases of 9 heterozygous cases and 1 compound heterozygous case in 70 deaf patients by Bukhari et al. [31], demonstrates that this is the most frequently occurring mutation in Pakistani deafness families and therefore becomes important in genetic counseling of Pakistani deaf patients.

In the current study *GJB2* mutations were found to be the most common, followed by *MYO15A* mutations. The overall frequency of the two most common nonsense variants c.71G>A (p.Trp24*) and c.231G>A (p.Trp77*) of *GJB2* in Pakistani deafness patients was obtained from the current (n = 125) as well as previously reported studies of Santos et al. [33] (n = 430) and Bukhari et al. [31] (n = 70). Using these data, the frequency was found to be 5.9% (p.Trp24*) and 4.3% (p.Trp77*) [31,33]. The variant p.Trp24* has a high prevalence in the Indian population as well [34], Pakistan and India have a shared genetic ancestry [35], which could be the reason of the presence of this variant in both populations. The third mutation p.Gly12Valfs*2 identified in the current study has previously been reported from Northern areas of Pakistan [31] and also in Caucasians and Turks [36], thus indicating a possible founder effect of this mutation. In the current cohort, 35% (60/173) individuals were found to be carriers of *GJB2* mutations. Therefore, as a preliminary screening of deaf families the sequencing of this gene is suggested in Pakistan. In the current study *MYO15A* was found to be the second leading cause of deafness in the Pakistani population, but still no recurrent mutation was identified in this gene.

A total of 7 nonsense mutations were identified in *GJB2*, *MYO15A* and *TMC1*, these nonsense mutations are likely to cause nonsense mediated decay (NMD) because they are either present in the middle or near the 5′end of the gene.

In *MYO15A* two splice site, a nonsense and a missense mutations were identified. The c.9948G>A (p.Gln3316Gln) mutation affects the last nucleotide of exon 61 and changes the consensus splice site sequence. Based on the results of the minigene assay the c.9948G>A mutation is expected to lead to skipping of exon 61, which would result in a frameshift and NMD can be expected to occur at least for part of the mRNAs. The second splice site mutation c.3866+1G>A is a canonical splice site change and is predicted to remove the splice donor site of exon 5. An alternative splice site is predicted at position +99 in intron 5, if this alternative site is used it would lead to a frameshift and a premature stop codon (encoded by nucleotide 2–4 of intron 5). Both splice site mutations are thus predicted to lead to a frameshift and NMD could occur for at least part of the mRNA transcripts. The two other novel mutations, c.8222T>C (p.Phe2741Ser) and c.8767C>T (p.Arg2923*), found in two different families, are located in the region of the gene that encodes the tail region of *MYO15A* and are likely to cause a loss of function of this region. The p.Arg2923* mutation is present in the SH3 domain, which is involved in the protein-protein interactions [37]. Most of the previously reported mutations of *MYO15A* causing congenital severe to profound deafness were found in the motor head and the tail domains [6,38]. Collectively these results indicate that the motor head and tail regions of *MYO15A* are essential in the hearing process and any mutation in these regions is thus critical [39].

*TMC1* encoding a transmembrane protein is expressed in the neurosensory hair cells of the mouse cochlea [40]. The recurrent nonsense mutation in exon 7 of *TMC1*, c.100C>T (p.Arg34*) is

**Table 3.** Recurrent mutations in known autosomal recessive non-syndromic hearing loss (ARNSHL) genes in 6 Pakistani families.

| Family ID | Size of Homozygous Region (Mb) | Chr. | Flanking SNPs | Chr. Position (In hg19) | Candidate Gene | Mutation (Predicted protein change) | Frequency in EVS | Ref. |
|---|---|---|---|---|---|---|---|---|
| DFR22 | 9.23 | 9 | rs4275319; rs2295861 | 68,513,625–77,745,424 | *TMC1*, (NM_138691.2) | Ex-15: c.1114G>A (p.Val372Met) | AA = 0, AG = 2, GG = 6501 | [23] |
| 19DFS | 11.96 | 9 | rs10867845;rs10867778 | 72252269–84222230 | *TMC1*, (NM_138691.2) | Ex-7: c.100C>T, (p.Arg34*) | Absent | [40] |
| DFR20 | 26.06 | 7 | rs10485886; rs2073791 | 78,057,840–104,122,989 | *HGF*, (NM_000601) | In-4: c.482+1991_2000delGATGATGAAA (p.?) | Absent | [25] |
| DFR37 | 37.85 | 7 | rs13234819; rs104869 | 44,342,969–82,197,469 | *HGF*, (NM_000601) | In-4: c.482+1986_1988delTGA (p.?) | Absent | [25] |
| DFR39 | 29.83 | 7 | rs2285507; rs10253693 | 92,989,228–122,825,956 | *SLC26A4*, (NM_000441.1) | Ex-11: c.1337A>G (p.Gln446Arg) | Absent | [26] |
| 26DF | 2652 | 3 | rs304838; rs536036 | 30806674–57326883 | *TMIE* (NM_147196) | Ex-3: c.241C>T (p.Arg81Cys) | Absent | [27] |

Acc. No., accession number of reference sequence; Chr, chromosome; Ex, exon; EVS, exome variant server; In, intron; SNPs, single nucleotide polymorphisms; Ref, references.

the most common *TMC1* mutation reported in Pakistan. It leads to a truncated protein and leads to congenital severe to profound hearing loss [40,41,42,43]. Ben Said et al. [42] have previously described that the p.Arg34* is an old founder mutation found in several populations including the Pakistani population. It is likely that the family described here carries the mutation on the founder haplotype. Also a novel intronic mutation in the *TMC1* gene, c.362+18A>G was identified in the current study (Table 2), which creates a novel splice donor site and the insertion of 17 nucleotides as demonstrated in the minigene approach.

*BSND* encodes the barttin protein, which is a vital subunit of the chloride and voltage-sensitive Ka (CLCNKA) and Kb (CLCNKB) channels in the inner ear and the kidney. Chloride channels and the barttin protein form heteromers which function in the recycling of the $K^+$ ions in the inner ear and salt reabsorption in the kidneys [44,45,46,47,48,49]. As predicted by *in silico* analysis, the currently identified *BSND* mutation p.Val33Leu residing in the transmembranal region might result in the malfunctioning of chloride channels CLCNKA and CLCNKB. However, in the current family there were no complaints of any renal problems.

Deafness caused by mutations in the *TMPRSS3* gene is bilateral and severe to profound with no defects of the middle ear and the vestibular system [50]. Mutations in *TMPRSS3* can also cause progressive hearing loss with a postlingual onset [51]. *TMPRSS3* mutation c.726C>G (p.Cys242Trp) in exon 8 affects the serine protease domain as predicted by 3D modeling. Previously another mutation in the same exon of *TMPRSS3*, c. 647G>T (p.Arg216Leu) has been shown to result in a failure of the protein to undergo proteolytic cleavage resulting in the inactivation of the sodium channel [52].

The homozygous variant p.Leu7Arg (c.20T>G) in *MSRB3* identified in the current study is located in the mitochondrial signal sequence and may result in mislocalization of the protein. Ahmed et al. [53] have shown the importance of the mitochondrial isoforms when they found a mutation c.55T>C (p.Arg19*) to underlie hearing impairment. This mutation also resides in the signal sequence for mitochondrial localization. However, the variant c.20T>G (p.Leu7Arg) was also found in heterozygous state in 3 out of 89 (1.7%) ethnically matched controls. The mutation might be a founder mutation in the corresponding population. However, currently it is uncertain whether this variant is the cause of hearing impairment in the family and further studies are necessary for a definite conclusion on the pathogenic effect of the variant.

## Conclusions

In the present study 53% (16/30) of the families were found to carry causative mutations in *GJB2* illustrating that the most frequently involved gene in deafness in the Pakistani population is *GJB2* followed by *MYO15A* (13%, 4/30) and *TMC1* (10%, 3/30). Based on these results it is therefore suggested that as an initial step for the genetic diagnosis of deafness, *GJB2* should be analyzed in Pakistani patients and if this gene is excluded then microsatellite markers flanking *MYO15A* and *TMC1* should be genotyped to exclude those genes or to indicate mutation analysis. Homozygosity mapping is an effective approach to determine the mutated genes in consanguineous families. Although a large number of deafness genes and mutations have already been identified, our study demonstrates that the full mutation spectrum in these genes is still not defined. Identification of novel mutations in these genes is important for genetic counseling and can provide handles for further studies on protein function. Genetic counseling of the families is important to better inform couples about the risk of their offspring to be hearing impaired. In addition, as can be seen in the current study, recurrent as well as novel mutations in known genes define the disease in the families which seem to have some population specificity. This information can be important in developing screening strategies.

## Supporting Information

**Figure S1 Multiple-alignment of the corresponding stretches of protein sequences across different species.** The blue color shading represents the intensity of conservation, where the dark blue shading represents highly conserved stretch while the light blue shading denotes moderate conservation of residues across different species. A) Amino acid sequence conservation of p.Gly200 across 9 species. B) Amino acid sequence conservation of p.Phe2741 across 11 species. C) Amino acid sequence conservation of p.Val33 across 7 species. D) Amino acid sequence conservation of p.Cys24 across 10 species. E) Non-conserved residue of p.Leu7 across 10 species.

**Table S1 Characteristics of 30 Pakistani families diagnosed with autosomal recessive non-syndromic hearing loss (ARNSHL).**

## Acknowledgments

We thank all the families for their cooperation in the current study. We thank Saskia van der Velde-Visser for excellent technical assistance.

## Author Contributions

Conceived and designed the experiments: S. Shafique S. Siddiqi MS JO TMS M. Azam HK RQ. Performed the experiments: S. Shafique S. Siddiqi MS JO HA AB M. Azam CZS TMS AM KM STAS AH M. Ajmal. Analyzed the data: S. Shafique S. Siddiqi MS JO HA AB M. Azam CZS TMS AM KM STAS AH M. Ajmal HK RQ. Contributed reagents/materials/analysis tools: MS TMS HK RQ. Wrote the paper: S. Shafique S. Siddiqi MS JO HA AB M. Azam CZS TMS AM KM STAS AH M. Ajmal HK RQ.

## References


1. Mustapha M, Salem N, Delague V, Chouery E, Ghassibeh M, et al. (2001) Autosomal recessive non-syndromic hearing loss in the Lebanese population: prevalence of the 30delG mutation and report of two novel mutations in the connexin 26 (GJB2) gene. J Med Genet 38: E36.
2. Van Camp G, Coucke PJ, Kunst H, Schatteman I, Van Velzen D, et al. (1997) Linkage analysis of progressive hearing loss in five extended families maps the DFNA2 gene to a 1.25-Mb region on chromosome 1p. Genomics 41: 70–74.
3. Morton NE (1991) Genetic epidemiology of hearing impairment. Ann N Y Acad Sci 630: 16–31.
4. Bayazit YA, Yilmaz M (2006) An overview of hereditary hearing loss. ORL J Otorhinolaryngol Relat Spec 68: 57–63.
5. Elahi MM, Elahi F, Elahi A, Elahi SB (1998) Paediatric hearing loss in rural Pakistan. J Otolaryngol 27: 348–353.
6. Hilgert N, Smith RJ, Van Camp G (2009) Forty-six genes causing nonsyndromic hearing impairment: which ones should be analyzed in DNA diagnostics? Mutat Res 681: 189–196.
7. Zelante L, Gasparini P, Estivill X, Melchionda S, D'Agruma L, et al. (1997) Connexin26 mutations associated with the most common form of non-syndromic neurosensory autosomal recessive deafness (DFNB1) in Mediterraneans. Hum Mol Genet 6: 1605–1609.
8. Estivill X, Fortina P, Surrey S, Rabionet R, Melchionda S, et al. (1998) Connexin-26 mutations in sporadic and inherited sensorineural deafness. Lancet 351: 394–398.
9. Kelley PM, Harris DJ, Comer BC, Askew JW, Fowler T, et al. (1998) Novel mutations in the connexin 26 gene (GJB2) that cause autosomal recessive (DFNB1) hearing loss. Am J Hum Genet 62: 792–799.
10. Bashir R, Fatima A, Naz S (2012) Prioritized sequencing of the second exon of MYO15A reveals a new mutation segregating in a Pakistani family with moderate to severe hearing loss. Eur J Med Genet 55: 99–102.
11. Sambrook J, Russell DW (2006) The condensed protocols from Molecular cloning: a laboratory manual. Cold Spring Harbor, N.Y.: Cold Spring Harbor Laboratory Press v, 800 p.p.
12. de Heer AM, Collin RWJ, Huygen PL, Schraders M, Oostrik J, et al. (2011) Progressive sensorineural hearing loss and normal vestibular function in a Dutch DFNB7/11 family with a novel mutation in TMC1. Audiol Neurootol 16: 93–105.
13. Schraders M, Lee K, Oostrik J, Huygen PL, Ali G, et al. (2010) Homozygosity mapping reveals mutations of GRXCR1 as a cause of autosomal-recessive nonsyndromic hearing impairment. Am J Hum Genet 86: 138–147.
14. Rozen S, Skaletsky H (2000) Primer3 on the WWW for general users and for biologist programmers. Methods Mol Biol 132: 365–386.
15. Seelow D, Schuelke M, Hildebrandt F, Nurnberg P (2009) HomozygosityMapper—an interactive approach to homozygosity mapping. Nucleic Acids Res 37: W593–599.
16. Hoffmann K, Lindner TH (2005) easyLINKAGE-Plus—automated linkage analyses using large-scale SNP data. Bioinformatics 21: 3565–3567.
17. Sim NL, Kumar P, Hu J, Henikoff S, Schneider G, et al. (2012) SIFT web server: predicting effects of amino acid substitutions on proteins. Nucleic Acids Res 40: W452–457.
18. Adzhubei IA, Schmidt S, Peshkin L, Ramensky VE, Gerasimova A, et al. (2010) A method and server for predicting damaging missense mutations. Nat Methods 7: 248–249.
19. Brunak S, Engelbrecht J, Knudsen S (1991) Prediction of human mRNA donor and acceptor sites from the DNA sequence. J Mol Biol 220: 49–65.
20. Petersen TN, Brunak S, von Heijne G, Nielsen H (2011) SignalP 4.0: discriminating signal peptides from transmembrane regions. Nat Methods 8: 785–786.
21. Venselaar H, Te Beek TA, Kuipers RK, Hekkelman ML, Vriend G (2010) Protein structure analysis of mutations causing inheritable diseases. An e-Science approach with life scientist friendly interfaces. BMC Bioinformatics 11: 548.
22. Gamundi MJ, Hernan I, Muntanyola M, Maseras M, Lopez-Romero P, et al. (2008) Transcriptional expression of cis-acting and trans-acting splicing mutations cause autosomal dominant retinitis pigmentosa. Hum Mutat 29: 869–878.
23. Santos RL, Wajid M, Khan MN, McArthur N, Pham TL, et al. (2005) Novel sequence variants in the TMC1 gene in Pakistani families with autosomal recessive hearing impairment. Hum Mutat 26: 396.
24. Searle C, Mavrogiannis LA, Bennett CP, Charlton RS (2012) The common TMC1 mutation c.100C>T (p.Arg34X) is not a significant cause of deafness in British Asians. Genet Test Mol Biomarkers 16: 453–455.
25. Schultz JM, Khan SN, Ahmed ZM, Riazuddin S, Waryah AM, et al. (2009) Noncoding mutations of HGF are associated with nonsyndromic hearing loss, DFNB39. Am J Hum Genet 85: 25–39.
26. Reardon W, O'Mahoney CF, Trembath R, Jan H, Phelps PD (2000) Enlarged vestibular aqueduct: a radiological marker of pendred syndrome, and mutation of the PDS gene. QJM 93: 99–104.
27. Naz S, Giguere CM, Kohrman DC, Mitchem KL, Riazuddin S, et al. (2002) Mutations in a novel gene, TMIE, are associated with hearing loss linked to the DFNB6 locus. Am J Hum Genet 71: 632–636.
28. Batissoco AC, Auricchio MT, Kimura L, Tabith-Junior A, Mingroni-Netto RC (2009) A novel missense mutation p.L76P in the GJB2 gene causing nonsyndromic recessive deafness in a Brazilian family. Braz J Med Biol Res 42: 168–171.
29. Minarik G, Ferak V, Ferakova E, Ficek A, Polakova H, et al. (2003) High frequency of GJB2 mutation W24X among Slovak Romany (Gypsy) patients with non-syndromic hearing loss (NSHL). Gen Physiol Biophys 22: 549–556.
30. Padma G, Ramchander PV, Nandur UV, Padma T (2009) GJB2 and GJB6 gene mutations found in Indian probands with congenital hearing impairment. J Genet 88: 267–272.
31. Bukhari I, Mujtaba G, Naz S (2013) Contribution of GJB2 mutations to hearing loss in the Hazara Division of Pakistan. Biochem Genet 51: 524–529.
32. Matos TD, Simoes-Teixeira H, Caria H, Rosa H, O'Neill A, et al. (2010) The controversial p.Arg127His mutation in GJB2: report on three Portuguese hearing loss family cases. Genet Test Mol Biomarkers 14: 141–144.
33. Santos RL, Wajid M, Pham TL, Hussan J, Ali G, et al. (2005) Low prevalence of Connexin 26 (GJB2) variants in Pakistani families with autosomal recessive non-syndromic hearing impairment. Clin Genet 67: 61–68.
34. Mani RS, Ganapathy A, Jalvi R, Srikumari Srisailapathy CR, Malhotra V, et al. (2009) Functional consequences of novel connexin 26 mutations associated with hereditary hearing loss. Eur J Hum Genet 17: 502–509.
35. Qamar R, Ayub Q, Mohyuddin A, Helgason A, Mazhar K, et al. (2002) Y-chromosomal DNA variation in Pakistan. Am J Hum Genet 70: 1107–1124.
36. Snoeckx RL, Huygen PL, Feldmann D, Marlin S, Denoyelle F, et al. (2005) GJB2 mutations and degree of hearing loss: a multicenter study. Am J Hum Genet 77: 945–957.
37. Weng Z, Rickles RJ, Feng S, Richard S, Shaw AS, et al. (1995) Structure-function analysis of SH3 domains: SH3 binding specificity altered by single amino acid substitutions. Mol Cell Biol 15: 5627–5634.

38. Belyantseva IA, Boger ET, Friedman TB (2003) Myosin XVa localizes to the tips of inner ear sensory cell stereocilia and is essential for staircase formation of the hair bundle. Proc Natl Acad Sci U S A 100: 13958–13963.
39. Anderson DW, Probst FJ, Belyantseva IA, Fridell RA, Beyer L, et al. (2000) The motor and tail regions of myosin XV are critical for normal structure and function of auditory and vestibular hair cells. Hum Mol Genet 9: 1729–1738.
40. Kitajiri SI, McNamara R, Makishima T, Husnain T, Zafar AU, et al. (2007) Identities, frequencies and origins of TMC1 mutations causing DFNB7/B11 deafness in Pakistan. Clin Genet 72: 546–550.
41. Sirmaci A, Duman D, Ozturkmen-Akay H, Erbek S, Incesulu A, et al. (2009) Mutations in TMC1 contribute significantly to nonsyndromic autosomal recessive sensorineural hearing loss: a report of five novel mutations. Int J Pediatr Otorhinolaryngol 73: 699–705.
42. Ben Said M, Hmani-Aifa M, Amar I, Baig SM, Mustapha M, et al. (2010) High frequency of the p.R34X mutation in the TMC1 gene associated with nonsyndromic hearing loss is due to founder effects. Genet Test Mol Biomarkers 14: 307–311.
43. Hilgert N, Alasti F, Dieltjens N, Pawlik B, Wollnik B, et al. (2008) Mutation analysis of TMC1 identifies four new mutations and suggests an additional deafness gene at loci DFNA36 and DFNB7/11. Clin Genet 74: 223–232.
44. Estevez R, Boettger T, Stein V, Birkenhager R, Otto E, et al. (2001) Barttin is a Cl- channel beta-subunit crucial for renal Cl- reabsorption and inner ear K+ secretion. Nature 414: 558–561.
45. Hayama A, Rai T, Sasaki S, Uchida S (2003) Molecular mechanisms of Bartter syndrome caused by mutations in the BSND gene. Histochem Cell Biol 119: 485–493.
46. Janssen AG, Scholl U, Domeyer C, Nothmann D, Leinenweber A, et al. (2009) Disease-causing dysfunctions of barttin in Bartter syndrome type IV. J Am Soc Nephrol 20: 145–153.
47. Kramer BK, Bergler T, Stoelcker B, Waldegger S (2008) Mechanisms of Disease: the kidney-specific chloride channels ClCKA and ClCKB, the Barttin subunit, and their clinical relevance. Nat Clin Pract Nephrol 4: 38–46.
48. Rickheit G, Maier H, Strenzke N, Andreescu CE, De Zeeuw CI, et al. (2008) Endocochlear potential depends on Cl- channels: mechanism underlying deafness in Bartter syndrome IV. EMBO J 27: 2907–2917.
49. Waldegger S, Jeck N, Barth P, Peters M, Vitzthum H, et al. (2002) Barttin increases surface expression and changes current properties of ClC-K channels. Pflugers Arch 444: 411–418.
50. Fasquelle L, Scott HS, Lenoir M, Wang J, Rebillard G, et al. (2011) Tmprss3, a transmembrane serine protease deficient in human DFNB8/10 deafness, is critical for cochlear hair cell survival at the onset of hearing. J Biol Chem 286: 17383–17397.
51. Weegerink NJ, Schraders M, Oostrik J, Huygen PL, Strom TM, et al. (2011) Genotype-phenotype correlation in DFNB8/10 families with TMPRSS3 mutations. J Assoc Res Otolaryngol 12: 753–766.
52. Elbracht M, Senderek J, Eggermann T, Thurmer C, Park J, et al. (2007) Autosomal recessive postlingual hearing loss (DFNB8): compound heterozygosity for two novel TMPRSS3 mutations in German siblings. J Med Genet 44: e81.
53. Ahmed ZM, Yousaf R, Lee BC, Khan SN, Lee S, et al. (2011) Functional null mutations of MSRB3 encoding methionine sulfoxide reductase are associated with human deafness DFNB74. Am J Hum Genet 88: 19–29.

# 3

# Objective Assessment of Spectral Ripple Discrimination in Cochlear Implant Listeners Using Cortical Evoked Responses to an Oddball Paradigm

**Alejandro Lopez Valdes[1]*, Myles Mc Laughlin[1,2], Laura Viani[3], Peter Walshe[3], Jaclyn Smith[3], Fan-Gang Zeng[2], Richard B. Reilly[1]**

**1** Trinity Centre for Bioengineering, Trinity College, Dublin, Ireland, **2** Hearing and Speech Laboratory, University of California Irvine, Irvine, California, United States of America, **3** National Cochlear Implant Programme, Beaumont Hospital, Dublin, Ireland

## Abstract

Cochlear implants (CIs) can partially restore functional hearing in deaf individuals. However, multiple factors affect CI listener's speech perception, resulting in large performance differences. Non-speech based tests, such as spectral ripple discrimination, measure acoustic processing capabilities that are highly correlated with speech perception. Currently spectral ripple discrimination is measured using standard psychoacoustic methods, which require attentive listening and active response that can be difficult or even impossible in special patient populations. Here, a completely objective cortical evoked potential based method is developed and validated to assess spectral ripple discrimination in CI listeners. In 19 CI listeners, using an oddball paradigm, cortical evoked potential responses to standard and inverted spectrally rippled stimuli were measured. In the same subjects, psychoacoustic spectral ripple discrimination thresholds were also measured. A neural discrimination threshold was determined by systematically increasing the number of ripples per octave and determining the point at which there was no longer a significant difference between the evoked potential response to the standard and inverted stimuli. A correlation was found between the neural and the psychoacoustic discrimination thresholds ($R^2 = 0.60$, $p<0.01$). This method can objectively assess CI spectral resolution performance, providing a potential tool for the evaluation and follow-up of CI listeners who have difficulty performing psychoacoustic tests, such as pediatric or new users.

**Editor:** Jyrki Ahveninen, Harvard Medical School/Massachusetts General Hospital, United States of America

**Funding:** This work was supported by a Higher Education Authority (HEA) Graduate Research Education Program in Engineering (GREP-Eng) scholarship to Alejandro Lopez Valdes, an EU FP7 Marie Curie International Outgoing Fellowship to Myles Mc Laughlin and the National Institutes of Health, the United States Department of Health and Human Services (P30 DC008369). The funders had no role in study design, data collection and analysis, decision to publish, or preparation of the manuscript.

**Competing Interests:** The authors have declared that no competing interests exist.

* E-mail: lopezvaa@tcd.ie

## Introduction

A cochlear implant (CI) can partially restore hearing in deaf individuals, allowing most listeners to obtain 70–80% correct sentence perception in quiet [1]. A CI is now the standard treatment for severe to profound deafness worldwide, with infants as young as 6 months being considered for implantation [2]. In spite of this success, there remains a large amount of variability in speech perception outcomes among CI listeners. While factors such as duration of deafness, age at onset of deafness or duration of CI use affect performance [3,4], they cannot completely account for all the observed variability [5–10]. Factors such as temporal and spectral processing capabilities also contribute to speech perception outcomes [11–14]. To help understand the causes of this performance variability, and to improve clinical evaluation and follow-up of CI listeners, there is a need for tests which can objectively quantify performance in both pediatric and adult populations.

Standardized sentence and word recognition tests are useful for directly measuring speech perception in CI listeners. However, they cannot be used with pre-lingual children (a rapidly expanding user group), nor do they directly asses underlying mechanisms of speech recognition (i.e. spectral resolution). A spectral ripple discrimination test is a non-linguistic psychoacoustic method for probing a normal hearing listener's spectral resolution [15]. A number of studies have now shown that spectral ripple discrimination correlates with different aspects of speech perception and music perception in CI users [13,14,16,17].

To measure spectral ripple discrimination thresholds in CI listeners, standard psychoacoustic threshold tracking methods are normally employed. CI listeners actively listen to a number of intervals containing either a standard stimulus or its ripple-phase inverted counterpart. They are requested to report which interval contained the inverted stimulus by, for example, pressing a button corresponding to the interval. This approach produces reliable results in adults. Although experienced researchers might be able to use an observer based psychoacoustic procedure to measure spectral ripple discrimination thresholds in infants [18], these standard psychophysical approaches are difficult to apply to special populations such as pediatric, pre-lingually deafened or non-compliant users in clinical practice.

An alternative to psychoacoustic methods is to employ an objective neural response to predict behavioral outcomes. An advantage of this approach is that listeners do not need to respond to the stimuli and often need not attend to the stimuli. Neural responses from the auditory nerve and brainstem in CI listeners have been shown to correlate reasonably well with threshold and comfort stimulation levels [19–22], while cortical evoked potentials have been shown to correlate with higher level outcomes such as speech perception [23–26], musical perception and auditory plasticity [27–32]. In particular, mismatch negativity (MMN) responses have been proposed as an objective index of auditory discrimination for different clinical conditions [33]. The MMN response can be obtained, via an unattended oddball paradigm, as the evoked potential difference between a frequently presented stimulus (standard) and a less frequently and randomly presented different stimulus (deviant or oddball).

The aim of this study was to use an unattended oddball paradigm to develop and validate a completely objective method for measuring spectral ripple discrimination thresholds in adult CI listeners. An objective method for measuring spectral ripple discrimination thresholds would potentially provide an additional tool when standard psychophysical approaches are difficult to apply to certain CI populations.

## Materials and Methods

### Subjects and Ethics Statement

**Subjects.** Nineteen adult CI listeners (6 male, 13 female) participated in the present study at two separate locations: Trinity Centre for Bioengineering, Trinity College Dublin (n = 15) and Hearing and Speech Laboratory, University of California Irvine (n = 4). One bilateral subject was evaluated separately for both ears yielding a total of 20 ears tested. Exclusion criteria applied to subjects under 18 years of age and subjects with cognitive or learning disabilities. There were no subjects withdrawn from this study. Subjects were aged between 31 and 79 years (mean 56, standard deviation 15). They used either a Cochlear (n = 17), Med-El (n = 1) or Advanced Bionics (n = 1) implants (device details on implant type and usage experience are shown in Table 1). All subjects used monopolar stimulation mode.

### Ethics Statement

Experimental procedures were approved by the Ethics (Medical Research) Committee at Beaumont Hospital, Beaumont, Dublin, the Ethical Review Board at Trinity College Dublin and The University of California Irvine's Institutional Review Board. Written informed consent was obtained from all subjects.

### Psychoacoustic Methods

**Psychoacoustic Stimuli.** Psychoacoustic spectral ripple discrimination thresholds were determined in all subjects using stimuli similar to that employed by Won et al. [14]. Stimuli were generated by summing 250 pure tones ranging from 250 to 5000 Hz. The amplitudes of the pure tones were determined by a full-wave rectified sinusoidal envelope on a logarithmic amplitude scale. The ripple peaks were spaced equally on a logarithmic frequency scale. The starting phases of the components were randomized for each presentation. The ripple stimuli were generated with 14 different densities, measured in ripples/octave. The ripple densities differed by ratios of 1.414 (0.125, 0.176, 0.250, 0.354, 0.500, 0.707, 1.000, 1.414, 2.000, 2.828, 4.000, 5.657, 8.000, and 11.314 ripples/octave). Standard and ripple-phase inverted stimuli were generated de novo in each trial run. For standard stimuli, the phase of the full-wave rectified sinusoidal spectral envelope was set to zero radians, and for phase-inverted stimuli, it was set to $\pi/2$. The stimuli were 500 ms in duration and 50 ms on and off cosine squared ramps were applied. Stimuli were filtered with a long-term, speech-shaped filter [34]. All stimuli were generated in MATLAB (MathWorks, Natick, MA) at 44.1 kHz and presented via a standard PC soundcard.

For both the psychoacoustic and evoked potential testing, stimuli were presented via the audio line-in on the CI at the most comfortable level, determined for each subject using a 0 (silence) to 10 (too loud) loudness scale, with 6 being the most comfortable level. To limit the effects of any unwanted background noise the CI microphone volume and sensitivity were set to the minimum allowable values. Subjects used their everyday speech processing strategy without any special adjustments other than changes to the microphone volume and sensitivity. Stimuli were always presented monaurally.

**Psychoacoustic Procedure.** A two-down, one-up, three-alternative forced-choice [35] paradigm was used to track the psychoacoustic spectral ripple discrimination threshold. Within one trial, two of the intervals were randomly selected to present the standard stimulus whilst the remaining interval presented the inverted stimulus, with all three intervals having stimuli with the same number of ripples/octave. If the subject's spectral resolution is sharp enough to resolve the spectral peaks and valleys, they should hear a difference in the standard and inverted stimuli [14,17]. The subject was asked to select the interval which was different by pressing a button on a graphical interface. After two consecutive correct responses, the number of ripples/octave was increased by a ratio of 1.414. As the number of ripples/octave increased the standard and inverted stimuli began to sound more similar. After one incorrect response the number of ripples/octave was decreased to the previously tested value. A run was terminated after 13 reversals. The psychoacoustic spectral ripple discrimination threshold was defined as the mean of the last eight reversals on the three-alternative forced-choice threshold tracking function [35]. All subjects completed at least five repetitions of the test to minimize any learning or attention effects. The final threshold was taken as the mean of all completed tests.

### Evoked Potential Methods

**Evoked Potential Stimuli.** The stimuli used in the evoked potential paradigm were similar to those used in the psychoacoustic paradigm except that 4000 pure tones ranging from 100 to 8000 Hz were used to cover the full frequency range of the CI filter bank. The lower pure tone range in the psychoacoustic stimuli allowed for the stimuli to be generated and presented faster while still presenting some energy to the highest CI high-frequency band.

Standard and ripple phase-inverted stimuli with durations of either 300 or 500 ms and with 0.125, 0.25, 0.5, 1, 2, 4 and 8 ripples/octave were generated and stored. Examples of the stimuli characterization at one and four ripples/octave can be seen in Fig. 1. There was no significant difference for the use of 300 or 500 ms stimuli with respect to the CI artifact, therefore, data from both stimuli duration were pooled together for analysis. The same set of stored stimulus tokens were used for all presentations to all subjects. In Trinity College Dublin stimuli were presented via a standard PC soundcard (44.1 kHz sampling rate) and in University of California, Irvine stimuli were presented using a USB digital to analog converter (DAC, 44.1 kHz sampling rate) (NI-USB 6221, National Instruments, Austin, TX).

**Evoked Potential Acquisition.** Fig. 2 shows a wideband, high-sampling rate, acquisition system that uses single-channel artifact attenuation to record late auditory evoked potentials in response to the spectral ripple stimuli presented in an oddball paradigm. The setup, along with the artifact attenuation

**Table 1.** Psychoacoustic and neural discrimination thresholds.

| Subject ID | Implant | Tested Ear | Years of CI Experience | Psychoacoustic Spectral Ripple Discrimination Threshold (RPO) | Neural Spectral Ripple Discrimination Threshold (RPO) | | |
|---|---|---|---|---|---|---|---|
| | | | | | Positive Area | Negative Area | Total Area |
| UCI 01 | Maestro | Left | 2 | 0.574 | 0.420 | 0.398 | 0.434 |
| UCI 02 | Freedom | Right | 5 | 1.403 | 1.008 | 0.900 | 0.989 |
| UCI 03 | Freedom | Left | 9 | 2.210 | 3.202 | 6.335 | 5.974 |
| UCI 03 | Freedom | Right | 1 | 1.542 | 2.085 | 1.188 | 2.407 |
| UCI 04 | Freedom | Right | 4 | 2.595 | 1.252 | 0.659 | 1.045 |
| TCD 01 | Freedom | Left | 3.5 | 1.158 | 1.793 | 0.665 | 0.763 |
| TCD 02 | Freedom | Left | 4 | 0.381 | 0.193 | 0.337 | 0.225 |
| TCD 03 | Clarion 1.2 | Right | 12 | 0.948 | 0.909 | 0.589 | 0.953 |
| TCD 04 | Freedom | Left | 7 | 0.618 | 0.248 | 0.221 | 0.237 |
| TCD 05 | Freedom | Left | 5 | 2.172 | 2.957 | 2.861 | 2.987 |
| TCD 06 | Freedom | Right | 1 | 0.658 | * | * | * |
| TCD 07 | Freedom | Right | 1 | 0.778 | * | 0.161 | 0.150 |
| TCD 08 | CI512 | Right | 1 | 0.400 | 0.473 | 0.239 | 0.409 |
| TCD 09 | Freedom | Left | 3.5 | 0.235 | 0.176 | * | 0.138 |
| TCD 10 | Freedom | Right | 3.5 | 0.312 | 0.821 | 0.546 | 0.739 |
| TCD 11 | CI24RE | Right | 9 | 1.113 | 0.489 | 0.833 | 0.782 |
| TCD 12 | Freedom | Right | 4 | 0.931 | 1.618 | 1.497 | 1.597 |
| TCD 13 | CI24R | Left | 8 | 0.463 | * | 0.461 | 0.482 |
| TCD 14 | CI24M | Right | 12 | 1.503 | 1.717 | 1.870 | 1.827 |
| TCD 15 | Freedom | Left | 5 | 0.240 | * | * | * |

RPO- Ripples per octave.
* Unable to estimate a neural spectral ripple discrimination threshold.

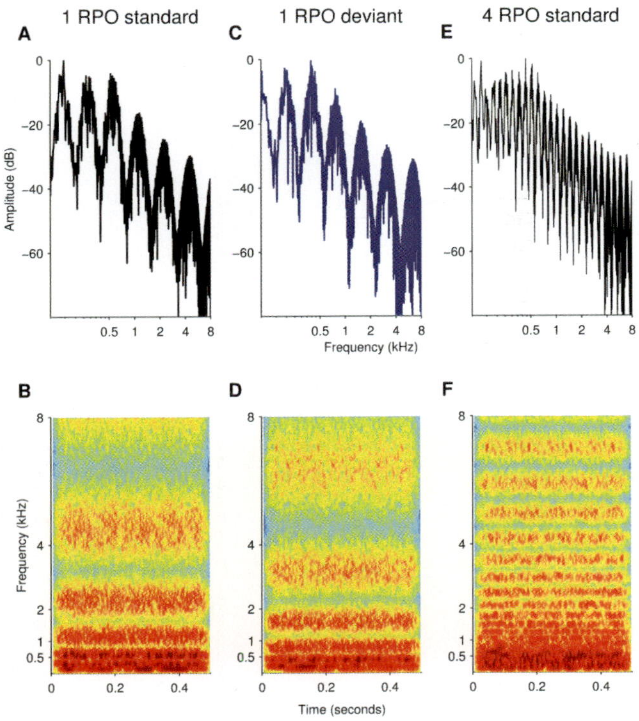


**Figure 1. Stimuli characterization.** (A) Frequency spectrum of a 500 ms standard stimulus with spectral peak density of one ripple per octave (RPO). Stimuli were composed of the sum of pure tones in a range of 0.25–5 kHz (psychoacoustic) or 0.1–8 kHz (electrophysiology). Spectral amplitudes were defined by a full-wave rectified sinusoidal envelope. One spectral peak can be clearly distinguished at the 0.5–1 kHz octave. Peak to valley amplitude of 30 dB as well as the high frequency attenuation of the speech-shaped filter can also be seen. (B) Spectrogram of the standard stimulus described, showing the frequency content of the stimulus along the 500 ms duration. Spectral peak density of one RPO can clearly be resolved in the 4–8 kHz octave. (C) Frequency spectrum of the corresponding phase-inverted, or deviant, stimulus employed along with the standard stimulus at one RPO in an oddball paradigm. The spectral envelope is shifted by $\pi/2$ with respect to the standard stimulus, as observed in the 0.5–1 kHz octave. (D) Spectrogram of the deviant stimulus, showing the inversed frequency content along the 500 ms duration with respect to the standard stimulus. (E) Frequency spectrum of a standard stimulus with spectral peak density of four RPO showing the increased spectral density with respect to the one RPO stimuli. (F) Spectrogram of the standard stimulus at four RPO. Spectral peak density of four RPO can clearly be resolved in the 4–8 kHz octave.

procedure, is described in detail elsewhere [36]. Briefly, the sampling rate on the analog to digital converter (ADC) (NI-USB 6221, National Instruments, Austin, TX) was set to 125 kHz, the amplifier (SRS 560, Stanford Research Systems, Sunnyvale, CA) gain was set to 2000, the amplifier high-pass filter was set to 0.03 and the low-pass filter to 100 kHz. Standard gold cup surface electrodes were placed at Cz, on the mastoid and on the collarbone, these last two electrodes were placed contralateral to the CI location. The positive end of the amplifier was connected to Cz, the negative end to the mastoid and the ground to the collarbone. Electrode impedances were always below 5 kΩ and care was taken to ensure that impedances were matched to within 1 kΩ to minimize low frequency artifacts [36]. The output of the amplifier was connected to one channel on the ADC. A trigger pulse generated simultaneously with the stimulus, and presented on a separate channel, was connected to a second channel on the ADC and used to synchronize stimulus presentation and acquisition.

**Evoked Potential Procedure.** Standard and ripple phase-inverted stimuli with the same number of ripples/octave were presented in an unattended oddball paradigm. The deviant stimulus was the ripple phase-inverted stimulus, having an occurrence probability of 10%, and the standard stimulus was the non-inverted stimulus. The inter-onset interval for each stimulus presentation was one second. One run began with 20 presentations of the standard stimulus after which the deviant randomly occurred at least once in every 10 stimulus presentations, with the additional condition that a deviant was never to be followed by another deviant. The paradigm was repeated at least four times for every subject, each time using stimuli with a different number of ripples/octave. Subjects were instructed to ignore the stimulus and to minimize movement to avoid movement artifacts in the recordings. Each oddball paradigm lasted approximately 12–15 minutes. Subjects watched a silent captioned film and rest breaks were provided after each run or upon subject's request. EEG data collection lasted approximately one hour per subject. At Trinity Centre for Bioengineering the acquisition sessions took place in a dedicated EEG room, while at the University of California Irvine, the sessions took place in a sound booth.

**Evoked Potential Epoching.** Raw EEG data were segmented into long epochs of 1100 ms, 300 ms pre- to 800 ms post-stimulus onset to avoid filter edge affects. Shorter epochs of 100 ms pre- to 500 ms post-stimulus were used for plotting the data. A baseline correction of 150 ms pre-stimulus was applied in all filtered epochs. Epochs were classified as response to standard or deviant stimuli and averaged across presentations. Online averaging and artifact attenuation allow the real time display of the evoked potential response to both standard and deviant stimuli. To speed up data collection a run was terminated when collecting more deviant responses did not significantly change the shape of the averaged deviant waveform. This change was evaluated by measuring the sum of squared differences of the averaged deviant epochs every time a new epoch was included, when the sum of squared differences stabilized at a low value it was determined that no significant change would be produced with the addition of more epochs. This was typically once 60 or 70 deviant responses were acquired, with a minimum of 50 deviants per run always being collected. A difference (or mismatch) waveform was calculated by subtracting the response to the standard stimuli from the response to the deviant stimuli. The oddball paradigm was repeated using stimuli with different numbers of ripples/octave, yielding one difference waveform for each ripple/octave stimulus.

**Evoked Potential Artifact Attenuation.** Mc Laughlin et al. [36] showed that with the wideband, high sampling-rate acquisition system, the CI related artifact consists of two components: a high frequency component which is a direct representation of the stimulation pulses and a low frequency component which is related to the envelope of the stimulation pulses. A 2$^{nd}$ order Butterworth band-pass filter (2–20 Hz, 12 dB/octave slope) was applied to the averaged standard and deviant responses (Fig. 3A and B single responses before filtering, Fig. 3C and D averaged responses after filtering). The low-pass edge of this filter attenuated the high frequency artifact component and the high-pass edge removed drift. The filter was applied using a zero-phase forward and reverse digital filtering method (filtfilt command, MATLAB).

It was observed that, within a subject, the signal envelopes derived from the CI stimulation pulse sequence associated to the standard and deviant stimuli were similar (compare Fig. 3A and B). A cross-correlation of 112 sets of standard and deviant CI

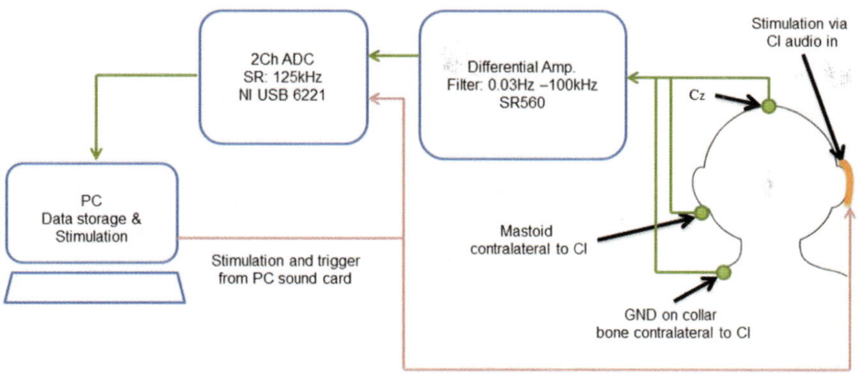


**Figure 2. Single-channel acquisition set-up.** Single-channel EEG acquisition system, featuring wideband and high-sampling rate recordings. EEG is recorded from electrode position Cz, referenced to the mastoid contralateral to the tested ear and grounded on the collar bone. The EEG signal is amplified with a biological differential pre-amplifier (SR560, Stanford Research System, Sunnyvale, CA) with filter settings at 0.03 Hz and 100 kHz. The signal is then digitized with an ADC (NI-USB 6221, National Instruments, Austin, TX) sampled at 125 kHz and recorded with a custom made software made in MATLAB (The MathWorks, Natick, MA). Stimulus and trigger presentation is done through the sound card of the computer. The trigger is fed to the ADC for event synchronization and the stimulus is presented via a personal audio cable to the auxiliary port of the subject's speech processor.

stimulation pulse sequences supported this observation (mean normalized correlation = 0.8871, standard deviation = 0.1597). With the result that any low frequency artifact component was equally present in both the response to the standard and the response to the deviant (compare onset and offset artifacts in Fig. 3C and D), calculating the difference waveform adequately attenuated any low frequency artifact components, leaving a difference waveform dominated by neural response (Fig. 3E).

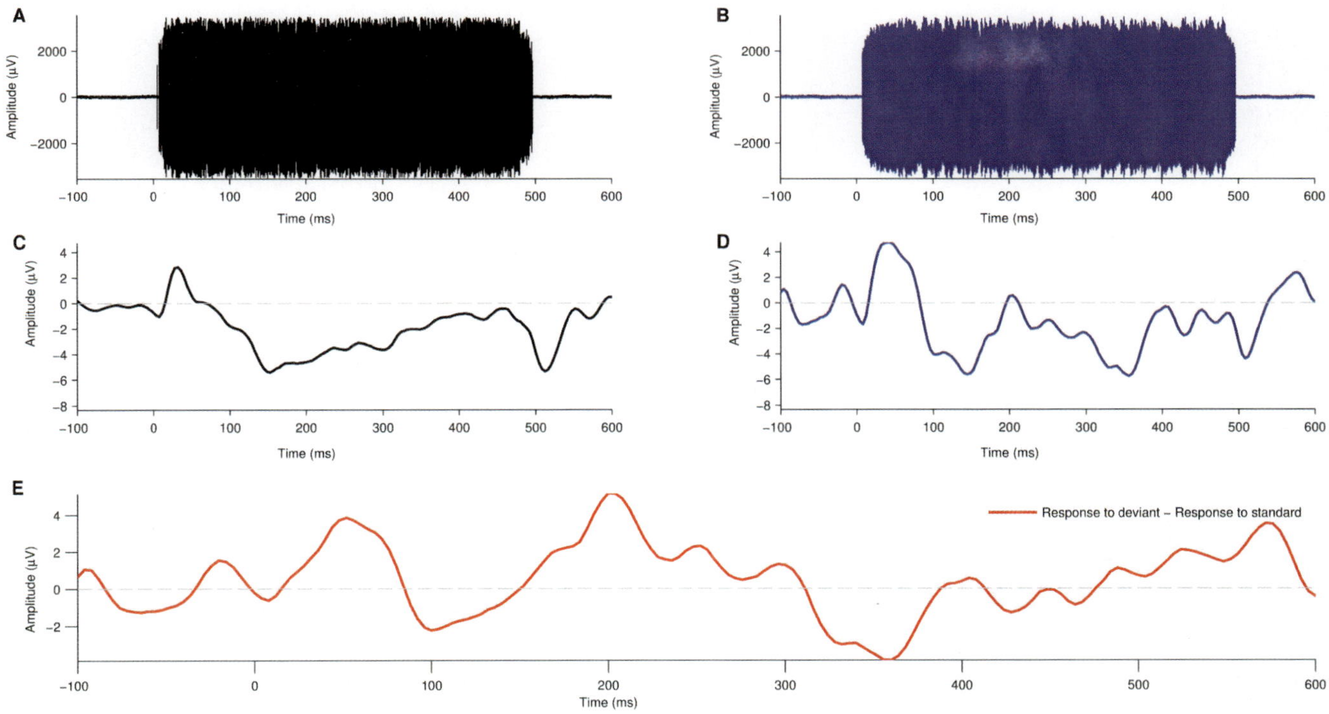


**Figure 3. Artifact attenuation and evoked potential extraction.** (A)–(B) Single EEG acquisition epoch of a 500 ms stimulus presented to a CI user. Data acquisition at a high-sampling rate (125 kHz) allows for the CI artifact to be clearly resolved from the recorded data as a high frequency and large amplitude component present during the 500 ms of stimulus duration (standard in black, deviant in blue). (C)–(D) Applying a 2nd order Butterworth band-pass filter (2–20 Hz) to the averaged epochs, recorded from an oddball paradigm, it is possible to attenuate the CI artifact and extract the evoked potential (EP) elicited to the each stimulus type (standard in black, deviant in blue). The N100, characteristic of auditory EPs can be identified in both standard (C) and deviant (D) stimuli types as a negative peak at around 100–150 ms. In some cases, after filtering, a low-frequency artifact is present at stimulus onset and offset with similar shape and amplitude in both standard and deviant responses. (E) A difference waveform is calculated by subtracting the neural response elicited to the standard stimuli from the neural response elicited to the deviant stimuli. This method allows further attenuation of residual low-frequency artifacts.

### Evoked Potentials: Spectral Ripple Discrimination Thresholds

**Hypothesis and Methodological Overview.** If a listener can acoustically perceive a difference between a standard and deviant stimulus, the evoked potential response to the deviant stimulus, when presented in an oddball paradigm, will differ in shape from that evoked by the standard stimulus [33,37]. This response is normally quantified by calculating a difference waveform, i.e. deviant response minus standard response and is often referred to as mismatch negativity. If the standard and deviant responses are the same, the difference waveform should be flat; while if they differ, the difference waveform will show oscillations. In practice the noise inherent in evoked potential recordings means that even if the underlying standard and deviant waveforms are identical the difference waveform will still show some oscillations. Therefore, to calculate a neural discrimination threshold it was necessary to first quantify the amount of noise in the difference waveform and then define what quantifies a significant difference waveform response.

**Calculating the Difference Waveform Noise Floor.** The noise present in one difference waveform was calculated by applying a bootstrap method to all the standard responses collected for that subject during that run. A randomly chosen sub-sample of 10% of all standard responses was chosen and averaged together to create a bootstrapped deviant response (Fig. 4A, blue line). The remaining 90% of the standard stimuli was then averaged together to create bootstrapped standard response (Fig. 4A, black line). The bootstrapped deviant was subtracted from the bootstrapped standard to give a bootstrapped difference waveform (Fig. 4B, red line). If no noise were to be present in the recording this bootstrapped difference waveform would be completely flat. Thus, oscillations present in the bootstrapped difference waveform quantify the noise present in the recording. The bootstrap procedure was repeated to generate 54 separate bootstrapped difference waveforms. The noise floor was defined as the standard deviation of all bootstrapped difference waveforms at each time point for positive and negative values (Fig. 4B, black lines).

**Defining a Significant Difference Waveform Response.** To quantify the difference waveform the area above the noise floor within a 90 to 450 ms time window was calculated. This time window allows for the expected evoked potential components such as N1, P2, N2, P3 or MMN to be included in the analysis. Given that the difference waveform is defined as microvolts in function of time in milliseconds, the area above the noise floor is defined as microvolts times milliseconds 'µVms'. A neural spectral ripple discrimination threshold was then defined as the point at which this area dropped below a predetermined significance level. As the aim of this study was to develop an objective evoked potential test to accurately predict the psychoacoustic spectral ripple discrimination threshold, the significance level was determined by calculating the neural threshold for a range of different significance levels and selecting the significance level which gave the best correlation with the psychoacoustic threshold across all subjects. The 'Defining a Significance Level' section presents details of how this procedure was applied together with results from a validation study where data from all 19 subjects were randomly partitioned into two groups. One group was used to estimate the significance level and the other group to test the accuracy of this significance level by predicting the psychoacoustic spectral ripple discrimination threshold.

## Results

### Psychoacoustic Spectral Discrimination Thresholds

Table 1 summarizes the individual spectral ripple discrimination thresholds for all ears tested. The range (0.235 to 2.595 ripples/octave) and mean (1.012 ripples/octave) are in general agreement with previously reported values for spectral ripple discrimination in CI listeners [13,14,38].

### Evoked Potential Spectral Ripple Discrimination Thresholds

**Evoked Potentials and Difference Waveform.** Fig. 5A shows an example of evoked potential waveforms recorded using an oddball paradigm in response to a 0.25 ripples/octave stimuli. The black line shows the response to the standard (standard spectral ripple stimulus) and the blue line the response to the deviant (inverted spectral ripple stimulus). This user reported hearing a difference between the standard and the deviant stimulus (psychoacoustic spectral ripple discrimination threshold of 2.210 ripples/octave) and correspondingly there was a marked difference in the response to the deviant. The deviant response has larger amplitude P2 than the standard response. It also contains a N3 and P4 component which are not present in the standard response. Fig. 5B shows the difference waveform calculated by subtracting the standard from the deviant response. The P2, N3 and P4 differences are apparent in the difference waveform and, importantly, their peaks are above or below the noise-floor indicating that the neural response to the deviant is significantly different than the neural response to the standard.

To determine a neural spectral ripple discrimination threshold, responses to spectral ripple stimuli with an increasing number of ripples/octave were measured in all subjects. The standard and deviant responses for one subject to stimuli with 0.25, 0.5, 1 and 2 ripples/octave are shown in Fig. 6A. The large positivity, around 40 ms, present in all standard and deviant responses is probably an onset artifact. The standard responses to the 0.25, 0.5, 1 and 2 ripples/octave stimuli are similar. However, the deviant responses change as the number of ripples/octave is increased. The deviant response to the 0.25 ripples/octave stimulus shows a large increase in the N1 and P2 component when compared with the standard response. As the number of ripples/octave increases (and the stimuli begin to sound more alike) this N1-P2 difference becomes smaller and delayed, until at 2 ripples per octave the response to the deviant is essentially the same as the response to the standard. This subject had a psychoacoustic spectral ripple discrimination threshold of 1.503 ripples/octave. Fig. 6B shows the difference waveforms. Since the onset artifact (around 40 ms) was equally present in both standard and deviant responses it is significantly attenuated in the difference waveform. Calculating the area above and below the noise floor (shaded) within a 90–450 ms time window allows a quantification of the difference in the neural response to the standard and deviant stimuli. This area is large for 0.25 ripples/octave where the subject perceives a clear difference between the standard and deviant stimuli and is negligible at 2 ripples/octave where the subject reports that the standard and deviant stimuli sound the same.

**Defining a Significance Level.** In Fig. 7, the area above and below the noise floor, and the total area, are plotted as a function of ripples/octave for the same subject shown in Fig. 6. It is clear that as the number of ripples/octave increases, the area above and below the noise floor decreases, i.e., the standard and deviant responses become similar. To allow the objective estimation of neural spectral ripple discrimination thresholds, a significance level (i.e. an area in microvolt times millisecond 'µVms') was defined as

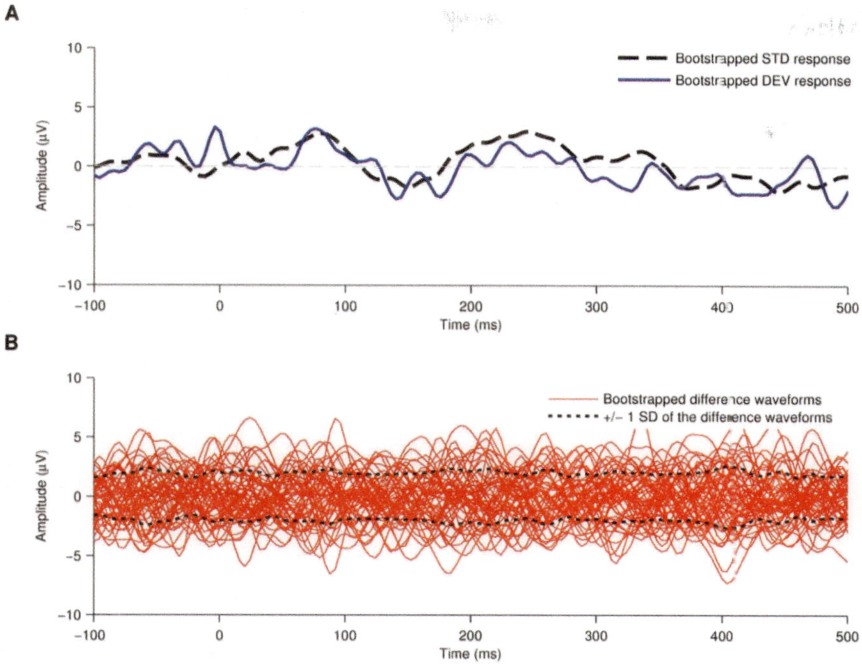


**Figure 4. Noise floor calculation of the neural response.** (A) The noise floor was calculated with a statistical bootstrap method. A random 10% sub-sample of epochs from the standard stimulus type was averaged to create a bootstrapped deviant response whilst the remaining epochs were averaged together to create a bootstrapped standard response. (B) A difference waveform was calculated by subtracting the bootstrapped standard response from the bootstrapped deviant response. This process was repeated 54 times, each time with a different randomly selected 10% sample of standard epochs. The noise floor of the signal was defined as +/− one standard deviation of the 54 resulting difference waveforms.

the threshold below which area differences between the standard and deviant response can be considered perceptually negligible.

A bootstrap method was employed to define and validate this significance level for the three different area measurements. The approach, described in detail below and in a flow chart in Fig. 8A,

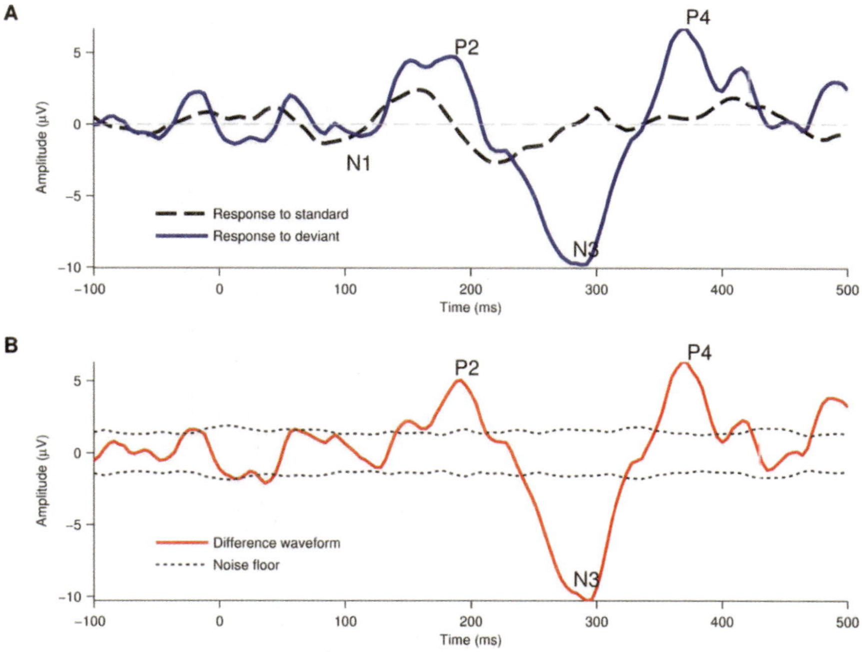


**Figure 5. Example of the difference waveform elicited using the oddball paradigm.** (A) Evoked potential responses elicited to 608 standard stimuli and 65 deviant stimuli at 0.25 RPO. When the standard and deviant stimuli are perceived as different sounds, the morphology of the neural response to the deviant stimuli (blue trace) is significantly different than the response to the standard stimuli (dashed, black trace). (B) The difference waveform represents the mismatch between the responses elicited to each stimulus type.

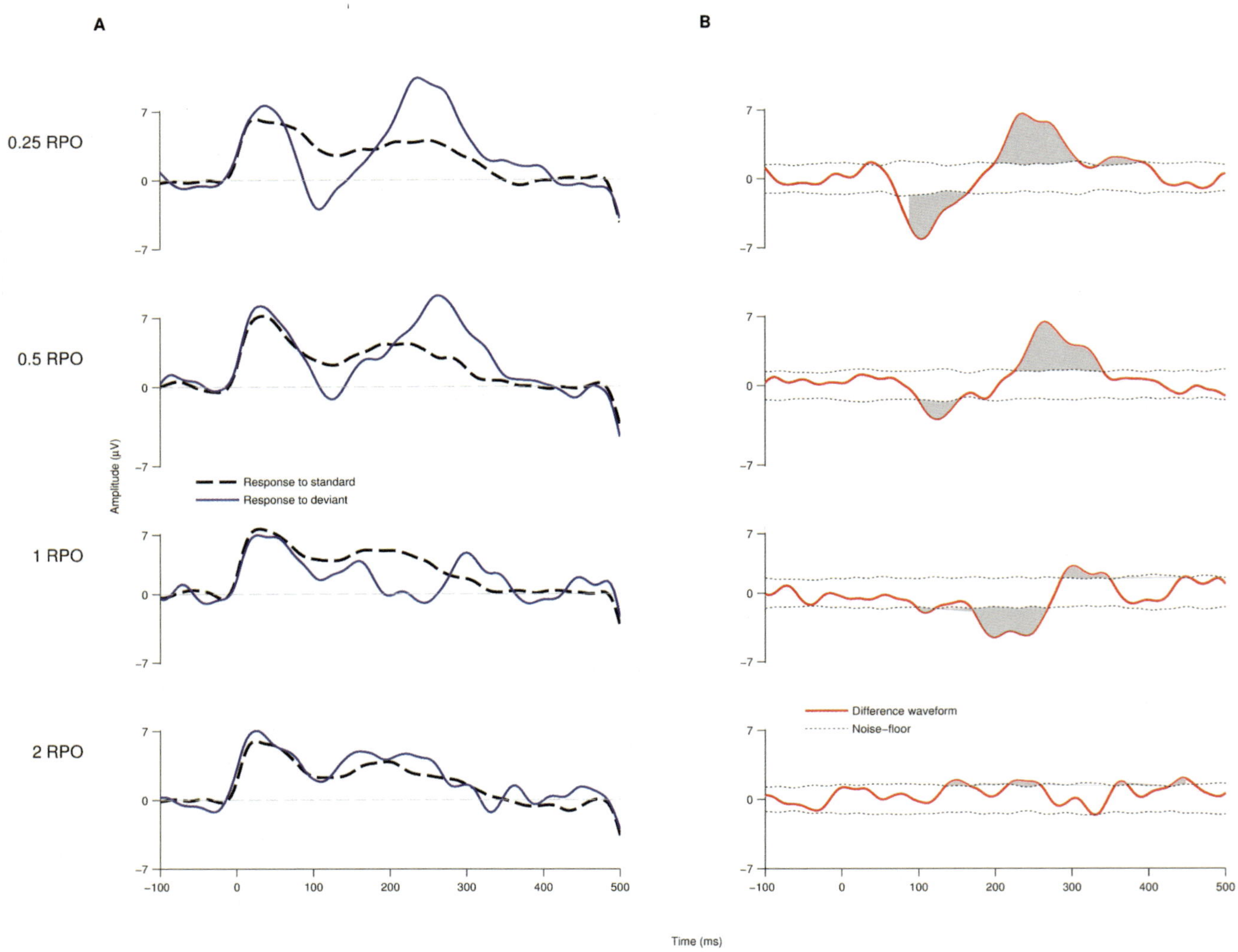


**Figure 6. Sequential decrease of the difference waveform's area above the noise floor.** (A) Evoked potential traces of standard and deviant stimuli elicited at 0.25, 0.5, 1 and 2 RPO. As the spectral density increases, the neural responses to the standard and deviant stimuli become more similar. (B) The difference waveform at each spectral density shows a sequential decrease of the mismatch between the responses elicited to each stimulus type. The area above the noise floor of the signal (shaded grey) is taken as an indicator of said mismatch decrease.

operated by first dividing the data into two groups. The first group (a determination group) was employed to determine one significance level, for all members, which gave the best correlation with the known psychophysical thresholds. The second group (an estimation group) was then employed to test how well this significance level could estimate the known psychophysical threshold.

Data from the 20 tested ears were separated in two groups: a determination and an estimation group. The determination group contained 12 randomly selected datasets whilst the estimation group contained the remaining 8 datasets. This partition ratio was chosen so that the estimation group represented more than a third of the total sample. Each dataset contained at least four measurements presenting stimuli with different ripples/octave. For the determination group, the neural spectral ripple discrimination threshold was calculated and linearly regressed with the measured psychoacoustic threshold for each subject. If the area never went below the significance level the dataset was excluded. This regression was tested for a range of 19 different predetermined significance levels, ranging from 10 µVms to 100 µVms at 5 µVms increments, yielding 19 different (determination) $R^2$ and p-values (Fig. 8B). Significance levels, for which the regression yielded a p-value greater than 0.01 or which excluded more than two datasets, were discarded. From the remaining significance levels, the one that yielded the greatest regression $R^2$ was selected (Fig. 8B, red dot). The selected significance level was applied to the estimation group to determine the neural spectral ripple discrimination threshold and then quantify, using linear regression, how well this predicted the psychophysical threshold (Fig. 8C). If this (estimation) regression yielded a p-value less than 0.05 with no dataset exclusions then the significance level was accepted. Otherwise, the significance level was rejected. One point on Fig. 8C represents one of the accepted estimation $R^2$ and p-values. Fig. 8C shows the p-values as a function of the regression $R^2$ value for the estimation group's linear regression.

This process was repeated, each time using a different random partitioning of the datasets into determination and estimation groups, until 20 significance levels that satisfied the criteria were generated (Fig. 8D). This shows that the significance level chosen performs accurately when estimating the psychoacoustic thresholds measured for each subject. The final significance levels defined for this study (and employed in Section 3.4) was the

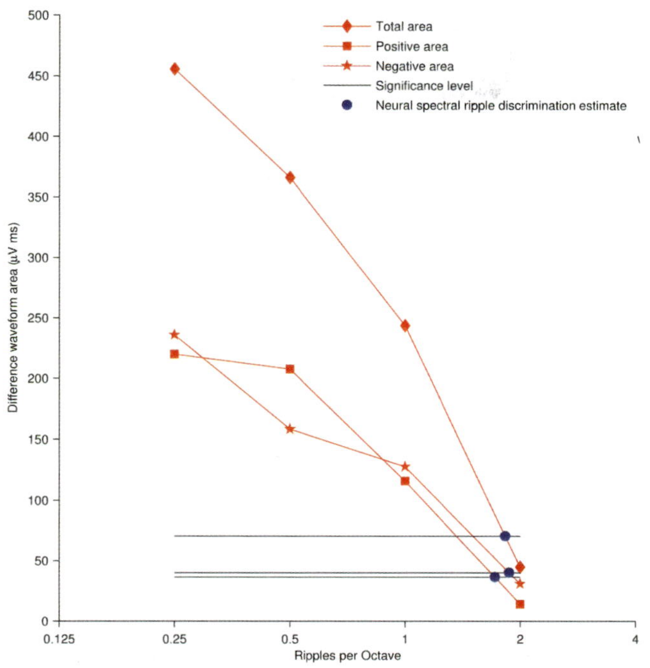


**Figure 7. Estimation of the spectral ripple discrimination threshold based on neural responses.** The neural spectral ripple discrimination threshold is estimated as the point where the mismatch between the neural responses dropped below a set significance level. Thresholds were estimated with three different area above the noise floor measurements: positive area, negative area and total area above the noise floor.

average of the accepted significance levels. The entire process was repeated for the positive, negative and total area measurements.

For the total area the mean significance level was determined to be 70.4 µVms (17.7 standard deviation). Two tested ears did not yield a neural threshold (Fig. 9A). For one tested ear (TCD 06 in Table 1) the area above the noise floor for all recordings was below the significance level defined, and for the remaining exclusion (TCD15 in Table 1), the area above the noise floor did not drop below significance level. The mean neural threshold across 18 datasets was 1.230 ripples/octave (1.386 standard deviation).

For the positive area the mean significance level was determined to be 36.3 µVms (13.8 standard deviation). Four datasets did not yield a neural threshold using the positive area (Fig. 9B). The area above the noise floor from two tested ears (TCD 13 and TCD 15 in Table 1) did not drop below the significance level in any of the four recordings. Contrastingly, the area above the noise floor from the remaining two exclusions (TCD 06 and TCD07 in Table 1) was below the significance level in all four recordings. Hence, it was not possible to estimate the neural spectral ripple discrimination threshold. The mean neural threshold for the remaining 16 datasets was 1.121 ripples/octave (0.920 standard deviation).

For the negative area the mean significance level was determined to be 40 µVms (3.9 standard deviation). Three datasets did not yield a neural threshold (Fig. 9C). The area above the noise floor of three tested ears (TCD 06, TCD 09 and TCD15 in Table 1) was below the significance level in every recording, making it not possible to estimate a neural spectral ripple discrimination threshold with the defined significance level. The mean neural threshold across 17 datasets was 1.116 ripples/octave (1.458 standard deviation). The individual neural thresholds for the positive, negative and total area are reported in Table 1.

## Correlation between Psychoacoustic and Neural Thresholds

Linear regression of the psychoacoustic spectral ripple discrimination thresholds with the neural spectral ripple discrimination thresholds produced a squared Pearson's correlation coefficient ($R^2$) of 0.60 and p-value$<$0.01 for total area (Fig. 9A), $R^2 = 0.65$ and p-value$<$0.01 for the positive area (Fig. 9B), and $R^2 = 0.50$ and a p-value$<$0.01 using the negative area (Fig. 9C).

Results from paired t-tests between psychoacoustic and neural thresholds, in all three area measurements, show no significant difference between the metrics: p-value = 0.75, t = 0.32 for positive area; p-value = 0.93, t = 0.09 for negative area; and p-value = 0.68, t = −0.41 for total area above the noise floor. A Steiger's Z test was employed to compare the correlations derived from the positive, negative and total area calculations. Results indicate that there is no significant difference between: the positive area and negative area correlations (Z = 1.51, p-value$>$0.05); the positive area and the total area correlations (Z = 1.14, p-value$>$0.05) and; the negative area and the total area correlation (Z = −1.34, p-value$>$0.05).

# Discussion

The present study developed and validated a method to objectively assess spectral ripple discrimination in a population of CI listeners using an oddball EEG paradigm. Using a clinically applicable single channel set-up [36], it was possible to acquire evoked potential responses to standard and deviant stimuli in CI listeners. Analysis of the difference waveform showed a strong correlation with behavioral spectral ripple discrimination thresholds, validating the utility of this approach as a clinical assessment tool.

## Artifact removal

It was possible to distinguish the expected N1-P2 complex from the evoked potential traces. The large positivity at around 40 ms and negativity at around 500 ms after stimulus onset found in some subjects (see Fig. 3C and Fig. 3D) are most likely on-set and off-set artifacts caused by high-pass filtering of the low frequency (or pedestal) artifact component identified by Mc Laughlin et al. [36] and others [39–42] related to the CI's response to the stimuli. The 40 ms delay in the on-set artifact is caused by a combination of the rise time of the stimuli (50 ms), the CI processor delay (~5 to 8 ms as observed in single stimulus presentations, see Fig. 3A and Fig. 3B) and the high-pass filter characteristics. When present, on-set and off-set artifacts where equally present in both standard and deviant responses. Thus, the subtraction operation, employed to obtain a difference waveform, attenuated these artifacts. The analysis time window (90 to 450 ms) also minimized any potential artifact influence on the area measurement used to determine the neural spectral ripple discrimination threshold.

## Objective assessment of neural thresholds

Judging the presence or absence of a neural response in cortical evoked potentials (or in a difference waveform) is generally a subjective task. This study developed and validated an objective statistical approach to determine the point at which a response in the difference waveform became perceptually non-significant. Parts of this approach are similar to the integrated mismatch negativity metric developed by Ponton et al. [43]. Measuring the peak amplitude of specific components in the spectral ripple

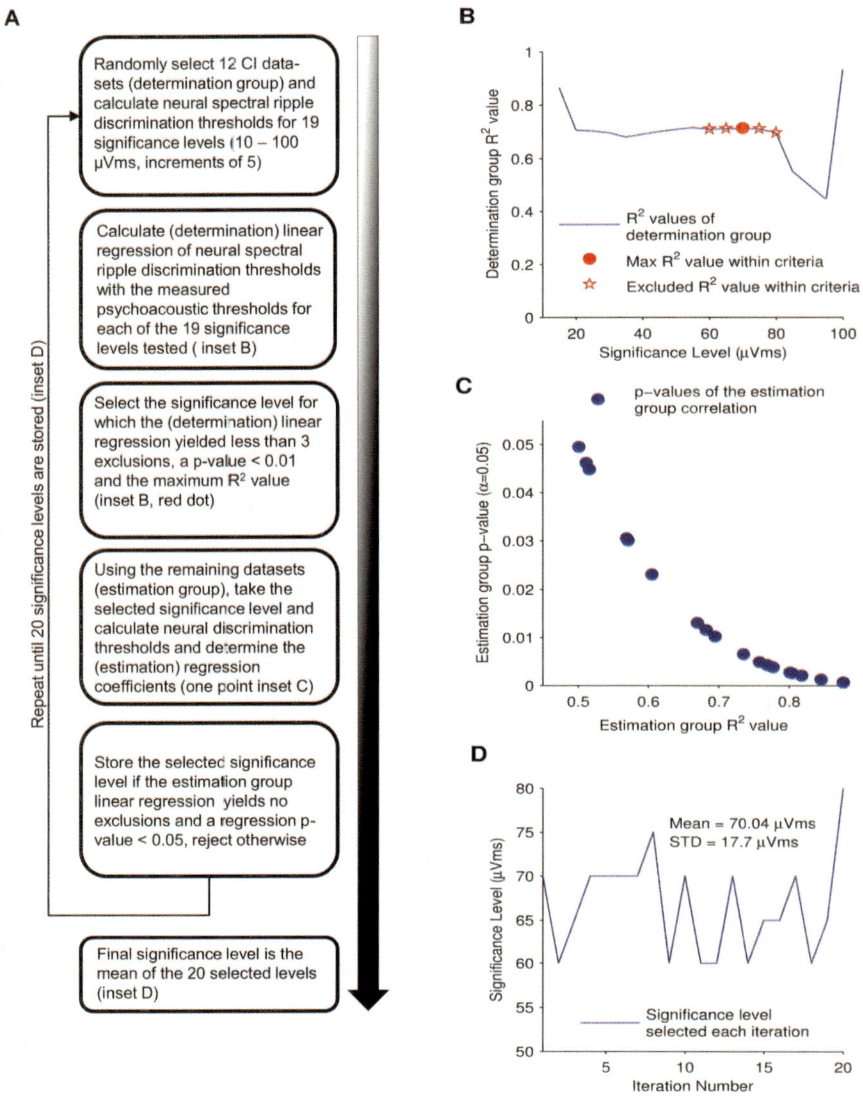


**Figure 8. Bootstrapped determination of the significance level.** (A) Describes the progression of the bootstrapping method employed to determine the level at which neural spectral ripple discrimination thresholds were estimated and regressed with the measured psychoacoustic thresholds. (B) The square of the Pearson's correlation factor ($R^2$) vs. the 19 significant levels tested on the determination group is plotted. The significance level that yields the maximum $R^2$ value within the selection criteria, identified as the red point in the plot, is selected to continue with the bootstrap method, the rest are excluded (hollow stars). (C) The selected significance level is evaluated with estimation group. The regression's p-value plotted vs. the regression's $R^2$ value resulting from the significance level evaluation on the estimation group for 20 bootstrap iterations. If the evaluation yields no exclusions and a p-value less than 0.05, the significance level is stored. (D) The bootstrap method is repeated to select 20 different significant levels. The mean of the selected values is employed as the final significance level.

difference waveform is difficult because not all subject's responses exhibit a similar morphology (compare Figs. 5 and 6). The more general approach taken in this study, of measuring the area above or below a bootstrapped determined noise floor, avoids this difficulty. An area-, as opposed to peak-, based metric has the added advantage of reducing noise, an important consideration when using difference waveforms which are by definition noisier than the responses from which they are derived. To define a significance level, below which a difference waveform area would be considered perceptually insignificant, a second bootstrap method was applied. Fig. 8C shows that, for 20 different data partitions, the selected significance level reasonably predicts the psychophysical thresholds of the estimation group. Additionally, variations of the significance level between around 20 and 80 μVms do not tend to produce large variations in the $R^2$ values (Fig. 8B), and most partitions of the data produce an estimate of the significance level close to 70 μVms (Fig. 8D). This shows that the good correlation between neural and psychophysical thresholds (Fig. 9) is robust and is not simply dependent on subjectively selecting the appropriate significance level. The use of the positive, negative or total area between the noise floor and the difference waveform did not yield a significant difference when estimating spectral discrimination thresholds. However, using the total area, above the positive and negative noise floor, succeeded to estimate a spectral ripple discrimination threshold in the largest number of tested ears.

In cases where the cortical responses were too small compared to the noise floor, such as TCD06 and TCD15, it was difficult to estimate a neural spectral ripple discrimination threshold. While monitoring the impedance levels accordingly during the recording

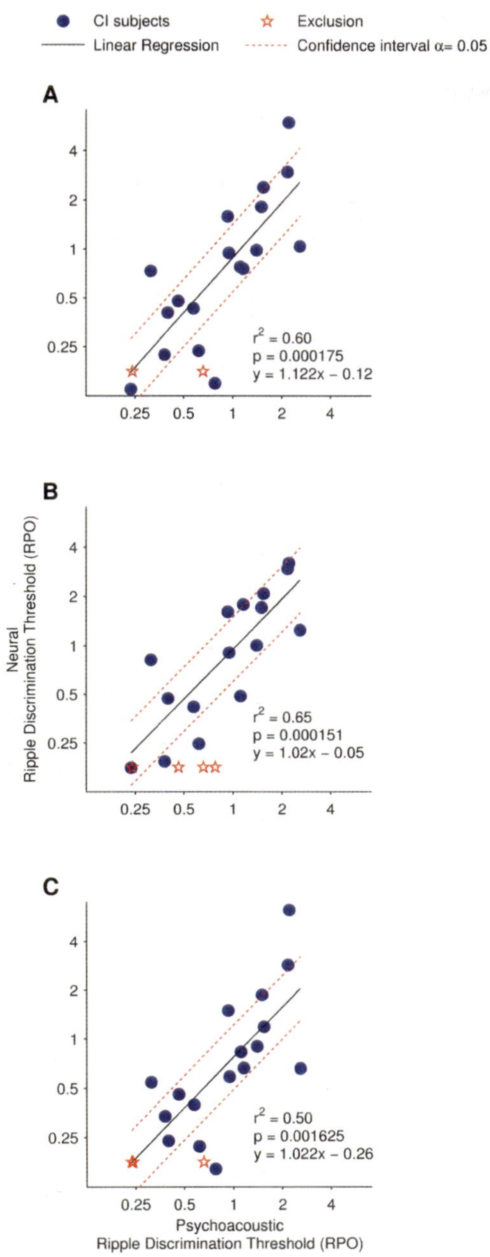


**Figure 9. Correlation of neural and psychoacoustic spectral ripple discrimination thresholds.** Linear regression of the psychoacoustic spectral ripple discrimination thresholds with the neural spectral ripple discrimination thresholds for each of the analyzed area above the noise floor measurements: (A) total area above the noise floor; (B) Positive area above the noise floor; and (C) negative area above the noise floor.

may reduce noise and CI artifact, small or unreliable cortical evoked potential responses from some subjects is a limitation when estimating neural spectral ripple discrimination thresholds. Reducing the noise in the signal as much as possible by limiting subject motion and external interference and increasing the stimulus presentation level may help get a better response in these subjects.

## Potential Clinical Applications

Previous work by our group [36] highlighted the elegance of single channel EEG acquisition and artifact attenuation in CI users. The simple, yet robust, approach makes it feasible for use within a clinical environment, with faster and more comfortable acquisition than with high density EEG set-ups. The results presented in this study suggest that the single channel EEG acquisition and artifact attenuation is a reliable method for measuring cortical responses to an oddball paradigm in CI users.

In addition to simply evaluating a CI subject's spectral resolution, it may also be possible to use the method to fine tune a subject's frequency map. Typically, a CI processor would be loaded with a standard frequency map, i.e. predefined frequency bands assigned to each electrode of the CI. An objective metric for spectral resolution, such as the one presented in this study, could allow the evaluation of customized frequency maps, in search of the map that allows the best spectral resolution. The time required to obtain spectral discrimination thresholds, approximately one hour, is a limiting factor for this potential application. However, being an objective metric, the possibility of an automated process may reduce the number of man-hours required for the task. Furthermore, the development of intra-cochlear recording methodologies that allow the recording of cortical evoked potentials without the additional EEG systems [44] may benefit from objective metrics as a building block for the development of automated frequency tuning processes.

Current efforts to enhance spectral resolution via different electrode stimulation modalities, i.e. partial bipolar stimulation (pBP), tripolar stimulation (TP) and partial tripolar stimulation (pTP), benefit from psychoacoustic evaluation of frequency resolution [45–47]. Objective assessment of spectral resolution using an oddball paradigm could be beneficial when evaluating different electrode stimulation modalities in CI populations where standard psychoacoustics cannot be performed such as young infants. The use of an oddball paradigm such as the mismatch negativity (MMN) has reported successful in normal hearing and cochlear implant infant populations [48–50]. Evidence in literature suggests that the pitch discrimination characteristics of the MMN in infants is developed between two and four months of age [49].

Clinical applications involving the use of cortical evoked potentials may be limited by the confounding factor of maturation changes during the longitudinal development of cortical potentials. The development of cortical auditory potentials can extend into adolescence [50] and even after prolonged acoustic deprivation, cortical auditory potentials can be re-developed over a period of time [30]. Changes in the morphology, latency and amplitude of potentials over time represents an impediment when performing a within subject cortical evoked potential assessment. Trainor et al. [51] identified changes in the EEG morphology of the MMN in young infants, with an age range of two, three, four and six months, suggesting that the difference at each age may be associated with layer-specific maturational processes in auditory cortex. However, the method developed in this study may overcome these limitations due to the robust nature of the oddball paradigm response and its applicability with different age populations as well as clinical conditions [33,49,50]. Despite maturational changes reflected by the EEG morphology of the MMN in young infants, the cognitive change detection mechanism associated with the MMN has been proposed to be developed between two and four months of age [49].

Provided that a spectral ripple discrimination threshold could be obtained with an oddball paradigm at any stage of the cortical auditory potential maturation process, a within subject assessment can be conducted regardless of the developmental changes presented during the duration of the assessment. Nonetheless, determining the applicability of spectral rippled stimuli as well as the complexity of the paradigms and the presentation rate for younger populations requires further investigation.

## Conclusions

In conclusion, the results presented in this study demonstrate that cortical responses to an oddball paradigm, utilizing complex stimuli, can be recorded with a single channel EEG acquisition set-up from a CI population. This cortical evoked potential based method can provide an estimated spectral ripple discrimination threshold in adult CI listeners. Further research is required to investigate the relationship of the objective assessment of spectral resolution with speech perception scores, as well as to investigate the applicability of the proposed objective method in a population of infant CI recipients.

## Acknowledgments

The authors would like to acknowledge the 19 cochlear implant participants, for their dedication and willingness during the experimental sessions.

## Author Contributions

Conceived and designed the experiments: ALV RBR MML FGZ LV JS PW. Performed the experiments: ALV MML. Analyzed the data: ALV MML RBR FGZ JS LV PW. Contributed reagents/materials/analysis tools: LV JS PW. Wrote the paper: ALV MML RBR FGZ JS LV PW. Critically revising the manuscript for important intellectual content; RBR FGZ LV PW JS ALV. Subject recruiting for research; LV JS PW ALV.

## References


1. Zeng F-G (2004) Trends in cochlear implants. Trends in Amplification 8: 1–34.
2. Waltzman SB, Roland JT (2005) Cochlear implantation in children younger than 12 months. Pediatrics 116: e487–e493.
3. van Dijk JE, van Olphen AF, Langereis MC, Mens LH, Brokx JP, et al. (1999) Predictors of cochlear implant performance. Audiology 38: 109–116.
4. Blamey P, Arndt P, Bergeron F, Bredberg G, Brimacombe J, et al. (1996) Factors affecting auditory performance of postlinguistically deaf adults using cochlear implants. Audiology and Neurotology 1: 293–306.
5. Clark JH, Yeagle J, Arbaje AI, Lin FR, Niparko JK, et al. (2012) Cochlear implant rehabilitation in older adults: literature review and proposal of a conceptual framework. Journal of the American Geriatrics Society 60: 1936–1945.
6. Loizou PC (1999) Introduction to cochlear implants. IEEE Engineering in Medicine and Biology Magazine 18: 32–42.
7. Zeng F-G, Rebscher S, Harrison W, Sun X, Feng H (2008) Cochlear implants: system design, integration, and evaluation. IEEE Reviews in Biomedical Engineering 1: 115–142.
8. Pisoni DB, Cleary M, Geers AE, Tobey EA (1999) Individual differences in effectiveness of cochlear implants in children who are prelingually deaf: New process measures of performance. The Volta Review 101(3): 111–164.
9. Zeng F-G, Grant G, Niparko J, Galvin J, Shannon R, et al. (2002) Speech dynamic range and its effect on cochlear implant performance. The Journal of the Acoustical Society of America 111: 377–386.
10. Lazard DS, Bordure P, Lina-Granade G, Magnan J, Meller R, et al. (2010) Speech perception performance for 100 post-lingually deaf adults fitted with Neurelec cochlear implants: comparison between Digisonic® Convex and Digisonic® SP devices after a 1-year follow-up. Acta Oto-Laryngologica 130: 1267–1273.
11. Friesen LM, Shannon RV, Baskent D, Wang X (2001) Speech recognition in noise as a function of the number of spectral channels: Comparison of acoustic hearing and cochlear implants. Journal of the Acoustical Society of America 110: 1150–1163.
12. Fu QJ (2002) Temporal processing and speech recognition in cochlear implant users. Neuroreport 13: 1635–1639.
13. Henry BA, Turner CW, Behrens A (2005) Spectral peak resolution and speech recognition in quiet: normal hearing, hearing impaired, and cochlear implant listeners. Journal of the Acoustical Society of America 118: 1111–1121.
14. Won JH, Drennan WR, Rubinstein JT (2007) Spectral-ripple resolution correlates with speech reception in noise in cochlear implant users. Journal of the Association for Research in Otolaryngology 8: 384–392.
15. Supin A, Popov VV, Milekhina ON, Tarakanov MB (1997) Frequency-temporal resolution of hearing measured by rippled noise. Hearing Research 108: 17–27.
16. Litvak LM, Spahr AJ, Saoji AA, Fridman GY (2007) Relationship between perception of spectral ripple and speech recognition in cochlear implant and vocoder listeners. Journal of the Acoustical Society of America 122: 982–991.
17. Jones GL, Drennan WR, Rubinstein JT (2011) Relationship between channel interaction and spectral-ripple discrimination in cochlear implant users. Journal of the Acoustical Society of America 133: 425–433.
18. Horn D, Werner L, Rubinstein JT, Won JH (2013). Spectral Ripple Discrimination in Infants: Effect of Ripple Depth and Envelope Phase Randomization. 36th Association for Research in Otolaryngology Annual MidWinter Meeting 36:289–290.
19. Abbas PJ, Brown CJ (1988) Electrically evoked brainstem potentials in cochlear implant patients with multi-electrode stimulation. Hearing Research 36: 153–162.
20. Brown CJ, Hughes ML, Luk B, Abbas PJ, Wolaver A, et al. (2000) The relationship between EAP and EABR thresholds and levels used to program the Nucleus 24 speech processor: data from adults. Ear and Hearing 21: 151–163.
21. Franck KH, Norton SJ (2001) Estimation of psychophysical levels using the electrically evoked compound action potential measured with the neural response telemetry capabilities of Cochlear Corporation's CI24M device. Ear and Hearing 22: 289–299.
22. Hughes ML, Brown CJ, Abbas PJ, Wolaver AA, Gervais JP (2000) Comparison of EAP thresholds with MAP levels in the nucleus 24 cochlear implant: data from children. Ear and Hearing 21: 164–174.
23. Dimitrijevic A, John MS, Picton TW (2004) Auditory steady-state responses and word recognition scores in normal-hearing and hearing-impaired adults. Ear and Hearing 25: 68–84.
24. Firszt JB, Chambers RD, Kraus, Reeder RM (2002) Neurophysiology of cochlear implant users I: effects of stimulus current level and electrode site on the electrical ABR, MLR, and N1-P2 response. Ear and Hearing 23: 502–515.
25. Ponton CW, Don M, Eggermont JJ, Waring MD, Masuda A (1996) Maturation of human cortical auditory function: differences between normal-hearing children and children with cochlear implants. Ear and Hearing 17: 430–437.
26. Sharma A, Nash AA, Dorman M (2009) Cortical development, plasticity and re-organization in children with cochlear implants. Journal of Communication Disorders 42: 272–279.
27. Brown CJ, Etler C, He S, O'Brien S, Erenberg S, et al. (2008) The electrically evoked auditory change complex: preliminary results from nucleus cochlear implant users. Ear and Hearing 29: 704–717.
28. Gilley PM, Sharma A, Dorman MF (2008) Cortical reorganization in children with cochlear implants. Brain Research 1239: 56–65.
29. Hofmann M, Wouters J (2010) Electrically evoked auditory steady state responses in cochlear implant users. Journal of the Association for Research in Otolaryngology 11: 267–282.
30. Pantev C, Dinnesen A, Ross B, Wollbrink A, Knief A (2006) Dynamics of auditory plasticity after cochlear implantation: a longitudinal study. Cerebral Cortex 16: 31–36.
31. Torppa R, Salo E, Makkonen T, Loimo H, Pykalainen J, et al. (2012) Cortical processing of musical sounds in children with Cochlear Implants. Clinical Neurophysiology 123: 1966–1979.
32. Won JH, Clinard CG, Kwon S, Dasika VK, Nie K, et al. (2011) Relationship Between Behavioral and Physiological Spectral-Ripple Discrimination. Journal of the Association for Research in Otolaryngology 12: 375–393.
33. Naatanen R, Kujala T, Escera C, Baldeweg T, Kreegipuu K, et al. (2012) The mismatch negativity (MMN)–a unique window to disturbed central auditory processing in ageing and different clinical conditions. Clinical Neurophysiology 123: 424–458.
34. Byrne D, Dillon H, Tran K, Arlinger S, Wilbraham K, et al. (1994) An international comparison of long-term average speech spectra. Journal of the acoustical society of America 96: 2108.
35. Levitt H (1971) Transformed up-down methods in psychoacoustics. Journal of the Acoustical Society of America 49: Suppl 2:467+.
36. McLaughlin M, Lopez Valdes A, Reilly RB, Zeng FG (2013) Cochlear Implant Artifact Attenuation in Late Auditory Evoked Potentials: A Single Channel Approach. Hearing Research 302:84–95.
37. Picton TW, Alain C, Otten L, Ritter W, Achim A (2000) Mismatch negativity: different water in the same river. Audiology and Neuro-otology 5: 111–139.
38. Henry BA, Turner CW (2003) The resolution of complex spectral patterns by cochlear implant and normal-hearing listeners. Journal of the Acoustical Society of America 113: 2861–2873.
39. Wong DD, Gordon KA (2009) Beamformer suppression of cochlear implant artifacts in an electroencephalography dataset. IEEE Transactions on Biomedical Engineering 56: 2851–2857.
40. Viola FC, Thorne JD, Bleeck S, Eyles J, Debener S (2011) Uncovering auditory evoked potentials from cochlear implant users with independent component analysis. Psychophysiology 48: 1470–1480.
41. Gilley PM, Sharma A, Dorman M, Finley CC, Panch AS, et al. (2006) Minimization of cochlear implant stimulus artifact in cortical auditory evoked potentials. Clinical Neurophysiology 117: 1772–1782.

42. Friesen LM, Picton TW (2010) A method for removing cochlear implant artifact. Hearing Research 259: 95–106.
43. Ponton CW, Don M, Eggermont JJ, Kwong B (1997) Integrated mismatch negativity (MMNi): a noise-free representation of evoked responses allowing single-point distribution-free statistical tests. Evoked Potentials-Electroencephalography and Clinical Neurophysiology 104: 143–150.
44. Mc Laughlin M, Lu T, Dimitrijevic A, Zeng F-G (2012) Towards a Closed-Loop Cochlear Implant System: Application of Embedded Monitoring of Peripheral and Central Neural Activity. IEEE Transactions on Neural Systems and Rehabilitation Engineering 20: 443–454.
45. Landsberger DM, Srinivasan AG (2009) Virtual channel discrimination is improved by current focusing in cochlear implant recipients. Hearing Research 254: 34–41.
46. Wu C-C, Luo X (2013) Current Steering with Partial Tripolar Stimulation Mode in Cochlear Implants. Journal of the Association for Research in Otolaryngology 14: 213–231.
47. Zhu Z, Tang Q, Zeng F-G, Guan T, Ye D (2012) Cochlear-implant spatial selectivity with monopolar, bipolar and tripolar stimulation. Hearing Research 283: 45–58.
48. Cheour M, Alho K, Ceponiene R, Reinikainen K, Sainio K, et al. (1998) Maturation of mismatch negativity in infants. International Journal of Psychophysiology 29: 217–226.
49. He C, Hotson L, Trainor LJ (2009) Maturation of cortical mismatch responses to occasional pitch change in early infancy: Effects of presentation rate and magnitude of change. Neuropsychologia 47: 218–229.
50. Ponton CW, Eggermont JJ, Don M, Waring MD, Kwong B, et al. (2000) Maturation of the mismatch negativity: Effects of profound deafness and cochlear implant use. Audiology and Neuro-Otology 5: 167–185.
51. Trainor L, McFadden M, Hodgson L, Darragh L, Barlow J, et al. (2003) Changes in auditory cortex and the development of mismatch negativity between 2 and 6 months of age. International Journal of Psychophysiology 51: 5–15.

# 4

# Massively Parallel DNA Sequencing Facilitates Diagnosis of Patients with Usher Syndrome Type 1


**Hidekane Yoshimura[1], Satoshi Iwasaki[2,3], Shin-ya Nishio[1], Kozo Kumakawa[4], Tetsuya Tono[5], Yumiko Kobayashi[6], Hiroaki Sato[6], Kyoko Nagai[7], Kotaro Ishikawa[8], Tetsuo Ikezono[9], Yasushi Naito[10], Kunihiro Fukushima[11], Chie Oshikawa[12], Takashi Kimitsuki[13], Hiroshi Nakanishi[14], Shin-ichi Usami[1]***

**1** Department of Otorhinolaryngology, Shinshu University School of Medicine, Matsumoto, Nagano, Japan, **2** Department of Hearing Implant Sciences, Shinshu University School of Medicine, Matsumoto, Nagano, Japan, **3** Department of Otorhinolaryngology, International University of Health and Welfare, Mita Hospital, Minatoku, Tokyo, Japan, **4** Department of Otolaryngology, Okinaka Memorial Institute for Medical Research, Toranomon Hospital, Minatoku, Tokyo, Japan, **5** Department of Otorhinolaryngology-Head and Neck Surgery, Miyazaki University School of Medicine, Miyazaki, Miyazaki, Japan, **6** Department of Otolaryngology-Head and Neck Surgery, Iwate Medical University, Morioka, Iwate, Japan, **7** Department of Otolaryngology-Head and Neck Surgery, Gunma University Graduate School of Medicine, Maebashi, Gunma, Japan, **8** Department of Otolaryngology, National Rehabilitation Center for Persons with Disabilities, Tokorozawa, Saitama, Japan, **9** Department of Otolaryngology, Saitama Medical University, Moroyama, Saitama, Japan, **10** Department of Otolaryngology, Kobe City Medical Center General Hospital, Kobe, Hyougo, Japan, **11** Department of Otorhinolaryngology, Head and Neck Surgery, Okayama University Postgraduate School of Medicine, Dentistry and Pharmaceutical Science, Okayama, Okayama, Japan, **12** Department of Otorhinolaryngology, Graduate School of Medical Sciences, Kyushu University, Fukuoka, Fukuoka, Japan, **13** Department of Otorhinolaryngology, Kyushu Central Hospital, Fukuoka, Fukuoka, Japan, **14** Department of Otorhinolaryngology, Hamamatsu University School of Medicine, Hamamatsu, Shizuoka, Japan



## Abstract

Usher syndrome is an autosomal recessive disorder manifesting hearing loss, retinitis pigmentosa and vestibular dysfunction, and having three clinical subtypes. Usher syndrome type 1 is the most severe subtype due to its profound hearing loss, lack of vestibular responses, and retinitis pigmentosa that appears in prepuberty. Six of the corresponding genes have been identified, making early diagnosis through DNA testing possible, with many immediate and several long-term advantages for patients and their families. However, the conventional genetic techniques, such as direct sequence analysis, are both time-consuming and expensive. Targeted exon sequencing of selected genes using the massively parallel DNA sequencing technology will potentially enable us to systematically tackle previously intractable monogenic disorders and improve molecular diagnosis. Using this technique combined with direct sequence analysis, we screened 17 unrelated Usher syndrome type 1 patients and detected probable pathogenic variants in the 16 of them (94.1%) who carried at least one mutation. Seven patients had the *MYO7A* mutation (41.2%), which is the most common type in Japanese. Most of the mutations were detected by only the massively parallel DNA sequencing. We report here four patients, who had probable pathogenic mutations in two different Usher syndrome type 1 genes, and one case of *MYO7A/PCDH15* digenic inheritance. This is the first report of Usher syndrome mutation analysis using massively parallel DNA sequencing and the frequency of Usher syndrome type 1 genes in Japanese. Mutation screening using this technique has the power to quickly identify mutations of many causative genes while maintaining cost-benefit performance. In addition, the simultaneous mutation analysis of large numbers of genes is useful for detecting mutations in different genes that are possibly disease modifiers or of digenic inheritance.



**Editor:** Klaus Brusgaard, Odense University hospital, Denmark

**Funding:** This study was supported by a Health and Labour Sciences Research Grant for Comprehensive Research on Disability Health and Welfare from the Ministry of Health, Labour and Welfare of Japan (S.U.), and by a Grant-in-Aid for Scientific Research from the (then) Ministry of Education, Science and Culture of Japan (http://www.mext.go.jp/english/) (S.U.). The funders had no role in study design, data collection and analysis, decision to publish, or preparation of the manuscript.

**Competing Interests:** The authors have declared that no competing interests exist.



* E-mail: usami@shinshu-u.ac.jp


## Introduction

Usher syndrome (USH) is an autosomal recessive disorder characterized by hearing loss (HL), retinitis pigmentosa (RP) and vestibular dysfunction. Three clinical subtypes can be distinguished. USH type 1 (USH1) is the most severe among them because of profound HL, absent vestibular responses, and prepubertal onset RP. USH type 2 (USH2) is characterized by congenital moderate to severe HL, with a high-frequency sloping configuration. The vestibular function is normal and onset of RP is in the first or second decade. The onset of the visual symptoms such as night blindness in USH usually occurs several years later than in USH1. USH type 3 (USH3) is characterized by variable onset of progressive HL, variable onset of RP, and variable impairment of vestibular function (normal to absent) [1,2].

To date, nine genetic loci for USH1(*USH1B-H*, *J*, and *K*) have been mapped to chromosomes 11q13.5, 11p15.1, 10q22.1, 21q21, 10q21-q22, 17q24-q25, 15q22-q23 (*USH1H* and *J*), and 10p11.21–q21.1 [2,3,4]. Six of the corresponding genes have been identified: the actin-based motor protein myosin VIIa

(*MYO7A*, USH1B) [5]; two cadherin-related proteins, cadherin 23 (*CDH23*, USH1D) [6] and protocadherin 15 (*PCDH15*, USH1F) [7]; and two scaffold proteins, harmonin (*USH1C*) [8] and sans (*USH1G*) [9]; the $Ca^{2+}$- and integrin-binding protein (*CIB2*, USH1J) [4]. In Caucasian USH1 patients, previous studies showed that mutations in *MYO7A*, *USH1C*, *CDH23*, *PCDH15*, and *USH1G*, were found in 39–55%, 7–14%, 7–35%, 7–11%, and 0–7%, respectively (the frequency of *CIB2* is still unknown) [10,11,12]. In Japanese, Nakanishi et al. showed that *MYO7A* and *CDH23* mutations are present in USH1 patients [13], however, the frequency is not yet known. In addition, mutations in three corresponding genes (usherin *USH2A* [14], G protein-coupled receptor 98; *GPR98* [15], and deafness, autosomal recessive 31; *DFNB31* [16]) have been reported so far in USH2, and USH3 is caused by mutations in the clarin 1 (*CLRN1*) [17] gene.

Comprehensive molecular diagnosis of USH has been hampered both by genetic heterogeneity and the large number of exons for most of the USH genes. The six USH1 genes collectively contain 180 coding exons [4,9,10] the three USH2 genes comprise 175 coding exons [15,16,18], and the USH3 gene has five coding exons [17]. In addition some of these genes are alternatively spliced ([4,7,8,16,17] and NCBI database: http://www.ncbi.nlm.nih.gov/nuccore/). Thus far, large-scale mutation screening has been performed using direct sequence analysis, but that is both time-consuming and expensive. We thought that targeted exon sequencing of selected genes using the Massively Parallel DNA Sequencing (MPS) technology would enable us to systematically tackle previously intractable monogenic disorders and improve molecular diagnosis.

Therefore, in this study, we have conducted genetic analysis using MPS-based genetic screening to find mutations in nine causative USH genes (except *CIB2*) in Japanese USH1 patients.

## Results

Mutation analysis of the nine USH genes in 17 unrelated USH1 patients revealed 19 different probable pathogenic variants, of which 14 were novel (Table 1).

All mutations were detected in only one patient each and sixteen of the 17 patients (94.1%) carried at least one mutation, while one patient had no mutations. Thirteen of the 16 mutation carriers each had two pathogenic mutations (Table 2).

Nonsense, frame shift, and splice site mutations are all classified as pathogenic, whereas missense mutations are presumed to be probable pathogenic variants based on results of prediction software for evaluation of the pathogenicity of missense variants (Table 1).

Of the 19 probable pathogenic mutations that we found, 17 were detected by MPS. The remaining two (p.Lys542GlnfsX5 in *MYO7A* and c.5821-2A>G in *CDH23*) were sequenced by direct sequence analysis.

Of our 17 USH patients, seven had *MYO7A* mutations (41.2%), three had *CDH23* mutations (17.6%), and two had *PCDH15* mutations (11.8%). We did not find any probable pathogenic mutations in *USH1C*, *USH1G*, and USH2/3 genes.

Four USH1 patients (Cases #3, 5, 8, 15) had probable pathogenic mutations in two different USH genes, with one being a biallelic mutation (Table 3). The other heterozygous/homozygous mutations were missense variants. Three of these patients (Cases #3, 5, 8) presented with earlier RP onset (night blindness) than in the other patients with two pathogenic mutations (Cases #1, 6, 7, 9, 11, 16) ($p = 0.007$) (Fig. 1).

One patient (Case #4) had heterozygote mutations in two USH1 genes (p.Ala771Ser in *MYO7A* and c.158-1G>A in *PCDH15*). His parents and one brother were found to also be carriers for these mutations. Another brother had no variants (Fig. 2).

## Discussion

For USH1, early diagnosis has many immediate and several long-term advantages for patients and their families [1]. However, diagnosis in childhood, based on a clinical phenotype, has been difficult because patients appear to have only non-syndromic HL in childhood and RP develops in later years. Although early diagnosis is now possible through DNA testing, performing large-scale mutation screening for USH genes in all non-syndromic HL children has been both time-consuming and expensive. Therefore, the availability of MPS, which facilitates comprehensive large-scale mutation screening [19] is a very welcome advance.

MPS technology enabled us to detect pathogenic mutations in USH1 patients efficiently, identifying one or two pathogenic/likely pathogenic mutations in 16 of 17 (94.1%) cases. This was comparable to previous direct sequence analysis results such as Bonnet et al. who detected one or two mutations in 24 out of 27 (89%) USH1 patients [11] and Le Quesne Stabej et al. who detected one or two mutations in 41 out of 47 (87.2%) USH1 patients [12].

In addition, MPS assists in the analysis of disease modifiers and digenic inheritance because it simultaneously investigates many causative genes for a specific disease, such as in our case, USH. Previous reports have described several USH cases with pathogenic mutations in two or three different USH genes [11,12,20]. In our study, four patients had two pathogenic mutations in one gene and missense variants in a different gene (Table 3). We considered the latter to possibly be a disease modifier. For example, *USH1C*:p.Tyr813Asp, which occurred in 0/384 control chromosomes and was predicted to be "probably damaging" by the Polyphen program, was found with a homozygous *CDH23* nonsense mutation (p.Arg2107X) (Case #15). As for what the variant "modifies", we speculate that for USH1 patients with a disease modifier, RP symptoms such as night blindness show an earlier onset. However, we think that profound HL and the absence of vestibular function in USH1 patients are not affected by modifiers as they are congenital and therefore not progressive.

Ebermann et al. described a USH2 patient with "digenic inheritance." a heterozygous truncating mutation in *GPR98*, and a truncating heterozygous mutation in PDZ domain-containing 7 (*PDZD7*), which is reported to be a cause of USH [20]. Our USH1 patient (Case #4) had segregated *MYO7A*:p.Ala771Ser and *PCDH15*:c.158-1G>A. Molecular analyses in mouse models have shown many interactions among the USH1 proteins [2]. In particular, *MYO7A* directly binds to *PCDH15* and both proteins are expressed in an overlapping pattern in hair bundles in a mouse model [21]. *PCDH15*:c.158-1G>A, predicted to alter the splice donor site of intron 3, has been classified as pathogenic. *MYO7A*:p.Ala771Ser is a non-truncating mutation, but was previously reported as disease-causing [13]. So, we consider the patient to be the first reported case of *MYO7A*/*PCDH15* digenic inheritance.

However, we should be aware of two limitations of MPS technology. First, the target region of MPS cannot cover all coding exons of USH genes. Actually, the coverage of the target exons was 97.0% in our study. So, it is impossible to detect a mutation in a region which is not covered using this system (Case #9: c.5821-2A>G). Secondarily, the MPS system used in this study, is not effective for detecting homo-polymer regions, for example poly C stretch [22] (Case #8: p.Lys542GlnfsX5). In addition, concerning

**Table 1.** Possible pathogenic variants found in this study.

| Gene | Mutation type | Nucleotide change | Amino acid change | exon/intron number | Domain | control (in 384 alleles) | SIFT Score | PolyPhen Score | Reference |
|---|---|---|---|---|---|---|---|---|---|
| *MYO7A* | Frameshift | c.1623dup | p.Lys542GlnfsX5 | Exon 14 | - | N/A | - | - | Le Quesne Stabej et al. (2012) |
| | | c.4482_4483insTG | p.Trp1495CysfsX55 | Exon 34 | - | N/A | - | - | This study |
| | | c.6205_6206delAT | p.Ile2069ProfsX6 | Exon 45 | - | N/A | - | - | This study |
| | Nonsense | c.1477C>T | p.Gln493X | Exon 13 | - | N/A | - | - | This study |
| | | c.1708C>T | p.Arg570X | Exon 15 | - | N/A | - | - | This study |
| | | c.2115C>A | p.Cys705X | Exon 18 | - | N/A | - | - | This study |
| | | c.6321G>A | p.Trp2107X | Exon 46 | - | N/A | - | - | This study |
| | Missense | c.2074G>A | p.Val692Met | Exon 17 | Motor domain | 0 | 0.09 | 0.982 | This study |
| | | c.2311G>T | p.Ala771Ser | Exon 20 | IQ 2 | 0.0026 | 0.01 | 0.825 | Nakanishi et al. (2010) |
| | | c.6028G>A | p.Asp2010Asn | Exon 44 | FERM 2 | 0 | 0 | 0.925 | Jacobson et al. (2009) |
| *CDH23* | Frameshift | c.3567delG | p.Arg1189ArgfsX5 | Exon 30 | - | N/A | - | - | This study |
| | | c.5780_5781delCT | p.Ser1927Cysfs16 | Exon 44 | - | N/A | - | - | This study |
| | Splicing | c.5821-2A>G | ? | Intron 44 | - | N/A | - | - | This study |
| | Nonsense | c.6319C>T | p.Arg2107X | Exon 48 | - | N/A | - | - | Nakanishi et al. (2010) |
| *PCDH15* | Splicing | c.158-1G>A | ? | Intron 3 | - | N/A | - | - | This study |
| | Nonsense | c.1006C>T | p.Arg336X | Exon 10 | - | N/A | - | - | This study |
| | | c.2971C>T | p.Arg991X | Exon 22 | - | N/A | - | - | Roux et al. (2006) |
| | | c.3337G>T | p.Glu1113X | Exon 25 | - | N/A | - | - | This study |
| | Missense | c.3724G>A | p.Val1242Met | Exon 28 | Cadherin 11 | 0 | 0 | 1 | This study |

Computer analysis to predict the effect of missense variants on MYO7A protein function was performed with sorting intolerant from tolerant (SIFT; http://sift.jcvi.org/), and polymorphism phenotyping (PolyPhen2; http://genetics.bwh.harvard.edu/pph2/).
N/A: not applicable.

**Table 2.** Details of phenotype and genotype of 17 USH1 patients.

| Sample No. | Age | Sex | Allele1 | Allele2 | Hereditary form | Onset of night blindness | Cataract | Hearing Aid | Cochlear Implant |
|---|---|---|---|---|---|---|---|---|---|
| *MYO7A* | | | | | | | | | |
| 1 | 37 | M | p.Gln493X | p.Trp1495CysfsX55 | sporadic | 13 | no | unilateral | unilateral |
| 2 | 41 | W | p.I2069fsX6 | p.I2069fsX6 | AR | unknown | both eyes | bilateral | no |
| 5 | 54 | M | p.Val692Met | p.Val692Met | AR | 5 | both eyes | no | no |
| 6 | 54 | W | p.Arg570X | p.Arg570X | sporadic | 6 | no | no | no |
| 8 | 14 | M | p.Lys542GlnfsX5 | p.Lys542GlnfsX5 | sporadic | 6 | no | unilateral | unilateral |
| 11 | 54 | M | p.Asp2010Asn | p.Trp2107X | sporadic | 13 | no | no | no |
| 17 | 56 | W | p.Cys705X | p.Cys705X | sporadic | unknown | no | no | no |
| *CDH23* | | | | | | | | | |
| 7 | 12 | W | p.Arg1189ArglfsX5 | p.Arg1189ArglfsX5 | sporadic | 12 | both eyes | no | bilateral |
| 9 | 9 | M | p.Ser1927Cysfs16 | c.5821-2A>G | sporadic | 8 | no | unilateral | unilateral |
| 15 | 16 | W | p.Arg2107X | p.Arg2107X | sporadic | unknown | no | no | no |
| *PCDH15* | | | | | | | | | |
| 3 | 47 | W | p.Glu1113X | p.Glu1113X | sporadic | 5 | both eyes | no | no |
| 16 | 28 | W | p.Arg991X | p.Arg991X | AR | 10 | no | no | no |
| 10 | 62 | M | p.Arg962Cys | unknown | sporadic | 9 | both eyes | no | no |
| 12 | 52 | M | p.Arg336X | unknown | sporadic | 3 | no | no | no |
| 13 | 51 | M | p.Val1242Met | unknown | sporadic | 10 | no | no | no |
| *MYO7A**1/*PCDH15**2 | | | | | | | | | |
| 4 | 21 | M | p.Ala771Ser*1 | c.158-1G>A*2 | sporadic | 10 | no | unilateral | unilateral |
| **unknown** | | | | | | | | | |
| 14 | 64 | W | unknown | unknown | sporadic | 15 | both eyes | unilateral | no |

*All subjects have congenital deafness and RP.

pathogenecity of mutations identified, functional analysis will be necessary to draw the final conclusion in the future.

In UK and US Caucasian USH1 patients, USH1B (*MYO7A*) has been reported as the most common USH1 genetic subtype [11,12], while USH1F (*PCDH15*) has been reported as the most common USH1 genetic subtype in North American Ashkenazi Jews [23]. In Japanese, our study revealed that the most common type was *MYO7A* (41.7%), which was similar to the frequency in the above Caucasian patients (46.8~55%) [11,12]. However, the small number of USH1 patients in our study might have biased the frequency and further large cohort study will be needed in the future.

In addition, most of our detected mutations were novel. We have previously reported genes responsible for deafness in Japanese patients and observed differences in mutation spectrum between Japanese (who are probably representative of other Asian populations) and populations with European ancestry [24].

In conclusion, our study was the first report of USH mutation analysis using MPS and the frequency of USH1 genes in Japanese. Mutation screening using MPS has the potential power to quickly identify mutations of many causative genes such as USH while maintaining cost-benefit performance. In addition, the simultaneous mutation analysis of large numbers of genes was useful for detecting mutations in different genes that are possibly disease modifiers or of digenic inheritance.

## Materials and Methods

### Subjects

We screened 17 Japanese USH1 patients (aged 9 to 64 years): three from autosomal recessive families (non-affected parents and two or more affected siblings), and 14 from sporadic families. There were 9 males and 8 females. None of the subjects had any other noteworthy symptoms. All subjects or next of kin on the behalf of the minors/children gave prior written informed consent for participation in the project, and the Ethical Committee of Shinshu University approved the study and the consent procedure.

### Amplicon Library Preparation

An Amplicon library of the target exons was prepared with an Ion AmpliSeq Custom Panel (Applied Biosystems, Life Technologies, Carlsbad, CA) designed with Ion AmpliSeq Designer (https://www.ampliseq.com/browse.action) for nine USH genes by using Ion AmpliSeq Library Kit 2.0 (Applied Biosystems, Life Technologies) and Ion Xpress Barcode Adapter 1–16 Kit (Applied Biosystems, Life Technologies) according to the manufacturers' procedures.

In brief, DNA concentration was measured with Quant-iT dsDNA HS Assay (Invitrogen, Life Technologies) and Qubit Fluorometer (Invitrogen, Life Technologies) and DNA quality was confirmed by agarose gel electrophoresis. 10 ng of each genomic DNA sample was amplified, using Ion AmpliSeq HiFi Master Mix (Applied Biosystems, Life Technologies) and AmpliSeq Custom primer pools, for 2 min at 99°C, followed by 15 two-step cycles of

**Table 3.** The patients with mutations in two different genes.

| Sample | Genes with two pathogenic mutations | Gene with one heterozygous mutation | Nucleotide change | Amino acid change | control | SIFT score | PolyPhen score | Referense |
|---|---|---|---|---|---|---|---|---|
| 5 | *MYO7A* | *CDH23* | c.C719T | p.P240L* | 0.26 | 0.06 | 0.999 | Wagatsuma et al. (2007) |
| 8 | *MYO7A* | *CDH23* | c.2568C>G | p.Ile856Met | 0 | 0.08 | 1 | This study |
| 15 | *CDH15* | *USH1C* | c.2437T>G | p.Tyr813Asp | 0 | 0.19 | 0.932 | This study |
| 3 | *PCDH15* | *USH1G* | c.28C>T | p.Arg10Trp | 0 | 0.19 | 1 | This study |

*homozygotes.

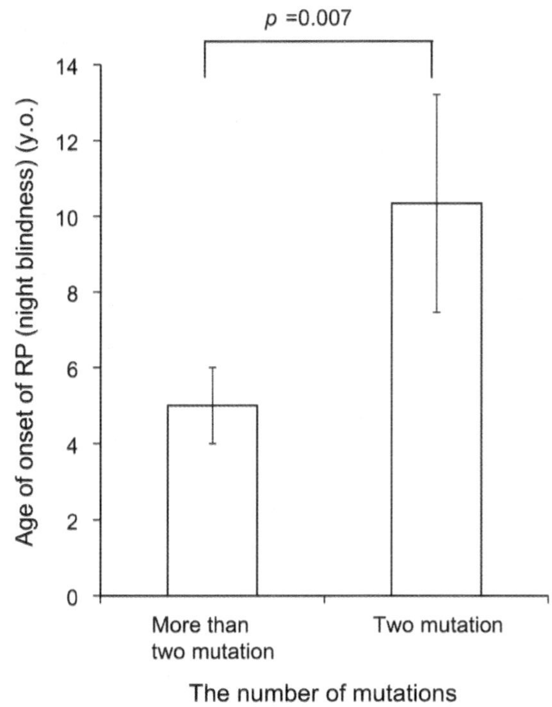


**Figure 1. The number of mutations and the age of RP onset in Usher syndrome type 1 patients.** The age of RP onset is earlier in the patients with more than two pathogenic mutations. RP: retinitis pigmentosa.

99°C for 15 sec and 60°C for 4 min, ending with a holding period at 10°C in a PCR thermal cycler (Takara, Shiga, Japan). After the Multiplex PCR amplification, amplified DNA samples were digested with FuPa enzyme at 50°C for 10 min and 55°C for 10 min and the enzyme was successively inactivated for 60°C for 20 min incubation. After digestion, diluted barcode adapter mix including Ion Xpress Barcode Adapter and Ion P1 adaptor were ligated to the end of the digested amplicons with ligase in the kit for 30 min at 22°C and the ligase was successively inactivated at 60°C for 20 min incubation. Adaptor ligated amplicon libraries were purified with the Agencourt AMPure XP system (Beckman Coulter Genomics, Danvers, MA). The amplicon libraries were quantified by using Ion Library Quantitation Kit (Applied Biosystems, Life Technologies) and the StepOne plus realtime PCR system (Applied Biosystems, Life Technologies) according to the manufacturers' procedures. After quantification, each amplicon library was diluted to 20 pM and the same amount of the 12 libraries for 12 patients were pooled for one sequence reaction.

## Emulsion PCR and Sequencing

The emulsion PCR was carried out with the Ion OneTouch System and Ion OneTouch 200 Template Kit v2 (Life Technologies) according to the manufacturer's procedure (Publication Part Number 4478371 Rev. B Revision Date 13 June 2012). After the emulsion PCR, template-positive Ion Sphere Particles were enriched with the Dynabeads MyOne Streptavidin C1 Beads (Life Technologies) and washed with Ion OneTouch Wash Solution in the kit. This process were performed using an Ion OneTouch ES system (Life Technologies).

After the Ion Sphere Particle preparation, MPS was performed with an Ion Torrent Personal Genome Machine (PGM) system

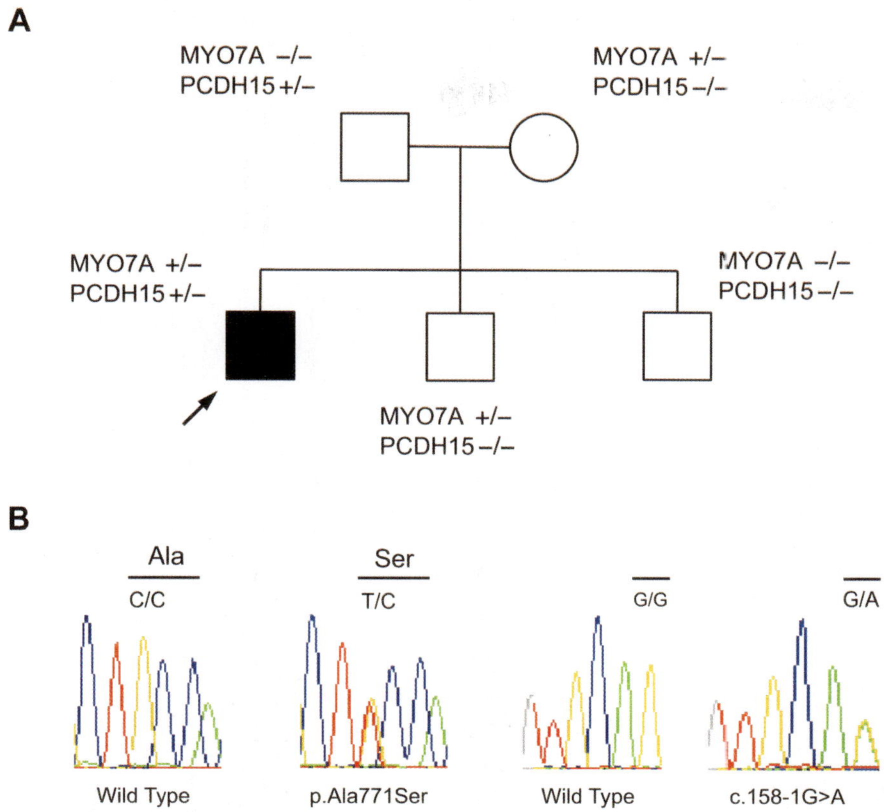


**Figure 2. Pedigree and sequence chromatograms of the patient with the p.Ala771Ser in *MYO7A* and c.158-1G>A in *PCDH15* mutations.** (A) The pedigree and sequence results of the proband and family. (B) Sequence chromatograms from wild-type and mutations. The proband, his mothor and one brother carried a heterozygous 2311G>T transition in exon 20, which results in an alanine to a serine (Ala771Ser) in *MYO7A*. Another variation, 158-1G>A in intron 3 of *PCDH15*, was derived from the proband and his father. Another brother had no variants.

using the Ion PGM 200 Sequencing Kit and Ion 318 Chip (Life Technologies) according to the manufacturer's procedures.

## Base Call and Data Analysis

The sequence data were processed with standard Ion Torrent Suite Software and Torrent Server successively mapped to human genome sequence (build GRCh37/hg19) with Torrent Mapping Alignment Program optimized to Ion Torrent data. The average of 562.33 Mb sequences with about 4,300,000 reads was obtained by one Ion 318 chip. The 98.0% sequences were mapped to the human genome and 94% of them were on the target region. Average coverage of depth in the target region was 314.2 and 93.8% of them were over 20 coverage.

After the sequence mapping, the DNA variant regions were piled up with Torrent Variant Caller plug-in software. Selected variant candidates were filtered with the average base QV (minimum average base quality 25), variant frequency (40–60% for heterozygous mutations and 80–100% for homozygous mutations) and coverage of depth (minimum coverage of depth 10). After the filtrations, variant effects were analyzed with the wANNOVAR web site [25,26] (http://wannovar.usc.edu) including the functional prediction software for missense variants: Sorting Intolerant from Tolerant (SIFT; http://sift.jcvi.org/), and Polymorphism Phenotyping (PolyPhen2; http://genetics.bwh.harvard.edu/pph2/). The sequencing data was available in the DNA databank of Japan (Accession number: DRA001273).

## Algorithm

Missense, nonsense, and splicing variants were selected among the identified variants. Variants were further selected as less than 1% of: 1) the 1000 genome database (http://www.1000genomes.org/), 2) the 5400 exome variants (http://evs.gs.washington.edu/EVS/), and 3) the in-house control. Candidate mutations were confirmed by Sanger sequencing and the responsible mutations were identified by segregation analysis using samples from family members of the patients. In addition, the cases with heterozygous or no causative mutation were fully sequenced by Sanger sequencing for USH1 genes in order to verify the MPS results.

## Direct Sequence Analysis

Primers were designed with the Primer 3 plus web server (http://www.bioinformatics.nl/cgi-bin/primer3plus/primer3plus.cgi). Each genomic DNA sample (40 ng) was amplified using Ampli Taq Gold (Life Technologies) for 5 min at 94°C, followed by 30 three-step cycles of 94°C for 30 sec, 60°C for 30 sec, and 72°C for 30 sec, with a final extension at 72°C for 5 min, ending with a holding period at 4°C in a PCR thermal cycler (Takara, Shiga, Japan). The PCR products were treated with ExoSAP-IT (GE Healthcare Bio, Buckinghamshire, UK) and by incubation at 37°C for 60 min, and inactivation at 80°C for 15 min. After the products were purified, we performed standard cycle sequencing reaction with ABI Big Dye terminators in an ABI 3130xl sequencer (Life Technologies).

### Accession numbers

*MYO7A*, [NM_000260.3]; *USH1C*, [NM_ 153676.3]; *CDH23*, [NM_ 022124.5]; *PCDH15*, [NM_ 033056.3]; *USH1G*, [NM_ 173477.2]; *USH2A*, [NM_206933.2]; *GPR98*, [NM_ 032119.3]; *DFNB31*, [NM_ 015404.3]; *CLRN1*, [NM_ 174878.2]; *PDZD7*, [NM_ 001195263.1].

## Acknowledgments

We thank A. C. Apple-Mathews for help in preparing the manuscript.

## Author Contributions

Conceived and designed the experiments: HY SI SN SU. Performed the experiments: HY SN. Analyzed the data: HY SN SU. Contributed reagents/materials/analysis tools: HY SI SN KK TT YK HS KN KI TI YN KF CO TK HN SU. Wrote the paper: HY SN SU.

## References

1. Kimberling WJ, Hildebrand MS, Shearer AE, Jensen ML, Halder JA, et al. (2010) Frequency of Usher syndrome in two pediatric populations: Implications for genetic screening of deaf and hard of hearing children. Genet Med 12: 512–516.
2. Yan D, Liu XZ (2010) Genetics and pathological mechanisms of Usher syndrome. J Hum Genet 55: 327–335.
3. Jaworek TJ, Bhatti R, Latief N, Khan SN, Riazuddin S, et al. (2012) USH1K, a novel locus for type I Usher syndrome, maps to chromosome 10p11.21-q21.1. J Hum Genet 57: 633–637.
4. Riazuddin S, Belyantseva IA, Giese AP, Lee K, Indzhykulian AA, et al. (2012) Alterations of the CIB2 calcium- and integrin-binding protein cause Usher syndrome type 1J and nonsyndromic deafness DFNB48. Nat Genet 44: 1265–1271.
5. Weil D, Blanchard S, Kaplan J, Guilford P, Gibson F, et al. (1995) Defective myosin VIIA gene responsible for Usher syndrome type 1B. Nature 374: 60–61.
6. Bork JM, Peters LM, Riazuddin S, Bernstein SL, Ahmed ZM, et al. (2001) Usher syndrome 1D and nonsyndromic autosomal recessive deafness DFNB12 are caused by allelic mutations of the novel cadherin-like gene CDH23. Am J Hum Genet 68: 26–37.
7. Ahmed ZM, Riazuddin S, Bernstein SL, Ahmed Z, Khan S, et al. (2001) Mutations of the protocadherin gene PCDH15 cause Usher syndrome type 1F. Am J Hum Genet 69: 25–34.
8. Verpy E, Leibovici M, Zwaenepoel I, Liu XZ, Gal A, et al. (2000) A defect in harmonin, a PDZ domain-containing protein expressed in the inner ear sensory hair cells, underlies Usher syndrome type 1C. Nat Genet 26: 51–55.
9. Mustapha M, Chouery E, Torchard-Pagnez D, Nouaille S, Khrais A, et al. (2002) A novel locus for Usher syndrome type I, USH1G, maps to chromosome 17q24-25. Hum Genet 110: 348–350.
10. Ouyang XM, Yan D, Du LL, Hejtmancik JF, Jacobson SG, et al. (2005) Characterization of Usher syndrome type I gene mutations in an Usher syndrome patient population. Hum Genet 116: 292–299.
11. Bonnet C, Grati M, Marlin S, Levilliers J, Hardelin JP, et al. (2011) Complete exon sequencing of all known Usher syndrome genes greatly improves molecular diagnosis. Orphanet J Rare Dis 6: 21.
12. Le Quesne Stabej P, Saihan Z, Rangesh N, Steele-Stallard HB, Ambrose J, et al. (2012) Comprehensive sequence analysis of nine Usher syndrome genes in the UK National Collaborative Usher Study. J Med Genet 49: 27–36.
13. Nakanishi H, Ohtsubo M, Iwasaki S, Hotta Y, Takizawa Y, et al. (2010) Mutation analysis of the MYO7A and CDH23 genes in Japanese patients with Usher syndrome type 1. J Hum Genet 55: 796–800.
14. Eudy JD, Yao S, Weston MD, Ma-Edmonds M, Talmadge CB, et al. (1998) Isolation of a gene encoding a novel member of the nuclear receptor superfamily from the critical region of Usher syndrome type IIa at 1q41. Genomics 50: 382–384.
15. Weston MD, Luijendijk MW, Humphrey KD, Moller C, Kimberling WJ (2004) Mutations in the VLGR1 gene implicate G-protein signaling in the pathogenesis of Usher syndrome type II. Am J Hum Genet 74: 357–366.
16. Aller E, Jaijo T, van Wijk E, Ebermann I, Kersten F, et al. (2010) Sequence variants of the DFNB31 gene among Usher syndrome patients of diverse origin. Mol Vis 16: 495–500.
17. Joensuu T, Hamalainen R, Yuan B, Johnson C, Tegelberg S, et al. (2001) Mutations in a novel gene with transmembrane domains underlie Usher syndrome type 3. Am J Hum Genet 69: 673–684.
18. Nakanishi H, Ohtsubo M, Iwasaki S, Hotta Y, Usami S, et al. (2011) Novel USH2A mutations in Japanese Usher syndrome type 2 patients: marked differences in the mutation spectrum between the Japanese and other populations. J Hum Genet 56: 484–490.
19. Miyagawa M, Nishio SY, Ikeda T, Fukushima K, Usami S (2013) Massively parallel DNA sequencing successfully identifies new causative mutations in deafness genes in patients with cochlear implantation and EAS. PLoS One.
20. Ebermann I, Phillips JB, Liebau MC, Koenekoop RK, Schermer B, et al. (2010) PDZD7 is a modifier of retinal disease and a contributor to digenic Usher syndrome. J Clin Invest 120: 1812–1823.
21. Senften M, Schwander M, Kazmierczak P, Lillo C, Shin JB, et al. (2006) Physical and functional interaction between protocadherin 15 and myosin VIIa in mechanosensory hair cells. J Neurosci 26: 2060–2071.
22. Loman NJ, Misra RV, Dallman TJ, Constantinidou C, Gharbia SE, et al. (2012) Performance comparison of benchtop high-throughput sequencing platforms. Nat Biotechnol 30: 434–439.
23. Ben-Yosef T, Ness SL, Madeo AC, Bar-Lev A, Wolfman JH, et al. (2003) A mutation of PCDH15 among Ashkenazi Jews with the type 1 Usher syndrome. N Engl J Med 348: 1664–1670.
24. Usami S, Wagatsuma M, Fukuoka H, Suzuki H, Tsukada K, et al. (2008) The responsible genes in Japanese deafness patients and clinical application using Invader assay. Acta Otolaryngol 128: 446–454.
25. Wang K, Li M, Hakonarson H (2010) ANNOVAR: functional annotation of genetic variants from high-throughput sequencing data. Nucleic Acids Res 38: e164.
26. Chang X, Wang K (2012) wANNOVAR: annotating genetic variants for personal genomes via the web. J Med Genet 49: 433–436.

5

# Novel and Recurrent *MYO7A* Mutations in Usher Syndrome Type 1 and Type 2

**Weining Rong[1]ᵑ, Xue Chen[2,3]ᵑ, Kanxing Zhao[4]ᵑ, Yani Liu[1], Xiaoxing Liu[2], Shaoping Ha[1], Wenzhou Liu[1], Xiaoli Kang[5], Xunlun Sheng[1]*, Chen Zhao[2,6]***

**1** Ningxia Eye Hospital, Ningxia People's Hospital, Ningxia, China, **2** Department of Ophthalmology, The First Affiliated Hospital of Nanjing Medical University, State Key Laboratory of Reproductive Medicine, Nanjing, China, **3** Department of Ophthalmology & Visual Sciences, The Chinese University of Hong Kong, Hong Kong, China, **4** Tianjin Medical University, Tianjin Eye Hospital, Tianjin Key Laboratory of Ophthalmology and Visual Science, Tianjin, China, **5** Department of Ophthalmology, Xinhua Hospital, Shanghai Jiao Tong University School of Medicine, Shanghai, China, **6** State Key Laboratory of Ophthalmology, Zhongshan Ophthalmic Center, Sun Yat Sen University, Guangzhou, China

## Abstract

Usher syndrome (USH) is a group of disorders manifested as retinitis pigmentosa and bilateral sensorineural hearing loss, with or without vestibular dysfunction. Here, we recruited three Chinese families affected with autosomal recessive USH for detailed clinical evaluations and for mutation screening in the genes associated with inherited retinal diseases. Using targeted next-generation sequencing (NGS) approach, three new alleles and one known mutation in *MYO7A* gene were identified in the three families. In two families with USH type 1, novel homozygous frameshift variant p.Pro194Hisfs*13 and recurrent missense variant p.Thr165Met were demonstrated as the causative mutations respectively. Crystal structural analysis denoted that p.Thr165Met would very likely change the tertiary structure of the protein encoded by *MYO7A*. In another family affected with USH type 2, novel biallelic mutations in *MYO7A*, c.[1343+1G>A];[2837T>G] or p.[?];[Met946Arg], were identified with clinical significance. Because *MYO7A*, to our knowledge, has rarely been correlated with USH type 2, our findings therefore reveal distinguished clinical phenotypes associated with *MYO7A*. We also conclude that targeted NGS is an effective approach for genetic diagnosis for USH, which can further provide better understanding of genotype-phenotype relationship of the disease.

**Editor:** Ludmila Prokunina-Olsson, National Cancer Institute, National Institutes of Health, United States of America

**Funding:** This work was supported by National Key Basic Research Program of China (973 Program, 2013CB967500); National Natural Science Foundation of China (81222009, 81170856, 81160124, 81260154, and 81170867); Thousand Youth Talents Program of China (to CZ); Jiangsu Outstanding Young Investigator Program (BK2012046); Jiangsu Province's Key Provincial Talents Program (RC201149); the Fundamental Research Funds of the State Key Laboratory of Ophthalmology (to CZ); Jiangsu Province's Scientific Research Innovation Program for Postgraduates (CXZZ13_05 to XC); Applied Research Program of the Science and Technology Commission Foundation of Tianjin (013111411 to KZ); and A Project Funded by the Priority Academic Program Development of Jiangsu Higher Education Institutions (PAPD). The funders had no role in study design, data collection and analysis, decision to publish, or preparation of the manuscript.

**Competing Interests:** The authors have declared that no competing interests exist.

* E-mail: dr.zhaochen@gmail.com (CZ); shengxunlun@163.com (XS)

ᵑ These authors contributed equally to this work.

## Introduction

Usher syndrome (USH) is a group of autosomal recessively inherited disorders characterized by bilateral sensorineural hearing loss (SNHL) and a gradual retinal degeneration typified as retinitis pigmentosa (RP). Some patients with USH may also manifest vestibular dysfunction [1]. USH is estimated to be responsible for the majority of deaf-blindness in human (accounting for over 50%) [2,3], with its prevalence ranging from 3.2 to 6.2 per 100,000 people in different populations [4,5].

USH is clinically and genetically heterogeneous. Three major clinical subtypes have been described called USH type 1, type 2, and type 3. They are mainly distinguished by the severity and progression of the deafness and the presence of vestibular defects [6,7]. Since the identification of the first USH-causative gene (*MYO7A*) in 1995 [8], by far, mutations in twelve genes have been implicated in the etiology of USH. USH type 1, accounting for 30% to 40% of total USH, is the most severe clinical form typified by profound congenital deafness, early onset of visual impairment (usually within the first decade of life), and vestibular dysfunction [9]. USH type 1 has been associated with nine genetic loci (USH1B-1H, 1J and 1K), among which six corresponding genes were identified including *MYO7A* (USH1B) [8], *USH1C* (USH1C) [10], *CDH23* (USH1D) [11], *PCDH15* (USH1F) [12], *USH1G* (USH1G) [13], and *CIB2* (USH1J) [14]. USH type 2, the most common form of USH, is presented with much less severer phenotypes than USH type 1 [9]. Typical clinical manifestations include normal vestibular functions, and moderate to severe congenital hearing impairments rather than totally deafness. RP usually occurs in the 2$^{nd}$ decade. Three disease causing genes from distinct genetic loci have been reported, namely *USH2A* (USH2A) [15], *GPR98* (USH2C) [16], and *DFNB31* (USH2D) [17]. Patients with Usher type 3 are manifested by variable onset of progressive hearing loss, variable vestibular dysfunction, and also variable onset of visual impairment [3]. Mutations in *CLRN1* [18] have been pinpointed to cause USH type 3. Other than all above mentioned USH causative genes, the *PDZD7* gene encodes a protein which would interact with proteins encoded by *DFNB31* and *USH1C*, and may modify other Usher syndrome relevant mutations, we therefore have included *PDZD7* as another putative disease causative gene for Usher syndrome [19].

Mutations in *MYO7A* are the most common causes for patents with USH type 1 globally, accounting for 29% to 50% of total [5,20,21,22,23]. In the present study, we report three novel mutations and a recurrent one in *MYO7A* gene identified in three Chinese families with autosomal recessive USH type 1 and type 2 using targeted gene approaches. We have also identified genotype-phenotype correlation between *MYO7A* mutations and USH type 2, which, to the best of our knowledge, has not been previously characterized in details.

## Materials and Methods

### Participants and Clinical Investigations

This study was approved by the Ethics Committee on Human Research of the People's Hospital of Ningxia Hui Autonomous Region, and conformed to the tenets of the Declaration of Helsinki. Written informed consents were obtained from all participants. Seven individuals, including four patients and three unaffected family members, of three unrelated families were recruited from Ningxia Hui Autonomous Region. Each participant underwent detailed pure tone audiometry testing and ophthalmic examinations, including best-corrected visual acuities (BCVAs) measurements, slit-lamp biomicroscopy, intraocular pressure (IOP) test, funduscopy, visual field (VF) test, and electroretinography (ERG) test. Detailed vestibular tests were further conducted on patients USH01-III:1 and USH01-III:2 as detailed previously [24]. Additionally, 100 controls over 60-year-old free of retinal dystrophies or other major eye diseases were included. Peripheral blood samples were obtained from all participants. Genomic DNA was extracted from leukocytes using a QIAmp DNA Blood kit (Qiagen, Valencia, CA) per the manufacturer's instructions.

### Targeted Gene Capture and Next-generation Sequencing

Two similar targeted sequence capture microarrays were used in this study. Microarray #1, the RDs189-Array, has been previously described and validated [25]. This chip was designed to capture the coding sequences with at least 100 base pairs (bps) of flanking intronic sequences, and 5′- and 3′- untranslated regions (UTR) of 179 genes associated with HRDs and 10 candidate genes including all USH-related genes. Probes of 250–300 bps were designed accordingly for sequence capture. Targeted gene approach using the RDs189-Array was performed on the two affected members in family USH01, USH01-III:1 and USH01-III:2. Microarray #2 was a commercial sequence capture array (BGI-Shenzhen, Shenzhen, Guangdong, China) that could capture the coding sequences of 316 genes with all known USH causative genes included. Patient USH02-II:1 and USH03-II:1 were screened using microarray #2. Information of the targeted genes of the commercial array has been previously described [26]. Sequence capture, enrichment, elution, and NGS were conducted in collaboration with the BGI-Shenzhen as previously stated [27].

### Bioinformatics Analysis and Mutation Validation

The NCBI human reference genome (NCBI build 37.1) was obtained from the UCSC database (http://hgdownload.cse.ucsc.edu/goldenPath/hg19/bigZips/). Bioinformatics analysis was performed as described previously [25]. Briefly, reads were aligned to the reference genome using Short Oligonucleotide Alignment Program (SOAP, http://soap.genomics.org.cn) for SNP analysis [28], and Burrows-Wheeler Aligner (BWA, http://bio-bwa.sourceforge.net/) for Indel detection [29]. Coverage and depth calculations were only performed on aligned reads. All detected variants were further filtered against the following 5 SNPs databases, including dbSNP137 (http://hgdownload.cse.ucsc.edu/goldenPath/hg19/database/snp137.txt.gz.), HapMap Project (ftp://ftp.ncbi.nlm.nih.gov/hapmap), 1000 Genome Project (ftp://ftp.1000genomes.ebi.ac.uk/vol1/ftp), YH database (http://yh.genomics.org.cn/), and Exome Variant Server (http://evs.gs.washington.edu/EVS/). Variants found homozygous in those databases or with minor allele frequency (MAF) >0.01 were filtrated. Datasets of NGS were deposited in National Institutes of Health (NIH) Short Read Archive (http://www.ncbi.nlm.nih.gov/sra). Sanger sequencing was subsequently performed for validation of variants in all USH causative genes and prevalence test in 100 unrelated controls, using a previously defined protocol [30]. Primer information was detailed in **Table S1**.

### *In silico* Analyses

Vector NTI Advance 11 software (Invitrogen, Grand Island, NY) was applied to evaluate the evolutionary conservation of the mutated amino acids through alignment of the *MYO7A* orthologous protein sequences of the following species: *Homo sapiens* (ENSP00000386331), *Pan troglodytes* (ENSPTRP00000007055), *Canis lupus familiaris* (ENSCAFP00000007721), *Bos taurus* (ENSBTAP00000005191), *Sus scrofa* (ENSSSCP00000015796), *Mus musculus* (ENSMUSP00000102745), *Gallus gallus* (ENSGALP00000001044), *Danio rerio* (ENSDARP00000083378), *Drosophila melanogaster* (FBpp0080282), and *Caenorhabditis elegans* (T10H10.1). The possible impacts of the mutation were indicated by three online software, including SIFT Human Protein DB (http://sift.bii.a-star.edu.sg/), PolyPhen-2 (Polymorphism Phenotyping, version 2; http://genetics.bwh.harvard.edu/pph2/) [31], and CONDEL (http://bg.upf.edu/condel/analysis). The effect of alteration of splice site was predicted by Human Splicing Finder version 2.4.1 (http://www.umd.be/HSF/), NetGene2 sever (http://www.cbs.dtu.dk/services/NetGene2/), Splice Site Prediction by Neural Network (http://www.fruitfly.org/seq_tools/splice.html), and SROOGLE (http://sroogle.tau.ac.il/). SWISS-MODEL online server was used to predict the crystal structures of the wide type and mutant proteins [32,33]. Predicted structures were displayed using PyMol software (version 1.5).

## Results

### Clinical Manifestations

Four affected members and three unaffected individuals from 3 families with USH were included in this study (**Figure 1B–1D**). The clinical manifestations of the affected members were detailed in **Table 1**. In family USH01, the parents of the two affected patients were asymptomatic. The 24-year-old proband, USH01-III:1, was found to have hearing problems since childhood. Pure tone audiometry testing revealed bilateral moderate sensorineural hearing impairment in the proband, which were 56.67 and 66.67 dB for the right and left ear, respectively (**Figure 2A, 2B**). His speech was normal and the hearing impairment was non-progressive. No vestibular defect was detected. He developed night blindness at 15-year-old age. RP characteristics were indicated by fundus photo, including vessel attenuation, pallor of optic disc, and pigmentary migration (**Figure 3A, 3B**). VF was significantly constricted to tubular vision, and ERG was diminished in both rod and cone responses. His current BCVA was 0.8 in both eyes. Macular region was relatively preserved according to his fundus appearance and OCT results. The anterior segment and IOP were also normal. The disease symptoms of his younger brother were a bit severer. He had non-progressive moderate to severe hearing loss (73.33 dB and 78.33 dB for the right and the left ear, respectively, **Figure 2C, 2D**), and slight language barrier. Similar to his brother, his RP onset age was 13, and he was also manifested with typical RP symptoms (**Figure 3C, 3D**). Since the RP onset ages for the two patients were 15 and 13 years of age, both of which were in accordance with the typical clinical manifestations presented by Usher syndrome type 2, we therefore concluded that the two patients from family USH01 displayed USH type 2 phenotypes.

Unlike family USH01, patients USH02-II:1 and USH03-II:1 are presented with typical USH type 1 phenotypes. Both patients suffered from severe bilateral hearing loss and severe speech problems since childhood. They also had vestibular dysfunctions. RP developed within the first decade of their life. Typical RP fundus and other ophthalmic examination results were revealed in both patients (**Figure 3E, 3F**). The detailed clinical information was listed in **Table 1**.

## Targeted Gene Approach

As aforementioned, targeted gene approach was performed on patients USH01-III:1, USH01-III:2, USH02-II:1, and USH03-II:1. The detailed results underlying NGS are discussed in **Table S2**. Generally, an over 98.54% coverage of target region was processed by each sample, and the rate of nucleotide mismatch for each sample was equal to or below 0.25%. A total of 8939 variants were initially disclosed in all three families, including 8041 SNPs and 898 Indels. We deposited our dataset in NIH Short Read Archive, and have provided the accession numbers of BioProject, Biosamples, and Runs for each individual in **Table 1**. The identified variants were first annotated to the 5 SNPs databases. Variants found homozygous in any of the 5 databases or with MAF>0.01 were filtered. Synonymous and non-coding variants (with exception of intronic variants within 10 bp flanking exons) were further removed. Remaining variants in all USH causative genes (as listed in **Table S3**) were subsequently confirmed by Sanger sequencing, and also tested in all attainable family members within each individual family and 100 unrelated negative controls. In all, four putative pathogenic variants in *MYO7A* gene were identified in the three individual families, of which three were novel, and one was recurrent. All four detected mutations were absent in 100 unrelated negative controls.

## Novel Biallelic *MYO7A* Mutations in Family USH01 with USH Type 2

Novel biallelic heterozygous mutations, *MYO7A* c.[1343+1G>A];[2837T>G], were detected in the two patients from family USH01 affected with USH type 2 (**Figure 1A, 1E–1F**). All mutations identified in this manuscript were described according to the guidelines summarized on the Mutation Nomenclature Homepage at the HGVS website (http://www.hgvs.org/mutnomen/). The former one, c.1343+1G>A, refers to a G to A substitution at the first nucleotide of the intron 12, the absolutely conserved donor splice site, which is right adjacent to the coding nucleotide numbered as c.1343, the last nucleotide of exon 12. The consensus splice site was eliminated according to results from all four online prediction websites, while a potential novel one would be produced over 300 bps away from the previous site. The latter mutation would result in a substitution of methionine for arginine at condon 946 (p.Met946Arg), which was found to be deleterious as revealed by all three online prediction software, including Polyphen (0.942, possibly damaging), SIFT (0.00, deleterious), and CONDEL (0.678, deleterious). Conservational analysis further indicated that this position was highly conserved among all mammalian animals (**Figure 1I**). Cosegregation analysis revealed that the two patients inherited the c.1343+1G>A mutation paternally and the p.Met946Arg mutation maternally.

## Mutation Analyses in Family USH02 and USH03 with USH Type 1

In the consanguineous family USH02, a novel homozygous variant, *MYO7A* c.581_582del, was identified in the patient (**Figure 1G**). The framshift mutation indicated a deletion of two coding nucleotides at c.581 and c.582. This deletion was a frameshift mutation with introduction of a premature termination codon (PTC), and therefore, the protein change is theoretically p.Pro194Hisfs*13, a truncated protein with 205 amino acid. However, the truncated proteins may not exist *in vivo* due to NMD. The sporadic case from family USH03 was found to carry a recurrent homozygous variants in *MYO7A*, c.494C>T [34], which would lead to the amino acid change from threonine to methionine at condon 165 (p.Thr165Met) (**Figure 1H**). Severe functional impact of this variant was indicated by all three online prediction software. That was 1.000 (possibly damaging) for Polyphen, 0.00 (deleterious) for SIFT, and 1.000 (deleterious) for CONDEL. Consistently, this mutational spot was highly conserved among all species analyzed by multiple protein sequences alignment (**Figure 1I**). We conducted structural modeling of the myosin-VIIa (residues 3–769), the protein encoded by *MYO7A* gene, on the basis of the crystal structure of Q02440, the motor domain of the chicken myosin-Va showing the sequence identity of 39.51% with the human myosin-VIIa [35]. The model built revealed that the wild type Thr165 located in the ATP binding site (158–165) generated four hydrogen bonds and interacted with four amino acids including Thr168, Lys169, Ser211, and Asp437 (**Figure 4A, 4B**). The substitution of threonine to methionine at residue 165 resulted in the elimination of hydrogen bonds between residue 165 and Ser211, and between residue 165 and Asp437 (**Figure 4C**). The elimination of the two hydrogen bonds, which link an α-helix with β-sheets, would potentially change the tertiary structure of the protein. Thus, we conclude that the variants identified are very likely the disease-causing mutations of the corresponding family.

# Discussion

Mutations in *MYO7A* gene have long been implicated in the disease etiology of USH type 1. In the present study, three novel mutations and a recurrent one were revealed as disease-causing in three unrelated families. Noteworthy, in a Chinese family with USH type 2, novel biallelic heterozygous mutations in *MYO7A* were identified namely c.[1343+1G>A];[2837T>G]. The two mutations cosegregated with disease phenotypes and were absent in 100 normal controls. To our knowledge, *MYO7A* mutations have rarely been correlated with USH type 2. Only Bonnet et al has identified biallelic *MYO7A* mutations in a sporadic Caucasian patient [36], but with no clinical data provided in their paper in addition to diagnosis. In our manuscript, we have summarized the clinical findings of a Chinese family with USH type 2, in which we identified novel biallelic *MYO7A* mutations. Therefore, we have provided sufficient analysis of genotype-phenotype correlation between *MYO7A* mutations and USH type 2, which, to our understanding, has not been previously characterized in details. Located on 11q13.5, the *MYO7A* gene yields a transcript of 7.46 Kb encompassing 49 exons. The encoded protein, myosin-VIIa, is an actin-based motor protein that plays an important role in intracellular transport, endocytosis, and intercellular adhesion

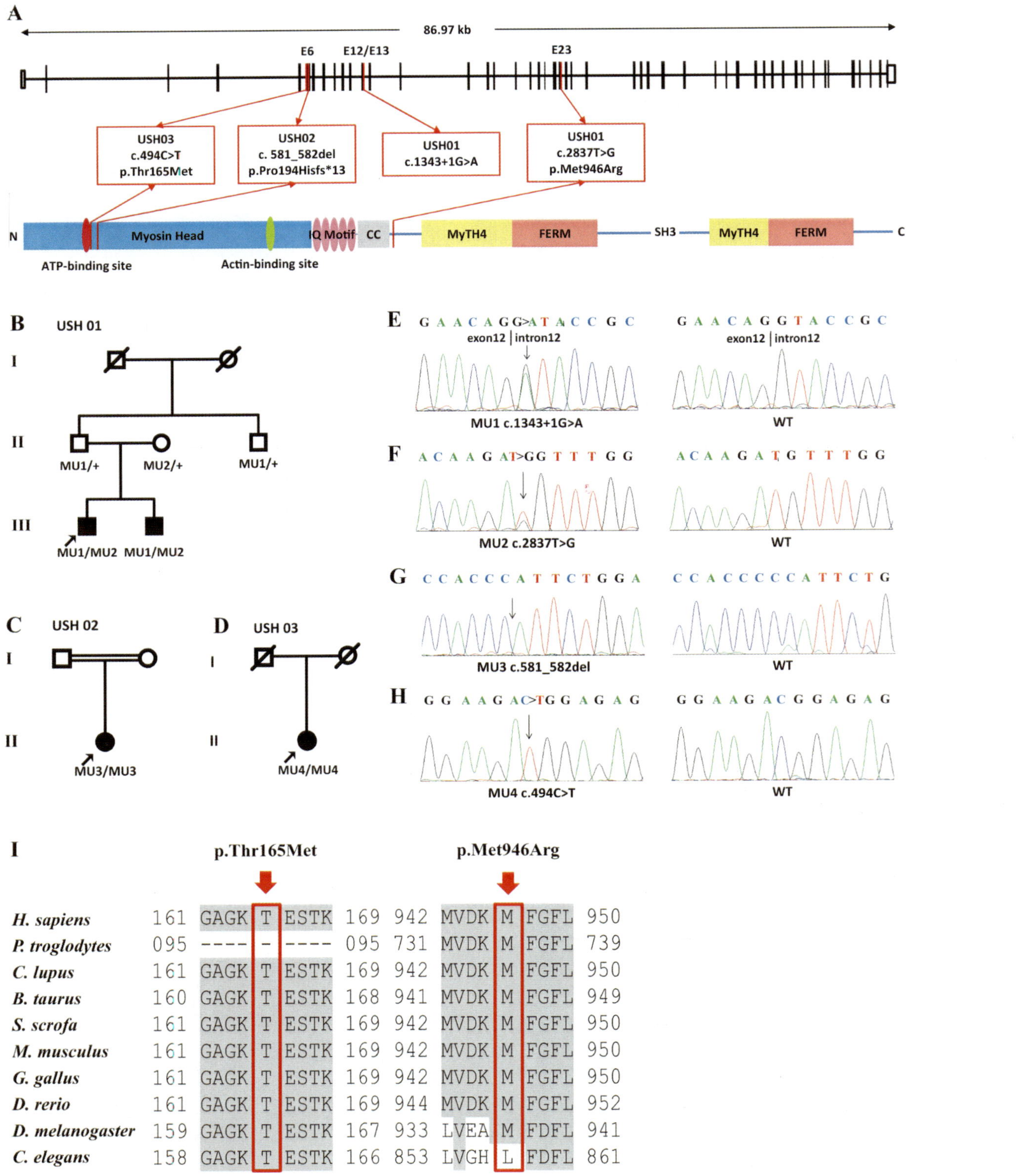


**Figure 1. Family pedigrees, DNA chromatogram sequences, and sequence alignment of the identified mutational spots.** (A) Schematic representation of the relative linear location of all four *MYO7A* mutations identified in the present study in context of genome structure (upper) and protein structure (below). (B–D) Pedigrees of families USH01 (B), USH02 (C), and USH03 (D). Filled and empty symbols represent affected and unaffected individuals, respectively. Probands (USH01-III1, USH02-II1, and USH03-II1) are indicated by arrows. Consanguinity exits in family USH02. (E–H) DNA sequencing profiles for the four identified disease-causing mutations (left panel) and the corresponding wide type forms (right panel). Biallelic heterozygous c.1343+1G>A (E, MU1) and c.2837T>G (F, MU2, p.Met946Arg) mutations are identified as disease causing mutations for family USH01. Homozygous c.581_582del (G, MU3, p.Pro194Hisfs*13) and c.494C>T (H, MU4, p.Thr165Met) mutations are indicated as disease causative for family USH02 and USH03, respectively. (J) The arrows indicate that the Thr165 and Met946 residues are evolutionary highly conserved among multiple species.

**Table 1.** Clinical Manifestations of Patients Carrying *MYO7A* Mutations.

| | USH01-III:1 | | USH01-III:2 | | USH02-II:1 | | USH03-II:1 | |
|---|---|---|---|---|---|---|---|---|
| | **O.D.** | **O.S.** | **O.D.** | **O.S.** | **O.D.** | **O.S.** | **O.D.** | **O.S.** |
| **Genotype (*MYO7A*)** | | | | | | | | |
| *Type of Mutation* | Biallelic | | Biallelic | | Homozygous | | Homozygous | |
| *Nucleotide Variation* | c.[1343+1G>A];[2837T>G] | | c.[1343+1G>A];[2837T>G] | | c.581_582del | | c.494C>T | |
| *Amino Acid Change* | p.[?];[Met946Arg] | | p.[?];[Met946Arg] | | p.Pro194Hisfs*13 | | p.Thr165Met | |
| *Novel or Recurrent* | Novel | | Novel | | Novel | | Recurrent | |
| **Frequency in Control Alleles** | 0/200 | | 0/200 | | 0/200 | | 0/200 | |
| **Accession Numbers in National Institutes of Health Sequence Read Archive** | | | | | | | | |
| *BioProject* | SRP040003 | | SRP040003 | | SRP040003 | | SRP040003 | |
| *BioSamples* | SRS579268 | | SRS579270 | | SRS569215 | | SRS579266 | |
| *Runs* | SRR1200449 | | SRR1200450 | | SRR1200411 | | SRR1200446 | |
| **Age (years)/Sex** | 24/M | | 22/M | | 50/F | | 60/F | |
| **Walking Age** | 12-month | | 12-month | | 20-month | | 24-month | |
| **Onset Age for Hearing Impairments** | since born | | since born | | since born | | since born | |
| **Onset Age for Visual Defects** | 15-year-old | | 13-year-old | | 7-year-old | | 6-year-old | |
| **BCVAs (logMAR)** | 0.8 | 0.8 | 0.6 | 0.7 | FC | FC | HM | HM |
| **IOP (mmHg)** | 14 | 13.8 | 13.2 | 14.5 | 14.5 | 18.5 | 17.5 | 16.5 |
| **Fundus Appearance** | | | | | | | | |
| *Macular Degeneration* | No | No | No | No | Yes | Yes | Yes | Yes |
| *Optic Disk* | Pale | Pale | Pale | Pale | Pale | Pale | Pale | Pale |
| *Artery Attenuation* | Yes | Yes | Yes | Yes | Yes | Yes | Yes | Yes |
| *Pigment Deposits* | Yes | Yes | Yes | Yes | Yes | Yes | Yes | Yes |
| **Visual Field** | TV | TV | TV | TV | NA | NA | NA | NA |
| **Electroretinography** | Diminished | Diminished | Diminished | Diminished | NA | NA | NA | NA |
| **Clinical Diagnosis** | USH type 2 | | USH type 2 | | USH type 1 | | USH type 1 | |

Abbreviations: USH: usher syndrome; O.D.: right eye; O.S.: left eye; SD: splice site mutation; M: male; F: female; BCVA: best-corrected visual acuities; FC: finger count; HM: hand move; IOP: intraocular pressure; TV: tubular vision; NA: not available.

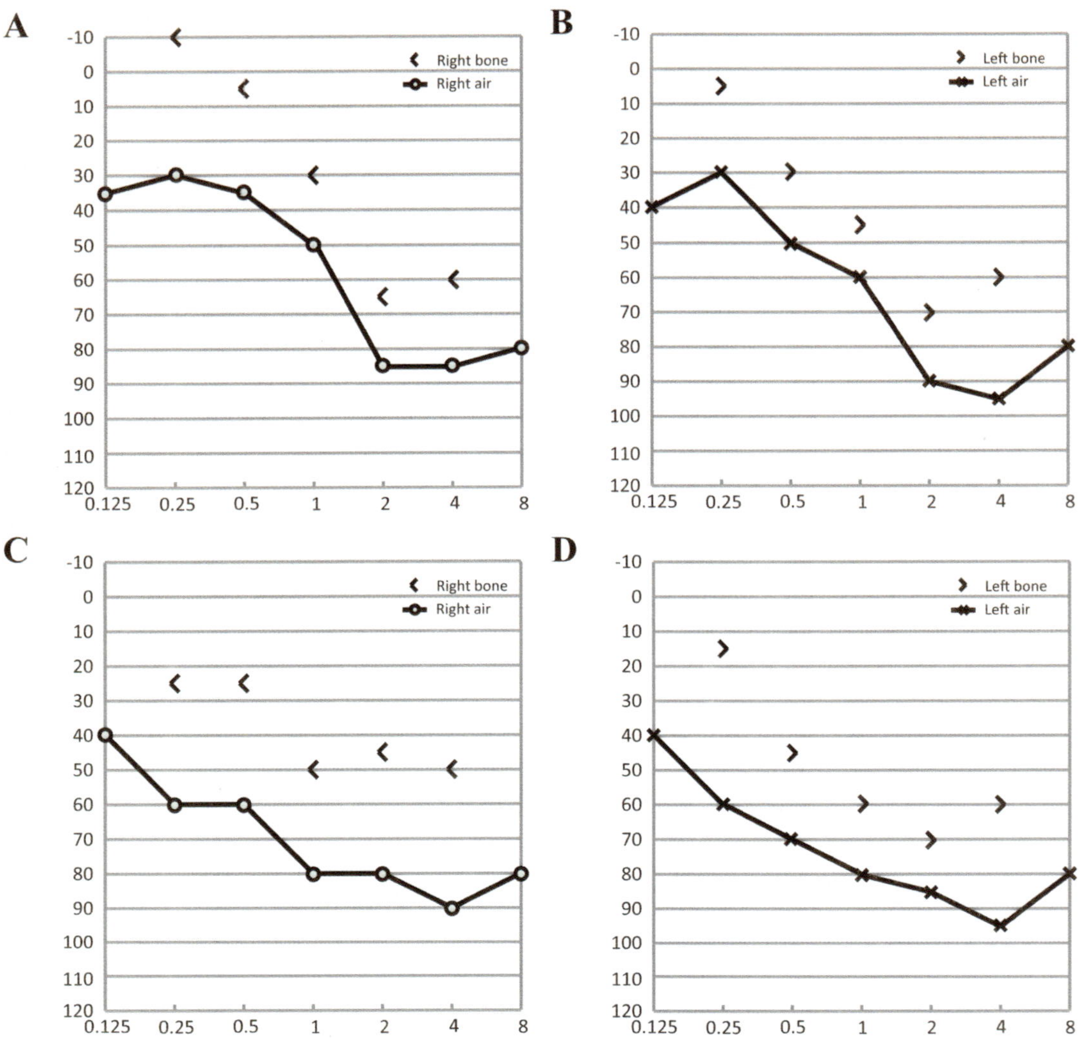


**Figure 2. Pure tone audiometry results of the two patients in family USH01.** (A–B) Pure tone audiometry results of patient USH01-III1 show moderate bilateral hearing impairments. (C–D) Moderate to severe bilateral sensorineural hearing loss is revealed in patient USH01-III2.

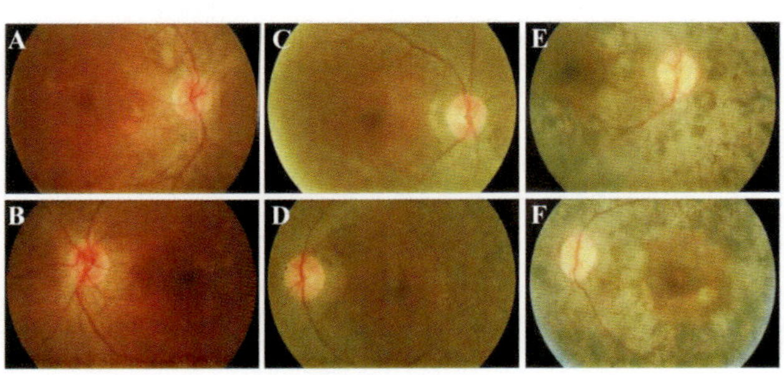


**Figure 3. Fundus photographs of the included patients.** (A–B) Fundus photographs of the 24-year-old proband of family USH01 reveal attenuation of retinal vessels, pallor of optic disc, and pigmentary migration, indicating an atypical RP fundus. Macular region is not affected in both eyes. (C–D) Fundus appearance of patient USH01-III2 (22-year-old) is similar to that of patient USH01-III1. Attenuated retinal vessels and pale optic disc are observed. Macular region is also preserved. (E–F) Typical RP fundus is shown by patient USH03-II1, including bone spicule-like pigmentation, retinal vascular attenuation, pallor of optic disk, and chorioretinal atrophy. Macular degeneration is observed in this patient.

[37]. Expressions of the myosin-VIIa protein in the cochlear hair cells, retinal photoreceptors, and retinal pigment epithelium (RPE) have been detected [38,39]. Although disagreements still exist regarding the subcellular localization of the myosin-VIIa protein, most studies support the association between the protein and the connecting cilium [40,41,42]. In rod photoreceptors, myosin-VIIa resides at the connecting cilium and functions in transporting rhodopsin to the rod outer segment (OS) discs [43,44]. In RPE, that protein localizes to the apical side [38,39], and deals with the proper localization of melanosomes to the RPE microvilli [45,46] and phagosome motility [47].

Since first identification in 1995, mutations in *MYO7A* gene have been reported to be implicated in causing a wide phenotypic spectrum, including USH type 1 [8], an atypical form of USH mimicking USH type 3 [34], two types of nonsyndromic deafness: autosomal dominant nonsyndromic deafness-11 (DFNA11) [48] and autosomal recessive nonsyndromic deafness-2 (DFNB2) [49,50], and even Leber congenital amaurosis [51]. Based on the great clinical and genetic heterogeneities, there has been hypothesis concerning the relationship between the localizations of the mutations and the diverse clinical phenotypes. The 2215 amino acids protein myosin-VIIa presents the following domains:

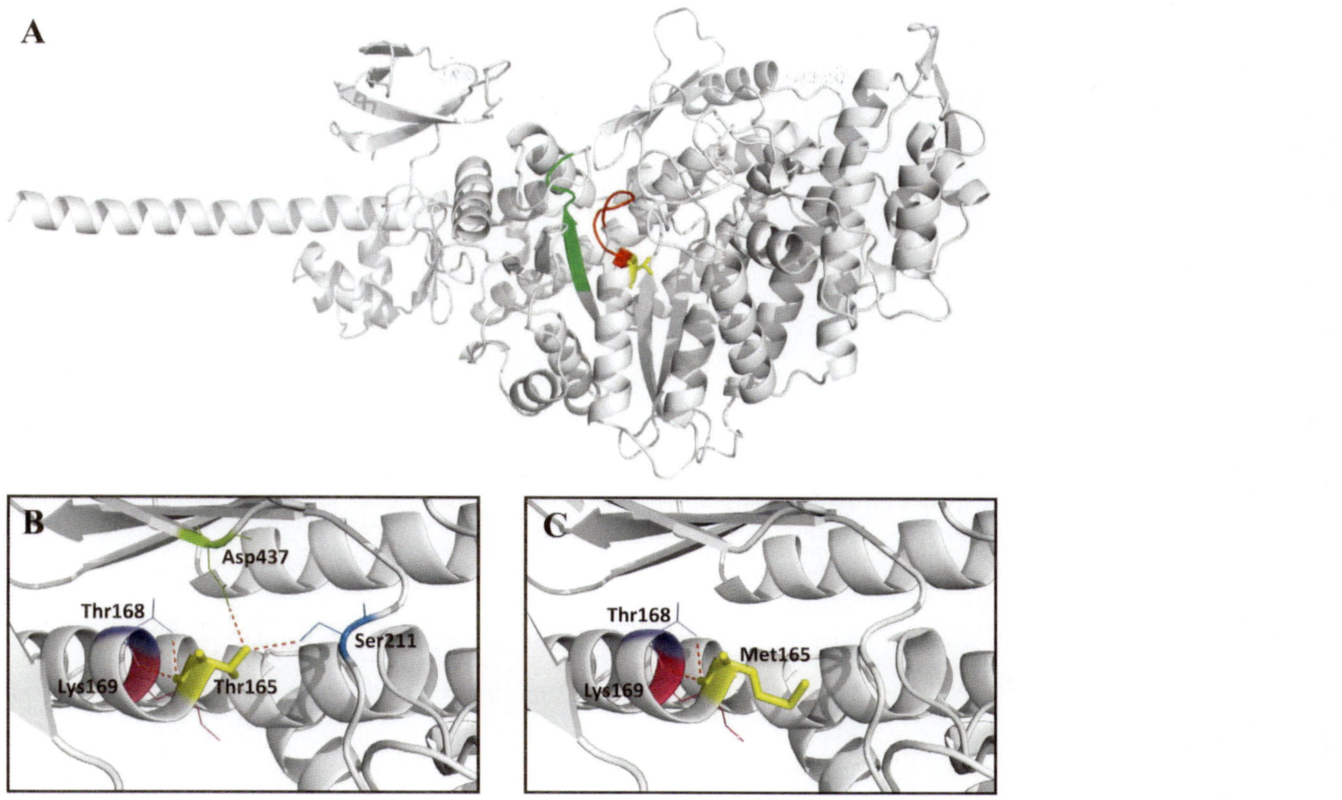


**Figure 4. Structural modeling of myosin-VIIa.** (A) Overview of the predicted structure of myosin-VIIa (3–769) covering the majority of the myosin head-like domain (1–729) and the first IQ motif (745–765). The ATP binding site (158–165) and the actin binding site (632–639) are included and are colored as red and green, respectively. The mutational spot identified in patient USH03-II:1 (Thr165) located in the ATP binding site is indicated in yellow. (B) A close view of the residue 165 highlighting the wide type amino acid threonine, the generated hydrogen bonds (in red), and their interacted amino acids, including Thr168, Lys169, Ser211, and Asp437. (C) Two previously indicated hydrogen bonds are eliminated due to the change of the wide type threonine into the mutant methionine.

a myosin head-like domain (1–729), which contains the crucial ATP-binding site (158–165) and actin-bind site (632–639), five IQ motifs (IQ1: 745–765, IQ2: 768–788, IQ3: 791–811, IQ4: 814–834, IQ5: 837–857), a coiled-coil region (858–935), two MyTH4 domains (1017–1253, and 1747–1896), two FERM domains (1258–1602, and 1902–2205), and an SH3 domain (1603–1672) [5].

Three of the four identified mutations are located within the myosin head-like domain. The recurrent missense mutation detected in patient USH03-II:1, p.Thr165Met, will lead to the amino acid change from the polar threonine to a nonpolar methionine. The Thr165 residue is located in the highly conserved ATP binding pocket region (161–165). Therefore, this mutation would obstruct the binding between the ATP and the protein, thus disturbing the motor function and preventing head movement. In addition, the mutational change from threonine to methionine would eliminate two hydrogen bonds. The two hydrogen bonds, which link an $\alpha$-helix with $\beta$-sheets according to the predicted crystal structure, are generally critical for the tertiary structure of the protein. Thus, the elimination of the two hydrogen bonds would potentially change the tertiary structure of the protein, and further disturb the internal interactions and reduce the stability of the protein. Noteworthy, one of the two eliminated hydrogen bonds was between resides Thr165 and Asp437, the latter of which has significance in the disease mechanism of Usher syndrome. For instance, the mutation p.Asp437N has previously been reported in patients with USH type 1 [52]. Residue Asp437 is located within the switch II loop of the myosin head-like domain, and is equivalent to residue Asp463 in chicken smooth muscle myosin and residue Asp454 in Dictyostelium. Residue Asp463 in chicken is recognized to form a hydrogen bond to the magnesium ion which coordinates the b- and g-phosphates of ATP [52,53], and a substitution in Dictyostelium, p.Asp454Ala, would abolish actin-activated Mg21ATPase activity thus inhibiting the myosin from moving actin filaments [52,54]. The p.Pro194Hisfs*13 identified in patient USH02-II:1 was also located within the myosin head-like domain. This novel frameshift variant would cause a PTC, and thus leading to nonsense mediated mRNA decay (NMD) [55] or the generation of a truncated protein containing 205 amino acids. However, the truncated proteins may not exist *in vivo* due to NMD.

The c.1343+1G>A affects a consensus donor splice site, which is essential for splicing of the intron 12. Similarly, multiple splice site mutations of the *MYO7A* gene have been reported previously [36,56,57], and two of those mutations were proved to alter the natural splicing through hybrid minigene assays [58]. In our case, in an attempt to understand the possible protein change resulted from c.1343+1G>A, we applied four online prediction software to evaluate the effect of c.1343+1G>A on splicing. As expected, all four programs similarly predicted that the DNA variant, c.1343+1G>A, would abolish the original splice donor site, resulting in the insertion of the beginning of intron 12 until a PTC, TAA, located at c.1343+50 to c.1343+52 in intron 12. Thus, the c.1343+1G>A allele is expected to lead to a NMD of the corresponding mRNA, which is not detectable by minigene assay, or, less likely, result into a truncated *MYO7A* proteins, p.Ser448Argfs*18.

Another mutation identified in patients USH01-III:1 and USH01-III:2 was a missense one, p.Met946Arg. That generates the amino acid change from the nonpolar methionine to an alkaline amino acid arginine at the highly conserved codon 946 between coiled coil region and the first MyTH4 domain. The two patients from family USH01 met the diagnostic criteria for USH type 2. The proband suffered from non-progressive moderate hearing impairments since childhood, while his younger brother had moderate to severe hearing loss and obstacles in communication. Ophthalmic examinations reveal RP phenotypes, including night blindness occurred in the 2$^{nd}$ generation, tubular vision, and RP fundus. The vestibular reflection of the two patients was normal. The Met946 residue avoids the important functional domains of myosin-VIIa, and that may help explain the atypical phenotypes. But that is not exclusive since previous reports have revealed mutations in near sites (p.Gly955Ser) in patients with USH type 1 [49].

Similar to our findings in the present study, previous study has also reported the identification of biallelic heterozygous *MYO7A* mutations, including p.Ala457Val and p.Lys269del, in a sporadic patient with USH type 2 [36]. Both residues Ala457 and Lys269 are located within the myosin head-like domain, and of note, the location of p.Ala457Val is quite close to that of mutation p.Ser448Argfs*18 identified in our study, which could possibly explain for the USH type 2 phenotypes they caused. USH type 2 are associated with three genes, namely *USH2A*, *GPR98*, and *DFNB31*, implying the potentially complicated genotype-phenotype correlations for USH type 2. Mutations in *USH2A* account for over 70% of cases affected with USH type 2. In particular, many patients carrying mutations in *USH2A* showed moderate to severe SNHL with no vestibular defects and progressive retinitis pigmentosa [15,59], all of which are very similar to the phenotypes observed in the present family USH01, and thus further confirm the clinical diagnosis of USH type 2 in this family. In addition, mutations in *USH2A* have been reported in causing nonsyndromic RP and nonsyndromic deafness [60], further indicating the clinical heterogeneity for USH causative mutations.

USH shows great clinical and genetic heterogeneities. Sometimes, it would be difficult for clinicians to make proper clinical diagnosis due to the atypical manifestations. Molecular diagnosis would definitely help with clinical diagnosis, and acts as the basis of prenatal testing and gene therapy. However, it would also be a huge job for mutation analysis using Sanger sequencing. At this point, our study proves that targeted gene approach is an efficient and economic tool in molecular diagnosis.

In conclusion, we here report biallelic novel heterozygous mutations in *MYO7A* gene leading to USH type 2 in a Chinese family. The genotype-phenotype correlation is discussed but the underlying mechanism needs further elucidations. Our study extends the spectrums of *MYO7A* mutations and its related clinical phenotypes. We also prove targeted gene approach as a valuable tool in molecular diagnosis.

## Supporting Information

**Table S1 Variants post filtration and primers used for mutation validation.**

**Table S2 Overview of data production.**

**Table S3 All variants in USH causative genes identified in the three families investigated.**

## Acknowledgments

We thank all patients and family members for their participation. We appreciate Liping Guan, Jingjing Xiao, and Jingjing Jiang from BGI-Shenzhen (Shenzhen, Guangdong, China) for technical support.

## Author Contributions

Conceived and designed the experiments: XS CZ KZ. Performed the experiments: WR XC YL XL SH WL. Analyzed the data: WR XC YL XL. Contributed reagents/materials/analysis tools: KZ XK. Wrote the paper: WR XC CZ.

## References

1. Friedman TB, Schultz JM, Ahmed ZM, Tsilou ET, Brewer CC (2011) Usher syndrome: hearing loss with vision loss. Adv Otorhinolaryngol 70: 56–65.
2. Boughman JA, Vernon M, Shaver KA (1983) Usher syndrome: definition and estimate of prevalence from two high-risk populations. J Chronic Dis 36: 595–603.
3. Yan D, Liu XZ (2010) Genetics and pathological mechanisms of Usher syndrome. J Hum Genet 55: 327–335.
4. Kimberling WJ, Hildebrand MS, Shearer AE, Jensen ML, Halder JA, et al. (2010) Frequency of Usher syndrome in two pediatric populations: Implications for genetic screening of deaf and hard of hearing children. Genet Med 12: 512–516.
5. Jaijo T, Aller E, Oltra S, Beneyto M, Najera C, et al. (2006) Mutation profile of the MYO7A gene in Spanish patients with Usher syndrome type I. Hum Mutat 27: 290–291.
6. Millan JM, Aller E, Jaijo T, Blanco-Kelly F, Gimenez-Pardo A, et al. (2011) An update on the genetics of usher syndrome. J Ophthalmol 2011: 417217.
7. Saihan Z, Webster AR, Luxon L, Bitner-Glindzicz M (2009) Update on Usher syndrome. Curr Opin Neurol 22: 19–27.
8. Weil D, Blanchard S, Kaplan J, Guilford P, Gibson F, et al. (1995) Defective myosin VIIA gene responsible for Usher syndrome type 1B. Nature 374: 60–61.
9. Hope CI, Bundey S, Proops D, Fielder AR (1997) Usher syndrome in the city of Birmingham–prevalence and clinical classification. Br J Ophthalmol 81: 46–53.
10. Bitner-Glindzicz M, Lindley KJ, Rutland P, Blaydon D, Smith VV, et al. (2000) A recessive contiguous gene deletion causing infantile hyperinsulinism, enteropathy and deafness identifies the Usher type 1C gene. Nat Genet 26: 56–60.
11. Bolz H, von Brederlow B, Ramirez A, Bryda EC, Kutsche K, et al. (2001) Mutation of CDH23, encoding a new member of the cadherin gene family, causes Usher syndrome type 1D. Nat Genet 27: 108–112.
12. Ahmed ZM, Riazuddin S, Bernstein SL, Ahmed Z, Khan S, et al. (2001) Mutations of the protocadherin gene PCDH15 cause Usher syndrome type 1F. Am J Hum Genet 69: 25–34.
13. Weil D, El-Amraoui A, Masmoudi S, Mustapha M, Kikkawa Y, et al. (2003) Usher syndrome type I G (USH1G) is caused by mutations in the gene encoding SANS, a protein that associates with the USH1C protein, harmonin. Hum Mol Genet 12: 463–471.
14. Riazuddin S, Belyantseva IA, Giese AP, Lee K, Indzhykulian AA, et al. (2012) Alterations of the CIB2 calcium- and integrin-binding protein cause Usher syndrome type 1J and nonsyndromic deafness DFNB48. Nat Genet 44: 1265–1271.
15. Eudy JD, Weston MD, Yao S, Hoover DM, Rehm HL, et al. (1998) Mutation of a gene encoding a protein with extracellular matrix motifs in Usher syndrome type IIa. Science 280: 1753–1757.
16. Weston MD, Luijendijk MW, Humphrey KD, Moller C, Kimberling WJ (2004) Mutations in the VLGR1 gene implicate G-protein signaling in the pathogenesis of Usher syndrome type II. Am J Hum Genet 74: 357–366.
17. Mburu P, Mustapha M, Varela A, Weil D, El-Amraoui A, et al. (2003) Defects in whirlin, a PDZ domain molecule involved in stereocilia elongation, cause deafness in the whirler mouse and families with DFNB31. Nat Genet 34: 421–428.
18. Joensuu T, Hamalainen R, Yuan B, Johnson C, Tegelberg S, et al. (2001) Mutations in a novel gene with transmembrane domains underlie Usher syndrome type 3. Am J Hum Genet 69: 673–684.
19. Schneider E, Marker T, Daser A, Frey-Mahn G, Beyer V, et al. (2009) Homozygous disruption of PDZD7 by reciprocal translocation in a consanguineous family: a new member of the Usher syndrome protein interactome causing congenital hearing impairment. Hum Mol Genet 18: 655–666.

20. Bharadwaj AK, Kasztejna JP, Huq S, Berson EL, Dryja TP (2000) Evaluation of the myosin VIIA gene and visual function in patients with Usher syndrome type I. Exp Eye Res 71: 173–181.
21. Ouyang XM, Yan D, Du LL, Hejtmancik JF, Jacobson SG, et al. (2005) Characterization of Usher syndrome type I gene mutations in an Usher syndrome patient population. Hum Genet 116: 292–299.
22. Roux AF, Faugere V, Le Guedard S, Pallares-Ruiz N, Vielle A, et al. (2006) Survey of the frequency of USH1 gene mutations in a cohort of Usher patients shows the importance of cadherin 23 and protocadherin 15 genes and establishes a detection rate of above 90%. J Med Genet 43: 763–768.
23. Oshima A, Jaijo T, Aller E, Millan JM, Carney C, et al. (2008) Mutation profile of the CDH23 gene in 56 probands with Usher syndrome type I. Hum Mutat 29: E37–46.
24. Pieke Dahl S, Kimberling WJ, Gorin MB, Weston MD, Furman JM, et al. (1993) Genetic heterogeneity of Usher syndrome type II. J Med Genet 30: 843–848.
25. Chen X, Zhao K, Sheng X, Li Y, Gao X, et al. (2013) Targeted sequencing of 179 genes associated with hereditary retinal dystrophies and 10 candidate genes identifies novel and known mutations in patients with various retinal diseases. Invest Ophthalmol Vis Sci 54: 2186–2197.
26. Chen X, Liu Y, Sheng X, Tam PO, Zhao K, et al. (2014) PRPF4 mutations cause autosomal dominant retinitis pigmentosa. Hum Mol Genet.
27. Zhang X, Lai TY, Chiang SW, Tam PO, Liu DT, et al. (2013) Contribution of SNRNP200 sequence variations to retinitis pigmentosa. Eye (Lond) 27: 1204–1213.
28. Li R, Yu C, Li Y, Lam TW, Yiu SM, et al. (2009) SOAP2: an improved ultrafast tool for short read alignment. Bioinformatics 25: 1966–1967.
29. Li H, Durbin R (2010) Fast and accurate long-read alignment with Burrows-Wheeler transform. Bioinformatics 26: 589–595.
30. Zhao C, Lu S, Zhou X, Zhang X, Zhao K, et al. (2006) A novel locus (RP33) for autosomal dominant retinitis pigmentosa mapping to chromosomal region 2cen-q12.1. Hum Genet 119: 617–623.
31. Adzhubei IA, Schmidt S, Peshkin L, Ramensky VE, Gerasimova A, et al. (2010) A method and server for predicting damaging missense mutations. Nat Methods 7: 248–249.
32. Arnold K, Bordoli L, Kopp J, Schwede T (2006) The SWISS-MODEL workspace: a web-based environment for protein structure homology modelling. Bioinformatics 22: 195–201.
33. Kiefer F, Arnold K, Kunzli M, Bordoli L, Schwede T (2009) The SWISS-MODEL Repository and associated resources. Nucleic Acids Res 37: D387–392.
34. Liu XZ, Hope C, Walsh J, Newton V, Ke XM, et al. (1998) Mutations in the myosin VIIA gene cause a wide phenotypic spectrum, including atypical Usher syndrome. Am J Hum Genet 63: 909–912.
35. Coureux PD, Sweeney HL, Houdusse A (2004) Three myosin V structures delineate essential features of chemo-mechanical transduction. EMBO J 23: 4527–4537.
36. Bonnet C, Grati M, Marlin S, Levilliers J, Hardelin JP, et al. (2011) Complete exon sequencing of all known Usher syndrome genes greatly improves molecular diagnosis. Orphanet J Rare Dis 6: 21.
37. Wolfrum U (2003) The cellular function of the usher gene product myosin VIIa is specified by its ligands. Adv Exp Med Biol 533: 133–142.
38. Hasson T, Heintzelman MB, Santos-Sacchi J, Corey DP, Mooseker MS (1995) Expression in cochlea and retina of myosin VIIa, the gene product defective in Usher syndrome type 1B. Proc Natl Acad Sci U S A 92: 9815–9819.
39. Gibbs D, Diemer T, Khanobdee K, Hu J, Bok D, et al. (2010) Function of MYO7A in the human RPE and the validity of shaker1 mice as a model for Usher syndrome 1B. Invest Ophthalmol Vis Sci 51: 1130–1135.
40. Liu X, Vansant G, Udovichenko IP, Wolfrum U, Williams DS (1997) Myosin VIIa, the product of the Usher 1B syndrome gene, is concentrated in the connecting cilia of photoreceptor cells. Cell Motil Cytoskeleton 37: 240–252.
41. Williams DS (2008) Usher syndrome: animal models, retinal function of Usher proteins, and prospects for gene therapy. Vision Res 48: 433–441.
42. Williams DS, Lopes VS (2011) The many different cellular functions of MYO7A in the retina. Biochem Soc Trans 39: 1207–1210.
43. Liu X, Udovichenko IP, Brown SD, Steel KP, Williams DS (1999) Myosin VIIa participates in opsin transport through the photoreceptor cilium. J Neurosci 19: 6267–6274.
44. Liu X, Williams DS (2001) Coincident onset of expression of myosin VIIa and opsin in the cilium of the developing photoreceptor cell. Exp Eye Res 72: 351–355.
45. Liu X, Ondek B, Williams DS (1998) Mutant myosin VIIa causes defective melanosome distribution in the RPE of shaker-1 mice. Nat Genet 19: 117–118.
46. Gibbs D, Azarian SM, Lillo C, Kitamoto J, Klomp AE, et al. (2004) Role of myosin VIIa and Rab27a in the motility and localization of RPE melanosomes. J Cell Sci 117: 6473–6483.
47. Gibbs D, Kitamoto J, Williams DS (2003) Abnormal phagocytosis by retinal pigmented epithelium that lacks myosin VIIa, the Usher syndrome 1B protein. Proc Natl Acad Sci U S A 100: 6481–6486.
48. Liu XZ, Walsh J, Tamagawa Y, Kitamura K, Nishizawa M, et al. (1997) Autosomal dominant non-syndromic deafness caused by a mutation in the myosin VIIA gene. Nat Genet 17: 268–269.
49. Liu XZ, Walsh J, Mburu P, Kendrick-Jones J, Cope MJ, et al. (1997) Mutations in the myosin VIIA gene cause non-syndromic recessive deafness. Nat Genet 16: 188–190.
50. Weil D, Kussel P, Blanchard S, Levy G, Levi-Acobas F, et al. (1997) The autosomal recessive isolated deafness, DFNB2, and the Usher 1B syndrome are allelic defects of the myosin-VIIA gene. Nat Genet 16: 191–193.
51. Wang X, Wang H, Cao M, Li Z, Chen X, et al. (2011) Whole-exome sequencing identifies ALMS1, IQCB1, CNGA3, and MYO7A mutations in patients with Leber congenital amaurosis. Hum Mutat 32: 1450–1459.
52. Riazuddin S, Nazli S, Ahmed ZM, Yang Y, Zulfiqar F, et al. (2008) Mutation spectrum of MYO7A and evaluation of a novel nonsyndromic deafness DFNB2 allele with residual function. Hum Mutat 29: 502–511.
53. Dominguez R, Freyzon Y, Trybus KM, Cohen C (1998) Crystal structure of a vertebrate smooth muscle myosin motor domain and its complex with the essential light chain: visualization of the pre-power stroke state. Cell 94: 559–571.
54. Kambara T, Rhodes TE, Ikebe R, Yamada M, White HD, et al. (1999) Functional significance of the conserved residues in the flexible hinge region of the myosin motor domain. J Biol Chem 274: 16400–16406.
55. Rio Frio T, Wade NM, Ransijn A, Berson EL, Beckmann JS, et al. (2008) Premature termination codons in PRPF31 cause retinitis pigmentosa via haploinsufficiency due to nonsense-mediated mRNA decay. J Clin Invest 118: 1519–1531.
56. Liu F, Li P, Liu Y, Li W, Wong F, et al. (2013) Novel compound heterozygous mutations in MYO7A in a Chinese family with Usher syndrome type 1. Mol Vis 19: 695–701.
57. Yoshimura H, Iwasaki S, Nishio SY, Kumakawa K, Tono T, et al. (2014) Massively parallel DNA sequencing facilitates diagnosis of patients with usher syndrome type 1. PLoS One 9: e90688.
58. Jaijo T, Aller E, Aparisi MJ, Garcia-Garcia G, Hernan I, et al. (2011) Functional analysis of splicing mutations in MYO7A and USH2A genes. Clin Genet 79: 282–288.
59. Yan D, Ouyang X, Patterson DM, Du LL, Jacobson SG, et al. (2009) Mutation analysis in the long isoform of USH2A in American patients with Usher Syndrome type II. J Hum Genet 54: 732–738.
60. Aller E, Jaijo T, Beneyto M, Najera C, Oltra S, et al. (2006) Identification of 14 novel mutations in the long isoform of USH2A in Spanish patients with Usher syndrome type II. J Med Genet 43: e55.

6

# A Lack of Immune System Genes Causes Loss in High Frequency Hearing but Does Not Disrupt Cochlear Synapse Maturation in Mice

**Melissa A. Calton[1], Dasom Lee[1], Srividya Sundaresan[1], Diana Mendus[1], Rose Leu[1], Felix Wangsawihardja[1], Kenneth R. Johnson[2], Mirna Mustapha[1]***

**1** Department of Otolaryngology-Head & Neck Surgery, Stanford University, Stanford, California, United States of America, **2** The Jackson Laboratory, Bar Harbor, Maine, United States of America

## Abstract

Early cochlear development is marked by an exuberant outgrowth of neurites that innervate multiple targets. The establishment of mature cochlear neural circuits is, however, dependent on the pruning of inappropriate axons and synaptic connections. Such refinement also occurs in the central nervous system (CNS), and recently, genes ordinarily associated with immune and inflammatory processes have been shown to play roles in synaptic pruning in the brain. These molecules include the major histocompatibility complex class I (MHCI) genes, *H2-K^b^* and *H2-D^b^*, and the complement cascade gene, *C1qa*. Since the mechanisms involved in synaptic refinement in the cochlea are not well understood, we investigated whether these immune system genes may be involved in this process and whether they are required for normal hearing function. Here we report that these genes are not necessary for normal synapse formation and refinement in the mouse cochlea. We further demonstrate that *C1qa* expression is not necessary for normal hearing in mice but the lack of expression of *H2-K^b^* and *H2-D^b^* causes hearing impairment. These data underscore the importance of the highly polymorphic family of MHCI genes in hearing in mice and also suggest that factors and mechanisms regulating synaptic refinement in the cochlea may be distinct from those in the CNS.

**Editor:** Olivia Bermingham-McDonogh, University of Washington, Institute for Stem Cells and Regenerative Medicine, United States of America

**Funding:** This work was supported by research and core grants from the National Institute in Deafness and other Communicative Disorders: R01 DC09590 (Dr. Mirna Mustapha), P30 DC010363 (Dr. Stefan Heller, Stanford University), R01 DC004301 (Dr. Kenneth R. Johnson, Jackson Laboratory) and by a Stanford Medical School Dean's Postdoctoral Fellowship (awarded to Melissa A. Calton). The funders had no role in study design, data collection and analysis, decision to publish, or preparation of the manuscript.

**Competing Interests:** The authors have declared that no competing interests exist.

* E-mail: mirnam@stanford.edu

## Introduction

In the sensory epithelium of organ of Corti, information about the timing, frequency and intensity of sounds is transmitted from and to the hair cells via highly organized synapses. While early brain development is characterized by an overabundant outgrowth of axons and dendrites that make connections with numerous targets, the formation of mature neural circuits requires activity-dependent axonal pruning and elimination of unnecessary axons and synapses. Similar synaptic refinement occurs in the cochlea as the murine organ of Corti matures into a fully functioning organ during the first two postnatal weeks.

The mature organ of Corti contains two types of sensory cells known as inner (IHC) and outer hair cells (OHCs) that are innervated by the spiral ganglion neurons (SGNs). The IHCs are considered the primary sensory cells responsible for transmitting neural signals via the afferent nerve, whereas the OHCs are responsible for signal amplification by virtue of their motor activity, which modulates IHC function [1–6]. Adult IHCs are innervated by 90% to 95% of type I SGNs, or SGI. About 15 to 20 unbranched myelinated SGIs connect with a single IHC while each neuron receives input from only one IHC [7,8]. The remaining 5 to 10% of SGNs are type II unmyelinated neurons, SGII, that project toward OHC and spiral toward the base to contact multiple OHC [8–12]. At birth, SGI project branched neurites that innervate several targets including IHCs and OHCs. OHCs are mainly innervated with afferent fibers at birth. The mature connectivity in the organ of Corti is established by pruning of inappropriate connections including the retraction of SGI branches and the death of excess SGII. Several growth factors and guidance cues such as neurotrophins and ephrins are involved in spiral ganglion outgrowth, attraction, and repulsion. Although these factors have been identified, the specific molecular cues necessary for afferent/efferent cochlear fiber refinement remain poorly understood and warrant further investigation.

Recently, genes ordinarily associated with immune and inflammatory processes have been shown to have roles in synaptic refinement, including the MHCI (major histocompatibility complex class 1) and *C1qa*, a member of the classical complement cascade. MHCI is a large and highly polymorphic family of over 50 genes. Down-regulation of MHCI was shown to prevent retinal refinement in a screen to identify factors involved in synapse pruning in the visual system, indicating a role for this protein in these processes [13]. Beta-2 microglobulin (*β2M*) gene expression is necessary for MHCI proteins to display on the cell surface and mice lacking the *β2M* gene retain immature patterns of innervation in the brain [13]. In the retina and cerebral Purkinje cells, MHCI proteins have been found at excitatory and inhibitory synapses [14,15]. Furthermore, a knockdown of the mouse MHCI genes *H2-K^b^* and *H2-D^b^* resulted in a dramatic increase of synapse number in the cerebellum, indicating a role in synaptic plasticity [14].

C1qa is a soluble, secreted protein, and is the initiating protein in the classical complement cascade that binds to foreign material marked for phagocytosis and clearance during an immune response. In the postnatal brain, C1qa is expressed by astrocyte-stimulated neurons [16]. Mice deficient in *C1qa* exhibit large sustained defects in CNS synapse elimination in the retina and in the cerebral cortex [16,17]. The function of *C1qa* in the CNS seems to be similar to its role in the immune systems, clearing cellular material marked for destruction [16]. Furthermore, a reactivation of *C1qa* expression in the brain has been associated with neuronal degenerative diseases. C1qa protein increases with aging in mouse and human brains in regions associated with neurodegenerative disease, whereas *C1qa*-deficient mice have less cognitive and memory loss [18].

A recent study found that MHCI genes $H2\text{-}K^b$ and $H2\text{-}D^b$ as well as *C1qa* are upregulated during the period of cochlear functional development [19]. In this study, we examined whether these genes play a role in synaptic maturation of the neonatal mouse cochlea.

## Materials and Methods

### Mice

All experiments were completed with national animal care guidelines and were approved by the Stanford University Administrative Panel on Laboratory Animal Care; APLAC 23001.

$H2\text{-}K^bD^{b-/-}$ double knockout mice on a C57BL/6 genetic background were obtained from Dr. Carla Shatz (Stanford) [15,20] and maintained as a homozygous breeding colony because both the targeted loci are now on the same chromosome [21]. C57BL/6 controls were purchased from The Jackson Laboratory (Bar Harbor, Maine) and were bred and maintained in our facility. *C1qa* knockout mice (hereafter referred to as $C1qa^{-/-}$) on C57BL/6 background were generously provided by Drs. Ben Barres and Marina Botto [22] and littermates were used as controls. Congenic $D2.B6\text{-}C1qa^{+/+}$, $D2.B6\text{-}C1qa^{+/-}$, and $D2.B6\text{-}C1qa^{-/-}$ mice were established by an intercross of $DBA/2J\text{-}C1qa^{+/+}$ and $D2.B6\text{-}C1qa^{-/-}$ F1 hybrids resulting in the F2 progeny with $C1qa^{+/+}$, $C1qa^{+/-}$, and $C1qa^{-/-}$ genotypes all on a DBA/2J background [23]. The study was carried out in strict accordance with recommendations in the Guide for the Care and Use of Laboratory Animals of the National Institutes of Health. All experiments were conducted under guidelines of the Stanford University Administrative Panel on Laboratory Animal Care. All hearing tests were performed under anesthesia, and all efforts were made to minimize suffering.

### Auditory Brainstem Responses (ABR)

ABR recordings were performed at the Auditory Core for Department of Otolaryngology, Stanford University. The presentation of stimuli, ABR acquisition, equipment control and data management were coordinated using the computerized Intelligent Hearing System (IHS; Miami, FL). Three needle electrodes were placed under the skin and animal body temperature was maintained at 37°C. Clicks and 8- 16- and 32-kHz tone-bursts were channeled through plastic tubes into the animal's ear canals. Sound levels were incremented in 5 dB steps from 10–20 dB below threshold to 80 dB (for 8 and 16 kHz) or 100 dB (for 32 kHz). Threshold for ABR was defined as the lowest stimulus level at which repetitive waves I and V could be identified in the response waveform. The amplitude analysis was done by peak-to-peak measurement of the ABR waveform and latency was

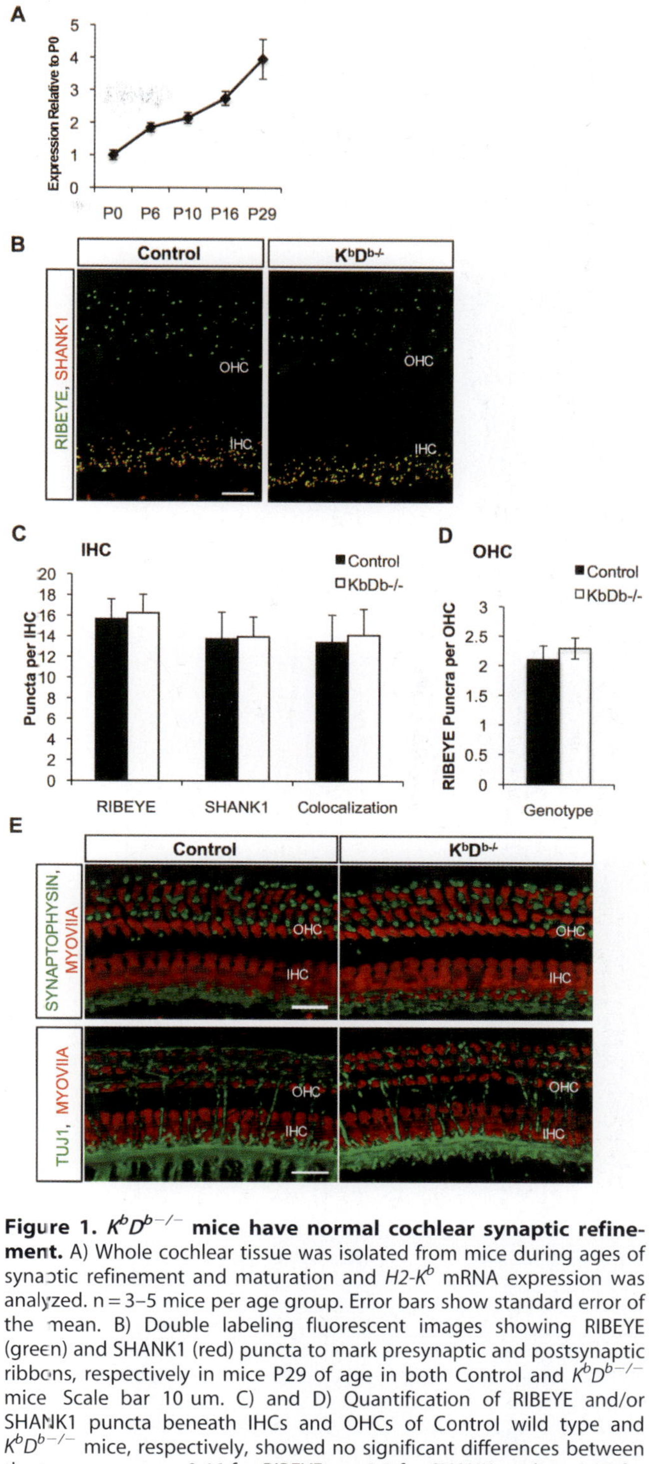


**Figure 1. $K^bD^{b-/-}$ mice have normal cochlear synaptic refinement.** A) Whole cochlear tissue was isolated from mice during ages of synaptic refinement and maturation and $H2\text{-}K^b$ mRNA expression was analyzed. n = 3–5 mice per age group. Error bars show standard error of the mean. B) Double labeling fluorescent images showing RIBEYE (green) and SHANK1 (red) puncta to mark presynaptic and postsynaptic ribbons, respectively in mice P29 of age in both Control and $K^bD^{b-/-}$ mice Scale bar 10 um. C) and D) Quantification of RIBEYE and/or SHANK1 puncta beneath IHCs and OHCs of Control wild type and $K^bD^{b-/-}$ mice, respectively, showed no significant differences between the two groups. $p = 0.46$ for RIBEYE, $p = 0.9$ for SHANK, and $p = 0.70$ for colocalized synaptic puncta in IHCs and $p = 0.06$ for RIBEYE in OHCs). E) Double labeling fluorescent images showing SYNAPTOPHYSIN (green) to mark efferent synapses or TUJ1 (green) for efferent and afferent fibers and MYOVIIa (red) to mark IHCs and OHCs in Control and $K^bD^{b-/-}$ mice at P29 of age. Scale bar 10 um.

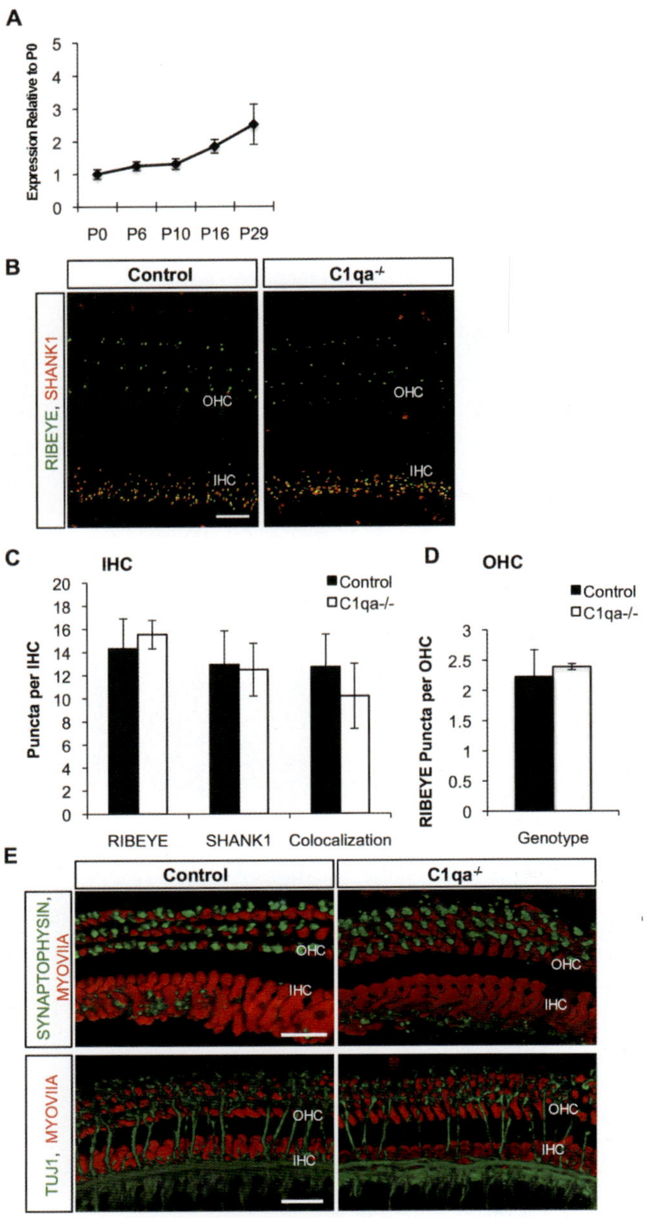


**Figure 2. *C1qa*$^{-/-}$ mice have no alteration in synaptic refinement.** A) Whole cochlea tissue was isolated from mice during ages of synaptic refinement and maturation and *C1qa* mRNA expression was analyzed. n = 3–5 mice per age group. Error bars show standard error of the mean. B) Double labeling fluorescent images showing RIBEYE (green) and SHANK1 (red) puncta to mark presynaptic and postsynaptic ribbons, respectively in mice P29 of age in both Control and *C1qa*$^{-/-}$ mice. Scale bar 10 um. C) and D) Quantification of RIBEYE and/or SHANK1 puncta beneath IHCs and OHCs of Control wild type and *C1qa*$^{-/-}$ mice, respectively, showed no significant differences between the two groups. $p = 0.27$ for RIBEYE, $p = 0.8$ for SHANK, and $p = 0.22$ for colocalized synaptic puncta in IHCs and $p = 0.517$ for RIBEYE in OHCs. E) Double labeling fluorescent images showing SYNPATOPHYSIN (green) to mark efferent synapses or TUJ1 (green) for efferent and afferent fibers and MYOVIIa (red) to mark IHCs and OHCs in Control and *C1qa*$^{-/-}$ mice at P29 of age. Scale bar 10 um.

calculated as time delay from the onset of the stimulus (0 ms) until the occurrence of the ABR response peak. ABR waveform amplitude and latency analysis was performed at the 16 kHz frequency at 40 dB.

## Distortion-Product Otoacoustic Emission (DPOAE)

To test the function of outer hair cells we measured DPOAEs as previously described [24], using the computerized National Hearing Instruments conducted in a sound-attenuating room at the Auditory Core for Department of Otolaryngology, Stanford University. DPOAE thresholds were calculated by interpolating the data and identifying when the signal was $> -5$ dB SPL and greater than two standard deviations above the noise floor. If no DPOAE response was detected even at our equipment limits of 80 dB SPL, we arbitrarily defined the threshold to be 80 dB.

## Immunofluorescence

The cochleae were dissected and perfused with 4% paraformaldehyde in PBS and were left in fixative solution for an additional 10 minutes in case of RIBEYE and SHANK1 staining, or for 1 h in case of staining for MYOVIIa, TUJ1, SYNAPTOPHYSIN, or PRESTIN. Samples were washed in PBS for 10 minutes and then blocked in 0.5% Triton X-100 plus 5% bovine serum albumin in PBS for 30 minutes at room temperature. Same blocking buffer was used for diluting antibodies. Primary antibodies were incubated at 4°C for 36 hours with light shaking on orbital shaker followed by three washes in 0.1% PBS-Tween with a final wash in PBS. Secondary antibodies were added for 1 hour at room temperature, followed by three washes in 0.1% PBS-Tween and PBS. The following antibodies were used primary - goat anti-CtBP2 (1:200, Santa Cruz Biotechnology), rabbit anti-SHANK1 (1:200, Neuromics), rabbit anti-MYOVIIa (1:300, Proteus), mouse anti-TUJ1 (1:200, Neuromics), anti-SYNAPTOPHYSIN (1:200, Synaptic System), anti-PRESTIN (1:300, clone N-20, Santa Cruz Biotechnology), and secondary – Alexa flour 488-conjugated anti-goat, Alexa flour 546-conjugated anti-rabbit, Alexa flour 488-conjugated anti-mouse (1:500, Invitrogen). Cochleae were decalcified and in case of RIBEYE and SHANK1 markers further fixed in 4% paraformaldehyde in PBS for 15 minutes. Cochleae were washed in PBS and dissected into 2–3 pieces and mounted on microscopic slides in ProLong (Invitrogen) anti-fading media.

## Confocal Analysis of Synapse and Fiber Number

Images were collected on a Zeiss AxioVert confocal inverted microscope. For RIBEYE or SHANK1 analysis, cochlear frequency map [25] was estimated for every sample in order to localize hair cells from different frequency regions. Cochlear z-stacks from a selected frequency region were taken for each sample. Each stack contained the entire synaptic pole of 15–20 inner hair cells. Synapses were automatically counted through a series of optical sections using the Volocity 3D Image Analysis Software. The number of fibers crossing the tunnel of Corti was counted by hand per 500 um area using Z-stack images using Volocity 3D Image Analysis Software.

## RNA Extraction and Quantitative RT-PCR (qPCR)

RNA was extracted from whole cochlea dissected from wildtype mice at the postnatal day(s): P0 (n = 5), P6 (n = 3), P10 (n = 4), P15 (n = 3) and P29 (n = 4) using an Ambion RNAqueous Micro Kit (Thermo Fisher Scientific Inc., Waltham, MA) according to the protocol of the manufacturer. Extracted RNA was converted to cDNA using a High Capacity RNA to cDNA kit from Applied Biosystems (Foster City, CA). cDNA was further used in PCR assays with Taqman (Applied Biosystems) proprietary probes and primers for *C1qa* (assay ID Mm00432142_m1) and *H2-K1* (assay ID Mm01612247_m1). *GAPDH* (assay ID Mm99999915_g1) was used as the internal standard. All Taqman qPCR assays were

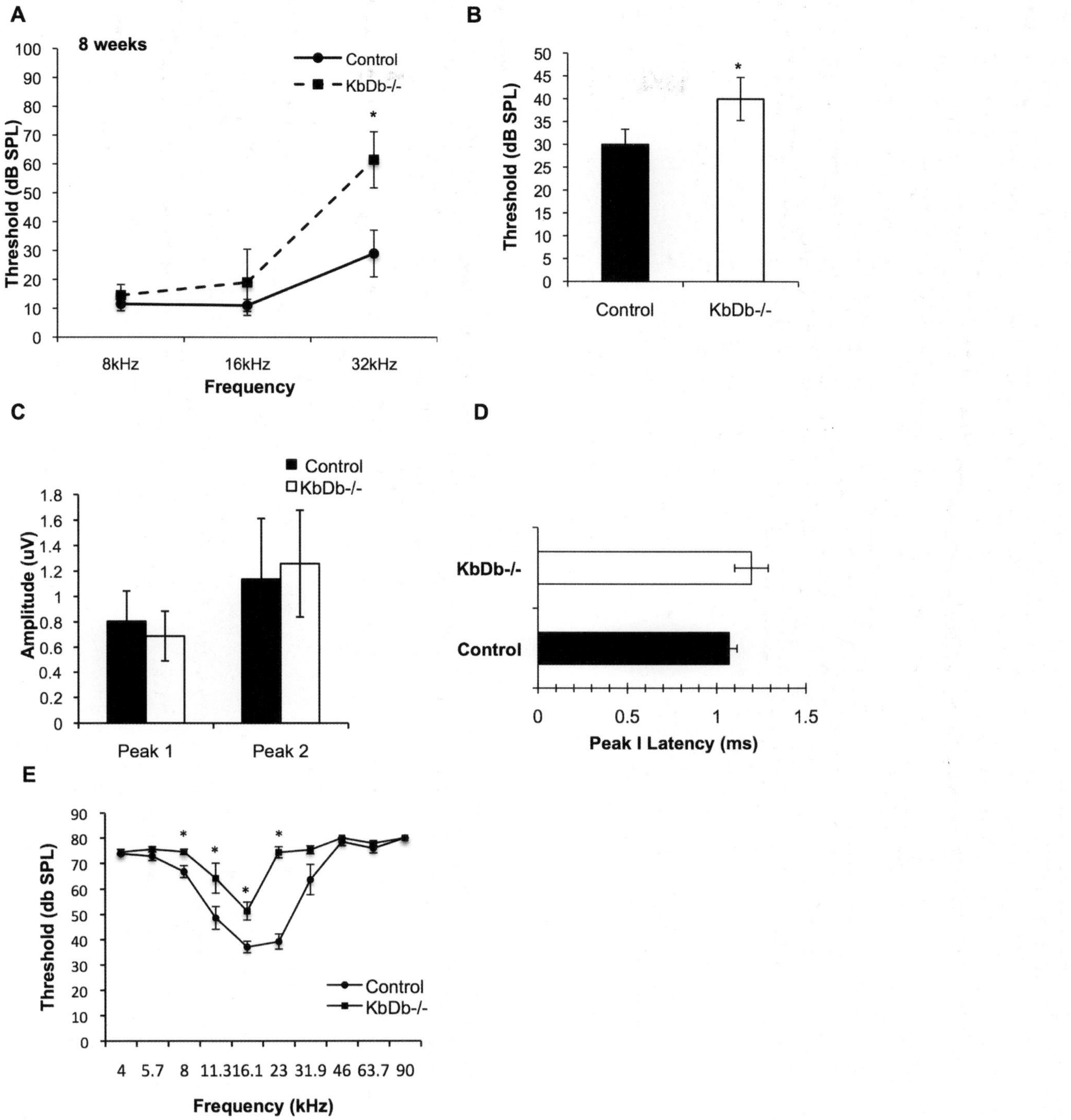


**Figure 3. ABR and DPOAE thresholds are increased in $K^bD^{b-/-}$ mice.** Average ABR (A–B) and DPOAE (E) thresholds are shown for mice at 8-weeks of age. Significantly increased ABR thresholds were recorded in $K^bD^{b-/-}$ mice with pure-tone 32 kHz stimuli (A) and with broad-band clicks (B). $^*p = 2.5E\text{-}07$ and $p = 0.0001$ for 32 kHz and broad-band clicks, respectively. ABR waveform amplitude of peaks 1 and 2 (C) and latency analysis of peak 1 (D) measured at the 16 kHz frequency stimulus and at 40 dB demonstrated no significant differences between Control and $K^bD^{b-/-}$ cohorts. $p = 0.44$, $p = 0.67$ and $p = 0.57$ for peak 1 and peak 2 amplitudes and peak 1 latency, respectively. Increased DPOAE thresholds were recorded at 8, 11.3, 16.1, and 23 kHz frequencies (E). n = 10 (Control) and 9 ($K^bD^{b-/-}$) mice per group. $^*p = 0.007$, $p = 0.04$, $p = 0.003$ and $p = 1.25E\text{-}07$ for 8, 11.3, 16 and 23 kHz, respectively. Error bars show SDs in (A), (B), (C), (D), and SEMs in (E). $^*p < 0.05$ for (E).

performed on a BIO-RAD CFX96™ Real-Time System (Bio-Rad, Hercules, CA) with accompanying software for data analysis. Expression of the gene of interest was normalized with respect to the internal standard, *GAPDH*. Expression levels at various ages tested are shown relative to expression at P0. Error bars represent standard error of the mean (SEM).

## Statistical Analysis

Analysis of variance (ANOVA) was performed to determine significant differences between control and test groups. Following the ANOVA, planned comparisons were performed using two-tailed Student's t-test. Values represent mean ± SEM, standard

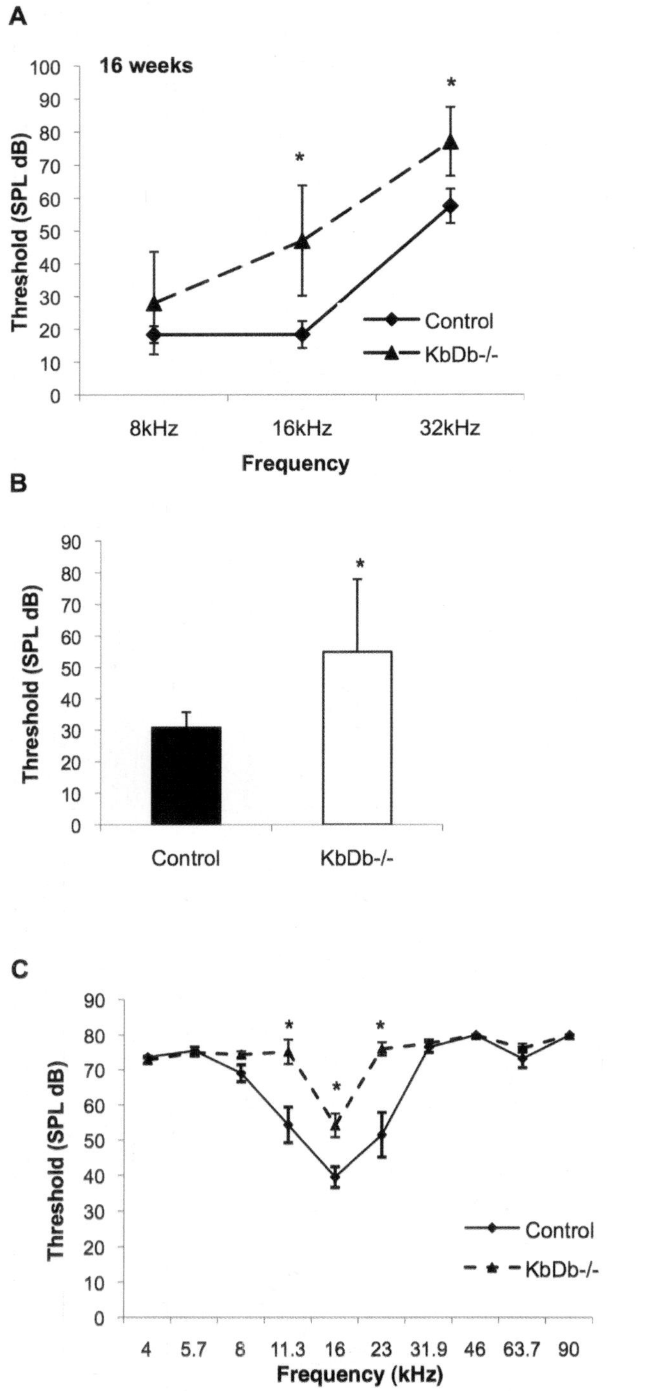


**Figure 4. Average ABR and DPOAE thresholds continue to elevate with age in $K^bD^{b-/-}$ mice.** Average ABR (A–B) and DPOAE (C) thresholds are shown for mice at 16-weeks of age. Significantly increased ABR thresholds were recorded in $K^bD^{b-/-}$ mice with pure-tone 16, and 32 kHz stimuli (A) and with broad-band clicks (B). $^*p = 0.017$, $p = 0.001$ and $p = 0.032$ for 16 kHz, 32 kHz and broad-band clicks, respectively. Increased DPOAE thresholds were recorded at 11.3, 16, and 23 kHz frequencies. $^*p = 0.006$, $p = 0.005$ and $p = 0.005$ for 11.3, 16 and 23 kHz, respectively. n = 6 (Control) and 5 ($K^bD^{b-/-}$) mice per group (C). Error bars show SDs in (A), (B) and SEMs in (C).

error of the mean, or ±SD, standard deviation, as specified in figure legends. Statistical analyses were conducted with SSPS software (IBM, Dublin, Ireland), Microsoft Excel (Microsoft Corp., Redmond, WA) or with Prism 6 (GraphPad Software Inc., La Jolla, CA). $p<0.05$ was considered to be statistically significant.

## Results

### Cochlear Afferent Synaptic Refinement is not Altered in *H2-K^bd^b* Double Knockout Mice

The age of onset of hearing in mice is around postnatal day 12 (P12), with synaptic refinement and functional maturation occurring during the first two postnatal weeks. Recent data demonstrates that $H2\text{-}K^b$ and $H2\text{-}D^b$ mRNAs are upregulated in the spiral ganglion at known times of synaptic refinement [19]. Our qPCR studies demonstrate that whole cochlear $H2\text{-}K^b$ mRNA expression increases from P0 to P29, as well as between P0 and P10 during the ages of synaptic refinement and maturation (Figure 1A). Because the knockdown of MHCI expression on the membrane of neurons results in a dramatic increase in synapse number in the cerebellum [14] we sought to determine if $K^bD^{b-/-}$ double knockout mice have immature cochlear synaptic morphology, or delays in refinement. We therefore analyzed afferent and efferent fiber and synaptic patterning at P15 (data not shown) and at P29. We focused on the 16 kHz area of the cochlea, which has the highest afferent synaptic density and hearing sensitivity in mice [26,27]. Pre- and post- synaptic puncta in the hair cells were visualized with immunostaining for afferent synapse markers RIBEYE/CtBP2 (presynaptic) and SHANK1 (postsynaptic). Quantification of pre- and post-synaptic puncta in both IHCs, displaying many afferent synapses, and OHCs, which have much less afferent synapses at P29 than IHCs, demonstrated no significant difference between $K^bD^{b-/-}$ and control mice (Figure 1B–D). In addition, we observed no significant difference in the colocalization of RIBEYE and SHANK1 in IHCs of control and $K^bD^{b-/-}$ animals: 15.7±1.9 RIBEYE puncta per IHC, 13.8±2.6 SHANK1 puncta per IHC (with 13.4±2.7 puncta colocalized) and 16.3±1.8 RIBEYE puncta per IHC, 14.0±1.9 SHANK1 puncta per IHC (with 14.1±2.6 puncta colocalized), respectively, which are expected values in an adult animal undergoing normal synaptic refinement [28]. SHANK1 immunofluorescence was absent in the OHCs at P29 in either group, which is consistent with the mature synaptic patterning. Consistently, there was no difference in RIBEYE staining in the OHCs between the $K^bD^{b-/-}$ and control adult mice (2.1±0.23 puncta per OHC cell vs. 2.3±0.20 puncta per OHC; respectively). Further, SYNAPTOPHYSIN staining for efferent synapses was not altered in $K^bD^{b-/-}$ mice in patterning or localization on the basal part of OHCs, suggesting proper efferent synapse formation (Figure 1E, Figure S1 in File S1). If proper refinement of the synapses in the OHCs did not occur, we would expect more fibers crossing the tunnel of Corti and innervating the OHCs. TUJ1 immunostaining for efferent and afferent fibers' synapses indicated that innervation patterns were grossly normal in mutants compared to controls (Figure 1E). The data presented above suggest that the number and structure of efferent and afferent fibers and synapses are comparable in the $K^bD^{b-/-}$ mice and controls.

### *C1qa*$^{-/-}$ Mice do not Have a Disruption in Cochlear Synaptic Refinement

qRT-PCR demonstrated that *C1qa* mRNA expression in the normal mouse cochlea increased in the first two postnatal weeks and continued to increase past this age (Figure 2A). Because *C1qa*$^{-/-}$ mice exhibit large sustained defects in CNS synapse elimination in the retina and in the cerebral cortex, we quantitatively and qualitatively analyzed cochlear synapses at

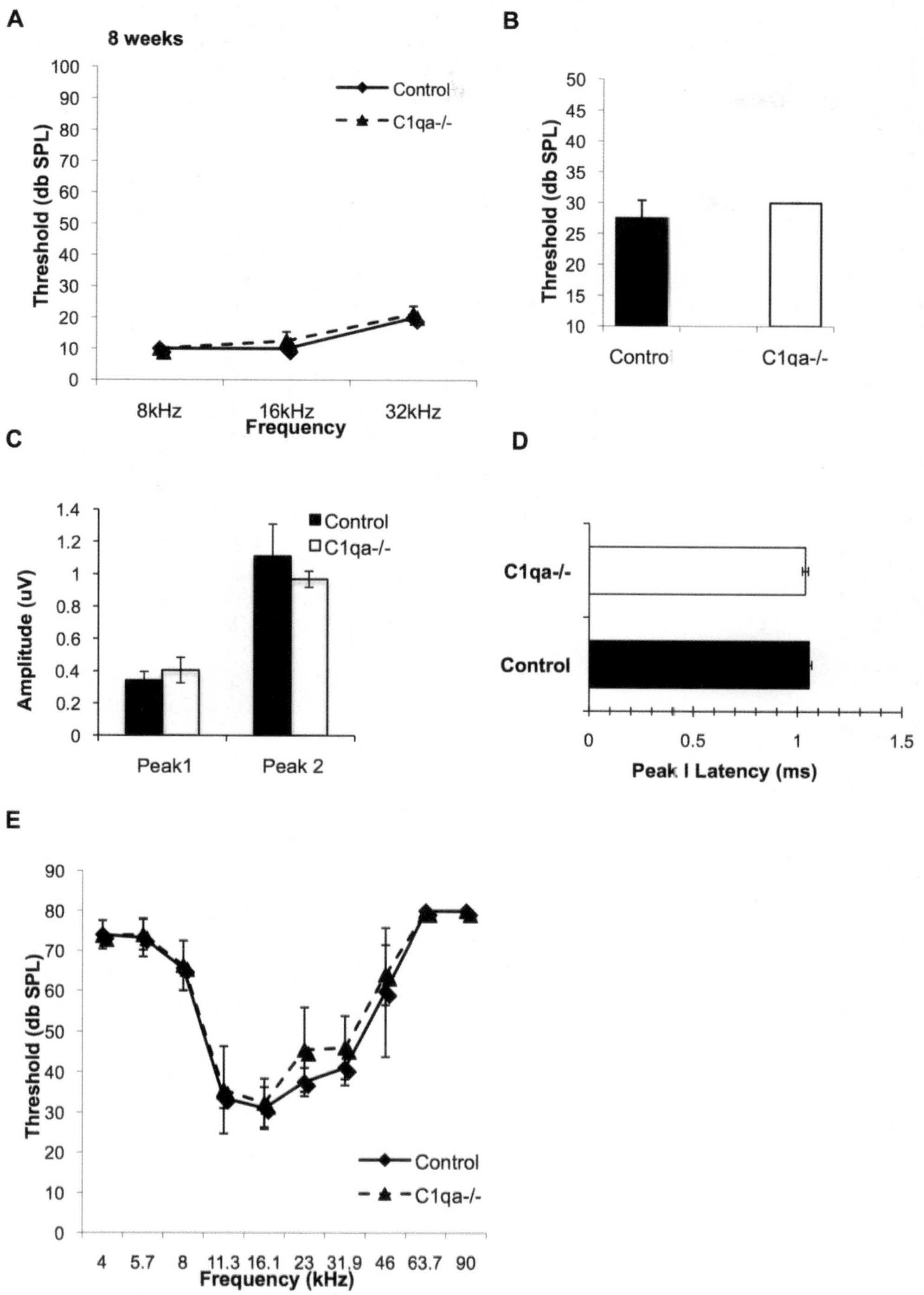


**Figure 5. ABR and DPOAE thresholds are not altered in** ***C1qa***$^{-/-}$ **mice.** Average ABR (A–B) and DPOAE (D) thresholds are shown for mice at 8-weeks of age. Student's t-test did not reveal significant differences in ABR thresholds that were recorded in *C1qa*$^{-/-}$ mice with pure-tone 8, 16, and 32 kHz stimuli (A) or broad-band clicks (B) compared to controls. ABR waveform amplitude of peaks 1 and 2 (C) and latency analysis of peak 1 (D) measured at the 16 kHz frequency stimulus and at 40 dB demonstrated no significant differences between Control and *C1qa*$^{-/-}$ cohorts. There were no differences in DPOAE thresholds at any frequency tested between the cohorts (E). $p>0.05$ for all comparisons. n = 4 mice per group. Error bars show SDs.

P29 in order to detect differences in the mutants with respect to wild type controls. Quantification of pre- and post-synaptic puncta beneath the IHCs, with markers RIBEYE and SHANK1 respectively, did not show significant differences between *C1qa*$^{-/-}$ and control mice (Figure 2B–D). We next quantified the colocalization of RIBEYE and SHANK1 in these mice as a reflection of synapse formation and function. We observed 12.7±2.8 colocalized RIBEYE and SHANK1 puncta per IHC in control mice and 10.18±2.8 colocalized RIBEYE and SHANK1 puncta per IHC in *C1qa*$^{-/-}$ animals. The number of observed puncta in our adult control animals was similar to expected values in an adult animal undergoing normal synaptic

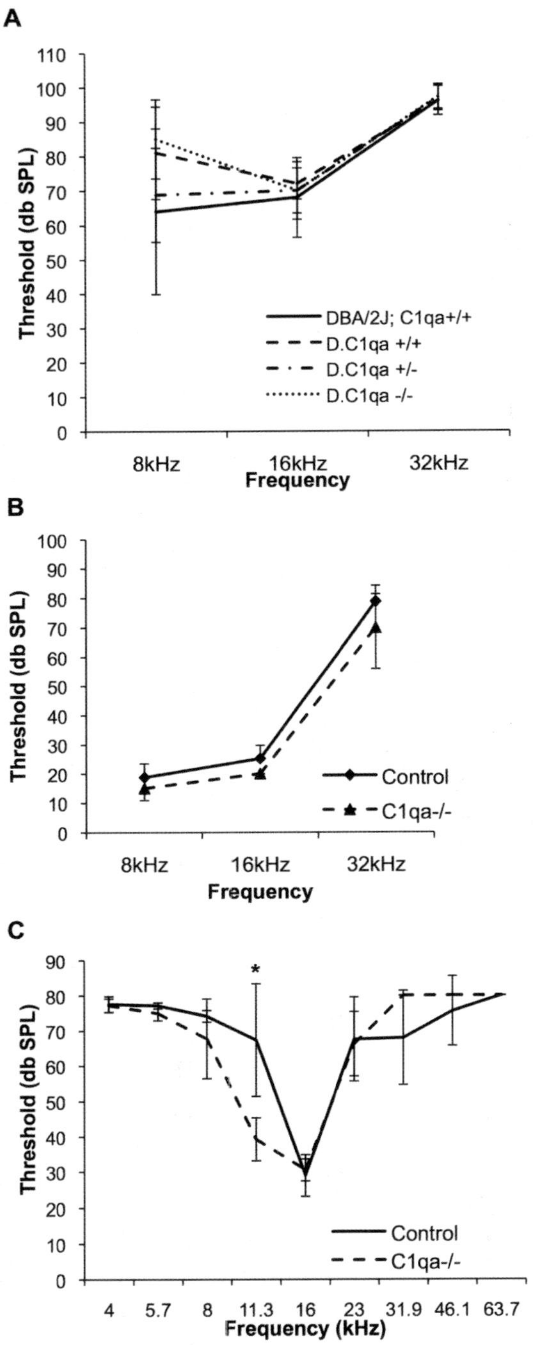


**Figure 6. *C1qa*$^{-/-}$ mice are not protected from progressive or age-related hearing loss.** A) Average ABR thresholds for *DBA/2J-C1qa*$^{+/+}$ controls (n = 5) and congenic *D2.B6-C1qa*$^{+/+}$ (n = 5), *D2.B6-C1qa*$^{+/-}$ (n = 8), and *D2.B6-C1qa*$^{-/-}$ (n = 9) mice at 1-month of age are shown. Average ABR (B) and DPOAE (C) thresholds are shown for *B6-C1qa*$^{-/-}$ (n = 4) and B6 control (n = 5) mice at 10-months of age. *($p$ = 0.01). Error bars show SDs.

refinement [28]. The *C1qa*$^{-/-}$ mice had a slight but non-significant decrease in the level of colocalization compared to controls, which is attributable to high variability and a slight increase in number of RIBEYE puncta (not significant when compared to controls; 14.3±3.58 puncta per IHC in controls vs. 15.5±1.2 puncta per IHC in mutants). Because IHC refinement and OHC refinement might be regulated by different mechanisms, we next analyzed OHC refinement in *C1qa*$^{-/-}$ compared to control mice. We did not observe SHANK1 expression in the OHC at P29 in either group, consistent with normal synaptic patterning. There was no difference in RIBEYE staining in the OHCs between and control and *C1qa*$^{-/-}$ adult mice (2.2±0.45 and 2.4±0.05 puncta per OHC respectively). Efferent synapse formation, as determined by SYNAPTOPHYSIN staining in the basal part of the OHCs, was also comparable in *C1qa*$^{-/-}$ and controls (Figure 2E). Efferent and afferent fibers crossing the tunnel of Corti, as determined by TUJ1 staining, were also not obviously different in *C1qa*$^{-/-}$ versus controls (Figure 2E). In summary, our data indicate that the efferent and afferent fiber patterning in *C1qa*$^{-/-}$ animals are not detectably different from controls. Similar to *H2-K*$^b$*D*$^b$ genes, *C1qa* expression does not appear to be necessary for proper afferent and/or efferent synapse formation and synaptic refinement, based on the parameters measured, occurs normally in mutant mice.

## Knockout of MHC Class I Genes Causes Hearing Impairment

Although our morphological data demonstrate normal synaptic refinement and development in the cochlea of mice lacking both *H2-K*$^b$ and *H2-D*$^b$ genes ($K^bD^{b-/-}$), whether MHC class I genes in play a role in auditory function is unknown. We analyzed auditory brain stem responses (ABRs) of $K^bD^{b-/-}$ mice at 8 weeks of age and found significant hearing impairment as demonstrated by an increase in frequency threshold compared to age/sex-matched C57BL/6 controls (Figure 3A–B, Figure S2 in File S1). A significant increase in thresholds was seen for click and 32 kHz stimuli. It has been shown that the ABR threshold does not always reflect subtle differences in the number of neurons that are firing [29–31]. Therefore, we decided to study the wave amplitude and latency to reveal differences in the average of all active synapses and firing neurons in control versus mutant animals. We measured the peak amplitude of wave 1, and also the time elapsed from the onset of stimulus to peak 1 (response latency). There were no differences in peak 1 amplitudes or peak 1 latencies between the two cohorts that would be suggestive of a possible deficiency in neural firing (Figure 3C–D) [29–31]. Previous work suggests that the complement cascade is involved in axonal but not dendrite synapse pruning in the CNS [16]. We assumed that a lack of refinement of axonal synapses would result in the retention of functional synapses, and this would lead to an increase in the number of firing synapses. Therefore, we analyzed the second wave amplitude (peak 2) as an estimate of the number of axonal synapses firing. Peak 2 amplitudes were also comparable between the $K^bD^{b-/-}$ mice and controls (Figure 3C). To determine whether the difference in average ABR thresholds at the higher frequency of 32 kHz is caused by alterations of OHC function, we tested the distortion-product otoacoustic emission (DPOAE) in these mice. We observed significant differences in the mutants as compared to controls at 8 kHz, 11.3 kHz, 16.1 kHz, and 23 kHz (Figure 3E). We also analyzed the hearing impairment phenotype at 16 weeks of age. Although the control mice had elevated thresholds due to their C57BL/6 background displaying early onset age-related hearing loss [32], we observed additional threshold elevations in both ABR and DPOAE thresholds in the $K^bD^{b-/-}$ mice (Figure 4A–C). Together, these data demonstrate that MHC class I genes are necessary for normal hearing when tested in adult mice of 8 and 16 weeks of age. To exclude other potential factors that might contribute to this phenotype, we examined the knockout mice for signs of inflammation in the middle and inner ear, suggesting an absence of middle ear infection. Further, the hearing impairment was not accompanied by gross morphological alterations in the cochlear duct as determined by examination of plastic-embedded sections (data not shown). However, we cannot rule out the possibility that elevated thresholds in the mutant mice are due to hearing loss involving conductive structures in the middle ear. Also, immunostaining with antibodies to PRESTIN, the motor protein expressed in outer hair cells, showed no apparent difference in morphology of outer hair cells in adult $K^bD^{b-/-}$ mice compared to controls (Figure S3 in File S1). Further investigations are needed to understand the hearing impairment caused by mutations in in these genes.

### *C1qa* Expression is not Necessary for Proper Hearing

We next sought to determine the role of the complement cascade in promoting proper hearing in the mouse cochlea. The ABR thresholds of 8-week-old $C1qa^{-/-}$ mice were compared to that of C1qa expressing control mice (Figure 5A–B). There was no difference in hearing thresholds at the 8, 16, and 32 kHz frequencies as well as in response to broadband click stimuli measured between the two genotypes. We analyzed the ABR data at 16 kHz, within the most sensitive frequency range for mice for peak 1 amplitudes and latencies. We did not observe a shift in peak 1 amplitude or latency in $C1qa^{-/-}$ mice compared to controls (Figure 5C–D). Since peripheral projections in the cochlea are considered long dendrites and may be C1qa independent, we analyzed the second wave amplitude (Peak 2) as an estimate of the number of axonal synapses firing and observed that it is also unaffected in $C1qa^{-/-}$ mice (Figure 5C). In addition, no difference in OHC function was revealed by DPOAE measurements between $C1qa^{-/-}$ and control mice (Figure 5E).

### Lack of *C1qa* Expression is not Protective in Progressive Hearing Loss

We next determined if a lack of *C1qa* expression would protect mice from progressive or age-related hearing loss (AHL) in two different mouse models. Mice from the DBA/2J strain suffer from early-onset, progressive hearing loss [33,34]. All of the genetic components contributing to the hearing loss phenotypes in DBA/2J mice have not been accounted for as of yet. The DBA/2J strain is also a well-known mouse model of glaucoma [35]. Retinal ganglion cell loss and degeneration of the optic nerve are characteristics of this neurodegenerative disease model. In early stages of glaucoma in this model, C1qa protein was re-expressed and localized to adult retinal synapses [16]. Further, *C1qa* deficiency on the DBA/2J background prevented damage to the retina and optic nerve and protected mice from glaucoma [23]. We hypothesized that the hearing loss observed in the DBA/2J mice is related to *C1qa*-regulated spiral ganglion cell loss. To test this hypothesis, we analyzed congenic mice that are deficient for *C1qa* on the DBA/2J mouse background ($D2.B6\text{-}C1qa^{-/-}$). ABR thresholds for DBA/2J mice with wild-type expression of *C1qa* ($DBA/2J\text{-}C1qa^{+/+}$) are shown in Figure 6C. We compared the one-month thresholds of the progeny from an intercross of $DBA/2J\text{-}C1qa^{+/+}$ and $D2.B6\text{-}C1qa^{-/-}$ F1 hybrids resulting in F2 progeny with $C1qa^{+/+}$, $C1qa^{+/-}$, and $C1qa^{-/-}$ genotypes all on a DBA/2J background. However, lack of *C1qa* failed to protect these mice from hearing loss (Figure 6A). C57/BL6 mice have an AHL mutation of *Cadherin 23* causing OHC degeneration and increasing the susceptibility to age-related hearing loss [32]. It has recently been shown that mice deficient in *C1qa* have less cognitive and memory loss with age compared to their littermate controls [18]. We hypothesized that *C1qa* synaptic re-expression in aging might mediate AHL and that a lack of *C1qa* expression in our $C1qa^{-/-}$ mice might protect against age-related hearing loss and OHC death. ABR thresholds of mice at 10 months of age were not different compared to control mice (Figure 6B), demonstrating the absence of a protective effect. A small reduction in DPOAE thresholds was seen at 11.3 kHz in mice lacking *C1qa* expression at 10 months of age but not at other frequencies (Figure 6C). In summary, these data suggest that although MHCI genes may be necessary for proper hearing function and a lack of *C1qa* in the brain exerts a protective effect in the central nervous system, its absence in the cochlea does not protect from AHL.

## Discussion

The cochlea is a good model system to study innervation and synaptic refinement because it contains only a few cell types that undergo a well-orchestrated developmental innervation and postnatal refinement program [28,36–40]. Microarray gene expression analysis by other groups has revealed a postnatal upregulation of MHC class I, MHC class II, and complement pathway genes in spiral ganglion neurons [19]. We extended the existing microarray studies with quantitative expression analyses over the course of postnatal refinement and found that $H2\text{-}K^b$ and complement component *C1qa* mRNA is increasingly expressed in the mouse cochlea during the first four postnatal weeks. The fact that MHCI and complement genes have recently been implicated in synaptic refinement such as synaptic elimination in development and aging [13–18] spurred our interest in investigating a potential role for these genes in the postnatal cochlea.

Interestingly, a lack of major histocompatibility genes $H2\text{-}K^b$ and $H2\text{-}D^b$, but not complement component *C1qa*, leads to an increase in hearing threshold at high frequency. This result leads to the question of whether sustained down-regulation of immune gene expression, leads to defective clearance of dead and dying cells that could become antigenic and drive organ-specific autoimmunity [41,42]. Assuming that the primary role of cochlear glial-like supporting cells, like that of other glial cells, is to support neuronal function, the challenge now is to determine what sort of pathological scenarios, like noise exposure or aging, could transform these supporting cells into auto aggressive effector cells that attack healthy neurons and cause neurodegeneration. In the CNS, glial cells are capable of performing both neuroprotective and neurodestructive functions [43]. Under physiological conditions, glial cells exhibit a deactivated phenotype that is associated with the production of anti-inflammatory and neurotrophic factors [44]. Microglia switch to an activated phenotype in response to pathogen invasion or tissue damage and thereby promote an inflammatory response that serves to further engage the immune system and initiate tissue repair. Glial cell dysfunction may become manifest in a number of ways, including a decreased ability to clear dead cells, decreased ability to produce neurotrophic factors, as well as increased neurotoxicity and synapse elimination. In our case, we hypothesized that *C1qa* knockout mice would lack the ability to clear out cellular debris caused by continuous noise exposure and this would lead to local autoimmunity in the cochlea. However, our aging ABR data suggests that this may not lead to hearing impairment. We also screened for *C1qa* playing a protective role in age-related hearing loss in the congenic *D2.B6-C1qa* model and found that a lack of *C1qa* does not prevent this condition. Because expression of MHCI proteins on the surface of cells may limit post-stress (post injury) synaptic loss and neuronal cell death, we might expect the $K^bD^{b-/-}$ mice to lack this protective function compared to controls. Noise exposure and/or aging may reveal an important protective role for these molecules. Further studies will need to be done to determine if autoimmunity has arisen mediating the hearing loss associated with $H2\text{-}K^b/H2\text{-}D^b$ deficiency.

Our study demonstrates that at an individual level these immune proteins are not necessary for proper synaptic refinement and lack of their expression is not sufficient to alter auditory circuit maturation. In gene families with many members, similar genes may functionally compensate for the deleted gene due to redundancy. Work ongoing in our laboratory aims to identify thyroid hormone-regulated gene profiles by microarray analysis in order to understand the genetic signature controlling auditory synaptic refinement and maturation at the spiral ganglion neuron level. We expect that along with MHC and complement pathways altered, we will also identify other genes involved in the "eat-me" signal of phagocytosis or clearance [45,46]. It is possible that many of the molecules in "eat-me" signaling are involved in the cochlea and only by deleting the pathways will we see a phenotype. It is also possible that these immune system pathways are not playing the main role in eliminating a weakened synapse or neuron but have a secondary function (like cleaning out debris) that will be compensated for by different pathways that remain to be elucidated. This study highlights the challenge of identifying the molecular mechanisms of synapse removal and refinement necessary for proper cochlear development. We performed a candidate gene based approach because these genes were associated with processes shared by the cochlea, brain and retina. Our study revealed that the individual genes regulating these processes in other neural tissues are not shared or regulated in the same manner in the cochlea as in the CNS. Although increased expression of *H2-K^b^*, *H2-D^b^*, and *C1qa* genes coincides with ages of auditory synaptic refinement, their functions and roles in the developing cochlea remain unclear.

## Acknowledgments

The authors thank Drs. Ben Barres and Alexander Stephan for providing C1qa mice and for discussions; Dr. Carla Shatz for providing $K^bD^b$ mice. Dr. Gareth Howell for providing D2.B6-C1qa mice.

## Author Contributions

Conceived and designed the experiments: MAC DL SS DM KRJ MM. Performed the experiments: MAC DM DL RL FW SS KRJ MM. Analyzed the data: MAC DL RL FW SS KRJ MM. Contributed reagents/materials/analysis tools: MAC DL SS KRJ MM. Wrote the paper: MAC DM DL SS KRJ MM.

## References

1. Lenoir M, Shnerson A, Pujol R (1980) Cochlear receptor development in the rat with emphasis on synaptogenesis. Anat Embryol 160: 253–262.
2. Bruce LL, Kingsley J, Nichols DH, Fritzsch B (1997) The development of vestibulocochlear efferents and cochlear afferents in mice. Int J Dev Neurosci 15: 671–692.
3. Simmons DD, Moulding HD, Zee D (1996) Olivocochlear innervation of inner and outer hair cells during postnatal maturation: an immunocytochemical study. Brain Res Dev Brain Res 95: 213–226.
4. Simmons DD, Mansdorf NB, Kim JH (1996) Olivocochlear innervation of inner and outer hair cells during postnatal maturation: evidence for a waiting period. J Comp Neurol 370: 551–562. doi:10.1002/(SICI)1096-9861(19960708)370: 4<551::AID-CNE10>3.0.CO;2-M.
5. Cole KS, Robertson D (1992) Early efferent innervation of the developing rat cochlea studied with a carbocyanine dye. Brain Res 575: 223–230.
6. Bruce LL, Christensen MA, Warr WB (2000) Postnatal development of efferent synapses in the rat cochlea. J Comp Neurol 423: 532–548.
7. Liberman MC (1980) Efferent synapses in the inner hair cell area of the cat cochlea: an electron microscopic study of serial sections. Hear Res 3: 189–204.
8. Liberman MC (1980) Morphological differences among radial afferent fibers in the cat cochlea: an electron-microscopic study of serial sections. Hear Res 3: 45–63.
9. Romand MR, Romand R (1990) Development of spiral ganglion cells in mammalian cochlea. J Electron Microsc Tech 15: 144–154. doi:10.1002/jemt.1060150206.
10. Hafidi A, Després G, Romand R (1993) Ontogenesis of type II spiral ganglion neurons during development: peripherin immunohistochemistry. Int J Dev Neurosci 11: 507–512.
11. Brown MC (1987) Morphology of labeled afferent fibers in the guinea pig cochlea. J Comp Neurol 260: 591–604. doi:10.1002/cne.902600411.
12. Brown MC (1987) Morphology of labeled efferent fibers in the guinea pig cochlea. J Comp Neurol 260: 605–618. doi:10.1002/cne.902600412.
13. Goddard CA, Butts DA, Shatz CJ (2007) Regulation of CNS synapses by neuronal MHC class I. Proc Natl Acad Sci USA 104: 6828–6833. doi:10.1073/pnas.0702023104.
14. McConnell MJ, Huang YH, Datwani A, Shatz CJ (2009) H2-K(b) and H2-D(b) regulate cerebellar long-term depression and limit motor learning. Proceedings of the National Academy of Sciences 106: 6784–6789. doi:10.1073/pnas.0902018106.
15. Datwani A, McConnell MJ, Kanold PO, Micheva KD, Busse B, et al. (2009) Classical MHCI molecules regulate retinogeniculate refinement and limit ocular dominance plasticity. Neuron 64: 463–470. doi:10.1016/j.neuron.2009.10.015.
16. Stevens B, Allen NJ, Vazquez LE, Howell GR, Christopherson KS, et al. (2007) The classical complement cascade mediates CNS synapse elimination. Cell 131: 1164–1178. doi:10.1016/j.cell.2007.10.036.
17. Chu Y, Jin X, Parada I, Pesic A, Stevens B, et al. (2010) Enhanced synaptic connectivity and epilepsy in C1q knockout mice. Proceedings of the National Academy of Sciences 107: 7975–7980. doi:10.1073/pnas.0913449107.
18. Stephan AH, Madison DV, Mateos JM, Fraser DA, Lovelett EA, et al. (2013) A Dramatic Increase of C1q Protein in the CNS during Normal Aging. Journal of Neuroscience 33: 13460–13474. doi:10.1523/JNEUROSCI.1333-13.2013.
19. Lu CC, Appler JM, Houseman EA, Goodrich LV (2011) Developmental profiling of spiral ganglion neurons reveals insights into auditory circuit assembly. Journal of Neuroscience 31: 10903–10918. doi:10.1523/JNEUROSCI.2358-11.2011.
20. Schott E, Bonasio R, Ploegh HL (2003) Elimination in vivo of developing T cells by natural killer cells. J Exp Med 198: 1213–1224. doi:10.1084/jem.20030918.
21. Vugmeyster Y, Glas R, Pérarnau B, Lemonnier FA, Eisen H, et al. (1998) Major histocompatibility complex (MHC) class I KbDb −/− deficient mice possess functional CD8+ T cells and natural killer cells. Proc Natl Acad Sci USA 95: 12492–12497.
22. Botto M (1998) C1q knock-out mice for the study of complement deficiency in autoimmune disease. Exp Clin Immunogenet 15: 231–234.
23. Howell GR, Macalinao DG, Sousa GL, Walden M, Soto I, et al. (2011) Molecular clustering identifies complement and endothelin induction as early events in a mouse model of glaucoma. J Clin Invest 121: 1429–1444. doi:10.1172/JCI44646.
24. Xia A, Visosky AMB, Cho J-H, Tsai M-J, Pereira FA, et al. (2007) Altered traveling wave propagation and reduced endocochlear potential associated with cochlear dysplasia in the BETA2/NeuroD1 null mouse. J Assoc Res Otolaryngol 8: 447–463. doi:10.1007/s10162-007-0092-9.
25. Müller M, Hünerbein von K, Hoidis S, Smolders JWT (2005) A physiological place-frequency map of the cochlea in the CBA/J mouse. Hear Res 202: 63–73. doi:10.1016/j.heares.2004.08.011.
26. Liu Q, Davis RL (2007) Regional specification of threshold sensitivity and response time in CBA/CaJ mouse spiral ganglion neurons. J Neurophysiol 98: 2215–2222. doi:10.1152/jn.00284.2007.
27. Meyer AC, Frank T, Khimich D, Hoch G, Riedel D, et al. (2009) Tuning of synapse number, structure and function in the cochlea. Nat Neurosci 12: 444–453. doi:10.1038/nn.2293.
28. Huang L-C, Barclay M, Lee K, Peter S, Housley GD, et al. (2012) Synaptic profiles during neurite extension, refinement and retraction in the developing cochlea. Neural Dev 7: 38. doi:10.1186/1749-8104-7-38.
29. Kujawa SG, Liberman MC (2009) Adding insult to injury: cochlear nerve degeneration after "temporary" noise-induced hearing loss. Journal of Neuroscience 29: 14077–14085. doi:10.1523/JNEUROSCI.2845-09.2009.
30. Liberman MC (1982) Single-neuron labeling in the cat auditory nerve. Science 216: 1239–1241.
31. Liberman MC (1982) The cochlear frequency map for the cat: labeling auditory-nerve fibers of known characteristic frequency. J Acoust Soc Am 72: 1441–1449.
32. Noben-Trauth K, Zheng QY, Johnson KR (2003) Association of cadherin 23 with polygenic inheritance and genetic modification of sensorineural hearing loss. Nat Genet 35: 21–23. doi:10.1038/ng1226.
33. Johnson KR, Longo-Guess C, Gagnon LH, Yu H, Zheng QY (2008) A locus on distal chromosome 11 (ahl8) and its interaction with Cdh23 ahl underlie the early onset, age-related hearing loss of DBA/2J mice. Genomics 92: 219–225. doi:10.1016/j.ygeno.2008.06.007.

34. Shin J-B, Longo-Guess CM, Gagnon LH, Saylor KW, Dumont RA, et al. (2010) The R109H variant of fascin-2, a developmentally regulated actin crosslinker in hair-cell stereocilia, underlies early-onset hearing loss of DBA/2J mice. Journal of Neuroscience 30: 9683–9694. doi:10.1523/JNEUROSCI.1541-10.2010.
35. Libby RT, Anderson MG, Pang I-H, Robinson ZH, Savinova OV, et al. (2005) Inherited glaucoma in DBA/2J mice: pertinent disease features for studying the neurodegeneration. Vis Neurosci 22: 637–648. doi:10.1017/S0952523805225130.
36. Uziel A, Pujol R, Legrand C, Legrand J (1983) Cochlear synaptogenesis in the hypothyroid rat. Brain Res 283: 295–301.
37. Rueda J, Prieto JJ, Cantos R, Sala ML, Merchán JA (2003) Hypothyroidism prevents developmental neuronal loss during auditory organ development. Neurosci Res 45: 401–408.
38. Fang Q, Giordimaina AM, Dolan DF, Camper SA, Mustapha M (2012) Genetic background of Prop1(df) mutants provides remarkable protection against hypothyroidism-induced hearing impairment. J Assoc Res Otolaryngol 13: 173–184. doi:10.1007/s10162-011-0302-3.
39. Barclay M, Ryan AF, Housley GD (2011) Type I vs type II spiral ganglion neurons exhibit differential survival and neuritogenesis during cochlear development. Neural Dev 6: 33. doi:10.1186/1749-8104-6-33.
40. Huang L-C, Thorne PR, Housley GD, Montgomery JM (2007) Spatiotemporal definition of neurite outgrowth, refinement and retraction in the developing mouse cochlea. Development 134: 2925–2933. doi:10.1242/dev.001925.
41. Nagata S, Hanayama R, Kawane K (2010) Autoimmunity and the Clearance of Dead Cells. Cell 140: 619–630. doi:10.1016/j.cell.2010.02.014.
42. Alexander JJ, Anderson AJ, Barnum SR, Stevens B, Tenner AJ (2008) The complement cascade: Yin-Yang in neuroinflammation - neuro-protection and - degeneration. J Neurochem 107: 1169–1187. doi:10.1111/j.1471-4159.2008.05668.x.
43. Neumann H, Kotter MR, Franklin RJM (2008) Debris clearance by microglia: an essential link between degeneration and regeneration. Brain 132: 288–295. doi:10.1093/brain/awn109.
44. Streit WJ (2002) Microglia as neuroprotective, immunocompetent cells of the CNS. Glia 40: 133–139. doi:10.1002/glia.10154.
45. Ravichandran KS (2011) Beginnings of a Good Apoptotic Meal:The Find-Me and Eat-Me Signaling Pathways. Immunity 35: 445–455. doi:10.1016/j.immuni.2011.09.004.
46. Chung W-S, Clarke LE, Wang GX, Stafford BK, Sher A, et al. (2013) Astrocytes mediate synapse elimination through MEGF10 and MERTK pathways. Nature. doi:10.1038/nature12776.

7

# Cross-Modal Re-Organization in Adults with Early Stage Hearing Loss

**Julia Campbell[1], Anu Sharma[1,2]***

1 University of Colorado at Boulder, Department of Speech, Language and Hearing Sciences, Boulder, Colorado, United States of America, 2 University of Colorado at Boulder, Institute of Cognitive Science, Boulder, Colorado, United States of America

## Abstract

Cortical cross-modal re-organization, or recruitment of auditory cortical areas for visual processing, has been well-documented in deafness. However, the degree of sensory deprivation necessary to induce such cortical plasticity remains unclear. We recorded visual evoked potentials (VEP) using high-density electroencephalography in nine persons with adult-onset mild-moderate hearing loss and eight normal hearing control subjects. Behavioral auditory performance was quantified using a clinical measure of speech perception-in-noise. Relative to normal hearing controls, adults with hearing loss showed significantly larger P1, N1, and P2 VEP amplitudes, decreased N1 latency, and a novel positive component (P2′) following the P2 VEP. Current source density reconstruction of VEPs revealed a shift toward ventral stream processing including activation of auditory temporal cortex in hearing-impaired adults. The hearing loss group showed worse than normal speech perception performance in noise, which was strongly correlated with a decrease in the N1 VEP latency. Overall, our findings provide the first evidence that visual cross-modal re-organization not only begins in the early stages of hearing impairment, but may also be an important factor in determining behavioral outcomes for listeners with hearing loss, a finding which demands further investigation.

**Editor:** Giuseppe Biagini, University of Modena and Reggio Emilia, Italy

**Funding:** This work was supported by the National Institutes of Health (RO106257 to A.S., F31DC011970 to J.C.). The funders had no role in study design, data collection and analysis, decision to publish, or preparation of the manuscript.

**Competing Interests:** The authors have declared that no competing interests exist.

* E-mail: anu.sharma@colorado.edu

## Introduction

A basic tenet of neuroplasticity is that central pathways will re-organize following long-term sensory deprivation. There is ample evidence from animal and human studies of cross-modal re-organization of the cortex that occurs in both blindness [1,2,3,4,5,6,7], and congenital deafness [8,9,10,11,12,13,14,15,16,17,18,19,20,21,22,23]. For example, congenitally deaf white cats show enhanced motion processing and localization in the visual periphery, and recruit higher-order auditory cortex for improved performance in these tasks [19,24]. Similarly, congenitally and post-lingually deaf humans (with and without cochlear implants) demonstrate activation of auditory cortical areas during processing of visual motion and complex visual pattern changes, which is not seen for normal hearing control subjects [15,17,25,26,27]. Although cross-modal recruitment serves to enhance behavioral performance for the recruiting modality [19,28], it has been linked to a decrease in performance of the recruited modality. In deaf adults fitted with cochlear implants, cross-modal recruitment (measured by event-related potentials) has been correlated with decreased performance on speech perception tasks [25,26,29]. All of the studies mentioned above have been conducted on individuals in the most advanced stage of hearing loss (i.e., profound deafness). However, most post-lingual deafened adults show a gradual decline in hearing, which typically progresses through the mild, moderate, severe and profound stages of hearing loss [30,31]. Thus, the degree of sensory deprivation necessary to induce cross-modal cortical plasticity remains unclear. Given the potential impact on clinical outcomes, it would be useful to determine whether cross-modal cortical changes begin during early stages of hearing decline or whether these changes are limited to the near-total sensory deprivation that accompanies deafness. In this study, we examined visual evoked potentials (VEP) using high-density electroencephalography and auditory behavioral outcome using a clinical test of speech perception in noise in persons with adult-onset mild-moderate hearing loss and normal hearing control subjects.

## Materials and Methods

### Participants and Ethics Statement

Seventeen adults between the ages of 37 to 68 years participated in this study. The study was approved by the University of Colorado at Boulder Institutional Review Board, and all participants provided written consent. Subjects were recruited via advertisements in the community, and hearing was tested for all subjects using standard clinical audiometric procedures prior to speech-in-noise and EEG measurements. Eight of the subjects (mean age and standard deviation: 50.5+/−6.2 years; range: 37.4–57 years) revealed clinically normal hearing thresholds (i.e., below 25 dB Hearing Level) for frequencies ranging from 250 Hz to 8000 Hz. Nine of the subjects demonstrated hearing loss (mean age and standard deviation: 56.9+/−8.9 years; range: 38.4–68.2 years). On average, this group showed normal hearing from 250 Hz through 1000 Hz and a mild-to-moderate sensorineural hearing loss bilaterally from 2000 Hz to 8000 Hz. Average audiograms for the two groups are shown in Figure 1. None of the participants with hearing loss were receiving clinical intervention at the time of enrollment. However, many participants suspected a possible hearing loss prior to diagnosis. Subjects who were diagnosed with hearing loss through the study received counseling from a state-licensed clinical audiologist (first author) and referrals to audiology clinics for possible consideration of amplification. EEG testing sessions took place on separate days for those diagnosed with hearing loss unless otherwise requested. The participants in the normal hearing (NH) group and hearing loss (HL) group showed no difference in age between groups ($t(15) = -1.69$, $p > 0.05$). All participants reported no issues with visual acuity and no neurological impairment.

## Auditory Behavioral Testing: Test of Speech Perception-in-noise

Speech perception in background noise was measured using the QuickSIN™ test [32], a clinical assessment of auditory acuity in background noise. Participants faced a speaker at 0° azimuth and were instructed to repeat two recorded sentence lists (six sentences each) presented at 65 dB Hearing Level (HL). Background noise was varied to determine the signal-to-noise ratio (SNR) required by the participant to accurately repeat 50% of the sentences. The SNR values began at 25 dB and decreased in 5 dB increments to 0 dB. The SNR score from the two lists was computed and averaged for each participant. Overall, the lower the SNR score, the better the performance on the test.

## EEG Procedures

**Visual stimuli.** Participants were shown a high contrast sinusoidal concentric grating that morphs into a radially modulated grating or circle-star pattern [25,33,34] on a 26-inch flat-screen LCD television at a viewing distance of approximately 42 inches. The circle and star figures were presented 150 times. The star figure was presented on the screen for 600 ms, then immediately followed by the circle figure, also lasting for 600 ms. This presentation method provided the percept of apparent motion and shape change to the viewer. A total of 300 stimulus presentations (sweeps) were presented, for a testing time of three minutes. The VEP was time-locked to the onset of each individual star and circle presentation. Participants were instructed to direct their gaze to the center of the star/circle at a black dot and to not shift gaze during the three minutes.

## EEG Recording and Analyses

Participants were fitted with a 128-channel EEG electrode recording net (Electrical Geodesic, Inc.) and seated in a comfortable reclining chair in an electro-magnetically shielded sound booth. All stimuli were presented via E-Prime® 2.0, stimulus software compatible with Net Station 4 (Electrical Geodesic, Inc). The sampling rate for the EEG recordings was 1 kHz, with a band-pass filter set at 0.1–200 Hz.

Data were band-pass filtered offline at 1–30 Hz and segmented according to the EEG activity surrounding the stimulus presentation (epochs), with 100 ms pre-stimulus and 495 ms post-stimulus time. EEG recordings were corrected to the pre-stimulus baseline, and eye-blink artifact recorded at designated eye channels was removed if greater than +/−100 μV, unless adjusted for individual subjects. Bad channels were removed from the recording and replaced with interpolated data from the remaining channels via a spline interpolation algorithm. Remaining data were averaged and re-referenced using common average reference. Individual waveform averages were averaged together for each of the two groups (i.e., the normal hearing and hearing loss group) to compute a grand-averaged waveform. Amplitudes and latencies for individual participants were recorded for all three obligatory visual evoked potential (VEP) peaks (i.e., P1, N1 and P2). The P1 peak component was observed as the first positive-going peak occurring approximately within a latency window of 90 to 130 ms, the N1 component was observed as the second peak or first negative-going peak occurring approximately between 135 ms to 200 ms, and the P2 component was observed as the third peak or second positive-going peak occurring approximately within 200

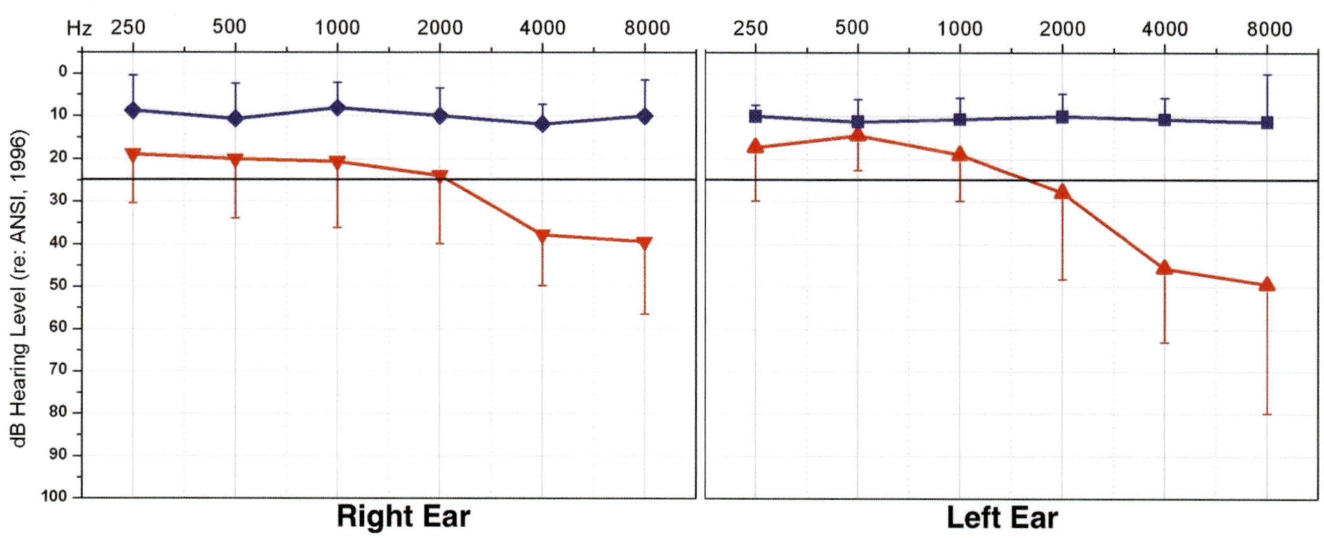


**Figure 1. Mean audiometric subject thresholds.** Auditory thresholds are shown for right and left ears for the standard audiometric frequencies from 250 Hz to 8000 Hz. Thresholds for the normal hearing (NH) group are depicted in blue; the hearing loss (HL) group in red. The positive-going blue bars illustrate the standard deviation for the average threshold at the designated frequency for the NH group, and negative-going red bars illustrate the standard deviation for the HL group. The solid black line illustrates the criterion for normal hearing, at 25 dB HL.

to 300 ms. If a peak component occurred outside of the described latency ranges, it was still marked and included according to the order of appearance (e.g., the first large positive component at 80 ms was marked as P1). P1 amplitudes were defined as the onset to peak value, N1 amplitudes as the peak of the N1 component to peak of the P2 component, and P2 amplitudes as peak of the P2 component to offset value. Latencies were chosen at the highest amplitude of the peak.

First we created a two-dimensional voltage map using Net Station 4 (Electrical Geodesic, Inc), which allowed us to examine regions of interest (ROI) around the occipital midline [25,29], focusing on the greatest group differences for visual stimuli. Using planned comparisons with the Bonferroni correction, electrodes within the ROI were then chosen for statistical analysis according to the largest mean group differences for the amplitude and latency of each VEP component.

### Source Localization Analysis (Current Density Reconstructions)

EEG data for individual participants were exported from Net Station and imported into EEGLAB [35] using MatLab® (The MathWorks®, Inc., 2010). The data were corrected to the baseline of a pre-stimulus interval of 100 ms and sweeps greater than +/− 100 μV were rejected as artifacts. The sampling rate was down-sampled to 250 Hz to reduce processing, altering the post-stimulus time to 492 ms. The first step in creating source models was to prune the concatenated EEG sweeps or trials for each subject through independent component analysis (ICA) [36,37]. This statistical procedure allows for observation of the spatially fixed and temporally independent components that underlie the evoked potential [38], and is useful in precise source modeling in EEG, including for deeper generators [37,39,40,41]. EEGLAB was chosen specifically for preliminary source localization analysis in order to utilize the ICA algorithm that provides for optimal cortical source localization, and to perform ICA on concatenated EEG sweeps [36,37,42]. Once the independent components that accounted for greatest percent variance in the evoked potential were identified in the designated timeframe for a peak component of interest (e.g., P1, N1, P2), the remaining independent components were regarded as artifact/noise and discarded. The pruned potential waveforms for each subject were then grand averaged for each group (NH and HL) and exported into CURRY® Scan 7 Neuroimaging Suite (Compumedics Neuroscan™) for source modeling. In CURRY®, an additional ICA was run on the VEP mean global field power (MGFP) (incorporating all 128 channel EEG data), with only components showing a signal-to-noise ratio (SNR) of 2.0 or greater accepted. The third VEP component in the HL group (P2') was pruned and averaged as an individual component as it was present in a subset of this group.

Peak components for the VEP MGFP waveforms were selected separately for current density reconstruction (CDR) via sLORETA, with no a-priori restrictions placed on the model. The selected head model was standardized using the boundary element method (BEM) [43]. sLORETA, or standardized low-resolution brain electromagnetic tomography, is a specific statistical method that estimates CDR [44,45]. The CDR is represented by a graded color scale image placed on an average MRI of 100 people. Sagittal MRI slices were selected to illustrate the greatest differences in cortical activation between the groups. Montreal Neurological Institute (MNI) co-ordinates (in millimeters) illustrate the three dimensional physical locations of each slice.

## Results

### Visual Evoked Potentials

Waveforms for the two groups across the whole head (128 channels) are shown in Figure 2. Three obligatory cortical VEP components elicited in response to the visual stimulus were analyzed: the P1 (occurring at approximately 100 ms), the N1 (occurring at approximately 150 ms), and the P2 (occurring at approximately 230 ms). We compared amplitude and latencies for these components between NH and HL groups at electrodes in the occipital ROI. A one-way ANOVA was computed to compare group differences. Post-hoc planned comparison of means using the Bonferroni correction was completed to describe significant differences between electrodes (see Figure 2).

P1 amplitude was larger for the HL group ($F(1, 285) = 6.265$, $\rho < 0.05$). N1 amplitude was larger for the HL group ($F(1, 285) = 9.865$, $\rho < 0.01$). N1 latency was decreased for the HL group ($F(1, 285) = 7.684$, $\rho < 0.01$). Finally, P2 amplitudes were increased for the HL group ($F(1, 285) = 8.983$, $\rho < 0.01$). Overall, this trend of decreased latencies and increased amplitudes for obligatory VEP components for HL listeners is consistent with previous results, which showed evidence of cross-modal recruitment in deaf subjects [13,25,26,46].

An unexpected finding was the visual identification of a positive component following the P2 (occurring between approximately 295 and 395 ms) in the HL group (see Figure 2C). We labeled this component P2'. While a possible component similar to this is observed by Doucet and colleagues [25], it was not analyzed or discussed in that study. Figure 2 shows the evoked potential waveforms for both groups at the described electrodes, with mean bar graphs illustrating significant differences.

### Cortical Source Localization

Cortical source localization, or current density reconstruction (CDR), was performed in order to visualize anatomical regions of possible cross-modal re-organization in the HL group. The sLORETA algorithm provided by CURRY® Scan 7 Neuroimaging Suite was applied to the three VEP peak components (Figure 3). The activations were superimposed on an average MRI (sagittal slice view) and the MNI co-ordinates are shown beneath each slice. The scale of the F distribution, indicating the strength of the activations, is also shown.

As expected, for the NH group, the visual stimuli elicited all three VEP components and activated visual processing regions, including multiple cerebellar areas, which have been shown to respond to visual motion [47,48] (Figure 3). Higher-order visual cortical regions such as Brodmann areas 18 and 19, and the fusiform region, were also activated. These findings are consistent with previous studies, which used stimuli generally similar to ours in NH subjects [34,47,48,49]. The P1 component showed similar cortical and cerebellar activation for both groups. However, for the N1 and P2 components, the HL group showed greater activation along the ventral visual stream in temporal areas, which are traditionally associated with auditory processing (including superior temporal gyrus (STG), medial temporal gyrus (MTG), and inferior temporal gyrus (ITG)). This result is consistent with previous reports of cross-modal activation of temporal areas in deaf subjects [15,17,27]. Figure 3 shows the current density reconstructions for the NH and HL groups. A table is provided in Figure 3 describing activated regions corresponding to each of the peak components. Interestingly, the P2' component (seen only in the HL group) showed activation of both cerebellar/occipital regions as well as temporal areas. This response pattern suggests

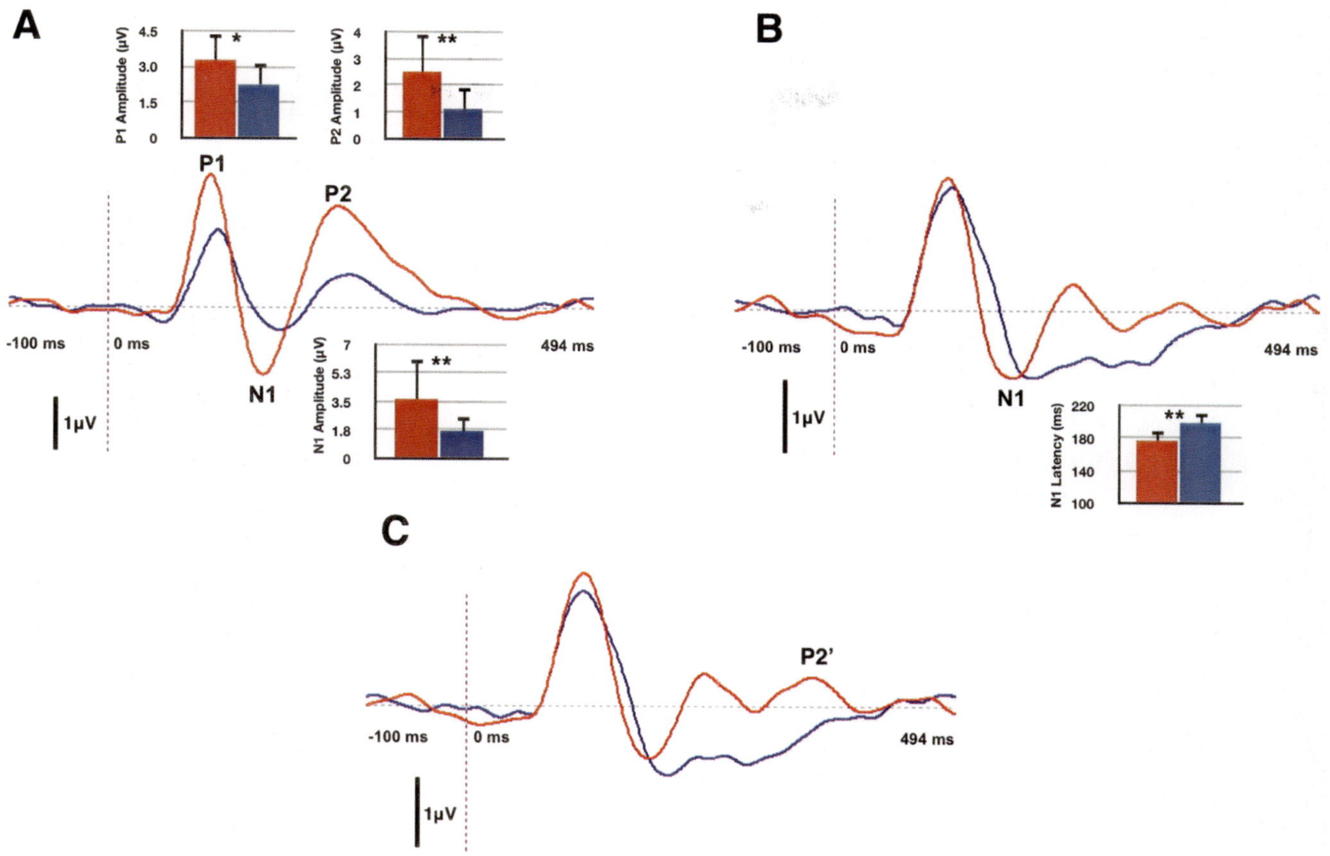


**Figure 2. Occipital Region of Interest (ROI) cortical visual evoked potentials (VEPs).** A. Peak components P1, N1, and P2 amplitudes are significantly larger for the adult Hearing Loss (HL) group (red) in comparison to the adult Normal Hearing group (blue). Mean group differences are illustrated in corresponding mean bar graphs for each component. One asterisk indicates significance at $p<0.05$; two asterisks indicate significance at $p<0.01$. B. The N1 component latency is significantly decreased in the HL group as compared to the NH group, also illustrated in the mean bar graph. C. A third positive peak component, denoted as P2′, has been found in a subset of the HL group.

that an additional processing step may take place within the ventral visual stream in listeners with hearing loss.

## Behavioral Performance

Speech perception-in-noise acuity was measured for both groups using the QuickSIN$^{TM}$ clinical test [32]. The results of the QuickSIN$^{TM}$ are reported as a signal-to-noise ratio (SNR) threshold; therefore a lower score reflects better performance. Mean scores for the NH and HL groups are shown in Figure 4A. A Mann-Whitney U Test revealed a significant difference between the two groups ($U=10.5$, $Z=-2.46$, $p<0.05$). This difference in auditory performance in background noise between normal hearing listeners and listeners with mild-to-moderate hearing loss is consistent with Killion et al. [32] and Wilson et al. [50].

The N1 VEP component has been suggested as a marker of cross-modal re-organization in deafness [13,26,46,51]. Therefore, we correlated the latency of the N1 with QuickSIN$^{TM}$ scores for the subjects. Due to hearing loss consisting of a gradual increase in auditory threshold from 0 dB HL, we included the N1 latency values and QuickSIN scores of all 17 participants in the correlation analysis. Mean QuickSIN$^{TM}$ scores and N1 VEP latencies were tested for normal distribution, and a Spearman's rank-order correlation was computed due to the non-normal distribution of the data. As seen in Figure 4B, a negative correlation was observed between N1 latency and QuickSIN scores ($r=-0.701$, $p=0.001$). That is, a shorter N1 latency was associated with higher scores (i.e., worse performance) on the QuickSIN$^{TM}$ test. Overall, our results reflecting differences in speech-in-noise perception between the NH and HL groups as a function of visual evoked potentials are consistent with previous studies in deaf subjects showing cross-modal re-organization in subjects with poor speech perception [25,26]. N1 latency changes also showed a significant negative correlation with the pure tone threshold averages (PTA) at 500, 1000, and 2000 Hz, which is a clinically relevant indicator of audiometric function (right ear, $r=-0.446$, $p<0.05$; left ear, $r=-0.540$, $p<0.05$). That is, as the degree of hearing loss increased, there was a corresponding decrease in N1 latency.

## Discussion

We sought to examine whether cross-modal recruitment is evident in early stages of hearing decline or whether cross-modal plasticity is limited to the near-total sensory deprivation that accompanies profound deafness. We recorded high-density EEG in response to a visual stimulus in adults with normal hearing in the low frequencies and a mild-to-moderate hearing loss in the high frequencies. A group of age-matched normal hearing adults served as the control group. All participants were administered the QuickSIN, a test of speech-in-noise perception which is used to document clinical outcomes in patients with hearing loss.

**A**

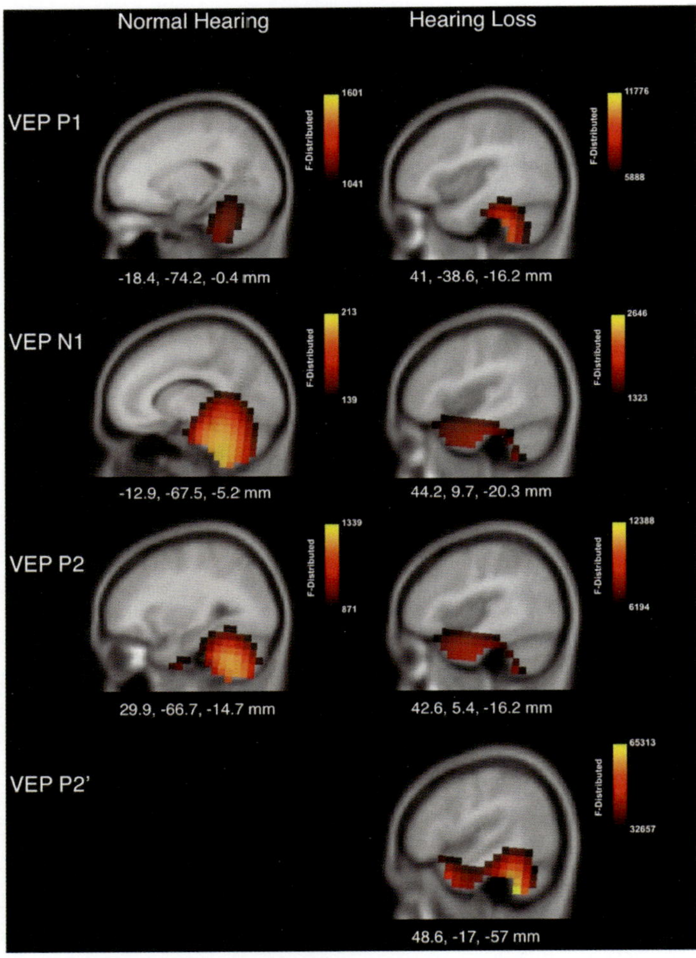


**B**

| | Normal Hearing | Hearing Loss |
|---|---|---|
| VEP P1 | Cerebellum, Brodmann Area 19 | Cerebellum, Brodmann Areas 20, 36, Fusiform gyrus |
| VEP N1 | Cerebellum, Brodmann Areas 18, 19, 30, Lingual Gyrus | Inferior Temporal Gyrus, Brodmann Area 20, Fusiform Gyrus, Medial Temporal Gyrus, Brodmann Area 21, Superior Temporal Gyrus, Brodmann Area 38, Cerebellum, Inferior Frontal Gyrus, Brodmann Area 47 |
| VEP P2 | Cerebellum, Brodmann Areas 36, 35, Fusiform Gyrus, Brodmann Areas 19, 20, 37, 38, Superior Temporal Gyrus | Inferior Temporal Gyrus, Brodmann Area 21, Medial Temporal Gyrus, Fusiform Gyrus, Brodmann Area 20, Superior Temporal Gyrus, Brodmann Area 38, Cerebellum, Inferior Frontal Gyrus, Brodmann Areas 36, 47 |
| VEP P2' | | Cerebellum, Brodmann Area 36, Superior Temporal Gyrus, Brodmann Area 38, Fusiform Gyrus, Brodmann Area 20, Medial Temporal Gyrus, Brodmann Areas 21, 37, Inferior Temporal Gyrus, Inferior Frontal Gyrus, Brodmann Area 47 |

**Figure 3. Current source density reconstructions for the NH and HL groups.** A. The cortical activation at the P1, N1 and P2 VEP peak components using sagittal magnetic resonance imaging (MRI) slices. The scale of the F Distribution is shown in a scale the upper right corner ranging from red to yellow (where yellow reflects the greater strength of activation). The Montreal Neurological Institute (MNI) coordinates are listed beneath each MRI slice. B. The table describing the activated cortical regions for the VEP components for the NH and HL groups, listed in approximate order of highest level of activation.

Relative to normal hearing controls, adults with mild-to-moderate hearing loss showed: (i) increased amplitude of the P1, N1 and P2 VEP components, (ii) presence of an additional positive VEP component (P2') occurring after the P2, (iii) decreased latency of the N1 VEP, (iv) cortical re-organization as evidenced by increased activation of auditory temporal areas elicited by visual stimulation, (iv) poorer speech perception scores in noise, (v) a significant negative correlation between the degree of hearing loss and N1 VEP latency, and (vi) a strong negative correlation between speech-in-noise perception and N1 VEP latency. Overall, this pattern of results in our listeners with mild hearing loss is consistent with previous findings in deaf subjects suggesting visual cross-modal recruitment in deafness [13,25,26,51].

Consistent with our findings, significantly increased amplitudes of N1 and P2 VEPs with hearing loss are well-documented in deafness [13,46,51]. More recently, changes in visual shift of form and motion have been shown to elicit larger N1 and P2 responses correlated with poor speech perception in deaf, cochlear-implanted adults, respectively [25,26]. Interestingly, smaller than normal amplitude of the visual P1 component has recently been reported in cochlear-implanted adults [29]. However, Sandmann and colleagues used a stimulus consisting of four separate checkerboard reversal patterns at varying luminance ratios, which is a more complex pattern of stimulation relative to the one used in this study. The checkerboard pattern is therefore more likely to tap into a different stage of visual processing than is evident in this study [29]. Typically, decreased latencies and increased amplitudes of evoked potential components are considered to be reflective of faster processing [52,53] suggesting that HL subjects recruit additional cortical areas to subserve processing speed and/or efficiency. To this end, we identified the P2' VEP component (following the P2) only in the HL group, possibly indicating a new or additional generator facilitating visual processing in the HL group.

Current source density reconstructions (CDR) were compared between NH and HL listeners. As expected, for the visual stimulus, NH listeners showed cerebellar/occipital activation for the P1, N1 and P2 VEP components (Figure 3). Responsive regions included Brodmann areas 18 and 19, which comprise higher-order visual cortex. Visual stimuli comparable in both shape and appearance of motion to the one used in the present study have been shown to

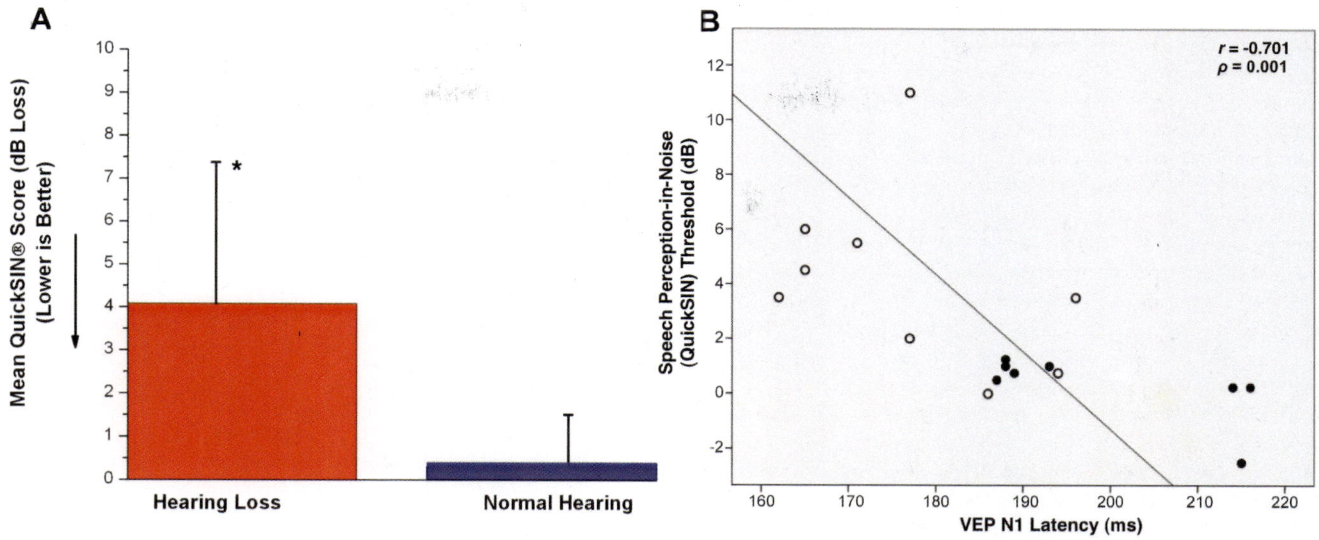


**Figure 4. Mean scores on the QuickSIN test for the NH and HL groups. (A).** Error bars are shown as vertical black lines. The asterisk reflects significant differences at $p < 0.05$. B. QuickSIN scores are shown on the vertical axis and N1 VEP component latencies on the horizontal axis. Values are shown as closed circles for the NH group and open circles for the HL group. The Spearman's rho value (−0.7) and significance at $p = 0.001$ are indicated on the upper right hand corner.

activate similar cortical regions in VEP and fMRI imaging studies [34,47,54].

The HL group showed occipital/cerebellar activation comparable to the NH group, as was evident in the CDR for the P1 response. However, higher-order processing as reflected by the CDR for the N1 and P2 components showed clear evidence of cortical re-organization. Cortical activation for these components showed an emphasis in ventral stream processing within temporal cortex, including temporal gyri (ITG, MTG and STG), which are typically associated with auditory cortical processing [55,56]. The P2' component, identified in only the HL group, showed underlying activation of both cerebellar/occipital areas and temporal areas, suggestive of a possible new generator in temporal cortex subserving visual processing.

In a recent study, Campbell and Sharma [57] examined cortical responses to auditory stimulation in adults with mild-moderate hearing loss. The authors reported a change in cortical resource allocation, including decreased temporal activation in STG and increased frontal activation in response to passive auditory stimulation in mild-moderate hearing loss. Taken together with the present results, this suggests that a decreased temporal activation to sound in mild-moderate hearing loss may be coincidental with the increased visual activation of temporal areas in this study.

Overall, the CDR findings are strongly suggestive of cortical re-organization facilitating cross-modal recruitment for visual processing in adults with mild-moderate hearing loss. The shift of activation to temporal cortex represents activation of the ventral visual stream, which is typically responsive to visual object form or shape changes, and is located within temporal cortex in proximity to auditory areas. The ventral stream has been implicated in the processing of facial and mouth movements [58,59]. Thus, our results may be suggestive of compensatory plasticity as HL listeners begin to rely on facial information as a strategy to compensate for their hearing impairment [60,61,62,63,64]. Because the ventral stream is largely responsible for processing object and face information, a heavier processing load may be imposed on this stream when listeners with hearing loss begin to pay more attention to lip and facial cues. Indeed, visual attention is a modulatory influence for compensatory plasticity, and congruent visual input has shown to enhance auditory speech perception performance in cochlear-implanted adults [18,65]. A recent study by Strelnikov and colleagues suggests that increased intra-modal compensatory activity in occipital cortex predicts better outcomes for post-lingually deaf adults after cochlear implantation, presumably due to the synergy of the visual system in deciphering auditory information and ultimately increasing the ability for auditory discrimination when sound is re-introduced via implantation [65]. However, similar to the present study, increased cross-modal re-organization in superior temporal sulcus (STS) appears to predict poor outcomes for both pre- and post-lingually deaf implant users [65,66,67].

Hearing loss is most consistently associated with poor outcomes in recognizing speech in background noise, a skill essential for everyday listening [30,68,69,70]. Consistent with previous research in hearing-impaired listeners, our results show that listeners with even mild-to-moderate hearing loss demonstrate a significant deficit when listening to speech in background noise [71,72]. A strong negative correlation was observed between speech perception-in-noise performance on the QuickSIN test and N1 VEP latency. That is, a shorter N1 latency was associated with higher scores (i.e., worse performance) on the QuickSIN™ test. While hearing loss is a well-known contributor to decreased speech in noise performance [73,74], our results suggest that cross-modal plasticity may also be an important factor that should be considered in the decreased auditory performance in background noise of listeners with hearing loss. If we assume that cross-modal plasticity implies a greater reliance on lip-reading, then it might possibly serve as a facilitatory compensation in noisy situations where congruent visual input enhances auditory processing [65]. A decrease in N1 latency was also correlated with higher audiometric thresholds, suggesting a possible increase in cross-modal recruitment as hearing loss gets worse. Future studies should systematically describe the extent of cross-modal recruitment as a function of hearing loss ranging from mild to profound, as well as investigate the possible contribution of cross-modal plasticity on speech perception performance.

Overall, the VEP and behavioral results that we describe are strongly indicative of visual cross-modal re-organization in adults with mild-moderate hearing loss. This is a new finding as previous reports of cross-modal plasticity have been confined to adults with deafness, which was congenital or pre-lingual, and/or in cochlear-implanted adults [13,25,27,51,65,75,76]. The mechanisms of cross-modal plasticity in both deafness and moderate hearing loss have been explored in animal studies. Recent studies suggest that only those cortical areas involved in the sharing of multi-modal information are recruited, and still maintain the functional specificity of the original sensory modality [19,24]. That is, higher-order, multi-modal areas are more susceptible to recruitment when a shared modality is no longer receiving appropriate input. Furthermore, this cross-modal plasticity has been found to take place as a result of moderate hearing loss, and not just profound sensory deprivation [77]. In humans, both audition and vision share object recognition functions in the ventral stream [78,79], and are thus primed for compensatory plasticity in hearing loss. When the listening environment becomes challenging, as in background noise, greater attention to visual objects in the form of processing of faces and lips, may facilitate auditory object recognition. Along these same lines, activation of the ventral stream in adults who have experienced late-onset blindness has been correlated with poor performance in an auditory spatial task [80]. Similarly, resting state studies of pre-lingually deaf cochlear implanted children and post-lingually deaf cochlear implanted children and adults showed ventral activation in patients who had poor speech perception outcomes [66,67]. Thus, it appears that compensatory activation, in either modality, of the cortical auditory-visual ventral stream may be associated with poorer auditory performance.

## Summary and Conclusion

Our study provides new evidence of cross-modal cortical re-organization in adult-onset mild-moderate hearing loss. Increased amplitudes of P1, N1 and P2 VEP components, decreased N1 latency, a novel P2' component and current source density reconstructions reflecting a ventral shift in activation were observed for adults with mild to moderate hearing loss relative to normal hearing controls. Furthermore, we observed a strong negative correlation between cross-modal re-organization (as reflected by decreased N1 latency) and speech perception in noise. Future studies are needed to outline the detailed trajectory of cross-modal changes as hearing declines from a mild hearing loss to deafness. Prospective longitudinal studies will provide important information concerning the timeline of cross-modal re-organization according to severity of hearing loss, including a quantification of the degree or severity of re-organization. In addition, such studies may indicate the effect of clinical interventions, such as amplification or cochlear implantation, in reversing cross-modal re-organization.

## Acknowledgments

We would like to acknowledge Teresa Mitchell, Ph.D, for her comments on a draft of the manuscript.

## Author Contributions

Conceived and designed the experiments: JC AS. Performed the experiments: JC. Analyzed the data: JC AS. Contributed reagents/materials/analysis tools: JC AS. Wrote the paper: JC AS.

## References

1. Kujala T, Alho K, Naatanen R (2000) Cross-modal reorganization of human cortical functions. Trends Neurosci 23(3): 115–20.
2. Roder B, Stock O, Bien S, Neville H, Rosler F (2002) Speech processing activates visual cortex in congenitally blind humans. Eur J Neurosci 16(5): 930–6.
3. Voss P, Gougoux FDR, Lassonde M, Zatorre RJ, Lepore F (2006) A positron emission tomography study during auditory localization by late-onset blind individuals. NeuroReport 17(4): 383–8.
4. Collignon O, Lassonde M, Lepore F, Bastien D, Veraart C (2007) Functional cerebral reorganization for auditory spatial processing and auditory substitution of vision in early blind subjects. Cereb Cortex 17(2): 457–65.
5. Collignon O, Vandewalle G, Voss P, Albouy G, Charbonneau G, et al. (2011) Functional specialization for auditory–spatial processing in the occipital cortex of congenitally blind humans. Proc Natl Acad Sci U S A 108(11): 4435–4440.
6. Watkins KE, Shakespeare TJ, O'Donoghue MC, Alexander I, Ragge N, et al. (2013) Early auditory processing in area V5/MT+ of the congenitally blind brain. J Neurosci 13; 33(46): 18242–18246.
7. Kupers R, Ptito M (2013). Compensatory plasticity and cross-modal reorganization following early visual deprivation. Neurosci Biobehav Rev S01497634(13)00191–197.
8. Sharma A, Dorman MF, Kral A (2005) The influence of a sensitive period on central auditory development in children with unilateral and bilateral cochlear implants. Hear Res 203(1–2): 134–143.
9. Sharma A, Gilley PM, Dorman MF, Baldwin R (2007) Deprivation-induced cortical reorganization in children with cochlear implants. Int J Audiol 46(9): 494–499.
10. Sharma A, Nash AA, Dorman M (2009) Cortical development, plasticity and re-organization in children with cochlear implants. J Commun Disord 42(4): 272–279.
11. Sharma A, Dorman M (2011) Central auditory system development and plasticity after cochlear implantation. In F-G Zeng et al. (Eds.), *Auditory Prostheses: New Horizons* (233–255). Springer Handbook of Auditory Research 39. New York: Springer.
12. Sharma A, Mitchell T (2013) The impact of deafness on the human central auditory and visual systems. In A Kral et al. (Eds.), *Deafness* (189–215). Springer Handbook of Auditory Research 47. New York: Springer.
13. Neville HJ, Lawson D (1987) Attention to central and peripheral visual space in a movement detection task: an event-related potential and behavioral study. II. Congenitally deaf adults. Brain Res 405(2): 268–83.
14. Bavelier D, Tomann A, Hutton C, Mitchell T, Corina D, et al. (2000) Visual attention to the periphery is enhanced in congenitally deaf individuals. J Neurosci 20(17): RC93.
15. Finney EM, Fine I, Dobkins KR (2001) Visual stimuli activate auditory cortex in the deaf. Nat Neurosci 4(12): 1171–3.
16. Neville HJ, Bavelier D (2001) Effects of auditory and visual deprivation on human brain development. Clin Neurosci Res 1(4): 248–57.
17. Finney EM, Clementz BA, Hickok G, Dobkins KR (2003) Visual stimuli activate auditory cortex in deaf subjects: evidence from MEG. NeuroReport 14(11): 1425–7.
18. Bavelier D, Hirshorn EA (2010) I see where you're hearing: how cross-modal plasticity may exploit homologous brain structures. Nat Neurosci 13(11): 1309–11.
19. Lomber SG, Meredith MA, Kral A (2010) Cross-modal plasticity in specific auditory cortices underlies visual compensations in the deaf. Nat Neurosci 13(11): 1421–7.
20. Kral A, Sharma A (2012) Developmental neuroplasticity after cochlear implantation. Trends Neurosci 35(2): 111–22.
21. Meredith MA, Allman BL (2012) Early hearing-impairment results in cross-modal reorganization of ferret core auditory cortex. Neural Plast 2012: 601591.
22. Gilley PM, Sharma A, Dorman MF (2008) Cortical reorganization in children with cochlear implants. Brain Res 1239: 56–65.
23. Kral A (2013) Auditory critical periods: a review from system's perspective. Neuroscience 5; 247: 117–133.
24. Meredith MA, Kryklywy J, McMillan AJ, Malhotra S, Lum-Tai R, et al. (2011) Crossmodal reorganization in the early deaf switches sensory, but not behavioral roles of auditory cortex. Proc Natl Acad Sci U S A 108(21): 8856–61.
25. Doucet ME, Bergeron F, Lassonde M, Ferron P, Lepore F (2006) Cross-modal reorganization and speech perception in cochlear implant users. Brain 129(Pt 12): 3376–83.
26. Buckley KA, Tobey EA (2011) Cross-modal plasticity and speech perception in pre- and postlingually deaf cochlear implant users. Ear Hear (1): 2–15.
27. Vachon P, Voss P, Lassonde M, Leroux J-M, Mensour B, et al. (2013) Reorganization of the auditory, visual and multimodal areas in early deaf individuals. Neuroscience 15; 245: 50–60.
28. Bosworth RG, Dobkins KR (2002) The effects of spatial attention on motion processing in deaf signers, hearing signers, and hearing nonsigners. Brain Cogn 49(1): 152–69.

29. Sandmann P, Dillier N, Eichele T, Meyer M, Kegel A, et al. (2012) Visual activation of auditory cortex reflects maladaptive plasticity in cochlear implant users. Brain 135(2): 555–68.
30. Lazard DS, Vincent C, Venail F, Van de Heyning P, Truy E, et al. (2012) Pre-, per- and postoperative factors affecting performance of postlinguistically deaf adults using cochlear implants: a new conceptual model over time. PLoS ONE 7(11): e48739.
31. Lazard DS, Innes-Brown H, Barone P (2014) Adaptation of the communicative brain to post-lingual deafness. Evidence from functional imaging. Hear Res 307: 136–143.
32. Killion MC, Niquette PA, Gudmundsen GI, Revit LJ, Banerjee S (2004) Development of a quick speech-in-noise test for measuring signal-to-noise ratio loss in normal-hearing and hearing-impaired listeners. J Acoust Soc Am 116(4 Pt 1): 2395–405.
33. Doucet ME, Gosselin F, Lassonde M, Guillemot JP, Lepore F (2005) Development of visual evoked potentials to radially modulated concentric patterns. NeuroReport 16(16): 1753–6.
34. Bertrand J-A, Lassonde M, Robert M, Nguyen DK, Bertone A, et al. (2012) An intracranial event-related potential study on transformational apparent motion. Does its neural processing differ from real motion? Exp Brain Res 216(1): 145–53.
35. Delorme A, Makeig S (2004) EEGLAB: an open source toolbox for analysis of single-trial EEG dynamics including independent component analysis. J Neurosci Methods 134(1): 9–21.
36. Debener S, Ullsperger M, Siegel M, Engel AK (2006) Single-trial EEG–fMRI reveals the dynamics of cognitive function. Trends Cogn. Sci 10(12): 558–63.
37. Debener S, Hine J, Bleeck S, Eyles J (2008) Source localization of auditory evoked potentials after cochlear implantation. Psychophysiology 45(1): 20–4.
38. Makeig S, Jung TP, Bell AJ (1997) Blind separation of auditory event-related brain responses into independent components Proc Natl Acad Sci U S A 94(20): 10979–10984.
39. Makeig S, Delorme A, Westerfield M, Jung TP, Townsend J, et al. (2004) Electroencephalographic brain dynamics following manually responded visual targets. PLoS Biol 2(6): e176.
40. Hine J, Debener S (2007) Late auditory evoked potentials asymmetry revisited. Clin Neurophysiol 118(6): 1274–85.
41. Joos K, Vanneste S, De Ridder D (2012) Disentangling depression and distress networks in the tinnitus brain. PLoS ONE 7(7): e40544.
42. Delorme A, Palmer J, Onton J, Oostenveld R, Makeig S (2012) Independent EEG sources are dipolar. PLoS ONE 7(2): e30135.
43. Fuchs M, Kastner J, Wagner M, Hawes S, Ebersole JS (2002) A standardized boundary element method volume conductor model. Clin Neurophysiol 113(5): 702–12.
44. Pascual-Marqui RD (2002) Standardized low-resolution brain electromagnetic tomography (sLORETA): technical details. Methods Find Exp Clin Pharmacol 24(Suppl. D): 5–12.
45. Grech R, Cassar T, Muscat J (2008) Review on solving the inverse problem in EEG source analysis. JNER 5: 25.
46. Armstrong BA, Neville HJ, Hillyard SA, Mitchell TV (2002) Auditory deprivation affects processing of motion, but not color. Brain Res Cogn Brain Res 14(3): 422–34.
47. Dupont P, Sary G, Peuskens H, Orban GA (2003) Cerebral regions processing first- and higher order motion in an opposed-direction discrimination task. Eur J Neurosci 17(7): 1509–17.
48. Kellermann T, Regenbogen C, De Vos M, Mößnang C, Finkelmeyer A, et al. (2012) Effective connectivity of the human cerebellum during visual attention. J Neurosci 32(33): 11453–60.
49. Wilkinson F, James TW, Wilson HR, Gati JS, Menon RS, et al. (2000) An fMRIstudy of the selective activation of human extrastriate form vision areas by radial and concentric gratings. Curr Biol 10(22): 1455–8.
50. Wilson RH, McArdle RA, Smith SL (2007) An Evaluation of the BKB-SIN, HINT, QuickSIN, and WIN Materials on Listeners With Normal Hearing and Listeners With Hearing Loss. J Speech Lang Hear Res 50(4): 844–56.
51. Neville HJ, Schmidt A, Kutas M (1983) Altered visual-evoked potentials in congenitally deaf adults. Brain Res 266(1): 127–32.
52. Tong Y, Melara RD, Rao A (2009) P2 enhancement from auditory discrimination training is associated with improved reaction times. Brain Res 1297: 80–8.
53. George EM, Coch D (2011) Music training and working memory: an ERP study. Neuropsychologia 49(5): 1083–1094.
54. Allison T, Puce A, Spencer DD, McCarthy G (1999) Electrophysiological studies of human face perception. I: Potentials generated in occipitotemporal cortex by face and non-face stimuli. Cereb Cortex 9(5): 415–30.
55. Andics A, McQueen JM, Petersson KM, Gál V, Rudas G, et al. (2010) Neural mechanisms for voice recognition. NeuroImage 52(4): 1528–40.
56. Pasley BN, David SV, Mesgarani N, Flinker A (2012) Reconstructing speech from human auditory cortex. PLoS biology 10(1): e1001251.
57. Campbell J, Sharma A (2013) Compensatory changes in cortical resource allocation in adults with hearing loss. Front Syst Neurosci 7: 71.
58. Puce A, Allison T, McCarthy G (1999) Electrophysiological studies of human face perception. III: Effects of top-down processing on face-specific potentials. Cereb Cortex 9(5): 445–458.
59. Nasr S, Tootell RBH (2012) Role of fusiform and anterior temporal cortical areas in facial recognition. NeuroImage 63(3): 1743–53.
60. McCullough S, Emmorey K, Sereno M (2005) Neural organization for recognition of grammatical and emotional facial expressions in deaf ASL signers and hearing nonsigners. Brain Res Cogn Brain Res 22(2): 193–203.
61. Sadato N, Okada T, Honda M, Matsuki K, Yoshida M, et al. (2005) Cross modal integration and plastic changes revealed by lip movement, random-dot motion and sign languages in the hearing and deaf. Cereb Cortex 15(8): 1113–22.
62. Woodhouse L, Hickson L (2009) Review of visual speech perception by hearing and hearing-impaired people: clinical implications. Int J Lang Commun Disord 44(3): 253–70.
63. Letourneau SM, Mitchell TV (2011) Gaze patterns during identity and emotion judgments in hearing adults and deaf users of American Sign Language. Perception 40: 563–575.
64. Rouger J, Lagleyre S, Démonet J-F, Fraysse B, Deguine O, et al. (2012) Evolution of crossmodal reorganization of the voice area in cochlear-implanted deaf patients. Hum Brain Mapp 33(8): 1929–40.
65. Strelnikov K, Rouger J, Demonet JF, Lagleyre S, Fraysse B, et al. (2013) Visual activity predicts auditory recovery from deafness after adult cochlear implantation. Brain 136(12): 3682–3695.
66. Giraud AL, Lee HJ (2007) Predicting cochlear implant outcome from brain organisation in the deaf. Restor Neurol Neurosci 25(3–4): 381–90.
67. Lee HJ, Giraud AL, Kang E, Oh SH, Kang H, et al. (2007) Cortical activity at rest predicts cochlear implantation outcome. Cereb Cortex 17(4): 909–17.
68. Souza PE, Boike KT, Witherell K, Tremblay K (2007) Prediction of Speech Recognition from Audibility in Older Listeners with Hearing Loss: Effects of Age, Amplification, and Background Noise. J AM Acad Audiol 18: 54–65.
69. Anderson S, Kraus N (2010) Sensory-Cognitive Interaction in the Neural Encoding of Speech in Noise: A Review. J AM Acad Audiol 21(9): 575–85.
70. Gifford RH, Revit LJ (2010) Speech perception for adult cochlear implant recipients in a realistic background noise: effectiveness of preprocessing strategies and external options for improving speech recognition in noise. J AM Acad Audiol 21(7): 441-51-quiz487-8.
71. Dubno JR (1984) Effects of age and mild hearing loss on speech recognition in noise. J Acoust Soc Am 76(1): 87–96.
72. Vermiglio AJ, Soli SD, Freed DJ, Fisher LM (2012) The relationship between high frequency pure-tone hearing loss, hearing in noise test (HINT) thresholds, and the articulation index. J AM Acad Audiol 23(10): 779–88.
73. Hornsby BW, Johnson EE, Picou E (2011) Effects of degree and configuration of hearing loss on the contribution of high- and low-frequency speech information to bilateral speech understanding. Ear Hear 32(5): 543–55.
74. Moore BC (1996) Perceptual consequences of cochlear hearing loss and their implications for the design of hearing aids. Ear Hear 17(2): 133–61.
75. Lazard DS, Lee HJ, Gaebler M, Kell CA, Truy E, et al. (2010) Phonological processing in post-lingual deafness and cochlear implant outcome. NeuroImage 49(4): 3443–51.
76. Lazard DS, Lee HJ, Truy E, Giraud AL (2013) Bilateral reorganization of posterior temporal cortices in post-lingual deafness and its relation to cochlear implant outcome. Hum Brain Mapp 34(5): 1208–1219.
77. Meredith MA, Keniston LP, Allman BL (2012) Multisensory dysfunction accompanies crossmodal plasticity following adult hearing impairment. Neuroscience 214: 136–48.
78. Rauschecker JP (2012) Ventral and dorsal streams in the evolution of speech and language. Front Evol Neurosci 4: 7.
79. Schirmer A, Fox PM, Grandjean D (2012) On the spatial organization of sound processing in the human temporal lobe: a meta-analysis. NeuroImage 63(1): 137–47.
80. Voss P, Gougoux F, Zatorre RJ, Lassonde M, Lepore F (2008) Differential occipital responses in early- and late-blind individuals during a sound-source discrimination task. NeuroImage 40: 746–758.

# Classification of Fricative Consonants for Speech Enhancement in Hearing Devices

**Ying-Yee Kong[1,2*], Ala Mullangi[2], Kostas Kokkinakis[3]**

**1** Department of Speech Language Pathology & Audiology, Northeastern University, Boston, Massachusetts, United States of America, **2** Bioengineering Program, Northeastern University, Boston, Massachusetts, United States of America, **3** Department of Speech-Language-Hearing, University of Kansas, Lawrence, Kansas, United States of America

## Abstract

***Objective:*** To investigate a set of acoustic features and classification methods for the classification of three groups of fricative consonants differing in place of articulation.

***Method:*** A support vector machine (SVM) algorithm was used to classify the fricatives extracted from the TIMIT database in quiet and also in speech babble noise at various signal-to-noise ratios (SNRs). Spectral features including four spectral moments, peak, slope, Mel-frequency cepstral coefficients (MFCC), Gammatone filters outputs, and magnitudes of fast Fourier Transform (FFT) spectrum were used for the classification. The analysis frame was restricted to only 8 msec. In addition, commonly-used linear and nonlinear principal component analysis dimensionality reduction techniques that project a high-dimensional feature vector onto a lower dimensional space were examined.

***Results:*** With 13 MFCC coefficients, 14 or 24 Gammatone filter outputs, classification performance was greater than or equal to 85% in quiet and at +10 dB SNR. Using 14 Gammatone filter outputs above 1 kHz, classification accuracy remained high (greater than 80%) for a wide range of SNRs from +20 to +5 dB SNR.

***Conclusions:*** High levels of classification accuracy for fricative consonants in quiet and in noise could be achieved using only spectral features extracted from a short time window. Results of this work have a direct impact on the development of speech enhancement algorithms for hearing devices.

**Editor:** Fan-Gang Zeng, University of California, Irvine, United States of America

**Funding:** This work was supported by NIH/NIDCD R01-DC-012300 to Y-YK. The funders had no role in study design, data collection and analysis, decision to publish, or preparation of the manuscript.

**Competing Interests:** The authors have declared that no competing interests exist.

* E-mail: yykong@neu.edu

## Introduction

A common configuration of hearing loss is high-frequency hearing loss, which affects the perception of speech sounds that have mostly high-frequency (2000–10000 Hz) energy, such as fricative consonants. There are a total of nine fricative consonants in English: /f, θ, s, ʃ, v, ð, z, ʒ, h/, and eight of them (all except for/h/) are produced by partially obstructing the airflow through the oral cavity. These fricative consonants differ in terms of the point of constriction in the vocal tract (i.e., place of articulation) – labiodental/f, v/; interdental/θ, ð/; alveolar/s, z/; and palatal/ʃ, ʒ/. Within each place, the fricatives differ in regard to the absence (voiceless) or presence (voiced) of the vocal fold vibration – voiceless/f, θ, s, ʃ/; and voiced/v, ð, z, ʒ/. Note also that the greatest spectral difference between voiced and voiceless phonemes is mainly at the low-frequency region below 1000 Hz where the voiced fricatives have higher energy at low frequencies compared to their voiceless counterparts. Given the large number of fricative consonants in the English language, perceptual deficits in this class of sounds could severely reduce oral communication especially in noisy listening environments.

### Effect of Hearing Loss on Fricative Perception

Previous studies have reported that there are multiple cues to the perception of fricatives, including the spectral differences in the fricative noise and lower frequency energy in the transition from fricative noise to the adjacent vowel [1–3]. Zeng and Turner [2] reported that adults with hearing loss rely primarily on fricative noise for the discrimination of voiceless fricatives, and their conclusion was further supported by recent work by Stelmachowicz et al. [4]. It has been shown that reduced audibility and spectral resolution at high frequency due to hearing loss significantly impaired listeners' ability to discriminate fricative consonants [5].

### Signal Processing to Enhance Perception of High-Frequency Speech Components

Signal processing techniques that increase the audibility of fricative sounds or spectral differences among fricatives could enhance speech perception performance in hearing-impaired listeners. To enhance listeners' ability to perceive high-frequency fricative content, recent research reported a significant benefit for speech recognition in hearing-impaired individuals with high-frequency amplification above 4 kHz compared to amplification only up to 4 kHz. For example, Stelmachowicz et al. [4] provided spectral cues up to 9 kHz to hearing-impaired adults and children with moderate to moderately severe hearing loss (i.e., between 40 and 70 dB HL) at 2 and 4 kHz. They reported that although the perception of the fricative/s/in quiet improved with increasing stimulus bandwidth, fricative perception performance remained significantly poorer for hearing-impaired than for normal-hearing listeners.

While extended high-frequency amplification could provide benefit for aidable hearing loss, for individuals who have severe-to-profound high-frequency hearing loss, signal processing strategies that lower high-frequency speech components to a lower-frequency region, such as frequency compression [6] or frequency transposition [7] have been recommended. While most algorithms utilized in hearing aids lower the high-frequency phonemes by a fixed ratio or by a constant for all speech sounds, others operate conditionally on nonsonorant consonants (i.e., fricatives, affricates, and stops) for frequency lowering [8–9].

Recent work in our laboratory [10–11] explored a method of frequency lowering that targets nonsonorant consonants and also enhances the spectral contrasts of the frequency-lowered fricatives. This speech enhancement method involves classification of fricative consonants followed by spectral shaping of the frequency-lowered signals based on the classification results. Here, we describe the conceptual framework of this algorithm, which prompted the investigation of fricative classification in the current study, along with a summary of the perceptual results from hearing-impaired listeners. The aforementioned frequency-lowering algorithm is described in more detail in Kong and Mullangi [11].

*A Vocoder-Based Frequency-Lowering System with Spectral Enhancement*: The vocoder-based frequency-lowering algorithm developed by Kong and Mullangi [10–11] is divided into analysis and processing stages. During the analysis stage, input signals are first bandpass-filtered into a number of frequency bands. The filtered signals are then subjected to an analysis that separates speech sounds into two classes, sonorants and nonsonorants. Only the nonsonorant sounds, which contain aperiodic high-frequency energy, will proceed to a second analysis that separates high-frequency frication sounds into three groups. Once classified, the nonsonorant sounds undergo frequency lowering via channel vocoding by which the amplitude of the high-frequency bands is used to amplitude modulate bands of low-frequency noise, which is added to the original speech signal. To enhance the spectral differences of the transposed signal for fricative perception, the spectrum of the low-frequency noise used in the system is determined by the classification results. With an earlier prototype of the system with fricative classification accuracy at about 88% on VCV syllables in quiet, Kong and Mullangi [11] reported that listeners with steeply-sloping high-frequency hearing loss received significant benefit for place-of-articulation perception for fricative consonants in quiet.

Since the spectral enhancement method described above selectively processes specific classes of phonemes, its success hinges on the accuracy of classification of speech sounds. The goal of this study is to further investigate acoustic features and classification methods that could separate fricative consonants into separate classes that differ in place of articulation with high levels of accuracy in quiet and also in noise. Although dynamic or relational features including relative amplitude between the fricative consonant and the adjacent vowel(s), duration of the fricative consonants, and relative amplitude of fricatives, have been shown to contribute to the correct classification of place of articulation in fricatives, only static acoustic features extracted within a very short time window were considered in the current study to allow for a real-time signal processing implementation in hearing devices. Previous research has shown that processing delay of less than 10 msec is necessary for hearing aids in order to preserve the sound quality and to prevent the user's perception of his or her own voice [12–13]. Thus, in this study, we used a short time window of 8 msec, which is well within the limit set by the industry. Among the static acoustic properties, combinations of spectral features including spectral slope, spectral peak location, and four spectral moments [14–17], were found to be robust features for separating fricatives into three groups. Previous studies and our own preliminary analyses did not find static features that could reliably separate the non-sibilant fricatives further into two groups (labiodental and inter-dental fricatives). It was shown that normal-hearing listeners use formant transition cues to perceptually discriminate labiodental and interdental fricatives. Also, at high frequencies, both voiced and voiceless fricatives have the similar patterns of spectral shape that are distinctive among fricatives differing in place of articulation. In addition, this work considers more realistic communication situations often encountered by users of listening devices, which include (1) speech recognition in quiet and in noisy situations at different signal-to-noise ratios (SNRs) and (2) variations of acoustic characteristics due to talker differences.

In this paper, we present and compare classification results of fricative sounds using a support vector machine (SVM) algorithm. Various acoustic static features, including the previously reported spectral features (i.e., spectral moments, peak, and slope), bandpass-filtered outputs, magnitude of fast Fourier Transform (FFT), and Mel-frequency cepstral coefficients (MFCCs) are investigated. Our results show high levels of fricative classification performance with spectral features extracted from a relatively short time frame. This suggests that the frication noise contains sufficient information about the identity of the fricative consonants, and that our classification methods have potential clinical applications on the future development of speech enhancement in hearing devices.

## Methods

### Speech materials

The classification experiments were performed on fricative consonants extracted from a TIMIT database [18], which contains a total of 6,300 continuous sentences spoken by 639 speakers from eight dialect regions in the United States. The sentences were recorded in a noise-free environment with a sampling rate of 16 kHz and 16-bit resolution. The TIMIT database is divided into training and testing sets. The core testing set in the database has a total of 168 speakers, resulting in a total of 1,344 sentences. In our experiments, the audio files were first scaled to have equal root-mean-squared (RMS) amplitude across all sentences in both the training and testing set. Additionally, the RMS-equalized TIMIT sentences were corrupted with two different types of noise. The level of the noise was adjusted depending on the pre-determined SNR test conditions for each experiment. For the training set, clean speech was corrupted with speech-shaped noise (SSN) at +10 dB SNR. To approximate the long-term average spectra of adult speech [19], the SSN was created by lowpass-filtering white noise with a first-order Butterworth filter using a cutoff frequency of 800 Hz. The use of this generic type of SSN allows for greater generalization of the classifier to other real-life listening situations. For the testing set, clean speech was corrupted with a 12-talker speech babble noise [20] at seven different SNRs (+20, +15, +10, +5, 0, −5, −10 dB). The rationale behind using different types of noise was to create a mismatch in the training and testing environments. The choice of multi-talker speech babble noise was motivated mainly by its ecological relevance. For each sentence and for each SNR condition, the clean speech was mixed with a different time segment of the speech babble noise. Each fricative was then extracted from the clean and noisy sentences using the TIMIT phone labels and transcription boundaries.

## Feature extraction for fricatives differing in place of articulation

Several types of static acoustic features have been shown to be different among the three classes of fricatives. Motivated by existing literature [14], [15], and [17], we examined six spectral features, including four spectral moments (i.e., mean [M1], variance [M2], skewness [M3], kurtosis [M4]), dominant spectral peak location (P), and spectral slope (S) for a subset of fricative tokens in the TIMIT training set, which were used for classification as will be described in the "Classification Procedure" section. Acoustical and statistical analyses were performed to confirm that these features are indeed discriminative among the fricative groups.

Spectral analyses on the six acoustic features were performed on clean speech using a 128-point FFT in the frequency range from 1kHz to 8 kHz. The upper frequency of 8 kHz was limited by the sampling rate of the recorded speech materials. Information was extracted from a randomly chosen 8-msec segment using a hamming window of the fricative tokens, and acoustical analyses were performed on each of these 8-msec segments. The mathematical description of the four moments can be found in Forrest et al. [21] and Maniwa & Jongman [17]. Spectral peak location (P) is defined as the frequency that corresponds to the highest amplitude peak of the FFT spectrum. Spectral slope is computed here as the difference between the highest and lowest amplitude of the FFT spectrum divided by the corresponding difference in the frequency. Each acoustic measurement was first examined to determine its contribution in the fricative classification using a Kruskal-Wallis test. This non-parametric test was used because the assumption of normality was not met for some of the acoustic features examined. Table 1 shows the measured median values for each feature for each fricative type along with statistical results. As indicated by the *p*-values in this table, the values of the acoustic features were significantly different between the three groups of fricatives. Hence, combinations of these features were included in the classification experiments.

Besides the well-documented acoustic features described above, we investigated additional three groups of features described below. Again, for training of the classifiers, the acoustic features were extracted from a randomly chosen 8-msec segment of the fricative tokens using a hamming window, and acoustical analyses were performed on each of the 8-msec segments. The upper frequency was restricted to 8 kHz limited by the sampling rate of the recorded speech.

**(1) Two versions of MFCCs – MFCC(3) and MFCC(13).** MFCC(3) denotes the first three coefficients of the 3 cepstra without derivatives and MFCC(13) denotes 13 cepstra without derivatives. MFCC(3) represents the first three coefficients of MFCC(13). The MFCCs were extracted using the VOICEBOX toolkit [22].

**(2) Gammatone filter outputs.** Two feature vectors of outputs of bands of Gammatone filters. One vector consisted of outputs of 14 filters [Gammatone(14)] at the high-frequency above 1 kHz, and the other consisted of 24 filter outputs [Gammatone(24)] for the wide frequency spectrum above 0.1 kHz. Gammatone(14) is a subset of Gammatone(24).

**(3) Magnitude spectrum of FFT.** The magnitudes of 128-point FFT at each frequency bin were calculated in the frequency range from 0.1 to 8 kHz.

Given that the numbers of dimensions are high for the Gammatone(24) and FFT feature vectors, dimensionality reduction techniques that project the high-dimensional feature vector onto a lower dimensional space were used to enable the classifier to achieve improved generalization through: (1) eliminating redundant dimensions that may not convey reliable information for the classification, (2) determining a manifold that exhibit maximal information about the class label, and (3) avoiding over-fitting from the classifier [23]. For signal processing in real-time, decreasing the number of dimensions of the feature vector could result in a considerable reduction of the overall processing time. For a high-dimensional feature vector $x \in R^n$, the aim is to determine a smooth mapping function $\boldsymbol{f}: \mathrm{R}^n \rightarrow \mathrm{R}^m$ where m<n such that the reduced dimensional feature vector is $y = \boldsymbol{f(x)}$. In this study, we investigated both linear and nonlinear projections to achieve the optimal manifold.

For linear dimensionality reduction (LDR), a commonly-used variable reduction technique referred to as principal component analysis (PCA) was used to map the data to a lower-dimensional space [24]. The data is transformed to orthogonal axes corresponding to the direction of the maximum variance in the original data space such that the first few dimensions of the new space account for the majority of variance in the data. For a random vector $x_k \in R^n$, the mean of each of the features is adjusted to 0 using Eq. (1):

$$\sum_{k=1}^{l} x_k = 0 \qquad (1)$$

where $l$ is the number of points in the dataset.

The covariance matrix of $x$ given by Eq. (2) is computed to obtain the eigenvalues and eigenvectors:

$$C = \frac{1}{l} \sum_{k=1}^{l} x_k \, x_k{}' \qquad (2)$$

To reduce the number of dimensions from $\boldsymbol{n}$ to $\boldsymbol{m}$, the eigenvectors corresponding to $\boldsymbol{m}$ largest eigenvalues of the covariance matrix are used for approximating the original $\boldsymbol{n}$-dimensional vector. $\boldsymbol{m}$ is determined by the number of eigenvalues that exceed a pre-determined threshold.

For nonlinear dimensionality reduction (NLDR), we adapted a projection technique using a kernel PCA [25]. A kernel PCA first

**Table 1. Median values and Kruskal-Wallis test results (*p*-values) for six acoustic features for the training set.**

| Measurements | /f, θ, v, ð/ | /s, z/ | /ʃ, ʒ/ | *p*-value |
|---|---|---|---|---|
| M1 (Hz) | 3,989 | 4,909 | 4,117 | < 0.0001 |
| M2 (MHz) | 3.89 | 2.47 | 2.55 | < 0.0001 |
| M3 | 0.31 | −0.11 | 0.58 | <0.0001 |
| M4 | −0.95 | −0.14 | −0.39 | <0.0001 |
| P (Hz) | 1,750 | 4,625 | 3,250 | <0.0001 |
| S | −0.008 | 0.011 | −0.006 | <0.0001 |

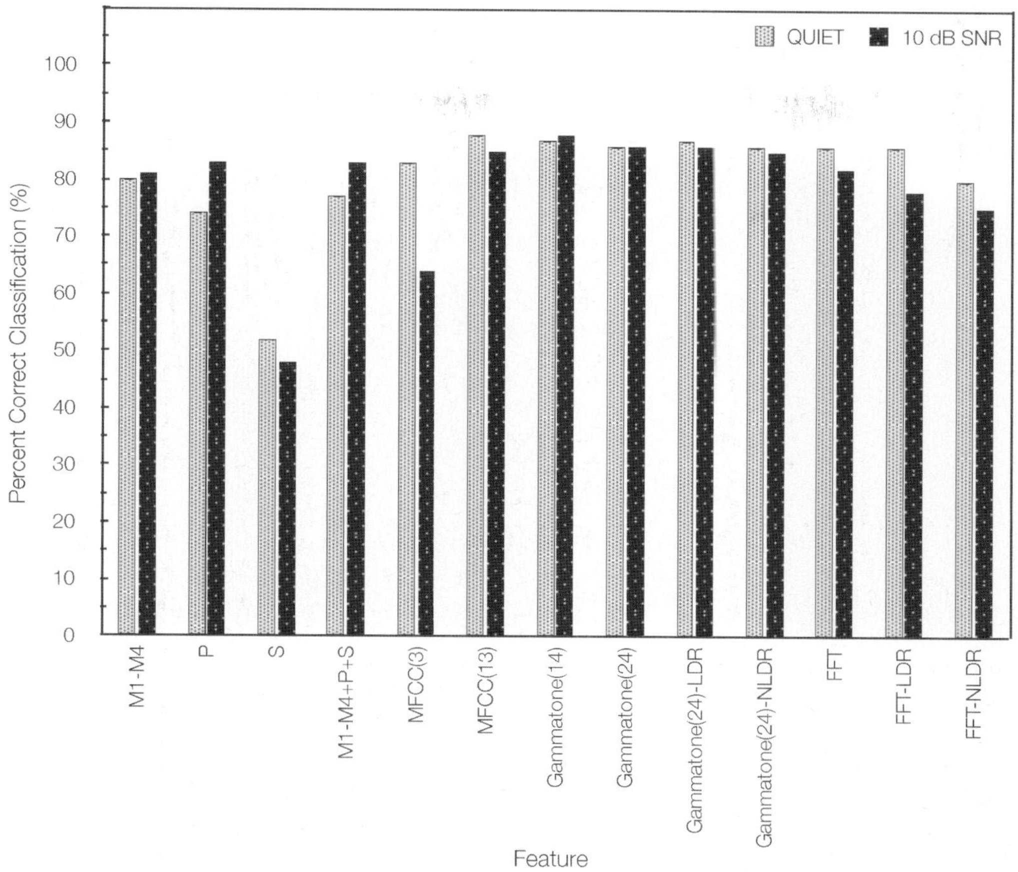


**Figure 1. Overall classification accuracy in quiet and at +10 dB SNR with different of features.**

projects the data into a feature space by calculating the kernel matrix (described below) such that a nonlinear function is applied to the original data with a reduced computational cost. A PCA can be then performed on the projected data. Let $\Phi$ be a nonlinear function that projects the random vector $\boldsymbol{x_k}$ into a feature space $F$ to obtain $\Phi(\boldsymbol{x_k})$. A kernel matrix ($K$) is calculated as in Eq. (3).

$$K = \Phi(x_i)\Phi(x_j) \tag{3}$$

where $i$ and $j$ index the row and the column in the matrix, respectively, and that both $i$ and $j$ vary from 1 to $l$.

To obtain a centered kernel matrix with a zero mean, a Gram matrix is computed using Eq. (4).

$$\hat{K} = K - 1_l K - K 1_l + 1_l K 1_l \tag{4}$$

where $1_l$ is an $l$x$l$ matrix with all elements equal to $1/l$.

Once projected to the nonlinear space, procedures for dimensionality reduction follow the principles of PCA as described above. The eigenvectors computed from the Gram matrix are taken as the kernel principal components.

## Classification Procedure

A one-stage classification procedure with a SVM algorithm was used for classifying fricatives into three groups. The MATLAB library LIBSVM described in Chang & Lin [26] was employed to perform a multi-class classification using a one-against-one strategy.

We used a subset of fricatives contained in the TIMIT training set to train the classifiers, and all fricatives in the TIMIT core testing set during the testing of the classifiers. The fricatives chosen for the training phase were sampled from a subset of speakers in all dialects in the TIMIT training set. The numbers of training tokens were similar across fricative groups. For training, acoustic information from a randomly chosen 8-msec segment of the fricative tokens was used. Given that the spectrum of the frication noise is relatively stable over the entire fricative consonant [14], random samples from each fricative token should provide a good representation of the fricatives for a large number of speakers while keeping the size of the training set manageable. The resulting numbers of fricative samples were 1,864 for the labio/inter-dental fricative group, 1,648 for the alveolar fricative group, and 1,455 for the palatal fricative group. Feature vectors were extracted from each of the 8-msec speech segments. During the training phase, the clean speech tokens and the tokens that were corrupted with SSN at +10 dB SNR in the training set were passed on as inputs to the SVM classifier.

In our preliminary study with a smaller number of speech tokens, we investigated a number of kernel types and kernel functions. We concluded that the C-support vector classification (C-SVC) kernel type and the radial basis kernel function (RBF) yielded the best performance. Thus, we used the C-SVC and RBF in this study. During a grid search in the training phase, the C parameter of the C-SVC and the gamma parameter of the RBF were selected using a cross validation procedure [27].

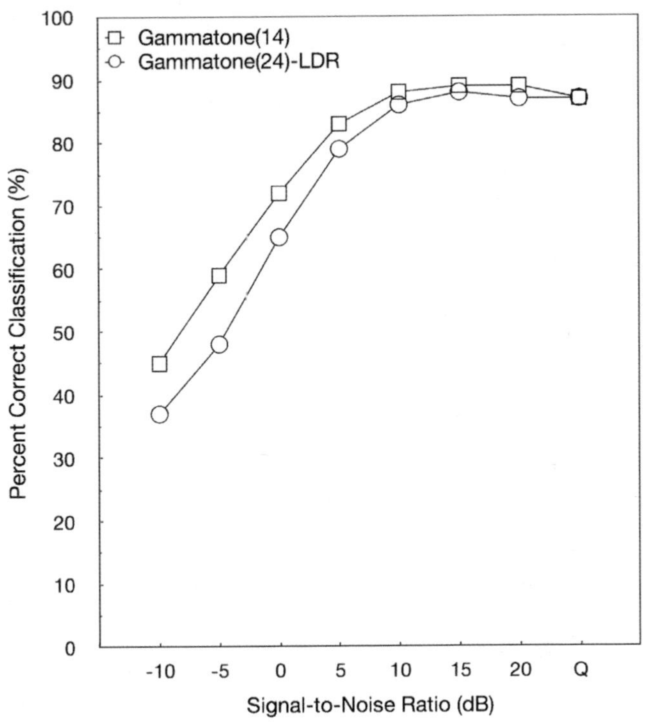


**Figure 2. Overall fricative classification accuracy in quiet and at seven SNRs ranging from +20 to −10 dB using Gammatone(14) and Gammatone(24)-LDR.**

After the SVM classifier was trained, classification was performed on all the fricative tokens in the TIMIT testing set. Similar to the training phase, classification was made for every 8-msec segment of the fricative consonants. Classification was performed on speech tokens in quiet, as well as on speech tokens corrupted with speech babble noise at different SNRs. To summarize the performance of the classifiers, classification accuracy reported below was determined on a consonant-by-consonant basis, in which the majority vote was taken as label for the sequence [28–30]. This means that the fricative group corresponding to the most frequently selected group across the 8-msec frames concluded the classification of the consonant. Overall classification accuracy for the fricative tokens in the testing set was calculated as the proportion of the fricatives correctly identified. This approach, as opposed to the calculation of the accuracy frame-by-frame, allows for a comparison of our results with findings from other studies [15], [28].

## Classification Results

### Comparisons of Features

Figure 1 shows the overall classification accuracy achieved using various features. As supported by the statistical results, the knowledge-based acoustic features (i.e., moments, peak location, and slope) yielded an above chance-level performance for both quiet and +10 dB SNR conditions. On the basis of Bernoulli fluctuations at the performance levels of 50%–90% and over 6,500 trials, the width of 95% confidence interval for each measure is less than 2.5 percentage points. The results showed that including the peak location and slope features did not significantly enhance the classification accuracy of moment features, as the M1-4+P+S condition (77% in Q and 83% in noise) produced similar percent correct scores to the M1-4 condition (80% in Q and 81% in noise).

There was no considerable difference in classification performance among the MFCC(13), Gammatone(14), Gammatone(24) features, with percent accuracy at 86%–88% in quiet and 85%–88% in noise. In comparison, classification accuracy using the FFT feature was slightly lower in noise (82%). The results of MFCC(3) were significantly lower in both quiet (83%) and noise (64%) conditions than those obtained by MFCC(13). For Gammatone(24), classification results were similar with and without dimensionality reduction, and the two reduction methods (linear vs. nonlinear) produced similar classification accuracy. It is noted that the resulting dimensions were 6 and 7 for the linear and nonlinear reduction, respectively. In contrast, dimensionality reduction decreased the classification accuracy for the FFT feature

**Table 2. Confusion matrices for fricative classification in quiet and at three SNRs using Gammatone(14).**

| **Clean speech: 87% accuracy** | **Detected as/f, θ, v, ð/** | **Detected as/s, z/** | **Detected as/ʃ, ʒ/** |
|---|---|---|---|
| /f, θ, v, ð/ | 85% | 11% | 4% |
| /s, z/ | 1% | 87% | 12% |
| /ʃ, ʒ/ | 1% | 10% | 89% |
| *+15 dB SNR: 89% accuracy* | Detected as/f, θ, v, ð/ | Detected as/s, z/ | Detected as/ʃ, ʒ/ |
| /f, θ, v, ð/ | 95% | 4% | 1% |
| /s, z/ | 3% | 89% | 8% |
| /ʃ, ʒ/ | 3% | 13% | 84% |
| *+10 dB SNR: 88% accuracy* | Detected as/f, θ, v, ð/ | Detected as/s, z/ | Detected as/ʃ, ʒ/ |
| /f, θ, v, ð/ | 97% | 2% | 1% |
| /s, z/ | 6% | 87% | 7% |
| /ʃ, ʒ/ | 5% | 15% | 80% |
| *+5 dB SNR: 83% accuracy* | Detected as/f, θ, v, ð/ | Detected as/s, z/ | Detected as/ʃ, ʒ/ |
| /f, θ, v, ð/ | 98% | 2% | 0% |
| /s, z/ | 14% | 81% | 5% |
| /ʃ, ʒ/ | 13% | 17% | 70% |

with the nonlinear reduction (reduced to 5 dimensions) showed a greater detrimental effect than linear reduction (reduced to 4 dimensions).

Overall classification accuracy was generally higher with MFCC, Gammatone, and FFT features when compared to that obtained with the spectral moments, peak, and slope features. For example, classification accuracy was higher with Gammatone(14) compared to the other six acoustic features combined (i.e., M1-4+P+S) by 10 percentage points in quiet and 5 percentage points in noise.

## Classification at Different Signal-to-Noise Ratios

Given that classification accuracy at +10 dB SNR was high for Gammatone features and Gammatone filters are commonly used in auditory modeling, a follow up classification experiment was performed using Gammatone(14) and Gammatone(24)-LDR on fricative consonants that were corrupted with speech babble noise at SNRs ranging from +20 down to -10 dB. Similar to the experiment described above, the SVM classifier was trained with both clean speech and speech materials that were corrupted with SSN at +10 dB SNR. Figure 2 plots the overall fricative classification accuracy. Results showed that classification performance was on average 9 percentage points higher for Gammatone(14) than for Gammatone(24)-LDR at lower SNRs from 0 dB to -10 dB, suggesting that the discriminative features for classification of three groups of fricatives are primarily centered at high frequencies above 1 kHz. Using the Gammatone(14) feature, classification accuracy remained greater than 80% for SNR conditions from +20 dB SNR down to +5 dB SNR, despite the fact that the noise for training (SSN) and testing (12-talker babble) were different. As the level of the noise increased, more sibilant fricatives/s, z, ʃ, ʒ/were identified as non-sibilant fricatives/f, v, θ, ð/. Table 2 shows the confusion matrices for each group of fricatives in quiet and for three noise levels (+15 dB SNR, +10 dB SNR, and +5 dB SNR) using the Gammatone(14) feature.

## Summary and Discussion

The present study examined acoustic features for classification of fricative consonants that differ in place of articulation. Among the features examined, MFCC(13), Gammatone(14), and Gammatone(24) produced similar classification results in quiet and at +10 dB SNR. A subsequent analysis showed that Gammatone(14) yielded a high level of classification accuracy even at challenging noise conditions, down to +5 dB SNR.

## Classification Accuracy

For clean (uncorrupted) speech, the MFCC(13), Gammatone, and FFT features achieved 86%–88% correct classification, a similar level of performance to that reported in the literature [14–

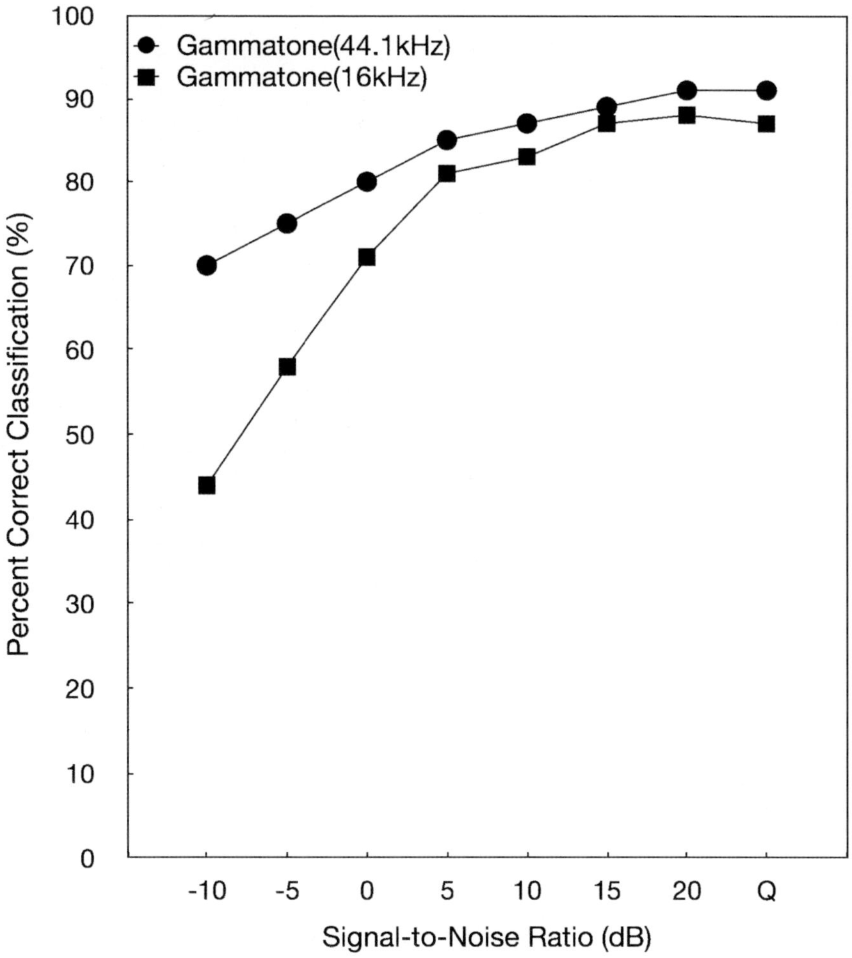


**Figure 3. Overall fricative classification accuracy observed in quiet and at seven SNRs ranging from +20 to −10 dB of speech materials with sampling rates equal to 16 kHz and 44.1 kHz.**

16]. For example, using a knowledge-based decision-tree-like algorithm, Ali et al. [15] reported 91% accuracy for classifying fricative consonants into three groups. Previous studies reported results similar to the present study using an artificial neural network [15] and a linear discriminant analysis [14], [16]. However, relational features, such as relative amplitude between the fricative consonant and the neighboring vowel were used in these studies. Without the relational feature, Ali et al. [15] reported an 87% correct classification for fricatives in quiet when the classifier was trained and tested on the same set of speech materials. Recently, Frid & Lavner [28] resorted to an SVM algorithm and a set of 15 features that included spectral peak, spectral moments, and MFCC(3) to classify fricatives into four groups and reported an accuracy of 85%. It is noted that only four voiceless fricatives/f, θ, s, ʃ/were considered in the Frid & Lavner [28] study, without including the voiced fricatives/v, ð, z, ʒ/.

For noisy speech, the SVM algorithm with the Gammatone(14) feature achieved correct classification greater than 80% for SNRs from +20 dB to +5 dB SNR. It is important to note that (1) both clean and noisy speech were used for the training, (2) the noise was different between training and testing, and (3) the classifier was trained with noisy speech at only one SNR condition (+10 dB SNR), but was tested on seven SNR conditions (from +20 to −10 dB SNR). In other words, the training and testing environments were mismatched.

### Effect of Dimensionality Reduction

Two methods of dimensionality reduction – linear and nonlinear projections – were investigated to lower the dimensions of the high-dimensional feature vectors for our dataset. The purpose of this was to determine the most discriminative dimensions and also reduce the processing time for classification. Our results showed that, depending on the feature vector, classification performance with nonlinear projection was either similar to that with linear projection [Gammatone(24)] or slightly lower than the classification accuracy obtained with linear projection (FFT).

When comparing performance with the feature vector containing only high frequencies, our results showed that classification performance was on average 9 percentage points higher for Gammatone(14) than for Gammatone(24)-LDR at lower SNRs from −10 dB to 0 dB, suggesting that the discriminative features for classification of three groups of fricatives in speech babble noise are primarily at high frequencies above 1 kHz.

### Importance of Spectral Information above 8 kHz

The TIMIT sentences used in the current study have a relatively low sampling rate of 16 kHz, which could have a negative effect on the fricative classification accuracy. Previous research reported spectral differences among three groups of fricatives for frequencies above 8 kHz [10], [16], and [31]. Thus, we hypothesize that classification accuracy would improve for speech materials with a higher sampling rate that allows for data analysis at high frequencies, because a possible cue for discrimination between alveolar and palatal fricatives is the high-frequency fall-off, which is usually above 8 kHz. Another cue for discrimination between sibilant and non-sibilant fricatives is the spectral slope above 8 kHz [10].

To demonstrate the importance of high-frequency information above 8 kHz on fricative classification, we conducted a small-scale classification study using speech materials with a sampling rate of 44.1 kHz. The recorded speech materials included 8 fricative stimuli in/vowel-consonant-vowel/utterances with three vowels (/a, i, u/), resulting in a total of 24 syllables. These stimuli were spoken three times (three repetitions) by each of 14 speakers (six male adults, six female adults, one male child age 11, and one female child age 11), resulting in a total of 1,008 tokens. The adult speakers were taken from the recordings in Shannon et al. [32] and the two child speakers were recorded in our laboratory. The RMS amplitude of all stimuli was equalized to the same value. We divided the stimuli into two sets: training set and test set. The training set contained speech stimuli from four adult males and four adult females. The test set contained the stimuli from the remaining speakers (two male adults, two female adults, one male child, and one female child). Similar to the experiments described above, the classifier was trained with clean and noisy speech with SSN at +10 dB SNR, and was tested with clean and noisy speech with multi-talker babble noise for a wide range of SNRs. Acoustic features used for the classifier included outputs of Gammatone filters above 1 kHz. In one condition, the recorded speech materials were down-sampled to 16 kHz, which limits the upper frequency for analysis to 8 kHz. In another condition, the originally recorded stimuli at a sampling rate of 44.1 kHz were used, which allows for acoustic analysis for frequencies above 8 kHz.

Figure 3 shows the percent classification accuracy in quiet and for SNRs from −10 dB to +20 dB for the two sampling rate conditions. Classification accuracy increased as the sampling rate increased from 16 to 44.1 kHz, and improvement was greater with an average increase of 17 percentage points for lower SNRs at 0, −5, and −10 dB.

### Application to Signal Processing for Hearing Devices

The results in the present study suggest that the proposed classification method that uses only static acoustic features extracted from an 8-msec time frame could potentially be implemented in real-time for potential use in hearing aid devices and other auditory prostheses. The earlier prototype of our frequency lowering algorithm [10], [11] used different methods (i.e., pre-determined thresholds, linear discriminant analysis) and different acoustic features to classify fricative consonants, and the classification accuracy was lower than that reported in the current study. In preliminary perceptual studies conducted with hearing-impaired listeners, discrimination of fricative consonants after frequency lowering improved with the spectral enhancement method [11]. In listening conditions with a low SNR, the perception of fricative consonants could be further improved by resorting to the features and classification method described here.

## Acknowledgments

The authors thank Dr. Tan Lee for his valuable comments.

## Author Contributions

Conceived and designed the experiments: Y-YK AM. Performed the experiments: Y-YK AM. Analyzed the data: Y-YK AM KK. Wrote the paper: Y-YK.

## References

1. Whalen DH (1981) Effects of vocalic formant transitions and vowel quality on the English [s]-[ʃ] boundary. J Acoust Soc Am 69: 275–282.
2. Zeng FG, Turner CW (1990) Recognition of voiceless fricatives by normal and hearing-impaired subjects. J Speech Hear Res 33: 440–449.

3. Nittrouer S, Miller ME, Crowther CS, Manhart MJ (2000) The effect of segmental order on fricative labeling by children and adults. Percept Psychophys 62: 266–284.
4. Stelmachowicz PG, Pittman AL, Hoover BM, Lewis DE (2001) Effect of stimulus bandwidth on the perception of/s/in normal- and hearing-impaired children and adults. J Acoust Soc Am 110: 2183–2190.
5. Lawrence DL, Byers VW (1969) Identification of voiceless fricatives by high frequency hearing impaired listeners. J Speech Hear Res 12: 426–434.
6. Simpson A, Hersbach AA, McDermott HJ (2006) Frequency-compression outcomes in listeners with steeply sloping audiograms. Int J Audiol 45: 619–629.
7. Kuk F, Keenan D, Korhonen P, Lau CC (2009) Efficacy of linear frequency transposition on consonant identification in quiet and in noise. J Am Acad Audiol 20: 465–479.
8. Posen MP, Reed CM, Braida LD (1993) Intelligibility of frequency-lowered speech produced by a channel vocoder. J Rehabil Res Dev 30: 26–38.
9. Robinson JD, Baer T, Moore BC (2007) Using transposition to improve consonant discrimination and detection for listeners with severe high-frequency hearing loss. Int J Audiol 46: 293–308.
10. Kong YY, Mullangi A (2012) On the development of a frequency-lowering system that enhances place-of-articulation perception. Speech Commun 54: 147–160.
11. Kong YY, Mullangi A (2013) Using a vocoder-based frequency-lowering method and spectral enhancement to improve place-of-articulation perception for hearing-impaired listeners. Ear Hear 34: 300–312.
12. Stone MA, Moore BC (1999) Tolerable hearing aid delays. I. Estimation of limits imposed by the auditory path alone using simulated hearing losses. Ear Hear 20: 182–192.
13. Dillon H (2001) Hearing Aids. New York, NY: Thieme.
14. Jongman A, Wayland R, Wong S (2000) Acoustic characteristics of English fricatives. J Acoust Soc Am 108: 1252–1263.
15. Ali AM, Van der Spiegel J, Mueller P (2001) Acoustic-phonetic features for the automatic classification of fricatives. J Acoust Soc Am 109: 2217–2235.
16. Fox RA, Nissen SL (2005) Sex-related acoustic changes in voiceless English fricatives. J Speech Lang Hear Res 48: 753–765.
17. Maniwa K, Jongman A, Wade T (2009) Acoustic characteristics of clearly spoken English fricatives. J Acoust Soc Am 125: 3962–3973.
18. Garofolo JS, Lamel LF, Fisher WM, Fiscus JG, Pallett DS, et al. (1993) The DARPA TIMIT acoustic-phonetic continuous speech corpus. Linguistic Data Consortium.
19. Byrne D, Dillon H, Tran K, Arlinger S, Wilbraham K, et al. (1994) An International Comparison of Long-Term Average Speech Spectra. J Acoust Soc Am 96: 2108–2120.
20. Bilger RC, Nuetzel JM, Rabinowitz WM, Rzeckowski C (1984) Standardization of a test of speech perception in noise. J Speech Hear Res 27: 32–48.
21. Forrest K, Weismer G, Milenkovic P, Dougall RN (1988) Statistical analysis of word-initial voiceless obstruents: preliminary data. J Acoust Soc Am 84: 115–123.
22 Brookes M. 1997. VOICEBOX: Speech Processing Toolbox for MATLAB.
23. Erdogmus D, Ozertem U, Lan T (2008) Information theoretic feature selection and projection. In: Prasad B, Prasanna SRM, editors. Speech, Audio, Image and Biomedical Signal Processing using Neural Networks, Berlin Heidelberg: Springer, pp. 1–22.
24. Jolliffe IT (1986) Principal Component Analysis. New York: Springer.
25. Scholkopf B, Smola A, Muller KR (1998) Nonlinear component analysis as a kernel eigenvalue problem. Neural Computation 10: 1299–1319.
26. Chang CC, Lin CJ (2001) LIBSVM: A library for support vector machines.
27. Hsu CW, Chang CC, Lin CJ (2003) A practical guide to support vector classification. Department of Computer Science, National Taiwan University. Available: http://www. http://www.csie.ntu.edu.tw/~cjlin/papers/guide/guide.pdf. Accessed 2 January 2013.
28. Frid A, Lavner Y (2010) Acoustic-phonetic analysis of fricatives for classification using SVM based algorithm. 26th IEEE Convention of Electrical and Electronics Engineers in Israel (IEEEI'10). Eilat, Israel751755doi: 10.1109/EEEI.2010.5662110.
29. Genussov M, Lavner Y, Cohen I (2010) Classification of unvoiced fricative phonemes using geometric methods. 12th International Workshop on Acoustic Echo and Noise Control (IWAENC'12), Tel-Aviv, Israel. Available: http://www.iwaenc.org/proceedings/2010/HTML/Uploads/960.pdf
30. Joder C, Schuller B (2012) Exploring nonnegative matrix factorisation for audio classification: application to speaker recognition. IEEE Proceedings of 10th ITG Conference on Speech Communication–.Braunschweig, Germany14
31. Onaka A, Watson CI (2000) Acoustic comparison of child and adult fricatives. 8th Australian International Conference on Speech Science and Technology–.Canberra, Australia134139
32. Shannon RV, Jensvold A, Padilla M, Robert ME, Wang X (1999) Consonant recordings for speech testing. J Acoust Soc Am 106: L71–74.

# A Functional Ser326Cys Polymorphism in *hOGG1* Is Associated with Noise-Induced Hearing Loss in a Chinese Population

**Huanxi Shen[1,2], Jinglian Cao[2,3], Zhiqiang Hong[1], Kai Liu[4], Jian Shi[1], Lu Ding[2,3], Hengdong Zhang[3], Cheng Du[1], Qian Li[6], Zhengdong Zhang[2,5]*, Baoli Zhu[2,3]***

**1** Kunshan Municipal Center for Disease Prevention and Control, Kunshan, China, **2** Department of Environmental Genomics, Jiangsu Key Laboratory of Cancer Biomarkers, Prevention and Treatment, Cancer Center, Nanjing Medical University, Nanjing, China, **3** Institute of Occupational Disease Prevention, Jiangsu Provincial Center for Disease Prevention and Control, Nanjing, China, **4** Department of Disease Prevention and Control of Yizheng Hospital, Drum Tower Hospital Group of Nanjing, Yizheng, China, **5** Department of Genetic Toxicology, the Key Laboratory of Modern Toxicology of Ministry of Education, School of Public Health, Nanjing Medical University, Nanjing, China, **6** The First People's Hospital of Kunshan, Kunshan, China

## Abstract

DNA damage to cochlear hair cells caused by 8-oxoguanine (8-oxoG) is essential for the development of noise-induced hearing loss (NIHL). Human 8-oxoG DNA glycosylase1 (hOGG1) is a key enzyme in the base excision repair (BER) pathway that eliminates 8-oxoG. Many epidemiological and functional studies have suggested that the *hOGG1* Ser326Cys polymorphism (rs1052133) is associated with many diseases. The purpose of this investigation was to investigate whether the *hOGG1* Ser326Cys polymorphism in the human BER pathway is associated with genetic susceptibility to NIHL in a Chinese population. This polymorphism was genotyped among 612 workers with NIHL and 615 workers with normal hearing. We found that individuals with the *hOGG1* Cys/Cys genotype had a statistically significantly increased risk of NIHL compared with those who carried the *hOGG1* Ser/Ser genotype (adjusted OR = 1.59, 95% CI = 1.13–2.25) and this increased risk was more pronounced among the workers in the 15- to 25- and >25-year noise exposure time, 85–92 dB(A) noise exposure level, ever smoking, and ever drinking groups, similar effects were also observed in a recessive model. In summary, our data suggested that the *hOGG1* Cys/Cys genotype may be a genetic susceptibility marker for NIHL in the Chinese Han population.

**Editor:** Giovanni Maga, Institute of Molecular Genetics IMG-CNR, Italy

**Funding:** This study was mainly supported by Jiangsu Province's Outstanding Medical Academic Leader program (LJ201130), and was partly supported by Natural Science Foundation of Jiangsu Province (BK2010080), the Key Program for Basic Research of Jiangsu Provincial Department of Education (08KJA330001). The funders had no role in study design, data collection and analysis, decision to publish, or preparation of the manuscript.

**Competing Interests:** The authors have declared that no competing interests exist.

* E-mail: zhubl@jscdc.cn (BZ); drzdzhang@gmail.com (ZZ)

These authors contributed equally to this work.

## Introduction

Noise-induced hearing loss (NIHL) is a common sensorineural impairment that is often caused by continuous and regular exposure to noise. NIHL is a leading occupational health risk in industrialised countries worldwide and the second most common form of sensorineural hearing impairment [1]. In the United States, 10 million people have noise-related hearing loss (http://www.cdc.gov/NIOSH/), and in China, the number of workers with NIHL has increased 77.8% in the last three years (2010–2012, http://www.aqsc.cn).

NIHL is a complex disease that is induced by a combination of environmental and genetic factors. It is well known that noise, chemicals such as organic solvents, ototoxic substances (e.g., aminoglycosides), heat, vibrations, smoking, and medical factors (increased blood pressure, cholesterol, and reduced iris pigmentation) are risk factors for NIHL [2,3]. To identify susceptible workers and to develop new therapies that prevent NIHL, increasing new research is focused on an understanding of NIHL at the molecular level.

In the last 20 years, several animal studies have demonstrated that knockout mice, including *SOD* −/− [4], *GPX* −/− [5], *PMCA2* −/− [6], and *CDH23* +/− [7], have shown more sensitivity to noise than their wild-type littermates. These studies have suggested that deficits in genes that disrupt different pathways (e.g., oxidative stress and potassium recycling) and critical structures of the cochlea (e.g., stereocilia) contribute to an increase in the susceptibility of the inner ear to noise [1]. However, in humans, the discovery of susceptibility genes to NIHL has encountered many difficulties; no formal heritability studies have been performed to date. Furthermore, it is difficult to collect data from families or twins in which all subjects have been exposed to similar noise environments. However, association studies adopting a candidate gene approach have opened the door to discovering NIHL susceptibility genes [1]. Over the last 10 years, several studies have found that potassium-recycling pathway genes [8,9], monogenic deafness genes [10,11], Hsp70 genes [11,12], and oxidative stress genes [13,14,15,16,17] have been associated with NIHL.

DNA damage to cochlear hair cells is essential for the development of NIHL, especially in the context of exposure to high noise levels [18]. The end result is cochlear hair death from a combination of necrosis and apoptosis. Correspondingly, several DNA repair pathways, including base excision repair (BER) [19,20,21], mismatch repair (MMR), nucleotide excision repair (NER), and DNA double-strain break repair [19], have evolved to maintain the genetic integrity of these cells and to prevent cell death. *Totonchy MB et al.* [22] also reported that DNA repair was important in the maintenance of hearing.

The 8-oxoguanine (8-oxoG) DNA lesion, caused by reactive oxygen species (ROS), is one of the most common forms of oxidative damage to DNA and leads to G: C to T: A transversions, causing carcinogenesis [23]. Human 8-oxoG DNA glycosylase1 (hOGG1) is a key enzyme in the BER pathway that eliminates 8-oxoG [19,24].

Many epidemiological and functional studies have suggested that the Ser326Cys polymorphism (rs1052133) in exon 7 of *hOGG1* gene may affect the activity of hOGG1 enzyme [25,26] and may therefore serve as a genetic marker for susceptibility to many diseases [27,28,29,30]; however, thus far, there have been no studies of association between the *hOGG1* Ser326Cys polymorphism and risk of NIHL.

To determine whether the *hOGG1* Ser326Cys polymorphism in the human BER pathway was associated with susceptibility to NIHL in the Chinese population, we genotyped 615 NIHL workers and 615 normal hearing workers and compared the genotype frequencies between these two groups.

## Materials and Methods

### 2.1 Subjects

This study included 615 NIHL workers and 615 normal hearing workers from the Datun Coal and Electricity Company (Xuzhou, China. 32 NIHL workers and 32 normal hearing workers were selected), Chenguang Machinery Manufacturing Group Corporation (Nanjing, China. 138 NIHL workers and 138 normal hearing workers were selected), and Yizheng Chemical Fiber Company Limited (Yizheng, China. 445 NIHL workers and 445 normal hearing workers were selected) between April 2010 and May 2011. All subjects (age range, 21–59 years) were Han Chinese. The detail population of information has been described in our previous study [16]. Briefly, these subjects had been continuously employed in these plants for at least one year, and all of them had their hearing tested once a year according to the Technical Specifications for Occupational Health Surveillance (2002) of China. We enrolled volunteers when workers exposed to occupational noise had their health examination; the inclusion criteria we used have been described in detail previously. In general, the selected workers had not been exposed commonly to chemical or physical factors associated with hearing loss (e.g., heat, vibrations, and organic solvents), had no record of military service, and had no medical factors or diseases that could affect hearing. The workers we selected did not regularly use hearing protection. The noise exposure time for each work was recorded according to their occupational health surveillance files which contained their exact noise exposure time. The subjects were recorded as ever smokers if they had smoked 100 cigarettes or more in their lifetimes. The subjects were recorded as ever drinkers if they had consumed three or more alcoholic drinks per week for at least one year [16]. This study protocol was approved by the institutional review board of Nanjing Medical University, and written informed consent was obtained from all participants.

### 2.2 Questionnaire

The structured questionnaires were administered in face-to-face interviews conducted by our topic-based group for each subject. The information requested in the questionnaire included informed consent, demographic characteristics, lifestyle habits (smoking and alcohol consumption), history of ototoxic drug use, work history, noise exposure, physical and chemical factor exposure, hearing protection use, disease history, family history of deafness, and so on. All of the workers had been interviewed, and 1,230 useable questionnaires were collected.

### 2.3 Audiological status assessment and environmental noise measurement

As we have described in a previous study [16], an otolaryngologist conducted 500, 1,000, 2,000, 3,000, 4,000, and 6,000 pure-tone air hearing threshold tests in a sound-attenuating chamber with a background noise level of less than 25 dB(A). The workers were required to avoid a noisy environment for 12–48 h before they were tested. According to the Diagnostic Criteria of Occupational Noise-Induced Hearing Loss (Chinese Occupational Health Standard, GBZ49-2002, http://www.zybw.net) and the Technical Specifications for Occupational Health Surveillance, an ascending method in 5 dB(A) steps was adopted to ascertain the hearing threshold levels of both ears. The final threshold value for each ear was defined as the lowest signal intensity that a subject detected with a minimum of 3 trials. Hearing thresholds of less than 25 dB in both high- and low-frequency ranges were defined as normal. Correspondingly, hearing thresholds worse than 25 dB in the high-frequency range or in both high- and low-frequency ranges were defined as NIHL. However, in our study a high-frequency hearing threshold worse than 25 dB was recorded only because NIHL workers (35 workers) with both low- and high-frequency hearing worse than 25 dB were required to be removed from noisy environments according to the Diagnostic Criteria of Occupational Noise-Induced Hearing Loss (GBZ49-2002).

We used individual sound pressure noise meters (Noise-Pro, Quest, Oconomowoc WI, USA) to detect noise exposure levels in the workplace; they were worn by 1 to 10 workers in each workplace during the work shift, three times a year, as mandated by the China National Criteria for Noise in the Workplace. Additionally, the Noise-Pro was used at 10 AM, 3 PM, and 5 PM for three consecutive days at each workplace to test the noise exposure levels.

In the final analysis, the normal hearing workers (615 workers) were matched with the NIHL workers (615 workers) by age, sex, and similarity of occupational exposures (including noise exposure time, noise exposure level and so on). All subjects donated 2 ml venous blood samples for DNA extraction.

### 2.4 Genotyping of hOGG1 Ser326Cys polymorphisms

Genomic DNA was isolated from the peripheral blood samples according to standard procedures using a TianGen DNA extraction kit (Beijing, China). The *hOGG1* Ser326Cys polymorphism was detected using the TaqMan SNP Genotyping assay and the 96-well ABI 7900HT Real Time PCR System (Applied Biosystems, Foster City, CA, USA). The primer sequences were 5′-CCTCCTACAGGTGCTGTTCAGTG-3′ and 5′-ACCCTTT-CTGCGCTT- TGCT-3′, and the probes were 5′-FAM-CCAATGCCGCCATG-MGB-3′ and 5′-HEX-CGCCAATC-CCGCCA-MGB-3′, which were designed and manufactured by

Applied Biosystems Inc. (Foster City, CA, USA). The final volume for each reaction was 10 μl, consisting of 2.5 μl ddH$_2$O, 5 μl TaqMan Master Mix, 0.5 μl F-prime, 0.5 μl R-prime, 0.25 μl FAM-probe, 0.25 μl HEX-probe (Applied Biosystems Inc.), and 10 ng DNA. The PCR profile consisted of an initial denaturation step at 50°C for 2 min, 95°C for 10 min, and 40 cycles of 95°C for 15 s and 60°C for 1 min. The fluorescence level was detected using an ABI 7900HT Real-Time PCR System. The allele frequencies were determined using ABI SDS 2.3 software.

The genotypes of 3 NIHL workers could not be determined, although 3 attempts were made. Therefore, 612 NIHL workers and 615 normal hearing workers were analysed in total. Two persons independently performed the genotyping in a blinded fashion. More than 10% of the samples were randomly selected for confirmation, and the reproducibility was 100%.

### 2.5 Statistical analysis

All of the data were reorganised and entered with EpiData 3.1, and the statistical analysis was performed using SAS statistical software (version 9.1.3; SAS Institute, Cary, NC, USA).

Continuous data were analysed by independent-sample two-sided t tests. Categorical data were computed by two-sided $\chi^2$ tests. Hardy-Weinberg equilibrium was tested by a goodness-of-fit $\chi^2$ test. Multivariate logistic regressions were used to compute odds ratios (ORs) and 95% confidence intervals (95% CIs) to test the associations of different genotypes with noise susceptibility. Adjusted ORs and 95% CIs were computed by multivariate logistic regression adjusted for age, sex, smoking status, and drinking status. Furthermore, the stratification analyses were performed according to the subsections of noise exposure time, noise exposure level, smoking status, and drinking status, to estimate the different combinations of *hOGG1* genetic variants between NIHL workers and normal hearing workers. Multivariate logistic regressions were also used to analyze gene-environment interactions. All of the tests were two-sided, and a *P*-value <0.05 was considered statistically significant.

## Results

### 3.1 Subject characteristics

The demographic and occupational characteristics of 612 NIHL workers and 615 normal hearing workers are shown in Table 1. Overall, there were no significant differences in the distribution of age, sex, smoking status, drinking status, exposure level, or exposure time between the NIHL and normal hearing workers. We did observe that the average threshold value of the NIHL workers was over two times greater than that of the normal hearing workers [37.2 dB(A) *vs.* 14.1 dB(A)]. The majority of the smokers and drinkers in our cohort were light smokers and light drinkers (the average was 4.8 cigarettes per day and 8.5 g of alcohol per day separately); we did not analyse the effects of smoking and drinking quantitatively.

### 3.2 Associations of the hOGG1 polymorphisms with the susceptibility to NIHL

The observed genotypes and allele frequencies of *hOGG1* among the NIHL workers and normal hearing workers and their associations with the risk of NIHL are presented in Table 2. The allele frequency of *hOGG1* Ser326Cys among the normal hearing workers was consistent with Hardy–Weinberg equilibrium ($P$=0.223). The frequency of the *hOGG1* Cys/Cys genotype in the normal hearing workers (12.7%), which is similar to that reported in a previous study in a Chinese population (the frequency of *hOGG1* Cys/Cys genotype is 13.4%) [31], was statistically lower than the frequency in the NIHL workers (17.9%, $P$=0.008). Multivariate logistic regression analyses also revealed that individuals with the *hOGG1* Cys/Cys genotype had a 1.59-fold risk of NIHL compared with individuals carrying a Ser/Ser genotype (adjusted OR = 1.59, 95% CI = 1.13–2.25). When we combined the Ser/Ser and Ser/Cys genotypes as a reference to conduct a recessive model, the number of workers with the Cys/Cys genotype was greater among the NIHL group than in the normal hearing worker group (17.9% *vs.* 12.7%, $P$=0.010); workers who carried the Cys/Cys genotype had a higher risk of NIHL (1.52, 1.11–2.08). We also found that there were more Cys allele individuals among the NIHL workers than among the normal hearing workers (41.9% *vs.* 37.2%, $P$=0.017). The multivariate logistic regression analysis revealed that the workers with the Cys allele had a higher risk of NIHL than the normal hearing workers (OR = 1.22, 95% CI = 1.04–1.43).

### 3.3 Stratification analysis between the hOGG1 polymorphism and risk of NIHL

The results of the stratification analysis are presented in Tables 3 and Table 4. In Table 3, we found that the individuals with the *hOGG1* Cys/Cys genotype were more susceptible to NIHL than those who carrying the *hOGG1* Ser/Ser genotype, both in the 15- to 25-year noise exposure group (adjusted OR = 1.67, 95% CI = 1.02–2.72) and in the >25-year noise exposure group (2.71, 1.16–6.36). Similar effects were also noted for smoking and drinking status; ever smoking or ever drinking subjects with the *hOGG1* Cys/Cys genotype were more susceptible to NIHL. But in the stratification of noise exposure level, we only found that the *hOGG1* Cys/Cys genotype carriers with 85 to 92 dB(A) exposure levels were at a significantly increased risk of NIHL (3.34, 1.59–7.02); no effects were observed in either the <85 dB(A) or >92 dB(A) noise-exposure levels.

A stratification analysis between the *hOGG1* recessive model and risk of NIHL is shown in Table 4. The subjects with the *hOGG1* Cys/Cys genotype had an increased risk of NIHL in the >25-year group (adjusted OR = 2.48, 95% CI = 1.20–5.14), the 85 to 92 dB(A) noise exposure level group (2.83, 1.46–5.49), the ever smoking group (1.68, 1.04–2.70), and the ever drinking group (1.78, 1.18–2.68).

Gene-environment interactions were also analyzed between the *hOGG1* Cys/Cys genotype and NIHL risk factors (noise exposure time, noise exposure level, smoking and drinking), but no gene-environment interactions were found in this study ($P$>0.05).

## Discussion

In this case-control study, we found that the *hOGG1* Cys/Cys genotype was statistically significantly associated with NIHL. Moreover, the synergistic effects of the *hOGG1* Ser326Cys polymorphism and noise exposure time, noise exposure level, smoking status, and drinking status on NIHL were observed in our study.

Several studies have reported that the *hOGG1* Ser326Cys polymorphism was associated with risk of cancers and various metabolic disorders [21,29,30,32]. However, there have been no studies published exploring the *hOGG1* Ser326Cys polymorphism and NIHL risk among noise exposure subjects. To the best of our knowledge, this study is the first to investigate the association between the *hOGG1* Ser326Cys polymorphism and NIHL risk in a Chinese population.

Caused by ROS, 8-oxoG in DNA is a major form of oxidative damage, which may lead to mutagenesis or carcinogenesis [23] and which can be repaired by the BER pathway. The hOGG1

**Table 1.** Demographic and occupational characteristics of the NIHL and normal hearing workers.

| Variables | NIHL workers (n = 612) | | Normal hearing workers (n = 615) | | $p^a$ |
|---|---|---|---|---|---|
| | N | % | N | % | |
| Age (years) | 40.4±6.3 | | 40.4±5.9 | | 0.979[b] |
| <35 | 122 | 19.9 | 120 | 19.5 | 0.963 |
| 35–45 | 368 | 60.2 | 369 | 60.0 | |
| >45 | 122 | 19.9 | 126 | 20.5 | |
| Sex | | | | | |
| Male | 565 | 92.3 | 564 | 91.7 | 0.692 |
| Female | 47 | 7.7 | 51 | 8.3 | |
| Smoking status | | | | | |
| Never | 366 | 59.8 | 359 | 58.4 | 0.611 |
| Ever | 246 | 40.2 | 256 | 41.6 | |
| Drinking status | | | | | |
| Never | 259 | 42.3 | 256 | 41.6 | 0.805 |
| Ever | 353 | 57.7 | 359 | 58.4 | |
| Exposure level [dB(A)] | 87.1±7.7 | | 87.0±7.6 | | 0.804[b] |
| <85 | 234 | 38.2 | 246 | 40.0 | 0.735 |
| 85–92 | 161 | 26.3 | 151 | 24.5 | |
| >92 | 217 | 35.5 | 218 | 35.5 | |
| Exposure time (years) | 18.6±7.6 | | 18.2±7.4 | | 0.403[b] |
| <15 | 189 | 30.9 | 194 | 31.5 | 0.645 |
| 15–25 | 308 | 50.3 | 318 | 51.7 | |
| >25 | 115 | 18.8 | 103 | 16.8 | |
| Threshold [dB] | 37.2±11.9 | | 14.1±4.1 | | **<0.001[b]** |

[a]Two-sided $\chi^2$ test was used for comparing the frequency distribution.
[b]Two-sided *t*-test was used for comparing the mean values of the continuous variables.

enzyme in the BER pathway, which is encoded by the *hOGG1* gene on chromosome 3p26, recognises the 8-oxoG lesions and catalyses the cleavage of the glycosidic bond between the modified base and sugar moiety, leaving an abasic, apurinic/apyrimidinic site (AP-site) in DNA, and the AP-endonuclease-1 (APEX/APE1) enzyme then acts upon it [19]. Multiple functional studies have revealed that the glycosylase activity of the Cys326 variant of the hOGG1 enzyme (Cys326-hOGG1 enzyme) is more sensitive to inactivation by oxidising agents compared with the Ser326-hOGG1 enzyme [25,33]. The activity for the repair of 8-oxoG was approximately 7-fold greater in the hOGG1-Ser326 protein than in the hOGG1-Cys326 protein in a complementation assay of an *E. coli* mutant defective in the repair of 8-oxoG [34]. Our study also found there were more individuals with the *hOGG1* Cys/Cys genotype among NIHL workers than among normal hearing workers, suggesting that subjects carrying the *hOGG1* Cys/Cys genotype may have

**Table 2.** Association of the *hOGG1* Ser326Cys polymorphism with the risk of NIHL.

| Genotypes | NIHL workers (n = 612) | | Normal hearing workers (n = 615) | | OR (95% CI) | Adjusted[a] OR (95% CI) | $p^b$ |
|---|---|---|---|---|---|---|---|
| | N | % | N | % | | | |
| Ser/Ser | 209 | 34.2 | 236 | 38.4 | 1.00 (reference) | 1.00 (reference) | |
| Ser/Cys | 293 | 47.9 | 301 | 48.9 | 1.10 (0.86–1.41) | 1.09 (0.86–1.40) | 0.451 |
| Cys/Cys | 110 | 17.9 | 78 | 12.7 | **1.59 (1.13–2.25)** | **1.59 (1.13–2.25)** | **0.008** |
| Ser/Ser+Ser/Cys | 502 | 82.1 | 537 | 87.3 | 1.00 (reference) | 1.00 (reference) | |
| Cys/Cys | 110 | 17.9 | 78 | 12.7 | **1.51 (1.10–2.07)** | **1.52 (1.11–2.08)** | **0.010** |
| Ser allele | 711 | 58.1 | 773 | 62.8 | 1.00 | | |
| Cys allele | 513 | 41.9 | 457 | 37.2 | **1.22 (1.04–1.43)** | | **0.017** |

[a]Adjusted for age, sex, smoking, and drinking status.
[b]Two-sided $\chi^2$ test for the frequency distributions of selected variables between the hearing loss workers and normal hearing workers.

**Table 3.** Stratified analysis of the *hOGG1* Ser326Cys polymorphism (Cys/Cys *vs.* Ser/Ser genotype) associated with NIHL risk.

| Variables | NIHL workers | | Normal hearing workers | | OR (95% CI) | Adjusted OR (95% CI)[a] | P[b] |
|---|---|---|---|---|---|---|---|
| | Ser/Ser (n = 209) | Cys/Cys (n = 110) | Ser/Ser (n = 236) | Cys/Cys (n = 78) | | | |
| | N (%) | N (%) | N (%) | N (%) | | | |
| Exposure time (years) | | | | | | | 0.130[c] |
| <15 | 69 (36.3) | 27 (14.2) | 69 (36.3) | 25 (14.2) | 1.08 (0.57–2.04) | 1.09 (0.57–2.07) | 0.813 |
| 15–25 | 103 (31.7) | 53 (16.3) | 129 (39.7) | 40 (12.3) | **1.66 (1.02–2.70)** | **1.67 (1.02–2.72)** | **0.040** |
| >25 | 37 (31.4) | 30 (25.4) | 38 (32.2) | 13 (11.0) | **2.37 (1.07–5.24)** | **2.71 (1.16–6.36)** | **0.031** |
| Exposure level [dB(A)] | | | | | | | 0.363[c] |
| <85 | 84 (31.9) | 47 (17.9) | 97 (36.9) | 35 (13.3) | 1.55 (0.92–2.62) | 1.53 (0.89–2.62) | 0.101 |
| 85–92 | 51 (30.7) | 36 (21.7) | 64 (38.6) | 15 (9.0) | **3.01 (1.49–6.10)** | **3.34 (1.59–7.02)** | **0.002** |
| >92 | 74 (36.3) | 27 (13.2) | 75 (36.8) | 28 (13.7) | 0.98 (0.53–1.81) | 0.98 (0.53–1.82) | 0.942 |
| Smoking status | | | | | | | 0.731[c] |
| Never | 128 (34.2) | 60 (16.0) | 142 (38.0) | 44 (11.8) | 1.51 (0.96–2.39) | 1.51 (0.96–2.39) | 0.075 |
| Ever | 81 (31.3) | 50 (19.3) | 94 (36.3) | 34 (13.1) | **1.71 (1.01–2.89)** | **1.73 (1.02–2.95)** | **0.046** |
| Drinking status | | | | | | | 0.318[c] |
| Never | 88 (34.0) | 40 (15.4) | 97 (37.5) | 34 (13.1) | 1.30 (0.76–2.23) | 1.33 (0.77–2.29) | 0.346 |
| Ever | 121 (32.3) | 70 (18.7) | 139 (37.2) | 44 (11.8) | **1.83 (1.17–2.86)** | **1.82 (1.16–2.86)** | **0.008** |

[a]Adjusted for age, sex, smoking, and drinking.
[b]Two-sided $\chi^2$ test for the frequency distributions of the selected variables between the NIHL workers and normal hearing workers.
[c]Gene-environment interaction *P* values for the *hOGG1* Ser326Cys polymorphism and NIHL risk factors.

**Table 4.** Stratified analysis of the *hOGG1* Ser326Cys polymorphism (Cys/Cys *vs.* Ser/Ser+Ser/Cys genotype) associated with NIHL risk.

| Variables | NIHL workers | | Normal hearing workers | | OR (95% CI) | Adjusted OR (95% CI)[a] | P[b] |
|---|---|---|---|---|---|---|---|
| | Ser/Ser+Ser/Cys (n = 502) | Cys/Cys (n = 110) | Ser/Ser+Ser/Cys (n = 537) | Cys/Cys (n = 78) | | | |
| | N (%) | N (%) | N (%) | N (%) | | | |
| Exposure time (years) | | | | | | | 0.072[c] |
| <15 | 162 (42.3) | 27 (7.1) | 169 (44.1) | 25 (6.5) | 1.13 (0.63–2.02) | 1.15 (0.64–2.08) | 0.689 |
| 15–25 | 255 (40.7) | 53 (8.5) | 278 (44.4) | 40 (6.4) | 1.45 (0.93–2.25) | 1.47 (0.94–2.29) | 0.104 |
| >25 | 85 (39.0) | 30 (13.8) | 90 (41.3) | 13 (5.9) | **2.44 (1.20–4.99)** | **2.48 (1.20–5.14)** | **0.013** |
| Exposure level [dB(A)] | | | | | | | 0.415[c] |
| <85 | 187 (39.0) | 47 (9.8) | 211 (44.0) | 35 (7.2) | 1.52 (0.94–2.45) | 1.50 (0.93–2.43) | 0.088 |
| 85–92 | 125 (40.1) | 36 (11.5) | 136 (43.6) | 15 (4.8) | **2.61 (1.36–5.00)** | **2.83 (1.46–5.49)** | **0.003** |
| >92 | 190 (43.7) | 27 (6.2) | 190 (43.7) | 28 (6.4) | 0.96 (0.55–1.70) | 0.95 (0.54–1.68) | 0.900 |
| Smoking status | | | | | | | 0.593[c] |
| Never | 306 (42.2) | 60 (8.3) | 315 (43.5) | 44 (6.1) | 1.40 (0.92–2.14) | 1.42 (0.93–2.16) | 0.112 |
| Ever | 196 (39.0) | 50 (10.0) | 222 (44.2) | 34 (6.8) | **1.67 (1.04–2.68)** | **1.68 (1.04–2.70)** | **0.035** |
| Drinking status | | | | | | | 0.231[c] |
| Never | 219 (42.5) | 40 (7.8) | 222 (43.1) | 34 (6.6) | 1.19 (0.73–1.95) | 1.21 (0.74–1.99) | 0.484 |
| Ever | 283 (39.8) | 70 (9.8) | 315 (44.2) | 44 (6.2) | **1.77 (1.18–2.67)** | **1.78 (1.18–2.68)** | **0.006** |

[a]Adjusted for age, sex, smoking, and drinking.
[b]Two-sided $\chi^2$ test for the frequency distributions of selected variables between the NIHL workers and normal hearing workers.
[c]Gene-environment interaction *P* values for the *hOGG1* Ser326Cys polymorphism and NIHL risk factors.

lower activity for repairing 8-oxoG damage, thereby increasing the risk of NIHL.

Notably, when the noise exposure time was combined with the *hOGG1* Cys/Cys genotype, the effects were more significant. NIHL is positively correlated with noise exposure time; when workers are exposed to noise for a longer time, the cumulative noise exposure (CNE) is greater, and they are more susceptible to NIHL [3]. Moreover, many workers with longer noise exposure times are older and may be influenced by age-related hearing impairment (ARHI). A previous study has also reported that there is a significantly age-associated decrease in DNA repair capacity [35].

Noise exposure levels are important for the activation of the antioxidant system. In chinchillas, *Jacono AA* [36] observed no increase in the antioxidant system after a conditioning noise exposure of 90 dB SPL (0.5 kHz, 6 h per day for 6 days), but a large increase in the antioxidant system in response to 105 dB SPL (0.5 kHz, 4 h). Positively induced by ROS, 8-oxoG is correlated with noise exposure level and also has a positive correlation with the expression of DNA repair enzymes [37]. NIHL is a progressive, cumulative disease; most workers in the >92 dB(A) noise exposure group were often transferred to a no-noise exposure position after working for a few years, as we described previously [16]. The subjects in the <85 dB(A) and >92 dB(A) groups had low cumulative noise exposures, while individuals in the 85 to 92 dB(A) group were assumed to have had sufficient cumulative noise exposure.

Smoking may accelerate NIHL; some studies have reported the adverse effects of smoking on hearing [38,39]. However, a few studies have not identified any associations between smoking and hearing loss [40]. Our study showed that smoking was associated with NIHL. Workers with the *hOGG1* Cys/Cys genotype had a 1.68-fold increased risk of NIHL than workers who carried the *hOGG1* Ser/Ser genotype among ever smokers. The effect was less pronounced when all subjects were included in the analysis (adjusted OR = 1.59, less than 1.68). In the recessive model, a similar phenomenon was also observed. A possible explanation for the underlying pathogenic mechanism may be the well-known vascular changes and the consequent cochlear hypoxia related to both smoking and noise exposure. Adverse effects were also observed between drinking and NIHL in this study, which was consistent with previous studies [41,42]. However, some studies have reported that drinking alcohol may not either influence hearing or be a protective factor [43,44]; more study is required to confirm this possibility.

Compared with other studies, ours was the first to investigate the association between the functional *hOGG1* Ser326Cys polymorphism and NIHL risk. Moreover, thousands of workers who had been exposed to steady noise for up to 20 years or more but who were less exposed to other occupational hazards were enrolled in our study. Furthermore, all of our NIHL workers were in an early stage of NIHL according to GBZ49-2002; additionally, individual noise meters were used to assess the noise environment so that the results would reflect real exposure levels. One limitation of this study was that the NIHL workers with both low- and high-frequency hearing ranges worse than 25 dB were all transferred from noisy environments; therefore, selection bias may exist in our study.

In conclusion, our data suggested that the *hOGG1* Cys/Cys genotype may be a genetic susceptibility marker for NIHL in the Han Chinese population, especially in the 15- to 25-year and >25-year noise exposure time, 85 to 92 dB(A) noise exposure level, ever smoking, and ever drinking groups. To confirm our findings, further case-control or cohort studies with more subjects (enrolling all NIHL workers) and *in vivo* functional evaluations are needed in the future.

## Author Contributions

Conceived and designed the experiments: BZ ZZ. Performed the experiments: HS JC LD. Analyzed the data: HS ZH. Contributed reagents/materials/analysis tools: KL JS HZ CD QL. Wrote the paper: HS.

## References


1. Sliwinska-Kowalska M, Pawelczyk M (2013) Contribution of genetic factors to noise-induced hearing loss: a human studies review. Mutat Res 752: 61–65.
2. Sliwinska-Kowalska M, Zamyslowska-Szmytke E, Szymczak W, Kotylo P, Fiszer M, et al. (2004) Effects of coexposure to noise and mixture of organic solvents on hearing in dockyard workers. J Occup Environ Med 46: 30–38.
3. Konings A, Van Laer L, Van Camp G (2009) Genetic studies on noise-induced hearing loss: a review. Ear Hear 30: 151–159.
4. Ohlemiller KK, McFadden SL, Ding DL, Flood DG, Reaume AG, et al. (1999) Targeted deletion of the cytosolic Cu/Zn-superoxide dismutase gene (Sod1) increases susceptibility to noise-induced hearing loss. Audiol Neurootol 4: 237–246.
5. Ohlemiller KK, McFadden SL, Ding DL, Lear PM, Ho YS (2000) Targeted mutation of the gene for cellular glutathione peroxidase (Gpx1) increases noise-induced hearing loss in mice. J Assoc Res Otolaryngol 1: 243–254.
6. Kozel PJ, Davis RR, Krieg EF, Shull GE, Erway LC (2002) Deficiency in plasma membrane calcium ATPase isoform 2 increases susceptibility to noise-induced hearing loss in mice. Hear Res 164: 231–239.
7. Holme RH, Steel KP (2004) Progressive hearing loss and increased susceptibility to noise-induced hearing loss in mice carrying a Cdh23 but not a Myo7a mutation. J Assoc Res Otolaryngol 5: 66–79.
8. Van Laer L, Carlsson PI, Ottschytsch N, Bondeson ML, Konings A, et al. (2006) The contribution of genes involved in potassium-recycling in the inner ear to noise-induced hearing loss. Hum Mutat 27: 786–795.
9. Pawelczyk M, Van Laer L, Fransen E, Rajkowska E, Konings A, et al. (2009) Analysis of gene polymorphisms associated with K ion circulation in the inner ear of patients susceptible and resistant to noise-induced hearing loss. Ann Hum Genet 73: 411–421.
10. Konings A, Van Laer L, Wiktorek-Smagur A, Rajkowska E, Pawelczyk M, et al. (2009) Candidate gene association study for noise-induced hearing loss in two independent noise-exposed populations. Ann Hum Genet 73: 215–224.
11. Konings A, Van Laer L, Michel S, Pawelczyk M, Carlsson PI, et al. (2009) Variations in HSP70 genes associated with noise-induced hearing loss in two independent populations. Eur J Hum Genet 17: 329–335.
12. Yang M, Tan H, Yang Q, Wang F, Yao H, et al. (2006) Association of hsp70 polymorphisms with risk of noise-induced hearing loss in Chinese automobile workers. Cell Stress Chaperones 11: 233–239.
13. Rabinowitz PM, Pierce Wise J Sr, Hur Mobo B, Antonucci PG, Powell C, et al. (2002) Antioxidant status and hearing function in noise-exposed workers. Hear Res 173: 164–171.
14. Fortunato G, Marciano E, Zarrilli F, Mazzaccara C, Intrieri M, et al. (2004) Paraoxonase and superoxide dismutase gene polymorphisms and noise-induced hearing loss. Clin Chem 50: 2012–2018.
15. Konings A, Van Laer L, Pawelczyk M, Carlsson PI, Bondeson ML, et al. (2007) Association between variations in CAT and noise-induced hearing loss in two independent noise-exposed populations. Hum Mol Genet 16: 1872–1883.
16. Shen H, Huo X, Liu K, Li X, Gong W, et al. (2012) Genetic variation in GSTM1 is associated with susceptibility to noise-induced hearing loss in a Chinese population. J Occup Environ Med 54: 1157–1162.
17. Li XT, Li X, Hu FF, Shen HX, Cao JL, et al. (2013) Association between Paraoxonase 2 Gene Polymorphisms and Noise-induced Hearing Loss in the Chinese Population. J Occup Health 55: 56–65.
18. Henderson D, Bielefeld EC, Harris KC, Hu BH (2006) The role of oxidative stress in noise-induced hearing loss. Ear Hear 27: 1–19.
19. Christmann M, Tomicic MT, Roos WP, Kaina B (2003) Mechanisms of human DNA repair: an update. Toxicology 193: 3–34.
20. Dahle J, Brunborg G, Svendsrud DH, Stokke T, Kvam E (2008) Overexpression of human OGG1 in mammalian cells decreases ultraviolet A induced mutagenesis. Cancer Lett 267: 18–25.
21. Hung RJ, Hall J, Brennan P, Boffetta P (2005) Genetic polymorphisms in the base excision repair pathway and cancer risk: a HuGE review. Am J Epidemiol 162: 925–942.

22. Totonchy MB, Tamura D, Pantell MS, Zalewski C, Bradford PT, et al. (2013) Auditory analysis of xeroderma pigmentosum 1971–2012: hearing function, sun sensitivity and DNA repair predict neurological degeneration. Brain 136: 194–208.
23. Cheng KC, Cahill DS, Kasai H, Nishimura S, Loeb LA (1992) 8-Hydroxyguanine, an abundant form of oxidative DNA damage, causes G----T and A----C substitutions. J Biol Chem 267: 166–172.
24. Hill JW, Evans MK (2006) Dimerization and opposite base-dependent catalytic impairment of polymorphic S326C OGG1 glycosylase. Nucleic Acids Res 34: 1620–1632.
25. Yamane A, Kohno T, Ito K, Sunaga N, Aoki K, et al. (2004) Differential ability of polymorphic OGG1 proteins to suppress mutagenesis induced by 8-hydroxyguanine in human cell in vivo. Carcinogenesis 25: 1689–1694.
26. Collins AR, Gaivao I (2007) DNA base excision repair as a biomarker in molecular epidemiology studies. Mol Aspects Med 28: 307–322.
27. Kim JI, Park YJ, Kim KH, Song BJ, Lee MS, et al. (2003) hOGG1 Ser326Cys polymorphism modifies the significance of the environmental risk factor for colon cancer. World J Gastroenterol 9: 956–960.
28. Okasaka T, Matsuo K, Suzuki T, Ito H, Hosono S, et al. (2009) hOGG1 Ser326Cys polymorphism and risk of lung cancer by histological type. J Hum Genet 54: 739–745.
29. Jiao X, Huang J, Wu S, Lv M, Hu Y, et al. (2007) hOGG1 Ser326Cys polymorphism and susceptibility to gallbladder cancer in a Chinese population. Int J Cancer 121: 501–505.
30. Li Q, Huang L, Rong L, Xue Y, Lu Q, et al. (2011) hOGG1 Ser326Cys polymorphism and risk of childhood acute lymphoblastic leukemia in a Chinese population. Cancer Sci 102: 1123–1127.
31. Xing DY, Tan W, Song N, Lin DX (2001) Ser326Cys polymorphism in hOGG1 gene and risk of esophageal cancer in a Chinese population. Int J Cancer 95: 140–143.
32. Xu J, Zheng SL, Turner A, Isaacs SD, Wiley KE, et al. (2002) Associations between hOGG1 sequence variants and prostate cancer susceptibility. Cancer Res 62: 2253–2257.
33. Bravard A, Vacher M, Moritz E, Vaslin L, Hall J, et al. (2009) Oxidation status of human OGG1-S326C polymorphic variant determines cellular DNA repair capacity. Cancer Res 69: 3642–3649.
34. Kohno T, Shinmura K, Tosaka M, Tani M, Kim SR, et al. (1998) Genetic polymorphisms and alternative splicing of the hOGG1 gene, that is involved in the repair of 8-hydroxyguanine in damaged DNA. Oncogene 16: 3219–3225.
35. Goukassian D, Gad F, Yaar M, Eller MS, Nehal US, et al. (2000) Mechanisms and implications of the age-associated decrease in DNA repair capacity. FASEB J 14: 1325–1334.
36. Jacono AA, Hu B, Kopke RD, Henderson D, Van De Water TR, et al. (1998) Changes in cochlear antioxidant enzyme activity after sound conditioning and noise exposure in the chinchilla. Hear Res 117: 31–38.
37. Peng T, Shen HM, Liu ZM, Yan LN, Peng MH, et al. (2003) Oxidative DNA damage in peripheral leukocytes and its association with expression and polymorphisms of hOGG1: a study of adolescents in a high risk region for hepatocellular carcinoma in China. World J Gastroenterol 9: 2186–2193.
38. Palmer KT, Griffin MJ, Syddall HE, Coggon D (2004) Cigarette smoking, occupational exposure to noise, and self reported hearing difficulties. Occup Environ Med 61: 340–344.
39. Mizoue T, Miyamoto T, Shimizu T (2003) Combined effect of smoking and occupational exposure to noise on hearing loss in steel factory workers. Occup Environ Med 60: 56–59.
40. Karlsmose B, Lauritzen T, Engberg M, Parving A (2000) A five-year longitudinal study of hearing in a Danish rural population aged 31–50 years. Br J Audiol 34: 47–55.
41. Itoh A, Nakashima T, Arao H, Wakai K, Tamakoshi A, et al. (2001) Smoking and drinking habits as risk factors for hearing loss in the elderly: epidemiological study of subjects undergoing routine health checks in Aichi, Japan. Public Health 115: 192–196.
42. Nakamura M, Aoki N, Nakashima T, Hoshino T, Yokoyama T, et al. (2001) Smoking, alcohol, sleep and risk of idiopathic sudden deafness: a case-control study using pooled controls. J Epidemiol 11: 81–86.
43. Popelka MM, Cruickshanks KJ, Wiley TL, Tweed TS, Klein BE, et al. (2000) Moderate alcohol consumption and hearing loss: a protective effect. J Am Geriatr Soc 48: 1273–1278.
44. Curhan SG, Eavey R, Shargorodsky J, Curhan GC (2011) Prospective study of alcohol use and hearing loss in men. Ear Hear 32: 46–52.

# CHD7 Deficiency in "*Looper*", a New Mouse Model of CHARGE Syndrome, Results in Ossicle Malformation, Otosclerosis and Hearing Impairment

**Jacqueline M. Ogier[1], Marina R. Carpinelli[1,2,3,4], Benedicta D. Arhatari[7], R. C. Andrew Symons[8], Benjamin T. Kile[3,4,5], Rachel A. Burt[1,2,3,5,6]***

**1** Murdoch Childrens Research Institute, Parkville, Victoria, Australia, **2** The HEARing Cooperative Research Centre, Parkville, Victoria, Australia, **3** Walter and Eliza Hall Institute of Medical Research, Parkville, Victoria, Australia, **4** Department of Medical Biology, University of Melbourne, Parkville, Victoria, Australia, **5** Department of Genetics, University of Melbourne, Parkville, Victoria, Australia, **6** Department of Paediatrics, University of Melbourne, Parkville, Victoria, Australia, **7** ARC Centre of Excellence for Coherent X-ray Science, Department of Physics, La Trobe University, Bundoora, Victoria, Australia, **8** Department of Ophthalmology, Royal Melbourne Hospital, Parkville, Victoria, Australia

## Abstract

CHARGE syndrome is a rare human disorder caused by mutations in the gene encoding chromodomain helicase DNA binding protein 7 (CHD7). Characteristics of CHARGE are varied and include developmental ear and hearing anomalies. Here we report a novel mouse model of CHD7 dysfunction, termed *Looper*. The *Looper* strain harbours a nonsense mutation (c.5690C>A, p.S1897X) within the *Chd7* gene. *Looper* mice exhibit many of the clinical features of the human syndrome, consistent with previously reported CHARGE models, including growth retardation, facial asymmetry, vestibular defects, eye anomalies, hyperactivity, ossicle malformation, hearing loss and vestibular dysfunction. *Looper* mice display an otosclerosis-like fusion of the stapes footplate to the cochlear oval window and blepharoconjunctivitis but not coloboma. Looper mice are hyperactive and have vestibular dysfunction but do not display motor impairment.

**Editor:** Michael G. Anderson, University of Iowa, United States of America

**Funding:** This work was supported by the HEARing CRC, established and supported under the Cooperative Research Centres Program – an Australian Government Initiative; the Garnett Passe and Rodney Williams Memorial Foundation (fellowship to MRC); the Australian Government's National Health and Medical Research Council (Program Grants 461219 and 1016647, and a fellowship to BTK); the Sylvia and Charles Viertel Foundation (fellowship to BTK); the Victorian State Government's Operational Infrastructure Support Program; the Australian Government's NHMRC IRIISS; and a National Collaborative Research Infrastructure Strategy grant to the Australian Phenomics Network. The funders had no role in study design, data collection and analysis, decision to publish, or preparation of the manuscript.

**Competing Interests:** The authors have declared that no competing interests exist.

* E-mail: rachel.burt@mcri.edu.au

## Introduction

Syndromic hearing loss accounts for approximately half of all inherited hearing impairment [1,2]. Over 400 syndromes involving hearing loss have been characterised [3], with most having an underlying genetic cause [1]. In 60% of reported cases a single point mutation is responsible for the disease [4]. CHARGE is a syndromic hearing impairment that is predominantly caused by mutations in the chromodomain helicase DNA binding protein 7 (*CHD7*) gene. CHARGE is an acronym describing some of the main clinical features of the disease (ocular **C**oloboma, **H**eart defects, choanal **A**tresia, **R**etarded growth, **G**enital hypoplasia and **E**ar anomalies). Numerous additional features are observed in the syndrome, including hyperactive behaviour [5], nerve anomalies, cleft palate, facial asymmetry and limb deformity [6]. The extent and variability of CHARGE characteristics exemplify the importance of CHD7 in multiple developmental pathways. The incidence of CHARGE syndrome is 1 in 8,500 to 10,000 live births [7].

CHD7 regulates gene expression, particularly that of transcription factor genes [8,9], through ATP-dependent nucleosome remodelling [10]. Whilst the timing and tissue-specific expression of CHD7 has been investigated [9,11,12] little is known about the precise genes and pathways that it regulates. CHD7 binds distally with over 10,000 enhancing regulators [13], co-binding with factors including PBAF [9] and Sox2 [8,14], potentially affecting numerous pathways driving early development. This explains to some extent the range of CHARGE characteristics [14].

Several *Chd7* mouse mutations have been reported, including two targeted, three gene-trapped, eleven chemically induced and one spontaneous allele (Table 1). Mutants exhibit relatively similar characteristics including a range of CHARGE-like anomalies with varying penetrance, although some differences between strains have been noted, and this may be due to allelic variation or differences in the genetic backgrounds on which these alleles have arisen [11]. Study of the phenotype of mice carrying nonsense mutations of *Chd7* indicates that the C-terminal NLS, BRK and SANT protein domains are functionally important. Similarly, nonsense mutations of *CHD7* lead to a more severe clinical presentation in patients [15]. We conducted a detailed phenotypic characterisation of a new mouse model of CHARGE, *Looper*, which carries an ethylnitrosourea (ENU)-induced point mutation in *Chd7*. We identified several phenotypic anomalies including growth retardation, facial asymmetry, eye anomalies and hyperactivity. The mice were hearing-impaired due to fusions of the stapes tubercle to the temporal bone, and of the footplate to the cochlear oval window. *Looper* mice also displayed hypoplasia of the semi-circular canals and vestibular dysfunction, but motor coordination appeared unimpaired. All of these phenotypic abnormalities have been previously observed in other CHARGE mutants. The coloboma observed in human patients has not been reported in mouse models. Herein, we provide evidence that CHD7-deficiency in mice does not result in coloboma in any structures of the eye.

## Materials and Methods

### Ethics Statement

The WEHI and MCRI animal ethics committees approved this work in project numbers 2011.016 and A726 respectively.

### Mice

Colonies of mice were maintained at the Walter and Eliza Hall Institute of Medical Research (WEHI) and the Murdoch Childrens Research Institute (MCRI). Animals were group-housed in individually ventilated micro-isolator cages (Airlaw, Smithfield, NSW, Australia) or (Tecniplast, Buguggiate, VA, Italy). All boxes were enriched with a plastic house/toy and animals had a 10–12 hour dark period. Mice had access to standard Barastoc mouse chow (Ridley AgriProducts, Melbourne, VIC, Australia) and sterilized water *ad libitum*.

### Mutagenesis Screen

Male BALB/c mice were injected intraperitoneally with 85 mg/kg ENU (Sigma-Aldrich, Castle Hill, NSW, Australia) weekly for 3 weeks as previously described [16,17]. After 12 weeks mice were mated with untreated BALB/c females to produce first generation ($G_1$) progeny. Animals were screened by acoustic startle response (ASR) testing at 8 weeks of age. Mice with an ASR below 200 mV in response to white noise bursts of 115 dB SPL were test-mated to determine heritability of the phenotype. Mutant strains were serially backcrossed to BALB/c for 9 generations before phenotypic analysis. Mice were genotyped for the *Chd7*$^{Looper}$ mutation using the Amplifluor SNPs HT genotyping system FAM-JOE (Merck Millipore, Kilsyth, VIC, Australia) and the primers GAAGGTGACCAAGTTCATGCTGCTCTACTGGCCGAACACGTC (forward wild-type), GAAGGTCGGAGTCAACGGATTGCTCTACTGGCCGAACACGTA (forward mutant) and CGCCGGTCCGTCTTCATTAG (reverse).

### Acoustic Startle Response

Acoustic startle response (ASR) was measured using an SR-LAB system (San Diego Instruments, San Diego, CA, USA). Testing was conducted in the light phase of the light cycle and the testing environment was illuminated. Mice were restrained in a Perspex chamber and acclimatized to background white noise of 70 dB SPL for 1 min. Trials were presented in pseudorandom order and separated by intervals of 3–8 sec. Mice underwent 6 trials each of 70, 85, 90, 95 and 100 dB SPL and 16 trials of 115 dB SPL. Each white noise pulse was presented for 40 msec. After deleting the largest and smallest values, the average startle amplitude for each stimulus was calculated and plotted using Prism v 6.0b software (GraphPad Software Inc, La Jolla, CA, USA).

**Table 1.** Published mutant alleles of *Chd7*.

| Allele | Background | Derivation | Mutation | Effect | Ref |
|---|---|---|---|---|---|
| *Coa1* | C57BL/6J | ENU | c.2155A>T | p.K719X | [35] |
| *Cycn* | BALB/c×C3H/HeN | ENU | c.4286T>A | p.L1429X | [11] |
| *Dz* | BALB/c×C3H/HeN | ENU | c.5536G>T | p.E1846X | [11] |
| *Edy* | BALB/c×C3H/HeN | ENU | c.307C>T | p.Q103X | [11] |
| *Flo* | C3HeB/FeJ | ENU | c.5635+2T>C (IVS27+2T>C) | p.S1864X | [11] |
| *Gt(RRR136)Byg* | 129P2/OlaHsd×C57BL/6 | gene trap | Insertion in intron 4 | reporter fusion | [36] |
| *Gt(S20-7E1)Sor* | 129S4/SvJae×C57BL/6J | gene trap | Insertion in exon 1 | reporter fusion | [12] |
| *Gt(XK403)Byg* | 129P2/OlaHsd×C57BL/6 | gene trap | Insertion in intron 36 | reporter fusion | [36] |
| *Lda* | BALB/c×C3H/HeN | ENU | c.3195T>A | p.Y1066X | [11] |
| *Looper* | BALB/c | ENU | c.5690C>A, | p.S1897X | |
| *Mt* | BALB/c×C3H/HeN | ENU | c.5021-2A>G (IVS22-2A>G) | p.V1688X | [11] |
| *Obt* | BALB/c×C3H/HeN | ENU | c.3945T>A | p.Y1315X | [11] |
| *Ome* | BALB/cByJ | Spontaneous | Deletion of exons 2 & 3 | No protein produced | [29] |
| *tm1.1Dmm* | 129S6/SvEvTac×129S1/Sv1mJ | Gene targeting | Floxed exon 2 | No effect | [37] |
| *tm1.2Dmm* | 129S6/SvEvTac×129S1/Sv1mJ×Swiss Webster | Gene targeting | Deletion of exon 2 | No protein produced | [37] |
| *Todo* | BALB/c×C3H/HeN | ENU | c.2208+2T>C (IVS3+2T>C) | p.H539X | [11] |
| *Vlk* | C3HeB/FeJ | ENU | c.4377T>A | p.Y1459X | [38] |
| *Whi* | C3HeB/FeJ | ENU | c.2918G>A | p.W973X | [11] |

Ref reference, ENU ethylnitrosourea. Build: GRCm38.p1, Reference: CCDS38689.1.

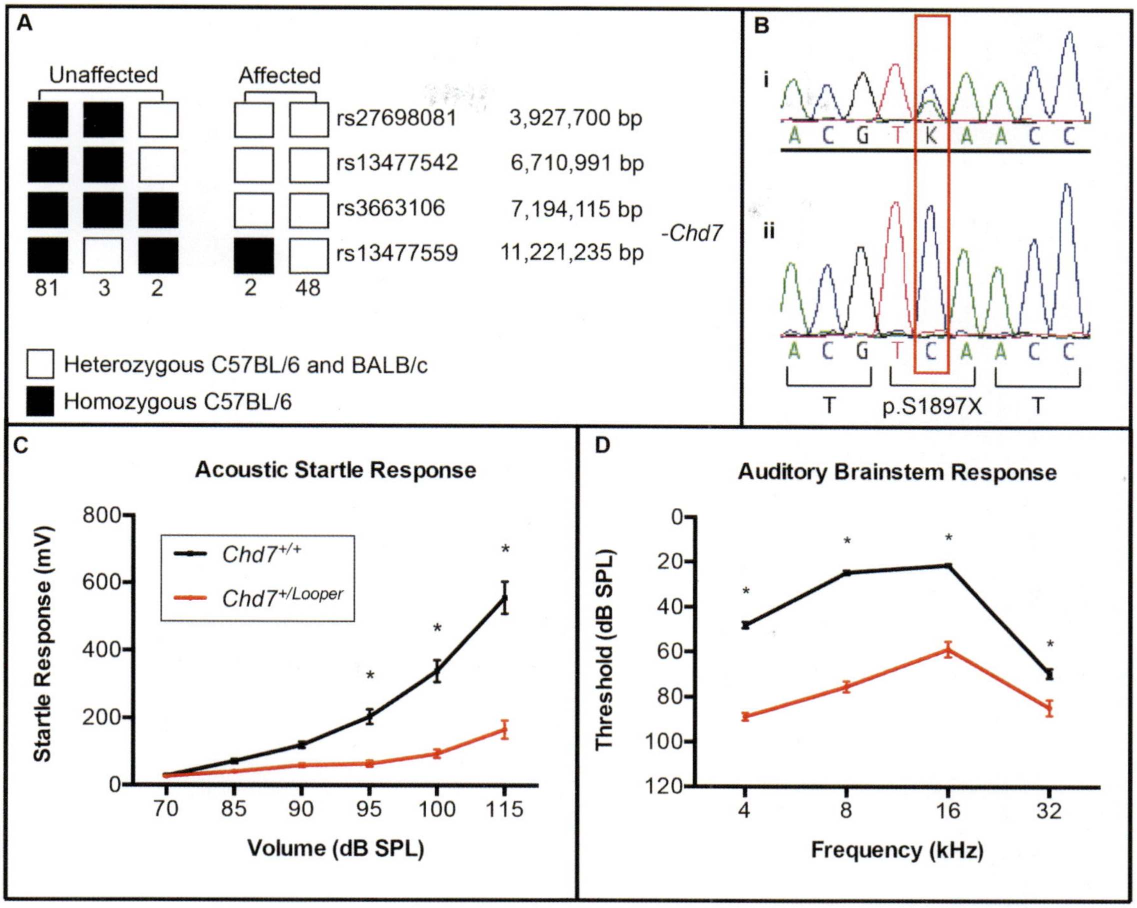


**Figure 1.** ***Looper* mice harbour a nonsense mutation in *Chd7*. A)** 136 $F_1N_1$ mice were click ABR-tested and classified as unaffected (threshold < 35 dB SPL) and affected (threshold >45 dB SPL). Haplotypes for a region of chromosome 4 are illustrated, with the numbers below each haplotype representing the number of mice observed with that haplotype. The region between rs13477542 and rs13477559 was homozygous C57BL/6 in all unaffected mice and heterozygous in all affected mice. This indicated that the *Looper* causative mutation was located between 6,710,991 bp and 11,221,235 bp. **B)** DNA sequence electropherograms of a region of *Chd7* exon 29 in (**i**) an affected *Looper* mouse and (**ii**) an unaffected littermate. The affected mouse was heterozygous for a c.5690C>A mutation, which was predicted to cause premature termination of translation at p.S1897. **C)** Average $Chd7^{+/Looper}$ acoustic startle responses (n = 19) were significantly lower than $Chd7^{+/+}$ controls (n = 20) at 95 to 115 dB SPL. **D)** Average $Chd7^{+/Looper}$ ABR thresholds (n = 18) were significantly elevated at all frequencies in comparison to $Chd7^{+/+}$ controls (n = 21). *$p<0.0001$ using two-way ANOVA and Fisher's Least Significant Difference test. Error Bars = SEM.

## Auditory Brainstem Response

The auditory brainstem response (ABR) of mice was tested using an evoked potentials workstation (Tucker Davis Technologies, Alachua, FL, USA) as described previously [16,18]. Briefly, mice were anaesthetized by intraperitoneal injection of 100 mg/kg ketamine and 20 mg/kg xylazine (BALB/c background) or 100 mg/kg ketamine, 10 mg/kg xylazine and 3 mg/kg acepromazine (mixed genetic background) and eyes moistened with lacrilube. In the latter case 2.5 mg/kg atipamezole hydrochloride was injected at the completion of testing to aid recovery. A free-field magnetic speaker (model FF1, Tucker Davis Technologies) was placed 10 cm from the left pinna. Computer-generated clicks (100 µsec duration, with a spectrum of 0–50 kHz) and 3 msec pure tone stimuli of 4, 8, 16 and 32 kHz were presented with maximum intensities of 100 dB SPL. ABRs were recorded differentially using subdermal needle electrodes (S06666-0, Rochester Electro-Medical, Inc., Lutz, FL, USA) positioned at the vertex of the skull (+ve), in the left cheek (−ve) and the hind left leg (ground). ABRs were averaged over 512 repetitions of each stimulus and traces were analysed to determine ABR threshold using BioSig software (Tucker Davis Technologies). The threshold was defined as the lowest intensity stimulus that reproducibly elicited an ABR.

## Mutation Identification

Exome sequencing of two $N_5$ $Chd7^{+/Looper}$ male mice was performed at the Australian Genome Research Facility (AGRF) using the 100803_MM9_exome_rebal_2_EZ_HX1 exome capture array (Roche Nimblegen, Madison, WI, USA), TruSeq Sample Preparation Kit (Illumina, San Diego, CA, USA) and HiSeq2000 Sequencing System (Illumina). Sequence analysis was performed by the Bioinformatics Unit of the Australian Phenomics Facility. A custom analysis pipeline was used to align the sequence reads with the reference genome (C57BL/6 NCBI m37), filter the raw single nucleotide variant (SNV) calls and generate a list of candidate SNVs as described [19]. Deep-sequencing datasets were deposited into the National Center for Biotechnology Information (NCBI) Sequence Read Archive (http://www.ncbi.nlm.nih.gov/sra) with the study accession number SRP020643. The $Chd7^{Looper}$ SNV was PCR-amplified and sequenced using primers TCCTCTGAGATCTAACGAGTCATC and CCAGCAGAGAAGGGAAGAGA under standard conditions and submitted

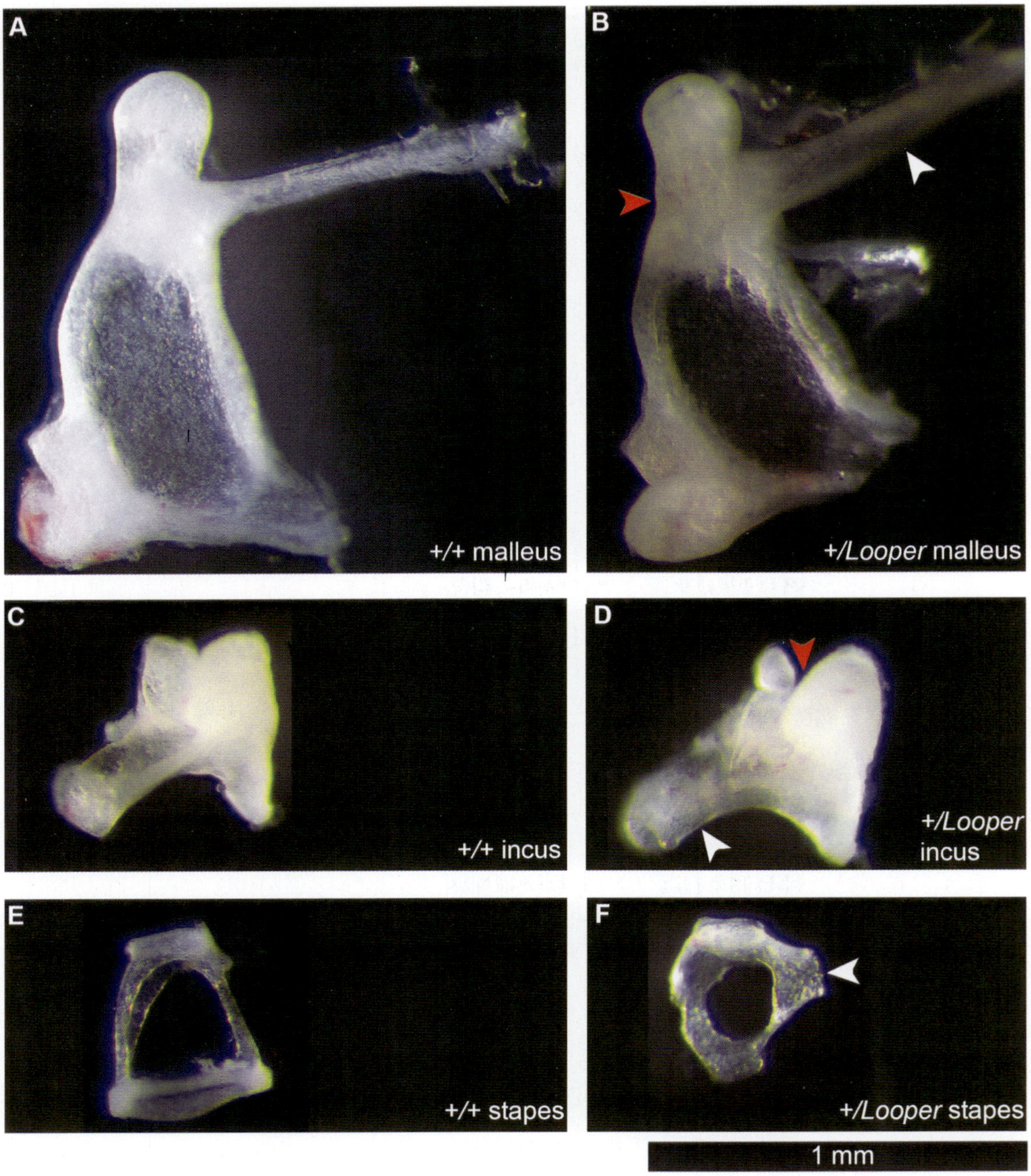


**Figure 2. *Looper* ossicles are malformed.** Light micrographs of whole mount ossicles. **A)** *Chd7*$^{+/+}$ malleus. **B)** *Chd7*$^{+/Looper}$ malleus with slight thickening of the neck (red arrowhead) and a manubrium (white arrowhead) protruding at an acute angle. **C)** *Chd7*$^{+/+}$ incus. **D)** *Chd7*$^{+/Looper}$ incus with deformed glenoid cavity (red arrowhead) and malformation of long process (white arrowhead). **E)** *Chd7*$^{+/+}$ stapes. **F)** *Chd7*$^{+/Looper}$ stapes, which was small and round with a bone bridge (arrowhead) extending from the tubercle to the otic capsule. Images are representative of 8 *Chd7*$^{+/+}$ and 10 *Chd7*$^{+/Looper}$ ears.

to the AGRF for capillary separation. Sequencing electropherograms were aligned using Seqman v 10.1 software (DNASTAR, Madison, WI, USA).

## Linkage Mapping

BALB/c-Chd7$^{+/Looper}$ mice were crossed to C57BL/6 and the resulting $F_1$ offspring were ABR-tested at 8 weeks of age. Those with a click ABR threshold above 40 dB SPL were backcrossed to C57BL/6 to generate 156 $F_1N_1$ offspring. These were ABR-tested at 8 weeks of age and liver DNA isolated as described [20]. Twenty-one affected $F_1N_1$ mice were genotyped for 660 SNPs spaced at 5–10 Mb intervals throughout the genome using the iPLEX Gold method [21], the MassARRAY System (Sequenom, San Diego, CA, USA) and an Autoflex MALDI-TOF mass spectrometer (Bruker, Billerica, MA, USA) at the AGRF. Haplotypes were constructed and regions of heterozygosity identified using Excel v 14.3.4 software (Microsoft, Redmond, WA, USA). $F_1N_1$ mice were genotyped for more finely spaced SNPs on chromosome 4 using the Amplifluor SNPs HT genotyping system FAM-JOE (Merck Millipore, Kilsyth, VIC,

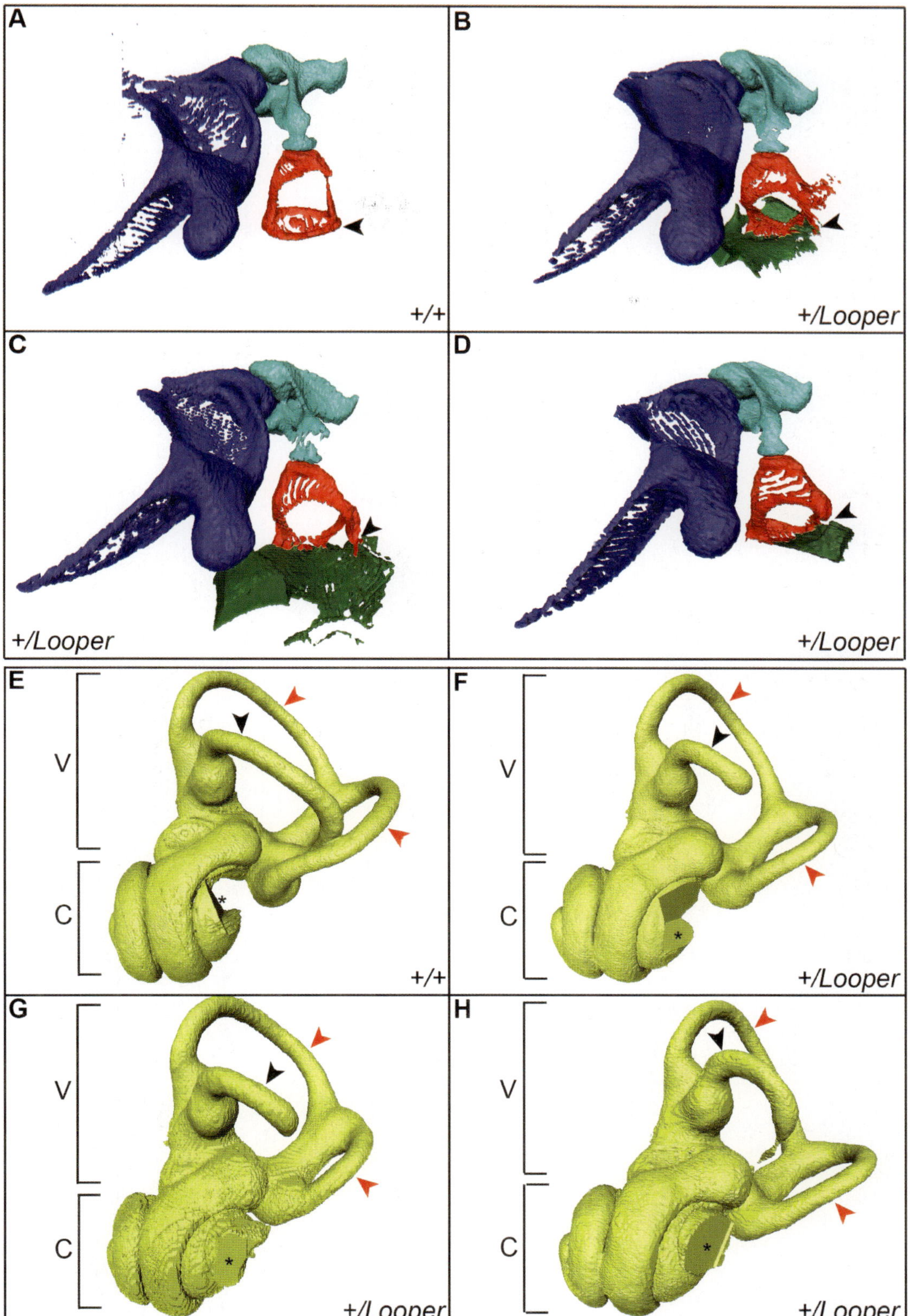


**Figure 3. The *Looper* stapes is fused to the oval window and semicircular canals are abnormal.** μCT images of left middle (A–D) and inner (E–H) ears of $Chd7^{+/+}$ and $Chd7^{+/Looper}$ mice. **A)** $Chd7^{+/+}$ and **B–D)** $Chd7^{+/Looper}$ malleus (purple), incus (aqua) and stapes (red). The stapes footplate (arrowhead) is fused to the oval window of the cochlea (green) in $Chd7^{+/Looper}$ mice. **E)** $Chd7^{+/+}$ and **F–H)** $Chd7^{+/Looper}$ vestibular apparatus (V) and cochlea (C). The lateral semicircular canal (black arrowhead) is incomplete and the posterior and anterior canals (red arrowheads) are hypoplastic in $Cdh7^{+/Looper}$ mice. The missing section in each cochlea (*) was an artifact of the imaging/reconstruction process. n = 1 $Chd7^{+/+}$ and 3 $Chd7^{+/Looper}$ mice.

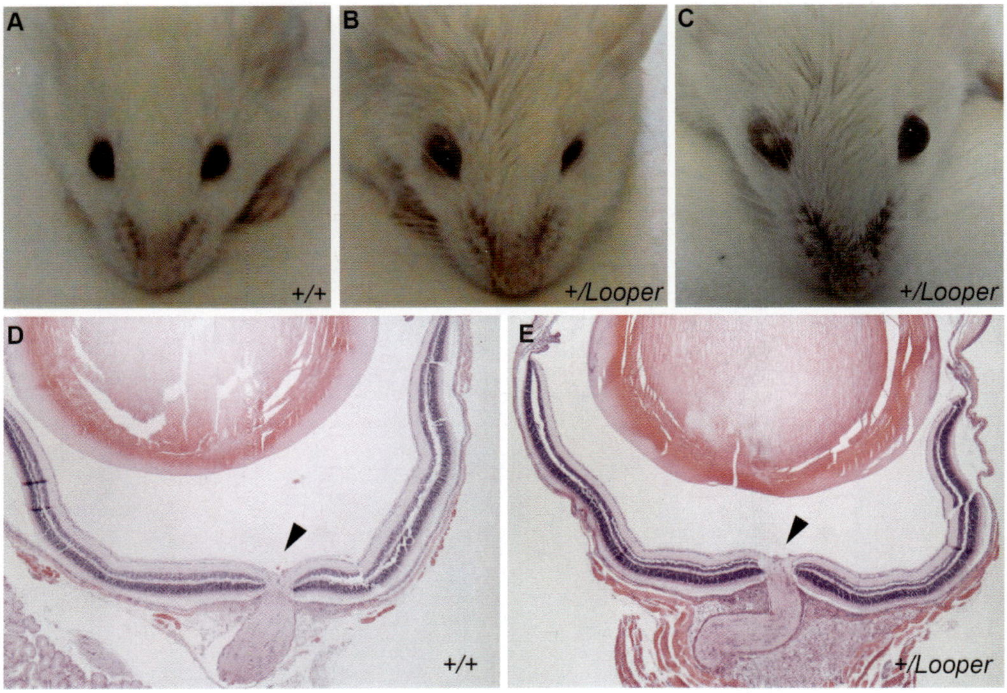


**Figure 4. Looper mice display blepharoconjunctivitis. A–C)** Photograph of the eyes of a *Chd7*$^{+/+}$ mouse compared with those of two affected *Chd7*$^{+/Looper}$ mice. *Chd7*$^{+/Looper}$ mice exhibited lid oedema, narrowed palpebral fissures (B) and blepharoconjunctivitis (C). Mice ages were 7.5 weeks (A, B) and 10 weeks (C). Images are representative of 11 affected *Chd7*$^{+/Looper}$ mice and 19 unaffected *Chd7*$^{+/+}$ mice. **D–E)** Light micrographs of H&E stained sagittal sections of the eye showing the optic nerve head (arrow) for *Chd7*$^{+/+}$ (D) and *Chd7*$^{+/Looper}$ (E) mice aged 6 weeks. Mag. 50x. Images representative of n = 4 per genotype.

Australia) and the primers listed in Table S1. Results were visualized and genotypes assigned using assayauditorEP.xls (Merck Millipore) and excel v 14.3.4 software (Microsoft).

## Histology

For cochlear and middle ear examination, mice were euthanized by intraperitoneal injection of 400 mg/kg ketamine and 80 mg/kg xylazine. After cessation of breathing, PBS was perfused through each animal via a cannula inserted into the left ventricle for 5 min, followed by 10% neutral buffered formalin for 5 min. Cochleae were dissected from the temporal bones and post-fixed for 1 hr at room temperature. Cochleae were washed in tris-buffered saline and decalcified in 10% EDTA for 5 days at 4°C with gentle rolling. Cochleae were oriented in 1% agarose in PBS in 10 mm×10 mm×5 mm cryomolds (Sakura Finetek, Torrance, CA, USA) and paraffin-embedded. 2 μm sections were cut parallel to the modiolus using a microtome and stained with hematoxylin and eosin (H&E). Sections of middle ear cavity were also examined for otitis media.

For eye examination, mice were euthanized via cervical dislocation and eyes fixed in 10% neutral buffered formalin before being embedded in paraffin. 2 μm sagittal sections were cut using a microtome and stained with H&E. Sections were imaged with a DM1000 compound microscope (Leica Microsystems, North Ryde, Australia) and DFC450 C camera (Leica Microsystems).

## X-ray Micro-Computed Tomography (μCT)

μCT was conducted using the Xradia machine MicroXCT-200 (Xradia Inc., Pleasanton, CA, USA), located in the Department of Physics, La Trobe University. An X-ray closed tube source with a Tungsten target was operated at 40 kV tube voltage and power of 10 W. The samples were placed 60–100 mm from the source and 30–50 mm from the detector. The imaging detector was a charge-coupled device camera coupled with a scintillator system and 4x objective lens. The sample was scanned by acquiring 361 projections at equal angles through an angular range of 180 degree using TXMController software (Xradia Inc.). Each projection image was recorded in 7–9 sec. Each image was corrected for the non-uniform illumination in the imaging system, determined by taking a reference image of the beam without sample. A filtered back projection algorithm was then used to reconstruct the acquisition data to create a three-dimensional image using TXMReconstructor software (Xradia Inc.). After the reconstruction process, the distribution of the linear attenuation coefficient was obtained along the section of the sample crossed by the radiation. The total reconstructed volume contained 512×512×512 voxels with the voxel size of 7–11 μm. Three-dimensional (3D) data was viewed with TXM3Dviewer software (Xradia Inc.) and segmented with Avizo-6.2 software (Mercury Computer Systems Inc., Merignac Cedex, France).

## Ocular Examination

Mice were anaesthetised as for ABR testing. To induce dilation of the pupils, 1% Mydriacyl (Alcon Laboratories, NSW, Australia) was applied to the eyes along with an eye lubricant, GenTeal (Novartis, NSW, Australia). A slit lamp was used to examine the anterior segments of each eye. Examination of the retina and optic discs was performed using the slit lamp by placing a cover slip over the cornea. GenTeal between the cornea and cover slip functioned as an ocular medium.

## Behavioural Testing

**Locomotor cell.** The TruScan photo beam activity monitoring system was used to monitor locomotor activity of mice over

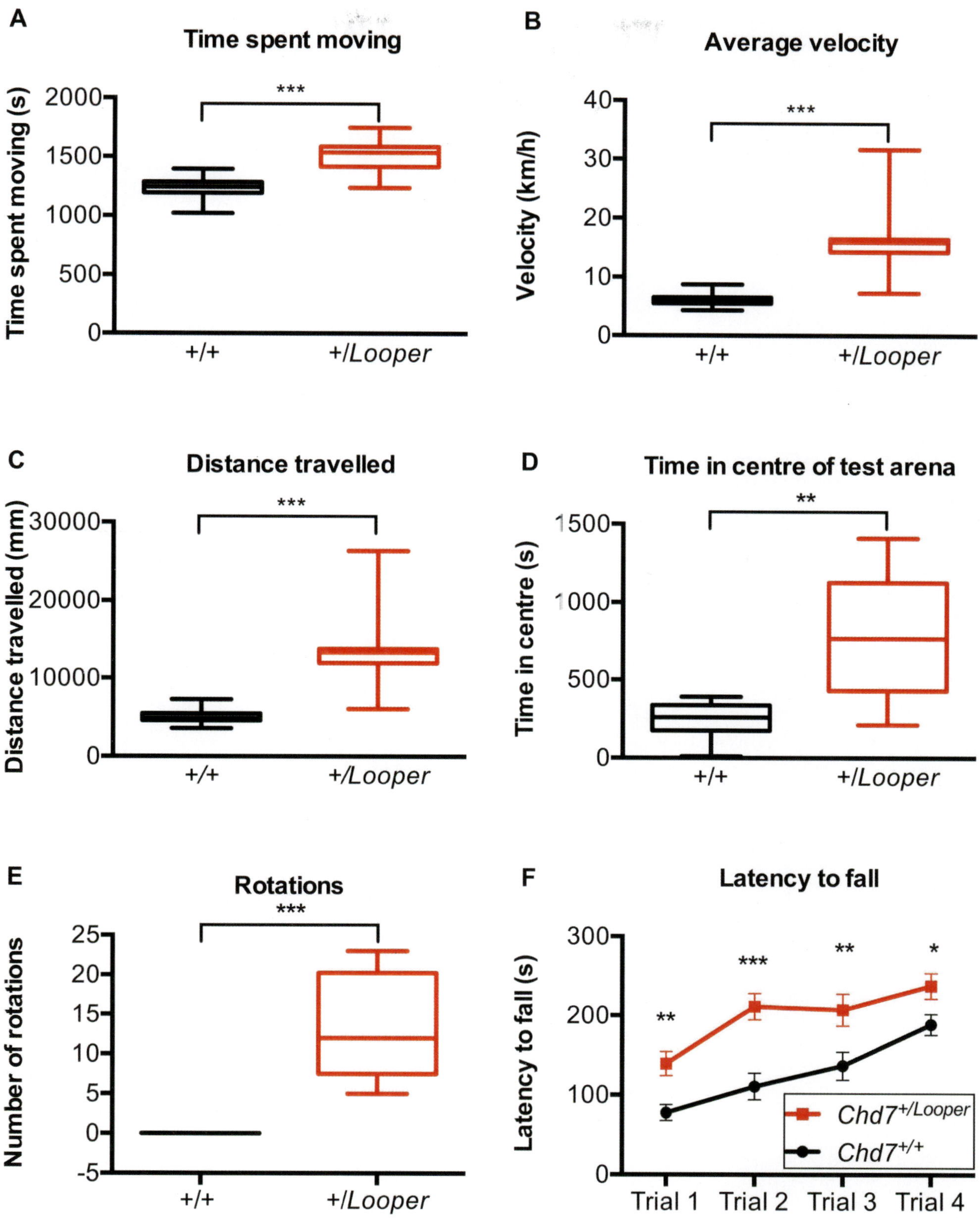


**Figure 5.** ***Looper* mice are hyperactive. A–E)** Box and whisker plots illustrating the mean and 1–99 percentile range for cohorts of *Chd7*$^{+/Looper}$ and *Chd7*$^{+/+}$ littermates for measures taken during Locomotor Cell and Swim testing. $^{**}p<0.001$, $^{***}p<0.0001$ calculated using the Mann Whitney test. **A)** Time spent moving. **B)** Average velocity. **C)** Distance travelled. **D)** Time spent in the centre of the test arena. **E)** Complete rotations made during 1 min of swimming. **F)** Plot of the average latency to fall off the rotor rod over the course of each of four trials, for cohorts of *Chd7*$^{+/Looper}$ and *Chd7*$^{+/+}$ littermates. Error Bars = SEM. $^{*}p<0.05$, $^{**}p<0.001$, $^{***}p<0.0001$ calculated using two-way ANOVA and post-hoc Fisher's Least Significant Difference test (F). n = 12 *Chd7*$^{+/+}$ and 12 *Chd7*$^{+/Looper}$ mice.

a 30 min period. Individual mice were placed in locomotor cells (40.6 cm wide×40.6 cm deep×40.6 cm high) in dim (10 lux) lighting. Photo-optic arrays encased the cell containing beams evenly spaced 2.5 cm apart to quantify mouse movements.

**Swim test.** Mice were placed in an inescapable beaker of 25°C water for 1 min. A ceiling-mounted colour CCTV camera (Sony, North Ryde, NSW, Australia) and a DMRES10 DVD recorder (Panasonic, Macquarie Park, NSW, Australia) were used to record behaviour including mobility, sinking and directional rotations.

**Rotarod.** Mice were placed on a rotarod (Ugo Basil, Comerio, VA, Italy) for 4 trials with 1 hr between trials. Trials were conducted under standard lighting of 300 lux. The rotarod speed gradually increased from 4 to 40 rpm during each 5 min trial. The time taken for the mouse to fall off the rotarod was recorded.

**Digigait.** Footprint analysis was conducted using the digigait computerised digital footprint analysis system (Mouse Specifics Inc., MA. USA). Mice were accustomed to a treadmill moving at increasing speeds prior to recording. Four complete step cycles at 15 cm/sec were recorded. Mice were placed in the Perspex chamber on the motorised transparent treadmill and the movement of the paws was captured from the ventral aspect using an A62 high-speed digital video recorder (Basler, Exton, PA, USA) mounted underneath. Gait parameters were calculated using Digigait analysis software.

### Statistical Analysis

Two-way ANOVA, post hoc t-tests, Mann Whitney tests and the Holm Sidak method for multiple testing were performed using Prism 6 software (GraphPad Software Inc.). The Chi-squared test was manually calculated.

## Results

### The *Looper* Phenotype is Caused by a Nonsense Mutation in *Chd7*

*Looper* arose in an ENU mutagenesis screen for deaf mice. The $G_1$ *Looper* founder mouse failed to startle in response to loud noise and this phenotype proved heritable in a dominant fashion. Meiotic mapping was undertaken to identify the genomic location of the *Looper* mutation. The ABR in response to clicks of 156 $F_1N_1$ mice was assessed, and mice were classified as affected (threshold >45 dB SPL) or unaffected (threshold <35 dB SPL). 20 mice had an intermediate click ABR threshold and were excluded from subsequent analysis. Genotyping of 21 affected $F_1N_1$ mice for 660 SNPs spaced every 5–10 Mb throughout the genome revealed a shared common haplotype between rs13477541 and rs32379175 of proximal chromosome 4 (data not shown). Genotyping of 136 $F_1N_1$ mice for SNPs within this region narrowed the minimal linkage interval to between rs13477542 at 6.7 Mb and rs13477559 at 11.2 Mb (Figure 1A).

Genomic DNA of two BALB/c-*Chd7*$^{+/Looper}$ $N_5$ male mice was subjected to exome enrichment and massively parallel DNA sequencing. 90% of the consensus coding sequence (CCDS) exome was sequenced at least 4-fold and the average depth of sequencing was 84 to 95 fold (Table S2). Between 10 and 14 SNVs were identified in each sample, with 7 SNVs present in both samples, in the following genes: *Ercc5*, *Ankrd44*, *Chd7*, *Mup20*, *Ric3*, *Txlnb* and *Kcnh4*. The only SNV within the minimal linkage interval was the *Chd7* SNV at 8.9 Mb on chromosome 4. Sanger sequencing of DNA from affected and unaffected littermates confirmed this SNV to be a point mutation that segregated with the *Looper* phenotype (Figure 1B). This c.5690C>A change in exon 29 is predicted to result in premature termination of translation of *Chd7* (c.5690C>A, p.S1897X, NCBI reference sequences NC_000070.6, NM_001081417.1, CCDS38689.1, NP_001074886.1).

### *Looper* Mice are Hearing-impaired

*Chd7*$^{+/Looper}$ mice startled less than *Chd7*$^{+/+}$ littermates in response to mixed frequency noise (Figure 1C). ABR thresholds of *Chd7*$^{+/Looper}$ mice were significantly elevated between 4 and 32 kHz (Figure 1D). An average threshold shift of 40–50 dB SPL was observed at 4, 8 and 16 kHz, while at 32 kHz, where BALB/c mice are prone to early onset age-related hearing loss [22], an average shift of 15 dB SPL was observed. Interestingly, the average click ABR threshold was significantly higher in *Chd7*$^{+/Looper}$ mice on the BALB/c genetic background than the mixed C57BL/6-BALB/c background (Figure S1).

### *Looper* Mice Display Middle Ear and Vestibular Defects

*Chd7*$^{+/Looper}$ ossicles displayed a range of malformations. The *Chd7*$^{+/Looper}$ malleus manubrium protruded at an abnormally acute angle while the neck was thickened and malformed (Figure 2A–B). The *Chd7*$^{+/Looper}$ incus exhibited incomplete development of the long and short process and malformation of the facet (Figure 2C–D). The most striking developmental anomaly was the *Chd7*$^{+/Looper}$ stapes, which was rounded and small with an ectopic bone bridge extending from the tubercle to the otic capsule (Figure 2E–F). μCT imaging revealed fusion of the

**Table 2.** Penetrance of *Looper* phenotypes.

| Phenotype | Number of *Chd7*$^{+/Looper}$ mice examined | Number of *Chd7*$^{+/+}$ mice examined |
|---|---|---|
| Circling | 5/6 | 0/10 |
| Low acoustic startle response (<200 mV at 115 dB SPL) | 15/17 | 0/22 |
| Hearing impairment (click ABR threshold >40 dB SPL) | 18/18 | 0/22 |
| Stapes malformation (whole mounts) | 5/5 | 0/4 |
| Semicircular canal malformation (microCT) | 3/3 | 0/1 |
| Swimming in circles | 12/12 | 0/12 |
| Hyperactivity (average velocity >10 km/hr) | 11/12 | 0/12 |
| Blepharoconjunctivitis | 11/16 | 0/19 |

stapedial footplate to the oval window of the cochlea in all 3 *Chd7*$^{+/Looper}$ samples examined (Figure 3A–D). μCT also revealed incomplete development of the lateral semicircular canal and various degrees of hypoplasia of the posterior and anterior canals (Figure 3E–H). Mid-modiolar sections of the cochlea were examined from four *Chd7*$^{+/+}$ and four *Chd7*$^{+/Looper}$ mice and revealed no morphological differences (data not shown).

### *Looper* Mice have Blepharoconjunctivitis but not Coloboma

*Chd7*$^{+/Looper}$ mice exhibited variable, narrowed palpebral fissures and lid oedema, often with one eye severely affected and one eye moderately affected or normal (Figure 4A–C). Eye irritation and probable blepharoconjunctivitis were observed in 11 of 16 *Chd7*$^{+/Looper}$ mice examined. Coloboma was not observed during retinal examination or by histological analysis of the eye (Figure 4D–E).

### *Looper* Mice are Hyperactive and Circle

*Looper* mice exhibited circling behaviour (Video S1). During Locomotor Cell testing, *Chd7*$^{+/Looper}$ mice spent significantly more time moving than *Chd7*$^{+/+}$ controls (Figure 5A). On average, *Chd7*$^{+/Looper}$ mice ran twice as quickly (Figure 5B) and travelled twice as far (Figure 5C) as *Chd7*$^{+/+}$ controls. This hyperactivity could be the reason for the observed growth delay of *Looper* mice, which were 30% lighter than controls (Figure S2). *Chd7*$^{+/Looper}$ mice were inclined to circle within the centre of the test arena, whilst *Chd7*$^{+/+}$ mice preferred the edges of the test arena (Figure 5D). Similar behaviours were observed during the swim test, with *Chd7*$^{+/+}$ mice occasionally floating motionless or seeking refuge at the outskirts of the test arena, whilst *Chd7*$^{+/Looper}$ mice swam in circles (Figure 5E, Video S2). *Chd7*$^{+/Looper}$ mice had a longer latency to fall from a rotating rod (Figure 5F) and scored normally in the digigait test (data not shown). These results indicate that directional control, but not motor coordination, is impaired in *Chd7*$^{+/Looper}$ mice.

## Discussion

The *Looper* mutation arose during an ENU mutagenesis screen for deaf mice. Linkage mapping and exome sequencing revealed the *Looper* allele to contain a nonsense mutation at codon 1897 of the *Chromodomain Helicase DNA binding 7* gene (*Chd7*). This nonsense mutation may mediate mRNA degradation (reviewed in [23]). Alternatively, a truncated CHD7 protein may be produced. Such a protein would lack two C-terminal BRK domains (www.ncbi.nlm.nih.gov/protein sequence NP_001264078.1) and may have reduced or dominant negative activity. However, the phenotypic similarity between *Chd7*$^{+/Looper}$ and *Chd7*$^{+/Edy}$ mice, which harbour a nonsense mutation at codon 103 [11], indicates that *Chd7*$^{Looper}$ is likely to be a null allele. The human and mouse amino acid sequences for CHD7 are 95% identical, and although there are no reported mutations that would truncate the human protein at the orthologous residue to *Looper* (p.S1907), multiple pathogenic nonsense mutations have been documented within 10 amino acids [24].

This is the 12$^{th}$ ENU-induced mutation reported for *Chd7*. The large size of the gene (>228,601 bp, 38 exons, reference sequence NC_000070.6) renders it prone to mutation. The same is true for the human orthologue *CHD7*, with 772 reported human mutations in the *CHD7* database (www.chd7.org) [24]. 75% of these mutations are nonsense or frameshift [25]. These pathogenic variants of *CHD7* result in CHARGE syndrome, a complex disease characterised by variable presentation of a range of developmental defects. The pattern of defects observed in human patients is largely reflected in the collection of reported mouse models bearing mutations in *Chd7*. In this manuscript we described in detail the hearing, eye and behavioural abnormalities of the *CHD7*-deficient *Looper* strain. Like other *Chd7* mutant mice, some phenotypes are incompletely penetrant in the *Looper* strain (Table 2). Characterisation of this, and other models of *CHD7*-deficiency will facilitate understanding of the role of this gene and the molecular pathways that it regulates during development.

*Chd7*$^{+/Looper}$ mice displayed an attenuated startle in response to white noise, indicating that they were not profoundly deaf. They had an average ABR threshold shift of 50.8 dB SPL at 8 kHz and an average 15.2 dB SPL threshold shift at 32 kHz. This is consistent with conductive hearing loss [26], with higher frequencies still detected due to bone conduction [27]. Cochlear histology was normal but ossicles were abnormal and the stapes fixed. Malformations of the ossicle chain were similar to those reported for other *Chd7* mutants [28]. μCT images of these ossicle abnormalities have not been published before. Unlike the *Chd7*$^{Ome}$ mouse [29], otitis media was not observed in *Looper* mice. *Looper* displayed severe hypoplasia of the lateral semicircular canal and variable hypoplasia of the other canals. This is consistent with malformation of the lateral semicircular canal in other *Chd7* mouse mutants [11,28] and in CHARGE patients, where the lateral canal is always affected and other canals are occasionally mildly affected [30].

*Chd7*$^{+/Looper}$ click ABR thresholds were more severely elevated on the BALB/c genetic background than on the BALB/c.C57BL/6 mixed genetic background. Furthermore, the severity of *Looper* hearing loss and ossicle malformation differed from that of published *Chd7* mutants on different genetic backgrounds [28,31]. These observations indicate that modifier genes affect the severity of the *Chd7*-deficient hearing phenotype.

An exact cause of the eye inflammation and discharge in *Chd7* mutant mice is yet to be identified. Other *Chd7* mutant mice have been reported to display keratoconjunctivitis sicca or "dry eye" [11]. In contrast, *Looper* mice display blepharoconjuctivitis, which may indicate increased susceptibility to infection or structural changes of the eye socket and lid. Bilateral asymmetry of *Looper* eye phenotypes correlates with CHARGE, but blepharoconjunctivitis does not [32]. Furthermore, ocular coloboma, one of the major diagnostic features of CHARGE was not observed in *Looper* mice.

*Looper* mice spend more time moving at high speed than controls. Hyperactivity has also been noted in CHARGE patients [5]. Vestibular deformity is most likely responsible for the circling behaviour of *Looper* mice. Surprisingly, *Looper* mice demonstrated an enhanced level of motor control during the rotarod test. It is possible the that the innate running behaviour of *Chd7*$^{+/Looper}$ mice may have lead to a higher level of physical conditioning, a confounding factor during this test. However, digigait analysis confirmed that *Looper* motor function was not impaired. Feng *et al.* described reduced neuronal differentiation and abnormal dendritic development of *Chd7*-deficient mice which returned to normal as a result of voluntary running [33]. It is possible that the excessive running of *Chd7*$^{+/Looper}$ mice has a positive effect on their neural pathways.

The excessive activity of *Chd7*$^{+/Looper}$ mice may cause growth delay through reduced food intake and increased energy expenditure. Alternatively, altered hormone levels may be a factor causing growth delay. Postnatal growth delay in CHARGE has been correlated with endocrine anomalies including gonadotrophin and growth hormone deficiencies [34], but the exact cause of growth delay is not understood. Whilst we did not observe heart anomalies or choanal atresia in Looper mice, this may have been due to pre-weaning deaths. 41% (68 of 167) of weaned mice had the *Chd7*$^{Looper/+}$ genotype. This is significantly different from the expected 50% ($p<0.05$ by Chi-squared test). Heart anomalies, cleft palate and choanal atresia have been identified in embryos of other *Chd7* mutant mice and attributed to early mortality [11].

## Conclusions

*Looper* mice carry an ENU-induced null mutation causing dominant *Chd7* haploinsufficiency. They display phenotypes related to those observed in human CHARGE syndrome including growth retardation, facial asymmetry, hyperactivity, hearing impairment, semicircular canal hypoplasia and fusion of the stapes to the otic capsule and cochlea. Further analysis of the *Looper* strain will facilitate elucidation of the function of *Chd7* and the pathology of CHARGE syndrome.

## Supporting Information

**Figure S1 *Looper* hearing loss is modified by genetic background.** Box and whisker plot illustrating the mean and 1–99 percentile range of ABR thresholds in response to clicks for cohorts of affected and unaffected littermates with different genetic backgrounds. Average ABR thresholds were lower for C57BL/6.BALB/c-*Chd7*$^{+/Looper}$ mice (n = 59) than for BALB/c-*Chd7*$^{+/Looper}$ mice (n = 18). ***$p<0.0001$ calculated using the Mann Whitney test. (C57BL/6.BALB/c-*Chd*$^{+/+}$ n = 87, BALB/c-*Chd7*$^{+/+}$ n = 21).
(TIFF)

**Figure S2 *Looper* mice are growth-delayed. A)** Graphs plotting the average weights of cohorts of male and female *Chd7*$^{+/+}$ (n = 14 female and 23 male) and *Chd7*$^{+/Looper}$ (n = 13 female and 12 male) mice each week from 3–12 weeks of age. *$p<0.05$ calculated using $t$ – tests. **B)** Photograph of 53 day old male *Chd7*$^{+/Looper}$ and *Chd7*$^{+/+}$ littermates illustrating the difference in size and length. Scale Bar = 5 cm.
(TIF)

**Table S1 Primers used in meiotic mapping.**

**Table S2 Massively parallel sequencing results.**

**Video S1 *Looper* mice run in circles.** Video of *Chd7*$^{+/+}$ (left) and *Chd7*$^{+/Looper}$ (right) littermates, documenting the circling behavior commonly observed for *Chd7*$^{+/Looper}$ mice.
(MP4)

**Video S2 *Looper* mice swim in circles.** Video of *Chd7*$^{+/+}$ (left) and *Chd7*$^{+/Looper}$ (right) littermates, documenting the swimming in circles commonly observed for *Chd7*$^{+/Looper}$ mice during the 1 min swim test. Representative of n = 12 *Chd7*$^{+/+}$ and n = 12 *Chd7*$^{+/Looper}$ mice.
(MP4)

## Acknowledgments

The authors wish to acknowledge technical assistance provided by Michael Manning, Anne Cooray, Elaine Major, Theresa Gibbs, Matthew Salzone, and Melanie Salzone.

## Author Contributions

Conceived and designed the experiments: RAB MRC JMO. Performed the experiments: JMO BDA BTK RCAS MRC RAB. Analyzed the data: JMO BDA BTK RCAS MRC RAB. Wrote the paper: JMO RAB MRC. Contributed to drafting of the manuscript: BTK BDA RCAS.

## References

1. Petit C (2006) From deafness genes to hearing mechanisms: harmony and counterpoint. Trends Mol Med 12: 57–64.
2. Dror AA, Avraham KB (2009) Hearing loss: mechanisms revealed by genetics and cell biology. Annu Rev Genet 43: 411–437.
3. Toriello H, Reardon W, Gorlin R (2004) Hereditary Hearing Loss and its Syndromes. New York: Oxford University Press.
4. Friedman LM, Dror AA, Avraham KB (2007) Mouse models to study inner ear development and hereditary hearing loss. Int J Dev Biol 51: 609–631.
5. Graham JM Jr, Rosner B, Dykens E, Visootsak J (2005) Behavioral features of CHARGE syndrome (Hall-Hittner syndrome) comparison with Down syndrome, Prader-Willi syndrome, and Williams syndrome. Am J Med Genet A 133A: 240–247.
6. Blake KD, Prasad C (2006) CHARGE syndrome. Orphanet J Rare Dis 1: 34.
7. Issekutz KA, Graham JM Jr, Prasad C, Smith IM, Blake KD (2005) An epidemiological analysis of CHARGE syndrome: preliminary results from a Canadian study. Am J Med Genet A 133A: 309–317.
8. Hurd EA, Micucci JA, Reamer EN, Martin DM (2012) Delayed fusion and altered gene expression contribute to semicircular canal defects in Chd7 deficient mice. Mech Dev 129: 308–323.
9. Bajpai R, Chen DA, Rada-Iglesias A, Zhang J, Xiong Y, et al. (2010) CHD7 cooperates with PBAF to control multipotent neural crest formation. Nature 463: 958–962.
10. Bouazoune K, Kingston RE (2012) Chromatin remodeling by the CHD7 protein is impaired by mutations that cause human developmental disorders. Proc Natl Acad Sci U S A 109: 19238–19243.
11. Bosman EA, Penn AC, Ambrose JC, Kettleborough R, Stemple DL, et al. (2005) Multiple mutations in mouse Chd7 provide models for CHARGE syndrome. Hum Mol Genet 14: 3463–3476.
12. Hurd EA, Capers PL, Blauwkamp MN, Adams ME, Raphael Y, et al. (2007) Loss of Chd7 function in gene-trapped reporter mice is embryonic lethal and associated with severe defects in multiple developing tissues. Mamm Genome 18: 94–104.
13. Schnetz MP, Handoko L, Akhtar-Zaidi B, Bartels CF, Pereira CF, et al. (2010) CHD7 targets active gene enhancer elements to modulate ES cell-specific gene expression. PLoS Genet 6: e1001023.
14. Puc J, Rosenfeld MG (2011) SOX2 and CHD7 cooperatively regulate human disease genes. Nat Genet 43: 505–506.
15. Bergman JE, Janssen N, van der Sloot AM, de Walle HE, Schoots J, et al. (2012) A novel classification system to predict the pathogenic effects of CHD7 missense variants in CHARGE syndrome. Hum Mutat 33: 1251–1260.
16. Carpinelli MR, Manning MG, Kile BT, Rachel AB (2013) Two ENU-induced alleles of Atp2b2 cause deafness in mice. PLoS One 8: e67479.
17. Carpinelli MR, Wise AK, Arhatari BD, Bouillet P, Manji SS, et al. (2012) Anti-apoptotic gene Bcl2 is required for stapes development and hearing. Cell Death Dis 3: e362.
18. Carpinelli MR, Wise AK, Burt RA (2011) Vitamin D-deficient diet rescues hearing loss in Klotho mice. Hear Res 275: 105–109.
19. Andrews TD, Whittle B, Field MA, Balakishnan B, Zhang Y, et al. (2012) Massively parallel sequencing of the mouse exome to accurately identify rare, induced mutations: an immediate source for thousands of new mouse models. Open Biol 2: 120061.
20. Laird PW, Zijderveld A, Linders K, Rudnicki MA, Jaenisch R, et al. (1991) Simplified mammalian DNA isolation procedure. Nucleic Acids Res 19: 4293.
21. Mendisco F, Keyser C, Hollard C, Seldes V, Nielsen AE, et al. (2011) Application of the iPLEX Gold SNP genotyping method for the analysis of Amerindian ancient DNA samples: benefits for ancient population studies. Electrophoresis 32: 386–393.
22. Willott JF, Turner JG, Carlson S, Ding D, Seegers Bross L, et al. (1998) The BALB/c mouse as an animal model for progressive sensorineural hearing loss. Hear Res 115: 162–174.
23. Schweingruber C, Rufener SC, Zund D, Yamashita A, Muhlemann O (2013) Nonsense-mediated mRNA decay - mechanisms of substrate mRNA recognition and degradation in mammalian cells. Biochim Biophys Acta 1829: 612–623.
24. van den Akker PC, Jonkman MF, Rengaw T, Bruckner-Tuderman L, Has C, et al. (2011) The international dystrophic epidermolysis bullosa patient registry: an online database of dystrophic epidermolysis bullosa patients and their COL7A1 mutations. Hum Mutat 32: 1100–1107.
25. Janssen N, Bergman JE, Swertz MA, Tranebjaerg L, Lodahl M, et al. (2012) Mutation update on the CHD7 gene involved in CHARGE syndrome. Hum Mutat 33: 1149–1160.
26. Qin Z, Wood M, Rosowski JJ (2010) Measurement of conductive hearing loss in mice. Hear Res 263: 93–103.
27. Chordekar S, Kriksunov L, Kishon-Rabin L, Adelman C, Sohmer H (2012) Mutual cancellation between tones presented by air conduction, by bone conduction and by non-osseous (soft tissue) bone conduction. Hear Res 283: 180–184.

28. Pau H, Hawker K, Fuchs H, De Angelis MH, Steel KP (2004) Characterization of a new mouse mutant, flouncer, with a balance defect and inner ear malformation. Otol Neurotol 25: 707–713.
29. Tian C, Yu H, Yang B, Han F, Zheng Y, et al. (2012) Otitis media in a new mouse model for CHARGE syndrome with a deletion in the Chd7 gene. PLoS One 7: e34944.
30. Abadie V, Wiener-Vacher S, Morisseau-Durand MP, Poree C, Amiel J, et al. (2000) Vestibular anomalies in CHARGE syndrome: investigations on and consequences for postural development. Eur J Pediatr 159: 569–574.
31. Hurd EA, Adams ME, Layman WS, Swiderski DL, Beyer LA, et al. (2011) Mature middle and inner ears express Chd7 and exhibit distinctive pathologies in a mouse model of CHARGE syndrome. Hear Res 282: 184–195.
32. Nishina S, Kosaki R, Yagihashi T, Azuma N, Okamoto N, et al. (2012) Ophthalmic features of CHARGE syndrome with CHD7 mutations. Am J Med Genet A 158A: 514–518.
33. Feng W, Khan MA, Bellvis P, Zhu Z, Bernhardt O, et al. (2013) The chromatin remodeler CHD7 regulates adult neurogenesis via activation of SoxC transcription factors. Cell Stem Cell 13: 62–72.
34. Tellier AL, Cormier-Daire V, Abadie V, Amiel J, Sigaudy S, et al. (1998) CHARGE syndrome: report of 47 cases and review. Am J Med Genet 76: 402–409.
35. Jiang X, Zhou Y, Xian L, Chen W, Wu H, et al. (2012) The mutation in Chd7 causes misexpression of Bmp4 and developmental defects in telencephalic midline. Am J Pathol 181: 626–641.
36. Randall V, McCue K, Roberts C, Kyriakopoulou V, Beddow S, et al. (2009) Great vessel development requires biallelic expression of Chd7 and Tbx1 in pharyngeal ectoderm in mice. J Clin Invest 119: 3301–3310.
37. Hurd EA, Poucher HK, Cheng K, Raphael Y, Martin DM (2010) The ATP-dependent chromatin remodeling enzyme CHD7 regulates pro-neural gene expression and neurogenesis in the inner ear. Development 137: 3139–3150.
38. Lenz DR (2010) The inner ear phenotype of Volchok (Vlk): An ENU-induced mouse model for CHARGE syndrome. Audiological Medicine 8: 110–119.

# 11

# Advanced Beamformers for Cochlear Implant Users: Acute Measurement of Speech Perception in Challenging Listening Conditions

**Andreas Buechner[1,2]*, Karl-Heinz Dyballa[1], Phillipp Hehrmann[3], Stefan Fredelake[3], Thomas Lenarz[1,2]**

**1** Department of Otolaryngology, Medical University Hannover, Hannover, Germany, **2** Cluster of Excellence hearing4all, Medical University Hannover, Hannover, Germany, **3** Advanced Bionics GmbH, European Research Center, Hannover, Germany

## Abstract

***Objective:*** To investigate the performance of monaural and binaural beamforming technology with an additional noise reduction algorithm, in cochlear implant recipients.

***Method:*** This experimental study was conducted as a single subject repeated measures design within a large German cochlear implant centre. Twelve experienced users of an Advanced Bionics HiRes90K or CII implant with a Harmony speech processor were enrolled. The cochlear implant processor of each subject was connected to one of two bilaterally placed state-of-the-art hearing aids (Phonak Ambra) providing three alternative directional processing options: an omnidirectional setting, an adaptive monaural beamformer, and a binaural beamformer. A further noise reduction algorithm (ClearVoice) was applied to the signal on the cochlear implant processor itself. The speech signal was presented from 0° and speech shaped noise presented from loudspeakers placed at ±70°, ±135° and 180°. The Oldenburg sentence test was used to determine the signal-to-noise ratio at which subjects scored 50% correct.

***Results:*** Both the adaptive and binaural beamformer were significantly better than the omnidirectional condition (5.3 dB±1.2 dB and 7.1 dB±1.6 dB ($p<0.001$) respectively). The best score was achieved with the binaural beamformer in combination with the ClearVoice noise reduction algorithm, with a significant improvement in SRT of 7.9 dB±2.4 dB ($p<0.001$) over the omnidirectional alone condition.

***Conclusions:*** The study showed that the binaural beamformer implemented in the Phonak Ambra hearing aid could be used in conjunction with a Harmony speech processor to produce substantial average improvements in SRT of 7.1 dB. The monaural, adaptive beamformer provided an averaged SRT improvement of 5.3 dB.

**Editor:** Meni Wanunu, Northeastern University, United States of America

**Funding:** Supported by the EU grant "Europa fördert Niedersachsen" (http://www.eufoerdert.niedersachsen.de/portal/live.php?navigation_id = 5562&article_id = 15298&_psmand = 18). The funders had no role in study design, data collection and analysis, decision to publish, or preparation of the manuscript.

**Competing Interests:** The authors have read the journal's policy and have the following conflicts: One co-author of the manuscript was employed by the MHH using 'no strings' funding supplied by Advanced Bionics. Additionally two co-authors hold scientific posts in the Advanced Bionics European Research Centre. The study protocol was developed in close cooperation between MHH and Advanced Bionics. All testing was conducted at MHH by MHH employees and all data were again analyzed in close cooperation between Advanced Bionics and MHH.

* E-mail: buechner@hoerzentrum-hannover.de

## Introduction

The performance of cochlear implant users continues to improve and many achieve good levels of speech perception, especially in quiet. Performance in noise however remains a challenge and manufacturers are constantly exploring different methods to improve it: Advances in the coding strategies used by the different devices, electrode design and the application of bilateral implants all contribute to improvements in performance [1–4]. However, technologies that have the ability to minimise the impact of noise in the incoming signal and improve the signal-to-noise ratio (SNR) have long been used in hearing aids and are now being explored in cochlear implants.

Cochlear implant manufacturers have used a number of different algorithms to reduce noise in the processing pathway such as Adaptive Dynamic Range Optimisation, used in recent versions of the Cochlear device [5] or ClearVoice, used in recent versions of the Advanced Bionics device [6]. Both these algorithms operate internally on a single-channel audio signal. More effective noise suppression techniques can be applied when signals from several microphones are available. Beamforming algorithms combine signals from multiple microphones to shape the directional response characteristics of the output. Rather than being equally sensitive to signals from all directions (omnidirectional), beamformers show highest sensitivity only for signals arriving from a limited range of angles. This directional selectivity can reduce the amount of noise drastically, if target and interfering signals are spatially separated in the environment. Despite being a standard feature in hearing aids for over a decade, the first beamforming algorithms for cochlear implant processors were commercially introduced in 2005 for users of the Cochlear Freedom sound processor [7–9].

Beamforming works by exploiting phase differences in the signal arriving at two or more spatially separated microphones from a particular direction of incidence. After applying an appropriate delay, the inputs can be subtracted from each other and different directionality patterns can thus be achieved. Beamformers can be used to produce a static pattern of directionality, where the point of maximum attenuation or null is fixed or an adaptive one, where the null follows dynamically the direction of noise incidence. That means adaptive systems have the advantage of being able to suppress moving noise sources.

In order for beamforming to work, a number of assumptions typically have to be met: the target should always be located within a narrow range on angles in front of the listener, and the target level should be identical at the two microphones. Well matched and calibrated microphones are essential and in reverberant rooms the performance has been shown to degrade, as both target and interfering noise become more spatially diffuse and consequentially more difficult to separate based on their directionality [10–13]. This limits the degree to which improvements measured in a highly controlled lab environment can be transferred to real life situations.

Directional microphones have been effectively employed in hearing aids to improve user performance in noise [14–17]. Ricketts and Henry (*2002*) compared fixed directional, adaptive, and omnidirectional microphone programs in 20 hearing impaired users of the Phonak Claro hearing aid (Phonak AG, Switzerland). They tested four noise conditions in a moderately reverberant room: (a) diffuse noise from 5 speakers at $75^0$ intervals, (b) noise from 2 speakers at $160^0$ and $200^0$ behind the listener, (c) noise from speakers at $70^0$ and $110^0$ to the side and (d) panning noise across all five speakers. Speech was always presented from 0° in front of the listener. The adaptive system was significantly better than the omnidirectional setting for all conditions, with a 2.9 dB improvement for sentences in diffuse noise. The fixed setting was only significantly better than the omnidirectional setting when the noise was presented from behind. The authors noted however that the fixed directional mode of the hearing aid used in the study was not optimised for diffuse noise, but noise coming from behind the listener. A systematic review of nine studies by Bentler in 2005 found evidence to support the effectiveness of directional microphones in current hearing aids [18]. McCreery (2012) identified seven paediatric studies, again indicating that directional microphones improve speech perception in controlled settings [19].

When hearing aids with adaptive directional microphone systems are fitted bilaterally, each system operates independently of the other. This situation was investigated by Mackenzie and Lutman: The authors found that although the adaptive systems worked independently, there were no detrimental effects, as measured by sentence recognitions scores in noise or quality ratings [20]. In fact, bilateral use of both the adaptive and the fixed system was consistently superior to the omnidirectional settings. However, in order to make the best use of a beamforming system using bilateral microphones the devices must communicate with each other [21]. The Phonak Ambra hearing aid (Phonak AG, Switzerland) implements such a system where the devices exchange audio data wireless between each other, effectively allowing beamforming to be performed using four microphones [22]. A different four-microphone spatial separation strategy was investigated by Kokkinakis et al. in five bilateral cochlear implant (CI) users [21]. The left and right audio signals were captured synchronously and processed together using a single processor, which was used to drive both CIs. However, the noise scenarios tested were limited, with speech shaped noise presented either from a single speaker at $90^0$ to the right or from three speakers placed at 30°, 60° and 90° to the right. Average improvements in percent correct scores over the unprocessed bilateral condition were 36% and 30% for the single and multiple noise sources respectively.

While several studies showed significant benefits of binaural beamformers for CI users [21,23,24], those studies were conducted using an experimental set-up that required a central body worn processing unit, which communicated continuously with both bilateral microphones as well as the CI system. The system investigated in our study was based on two hearing aids which can communicate with each other wirelessly and do not require a central processing unit. The major aim of this study was to compare the benefit of an adaptive monaural beamformer to the benefit of a wireless binaural beamformer for monaural CI users in a realistic set-up with noise presented from both, the frontal and rear, hemispheres.

### Study Objectives

This study investigated the performance of CI recipients using beamforming technology, as implemented in Phonak Ambra hearing aids, when combined with the Advanced Bionics Harmony speech processor (Advanced Bionics LLC, USA) in an experimental test setup. For this purpose the output signal of the Phonak Ambra hearing aid was galvanically coupled to the auxiliary input of the Harmony speech processor. The hearing aids used in this study implement a binaural beamformer using four microphones across the two hearing aids, producing a very narrow target beam and a monaural adaptive beamforming program called UltraZoom [22,25]. The steering of the adaptive monaural beamformer is frequency specific and based on an approach proposed by Elko and Pong [26]. The two types of beamforming (adaptive monaural and binaural) were compared to an omnidirectional microphone setting.

The effect of adding ClearVoice (CV) as a post-processing stage to all three microphone settings was also assessed. CV is a single-microphone noise reduction algorithm implemented in the Advanced Bionics speech processor [6]. It acts on the signal after it has been band-pass filtered into the frequency ranges associated with the different CI electrode contacts, and is based on the assumption that the speech envelope is modulated while the noise envelope is stationary. The SNR is estimated separately in each frequency band, based on the modulation content, and bands with low estimated SNRs are attenuated. Attenuation of bands which are dominated by noise improves the overall SNR across all channels in the pulse stream transmitted to the CI user.

The study showed that both the binaural beamformer and the monaural adaptive beamformer implemented in the Phonak Ambra hearing aid could be used in conjunction with a Harmony speech processor to produce substantial average improvements in SRT. ClearVoice added a further benefit.

## Method

### Ethics Statement

The study protocol was reviewed and approved by a registered ethics board (Freiburger Ethik-Kommission International). After explanation of the study protocol and the risks and benefits of participating, all subjects signed a consent form before taking part.

## Subject Demographics

12 postlingually deafened subjects with an Advanced Bionics HiRes90K or CII cochlear implant were recruited randomly at the Cochlear Implant Center to participate in the study. All subjects were regular users of the HiRes120 processing strategy and had a minimum experience with their current strategy and processor of three months. All subjects had word scores of more than 15% for sentences in noise in the last clinical test. There were no criteria for the contralateral ear and five subjects were bilaterally implanted. If a subject was bilaterally implanted, the side with the better speech intelligibility was used, determined by the routine sentence test data collected in the clinic. The other side was turned off. The contralateral ear was plugged in subjects with residual contralateral hearing.

The mean age of implantation was 57 years, ranging from 30 to 72 years. The mean duration of deafness was nine years, ranging from zero to 30 years, based on the age when a telephone call was no longer possible till the age of implantation. The mean duration of cochlear implant use was three years, ranging from one to five years. Subject demographics are shown in table 1.

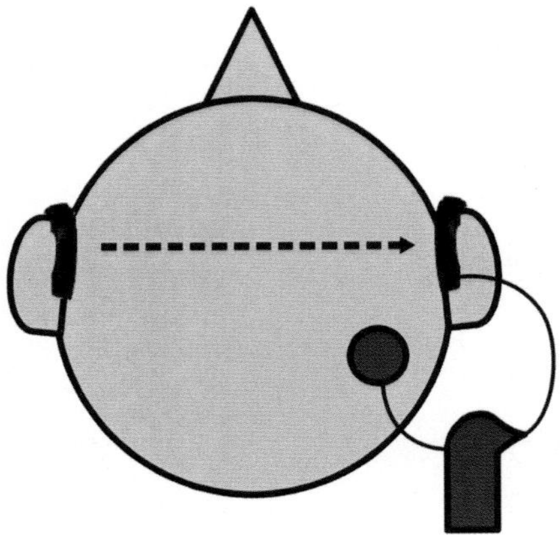

**Figure 1. Set-up of hearing aids and cochlear implant processor.** Subjects wearing Ambra behind-the-ear hearing aids on both sides communicating wirelessly; the hearing aid on the implanted side being connected to the cochlear implant speech processor.

## Test Set Up

Subjects were provided with an Ambra behind-the-ear (BTE) hearing aid which was placed ipsilaterally to the test side and connected to the speech processor, allowing the subjects to listen directly through the hearing aid. For the binaural beamformer condition a second hearing aid was placed on the contralateral ear, which was wirelessly linked to the other hearing aid connected to the speech processor (Figure 1). To connect the ipsilateral hearing aid with the speech processor, a technical modification had to be made: Instead of a hearing aid receiver a wire was attached to the output of the hearing aid to pick up the pulse-width modulated signal normally driving the miniature loudspeaker of the hearing aid. In order to generate an analogue audio signal from the hearing aid output as required by the speech processor, a low pass filter was applied using an LRC-circuit. This audio signal was delivered to the auxiliary input socket of the speech processor. With the hearing aid in omnidirectional mode, the frequency response of this experimental input configuration was confirmed to be equivalent to that of the regular omnidirectional BTE microphone of the speech processor.

Using the integrated pair of microphones of the modified hearing aid positioned at ear level, three different directional settings were programmed into the hearing aid:

1. Omnidirectional (omni): In this mode, the signal of the omnidirectional front microphone is transmitted to the speech processor without further processing.
2. The monaural adaptive beamformer (aBF): The aBF generates its directionality from one pair of microphones in the same device. It changes its directionality adaptively, based on the direction of noise.
3. The binaural beamformer (bBF): The bBF generates its directionality using two pairs of microphones on two separate

**Table 1.** Description of study participants.

| Age at implantation in years | Duration of deafness in years | Duration of implant use in years | ClearVoice user? |
|---|---|---|---|
| 71 | 16 | 2 | rarely |
| 62 | 17 | 4 | yes |
| 48 | 00 | 4 | yes |
| 30 | 30 | 1 | yes |
| 68 | 01 | 2 | rarely |
| 64 | 06 | 4 | no |
| 58 | 00 | 5 | yes |
| 58 | 16 | 4 | no |
| 58 | 06 | 2 | no |
| 57 | 00 | 2 | yes |
| 70 | 09 | 3 | yes |
| 72 | 01 | 2 | yes |

ears. Thus, when using the bBF, a second hearing aid was needed on the contralateral ear. The two hearing aids were wirelessly linked and one was connected to the CI as described above.

## CI Signal Processing

Generally, CIs deliver time-staggered, amplitude-modulated electric pulse trains to an electrode array in the inner ear, where they excite the fibers of the auditory nerve. Current amplitudes are derived from the envelopes of a filter bank by the externally-worn speech processor and transmitted to the implanted circuit using a radio frequency link. For a typical user of the HiRes 120 coding strategy with 16 active implant electrodes, the number of filter-bank channels is 15, spanning a frequency range of approximately 250 to 8000 Hz [27].

ClearVoice is a noise reduction algorithm optionally available for users of HiRes 120. It applies attenuation to the output of each filter bank channel depending on the estimated *a posteriori* signal-to-noise ratios (SNRs), such that channels dominated by noise are dynamically attenuated. The background noise level is estimated using a voice-activity-dependent minimum tracking procedure. Channel-specific attenuations are determined based on a perceptually-motivated sigmoidal gain function. The highest possible attenuation per channel thus applied can be set to 6, 12 or 18 dB during fitting.

## Speech Processor Fitting

During testing, input to the processor was provided solely from the auxiliary input connected to the hearing aids. Before testing the speech processor was set to a sensitivity of 0. The volume dial allowed the subjects to change their M-levels globally by ±50%. Two programs were created: i) the clinical program without CV, ii) the same program with CV medium and with the most comfortable listening levels raised by 5% (as described in 6). The medium setting of CV was used, limiting the maximum amount of attenuation to 12 decibels (dB). Prior to each test condition, the subject was allowed to adjust the volume for optimal perception.

## Adaptive beamformer

The adaptive beamformer is based on the approach proposed by Elko and Pong [26] and consists of two signal processing steps in order to achieve the adaptive time-varying behavior as shown in Figure 2. In the first step, the signals from both omnidirectional microphones in the device are processed with two static cardioid beamformers with one cardioid facing 0° and the other one facing 180° direction. This is achieved by applying a constant time delay T to one microphone signal before subtracting it from the other. In the second step, the output of the back-facing beamformer is added to that of the front-facing one with a time-varying weighting factor β, which is adjusted to minimise the expected short-term power of the summation signal. As a result, the null of the adaptive beamformer is placed towards the direction with the highest noise power in the back hemispherewhile preserving signals from front. This processing is frequency-specific, such that multiple noise sources with non-overlapping frequency content can be cancelled simultaneously even when they are located at different spatial positions.

## Binaural beamformer

The binaural beamformer requires two dual-microphone systems, one on each ear (Figure 3). First, a monaural beamforming algorithm is applied independently within each dual-microphone system. The two resulting audio signals are then transmitted wirelessly and concurrently to the respective contralateral device. There, they are combined with the contralateral dual-microphone output, effectively resulting in a 3rd order (i.e. four-microphone) beamformer. The combination of signals across ears yields in a narrower and more focussed frontal and lateral beam pattern especially in the low-frequencies.

Both microphone systems attenuate noise from rear and lateral angles while maintaining the signal level from 0° front, thus yielding in an improved signal-to-noise ratio compared to an omnidirectional microphone system. Since the binaural beamformer has a more focussed beam to the front, i.e., more attenuation of surrounding noise, more improvement of the signal-to-noise ratio is achieved than with the monaural adaptive beamformer.

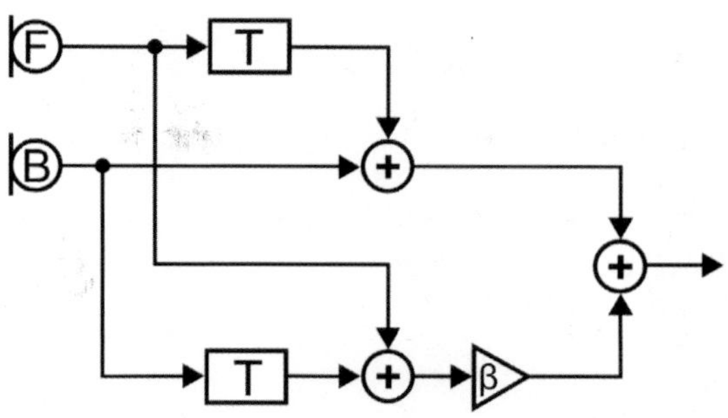


**Figure 2. Flow-chart of the adaptive beamformer.** The front (F) and back (B) microphone signals are added with a fixed delay to form the static cardioid beamformer. Afterwards, the beamformer outputs are added using a time-varying factor β for the adaptive beamformer. Not shown is the signal processing in different frequency bands.

## Objective comparison of microphone directionality

A quantitative measure of microphone directionality was derived from polar plots obtained for a hearing aid on the left ear of a KEMAR artificial head in an anechoic room using a single noise source from varying angles (Figure 4). The radius in a given direction of the polar contour signifies the amount of attenuation of the processed signal from that direction relative to a signal from 0°. In order to obtain meaningful and comparable polar patterns, the adaptive beamformer was switched to a static mode for this particular measurement. For the lateral angles, the binaural

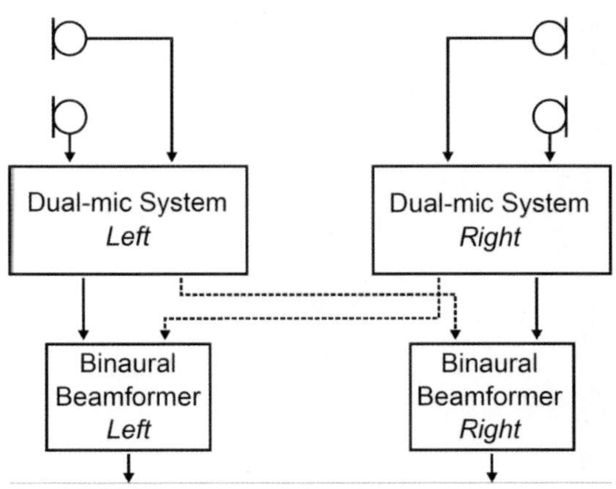


**Figure 3. Flow-chart of the binaural beamformer.** In the left and right device a dual-microphone beamformer is calculated and the audio signal is wirelessly transmitted to the opposite device yielding in the binaural beamformer.

beamformer attenuated sounds more than the monaural beamformer (by approximately 5 dB for a -60° angle, for example). Compared to the monaural beamformer, the maximum attenuation in the back hemisphere under anechoic conditions is less pronounced with the binaural beamformer. Nevertheless, the directivity index (i.e., the averaged attenuation from a microphone system for all angles relative to the attenuation for the front) reveals an overall attenuation of 3.4 and 4.6 dB for the monaural and binaural beamformer, respectively. In contrast, the omni directional microphone has a lower directivity index of −2.5 dB. In short, the binaural beamformer provides the highest directivity, i.e., a higher attenuation than the monaural beamformer, as characterised by a relative improvement in the directivity index of 1.2 dB.

As a further method to obtain an objective estimate of the prospective performance benefit for both beamforming algorithms,the relative attenuation of diffuse speech-shaped noise signals was determined in the particular spatial setup of this study: noise was simultaneously presented from the five noise speakers, and its speech-intelligibility weighted attenuation relative to a subsequent speech signal from the front was determined (Acoustical Society of America American National Standards for Calculation of Speech Intelligibility Index S3.5–1997). The SNR improvements thus estimated were 4.1 dB for the adaptive monaural and 7.6 dB for the binaural beamformer relative to the omnidirectional condition.

## Hearing Aid fitting

The hearing aid was programmed with a flat frequency response, providing 0 dB gain for all levels, and only the respective directional processing algorithm active. All other features were turned off. Furthermore, the hearing aid output level was matched to the input sensitivity of the CI system.

## Speech testing

Acute speech tests were carried out over the course of two sessions, one to six weeks apart, in a low-reverberant, sound-damped room. Each appointment typically lasted approximately two hours including two breaks. Six different conditions were tested and two were repeated at the following appointment, as shown in table 2. The order of conditions within each appointment, as well the order of the two appointments, was randomised. However, all conditions required for determination of the benefit of the aBF and its combination with CV were tested in a single appointment, while all conditions required to compare the aBF to the binBF as well as the maximal expected benefit of binBF and CV were covered in the other appointment. This distribution avoids additional spread of data due to differences in the physical or mental stage of subjects at the day of testing. Hence, appointment A investigated the difference between aBF and omni conditions and the additional effect of CV. Appointment B investigated the difference between aBF and bBF as well as measuring the benefit from bBF with CV.

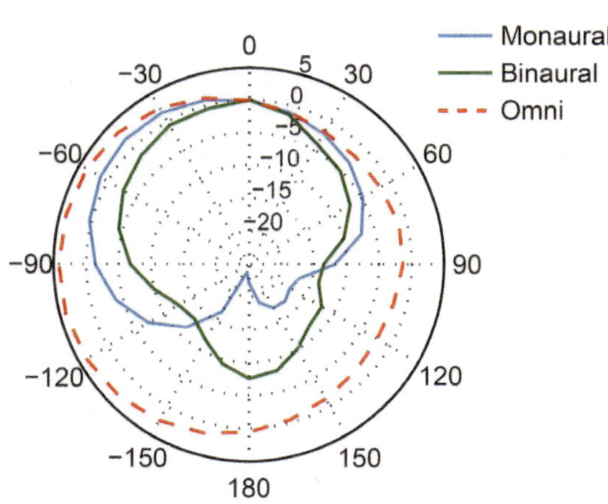


**Figure 4. Spatial characteristic of the monaural and binaural beamformer.** The polar plots are showing the microphone response for the omnidirectional microphone as well as monaural and binaural beamformers on a KEMAR dummy. Circles indicate the gain in decibels (dB) relative to the $0^0$ response.

The test set up was as shown in Figure 5. Six loudspeakers were located on a circle with a radius of 1.2 meters around the subject at angles of 0, ±70°, ±135° and 180°. The speech signal was presented from 0° while the noise was presented from ±70°, ±135° and 180°. Sounds were generated on a laptop connected to a RME Fireface 800 D/A converter, amplified with two Apart Champ Four amplifiers and finally presented via seven JBL Control 1 loudspeakers. To determine the speech intelligibility, the Oldenburg sentence test (OLSA) was used [28]. Sentences were presented in uncorrelated noise at an overall level of 65 dB SPL, with each loudspeaker calibrated for the same free-field presentation level. The OLSA noise is composed of an unintelligible, randomly-aligned superposition of all words in the test corpus, and thereby reflects the long-term spectrum of the speech material [29]. The speech level changed adaptively, depending on the answers of the subject, and the SNR determined where a speech intelligibility rating of 50% was scored (i.e., the speech reception threshold, SRT). Each test condition was assessed using a randomly chosen list and the consecutive list. The final individual SRT was calculated by averaging the two results for each condition. As training prior the test in the first condition, a minimum of four lists were presented.

## Study Design

A single-subject repeated measures design was used where each subject acted as their own control. Parametric statistics were applied. Data from appointment A was compared with a repeated measures two-way ANOVA, with the factors microphone directionality (omni vs. aBF) and noise reduction (CV on and off). Data from appointment B was compared using a one-way ANOVA to test for the effect of processing scheme only (omni, aBF, bBF, bBF+CV). Where a statistically significant effect was identified by the ANOVA, pairwise comparisons were made using two-tailed t-tests with Bonferroni corrected p-values. Following each ANOVA six pairs of data were compared, therefore a correction factor of 6 was applied and all p-values given in the text or graphs are the t-test p-value outcomes multiplied by 6. Means are quoted with 95% confidence intervals.

**Table 2.** Conditions tested in each session.

| Session A | Session B |
|---|---|
| Omnidirectional | Omnidirectional |
| Omnidirectional + ClearVoice | Adaptive Beamformer |
| Adaptive Beamformer | Binaural Beamformer |
| Adaptive Beamformer + ClearVoice | Binaural Beamformer + ClearVoice |

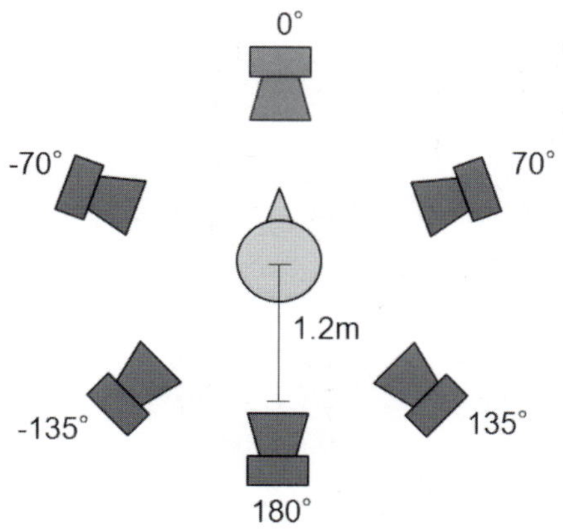


**Figure 5. Speaker set up for speech perception testing.** Six loudspeakers were positioned in a circle of 1.2 m radius. Speech was presented at $0^0$ and noise was presented simultaneously from the other five speaker locations.

## Results

Individual results from all 12 subjects are shown in Figure 6. Subject 44 did not attend for testing at appointment A and subject 43 was excluded because of significant residual hearing in the contralateral ear, which could not be successfully blocked with the ear plug. Statistical analysis was performed on the 10 remaining subjects, who had complete data sets for both sessions.

The results of the ANOVA are shown in table 3. The two-way ANOVA conducted for session A revealed a significant main effect of both microphone directionality ($p<0.001$) and noise reduction ($p = 0.005$) but there was no significant interaction between the two factors. The one-way ANOVA conducted for session B revealed a significant main effect of the processing scheme used ($p<0.001$). Post hoc testing conducted on both sets of data identified a number of significant differences of interest.

Figure 6 also shows the average SRT score for each condition tested in session A indicated by a short black line. The best performance was measured for the aBF+CV condition, with a large significant improvement over the omni condition of 6.1 dB±0.9 dB ($p<0.001$). The aBF condition without CV was also significantly better than the omni condition and the omni+CV condition (5.2 dB±0.7 dB ($p<0.001$), 4.3 dB±1.2 dB ($p<0.001$)).

Figure 7 shows the average SRT score for each condition tested in session B. The best performance in this session was achieved with the binaural beamforming plus CV condition, bBF+CV, with a significant improvement in SRT over the omni condition alone condition of 7.9 dB±2.4 dB ($p<0.001$). Both the aBF and bBF conditions alone were also significantly better than the omni condition (5.3 dB±1.2 and 7.1 dB±1.6, ($p<0.001$)) and were significantly different from each other by 1.9 dB±1.6 ($p<0.05$). However there was no significant advantage shown of adding CV to the bBF condition in the post hoc testing.

## Discussion

This study was conducted to investigate the performance benefit of monaural adaptive and binaural beamforming technology with an additional noise reduction algorithm in unilateral CI users. As still a significant number of CI users is unilaterally implanted and

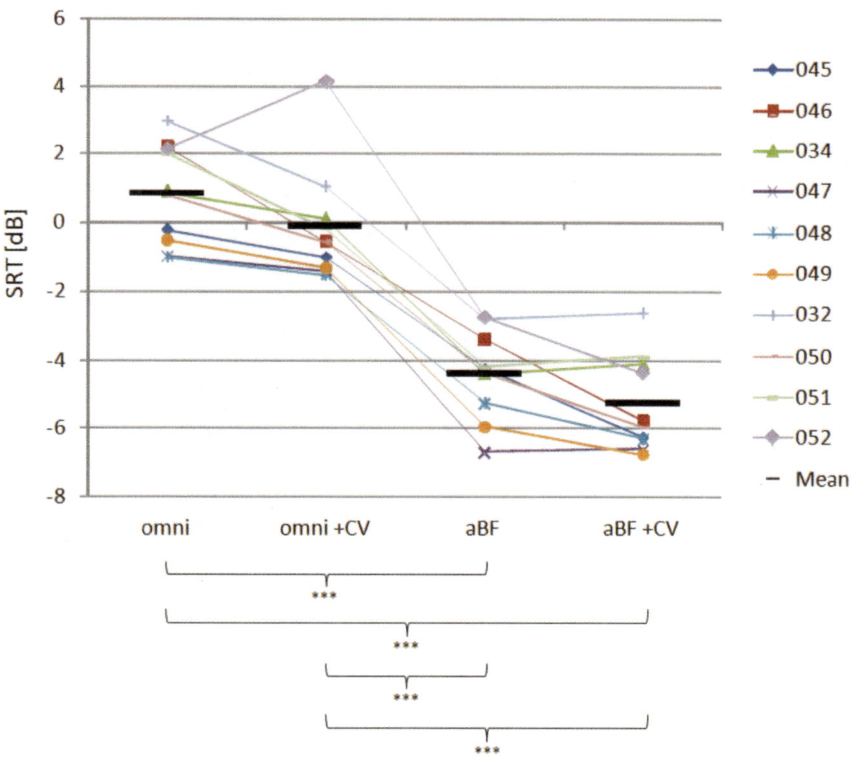


**Figure 6. Mean and individual speech reception thresholds for the monaural adaptive beamformer test session.** Speech reception thresholds (SRT) as measured for the OLSA sentences for each of the 10 subjects, in the four conditions tested during session A (omni – omnidirectional microphone; omni+CV – omnidirectional microphone with ClearVoice; aBF – monaural adaptive beamformer; aBF+CV – monaural adaptive beamformer mit ClearVoice). Short black lines indicate the mean of the study group; horizontal brackets indicate significant differences (*** at $p<0.001$).

**Table 3.** Results of the ANOVA for Sessions A and B.

| Factor | Processing Scheme | F Value | Degrees of Freedom (Hypothesis) | Degrees of Freedom (Error) | Significance |
|---|---|---|---|---|---|
| Session A | | | | | |
| Microphone directionality | aBF; omni | 665.7 | 1 | 9 | 0.000 |
| Noise reduction | CV; no CV | 13.2 | 1 | 9 | 0.005 |
| Interaction | omni; omni+CV; aBF; aBF+CV | 0.03 | 1 | 9 | 0.859 |
| Session B | | | | | |
| Processing scheme | Omni; aBF; binBF; binBF+CV | 83.2 | 3 | 7 | 0.000 |

generally unilateral hearing conditions do not allow spatial release from diffuse background noise [30], the study focussed on unilateral CI use. Due to subject availability, a number of bilaterally implanted subjects were also recruited. For those subjects, the side they generally rely on less was always deactivated during the test sessions in order to mimic the situation of a unilaterally implanted user. Performance was only compared between unilaterally tested conditions and no comparison to the usually worn condition was done. Therefore any effect of bilateral interaction on the results can be excluded. During the test sessions, six loudspeakers were distributed on a circle around the subject; all but the front one presented noise to create a field with diffuse noise except for a narrow lobe from the front. This is a fairly realistic situation corresponding e. g. to a class room or lecture hall where the signal of interest comes from the front but background noise from both sides and rear.

The results of this study show that the use of beamforming technology significantly improved performance over the omni setting in diffuse noise in all conditions. The largest SRT improvement of 7.9 dB over the omni setting was observed for the bBF+CV condition. When looking at the effect of microphone directionality only, an SRT improvement of 7.1 dB was found for bBF compared to omni.

The SNR improvements estimated by the speech-intelligibility weighted noise attenuation were 4.1 dB for the adaptive monaural and 7.6 dB for the binaural beamformer, which was broadly consistent with the differences in directivity indices relative to the omni directional condition (5.9 and 7.1 dB) and the improvements found in the study subjects in appointments A and B (5.2 dB and 7.1 dB, respectively). Note that speech-intelligibility weighted attenuation was measured in the room and loudspeaker setup in which the subjects were tested, whereas the directivity index was measured with one single loudspeaker from different angles in an anechoic room. Different rooms and loudspeaker setups led to slightly different results between predicted SNR improvements and directivity indices. Nevertheless, both objective technical measures reflect more attenuation of noise with the binaural beamformer than with the adaptive beamformer, which is consistent with results obtained in subject testing.

In comparison to the adaptive monaural beamformer, the binaural beamformer proved to be significantly more efficient. The SRT difference between the two algorithms was 1.9 dB, consistent with in-house testing at Phonak where, in hearing-impaired hearing aid users, a difference between binaural and adaptive algorithms of 2.4 dB ($p = 0.012$) was shown [25]. The binaural beamformer derives the output signal from four microphones, which are arranged in pairs on either side of the head; the monaural beamformer is only based on the information of one microphone pair worn on a single side. Therefore the binaural beamformer has significantly more spatial information available and thus yields better suppression of spatially distributed noise.Although a comparison of these results with other studies is difficult, some implications can be made: A 6 dB improvement was reported by Wolfe et al. using a monaural fixed directional microphone. However, there are key differences between the studies [9]. The authors used a single multi-talker babble noise source directly from the side only rather than a diffuse noise pattern as was used here; the use of diffuse noise creates a more realistic and challenging situation, especially with the positioning of the noise speakers in the frontal hemisphere [24]. However, in the Wolfe study the results were compared to a standard microphone setting which is already moderately directional, thereby reducing the amount of benefit that can be expected from adding the beamformer [31,32]. The SRT improvement of 7.1 dB reported here for the bBF condition compares favourably.

In the studies reported by Brockmayer et al [33], Hersbach et al [7] and Spriet et al [8], adaptive beamformers were tested in a laboratory situation. A gain of 6.5 dB was reported by Spriet et al. for three loudspeaker diffuse noise with loudspeakers positioned only in the back hemisphere at ±90° and 180° and 13.4 dB for a single loudspeaker positioned at +90°. However, adaptive beamforming is known to be most effective at reducing noise from the sides and behind the listener, with the source signal to the front. Studies using a single noise source placed either behind or at the side of the recipient, are likely to show the greatest improvement, while the setup itself is not realistic at all. Hersbach et al. reported gains of 6 dB but with a moving noise source, roving between seven speakers positioned at 30° intervals between 90° and 270° behind the listener. None of the above mentioned studies used noise sources in the frontal hemisphere, thus better performance than in our setup could be expected. Some studies have attempted to test beamforming in more realistic conditions [33,34]. With the R-SPACE set up, uncorrelated restaurant noise is presented simultaneously from eight speakers positioned at 45° intervals all around the subject, including from the direction of the speech signal. Using this configuration reduced the reported improvements to between 3.9 and 4.5 dB at 60 dB noise over the subject's standard setting. Taking into account the variations in the test setups as discussed above, the 5.2 dB SRT improvement reported for adaptive monaural beamforming in this study is a remarkable outcome.

The two-way ANOVA with the factors microphone directionality (omni vs. aBF) and noise reduction (CV on and off) revealed a significant main effect of 0.8 dB for CV which was independent from the microphone directionality. This means the CV benefit is additive to the beamformer benefit. The benefit is smaller than expected from previous studies[6]. This discrepancy may be explained by the test methodology. Due to the very good SRTs

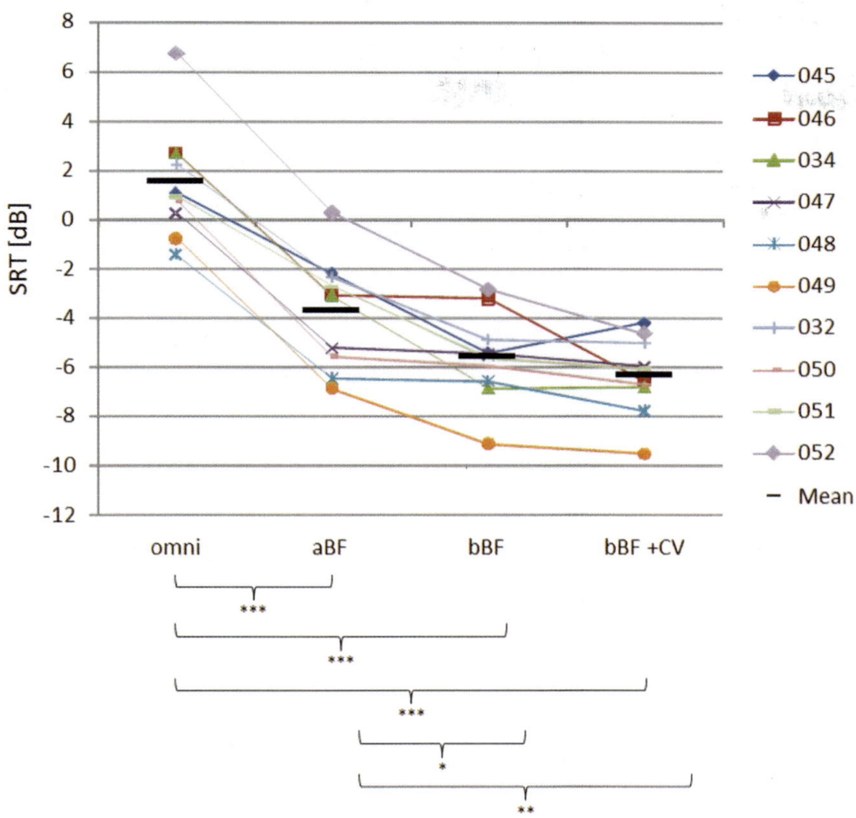


**Figure 7. Mean and individual speech reception thresholds for the binaural beamformer test session.** Speech reception thresholds (SRT) as measured for the OLSA sentences for each of the 10 subjects, in the four conditions tested during session B (omni – omnidirectional microphone; aBF – monaural adaptive beamformer; bBF – binaural beamformer; bBF+CV – binaural beamformer mit ClearVoice). Short black lines indicate the mean of the study group; horizontal brackets indicate significant differences (*** at $p<0.001$; ** at $0.001<p<0.01$; * at $0.01<p<0.05$).

obtained in this particular study group, even in the omnidirectional baseline condition (0.8 dB SNR in session 1), CV operated in an unfavourable SNR regime throughout the experiments, i.e. very close to zero.

According to the experiences in the hearing aid field, the benefit of beamformers is probably smaller in real life than in laboratory studies. On one hand, limitations of the experimental designs used so far may explain this discrepancy. On the other hand, reported problems from directional microphone studies in the hearing aid field are not directly applicable to the world of CIs: CI users still usually have little or no residual hearing and as a consequence, receive only the processed signal; no unprocessed, acoustic signals through an ear-mould venting can disturb the hearing like in hearing aid subjects, which commonly reduces the benefit of directional microphones in conventional hearing aids [35].

In order for beamforming to be used effectively the CI user must have a good understanding of when to use the beamformer. The narrow directional pattern of the binaural beamformer allows to focus on a single target source located opposite the listener, eliminating sounds from the back, sides and even off-centre frontal angles. This may be the appropriate configuration for a face-to-face conversation in a noisy bar or restaurant. If, however, the target speaker was to move positions constantly as in the case of a typical round-table discussion, the use of the adaptive beamformer is likely to be more advantageous. In situations where speech and noise are not sufficiently spatially separated, a single-channel noise reduction algorithm such as CV can still improve the listening performance.

When speech intelligibility is very difficult due to background noise and the talker is located in front of the CI user, then switching to a beamforming program will be appropriate. In contrast, for speech in quiet, the everyday program with omnidirectional microphone characteristic should be selected. In reality however, very few users change programs from their everyday settings and are often not used to seeking out noisy situations, but avoiding them [33]. Thus, a classifier that can detect acoustic situations and switch between programs and preprocessing algorithms would be highly desirable [36]. In case of a unilaterally worn CI system the binaural beamformer would not be available. Therefore the classifier only has to differentiate between noisy and quiet situations and accordingly switch between no preprocessing and adaptive beamformer in combination with ClearVoice. In case of a bilateral system more sophisticated rules are required. Based on similarities or differences between the raw signals at the four microphones the classifier has to decide whether the narrow beam of the binaural beamformer or the wider beam of the monaural adaptive beamformer is more appropriate. In principle, the available computational power of modern hearing systems is sufficient for the required algorithms. For the realization of a bilateral system, several options are conceivable; a unilaterally implanted CI user may use a satellite system on the contralateral ear which could look like a small light weighted hearing aid. This satellite may wirelessly transmit the two microphone signals to the contralaterally worn CI behind the ear processor. The CI processor would then perform all processing which was distributed between the hearing aids and the processor in our set-up. In case of bilaterally implanted CI users each processor on either side may integrate the required functionality for transmission and processing of all for microphone systems. As bimodal use with a CI on one side and a hearing aid on the other get more and more common the binaural beam former may also be realised by communication between a hearing aid and a linked CI processor. But in case of bimodal and bilateral CI use, further investigation is required to compare the binaural performance with the binaural beamformer to binaural performance with monaural or no beamformer. Binaural users have generally access to spatial cues which may become reduced or distorted with a binaural beamformer; their own physiological capability of spatial release from masking in many everyday life situations may be superior to a technical solution (as outlined above) that potentially interferes with their awareness for the room situation. However, also for those subjects a binaural beamformer is still of interest when selected intentionally for certain situations but not based on a classifier.

## Conclusions

The study showed that already the adaptive beamformer implemented in the Ambra hearing aid in conjunction with a Harmony speech processor produced a substantial improvement of 5.2 dB in SRT in a challenging noise setting with speech weighted noise compared to the omni-directional microphone. The binaural beamformer even produced SRT improvements of 7.1 dB over the omni-directional microphone. An overall trend towards better performance with CV was observed. Improvements of CV were likely limited in this particular study group, at least in parts, by the adaptive test methodology and the very good SRTs obtained, even without beamformer. The challenging test set up with noise sources also in the frontal hemisphere, aimed to produce a more realistic scenario compared to other studies, where noise was presented from one single speaker or within the rear hemisphere only. Even though the gain of the single-sided adaptive beamformer was remarkable, the results demonstrate that the potential performance benefits of a four-microphone binaural beamformer in challenging hearing situations are still large.

## Author Contributions

Conceived and designed the experiments: AB PH SF TL. Performed the experiments: AB KD. Analyzed the data: AB KD PH SF TL. Contributed reagents/materials/analysis tools: KD PH SF. Wrote the paper: AB KD SF PH TL. Preparation of measurement setup: PH SF.

## References

1. Firszt JB, Holden LK, Skinner MW, Tobey EA, Peterson A, et al. (2004) Recognition of speech presented at soft to loud levels by adult cochlear implant recipients of three cochlear implant systems. Ear Hear. 25(4):375–87.
2. Litovsky R, Parkinson A, Arcaroli J, Sammeth C (2006) Simultaneous bilateral cochlear implantation in adults: a multicenter clinical study. Ear Hear. 27(6):714–31.
3. Patrick JF, Busby PA, Gibson PJ (2006) The development of the Nucleus Freedom Cochlear implant system. Trends Amplif. 10(4):175–200.
4. Spahr A, Dorman M (2004). Performance of subjects fit with the Advanced Bionics CII and Nucleus 3G cochlear implant devices. Arch Otolaryngol Head Neck Surg. 130(5):624–8.
5. James CJ, Blamey PJ, Martin L, Swanson B, Just Y, et al. (2002) Adaptive dynamic range optimization for cochlear implants: a preliminary study. Ear Hear. 23(1 Suppl):49S–58S.
6. Buechner A, Brendel M, Saalfeld H, Litvak L, Frohne-Buechner C, et al. (2010) Results of a pilot study with a signal enhancement algorithm for HiRes120 cochlear implant users. Otol Neurotol. 31(9):1386–90.
7. Hersbach AA, Arora K, Mauger SJ, Dawson PW (2012) Combining directional microphone and single-channel noise reduction algorithms: a clinical evaluation in difficult listening conditions with cochlear implant users. Ear Hear. 33(4):e13–23.
8. Spriet A, Van Deun L, Eftaxiadis K, Laneau J, Moonen M, et al. (2007) Speech understanding in background noise with the two-microphone adaptive beamformer BEAM in the Nucleus Freedom Cochlear Implant System. Ear Hear. 28(1):62–72.
9. Wolfe J, Parkinson A, Schafer EC, Gilden J, Rehwinkel K, et al. (2012) Benefit of a commercially available cochlear implant processor with dual-microphone beamforming: a multi-center study. Otol Neurotol. 33(4):553–60.
10. Greenberg JE, Zurek PM (1992) Evaluation of an adaptive beamforming method for hearing aids. J Acoust Soc Am. 91(3):1662–76.
11. Kates JM (1993) Superdirective arrays for hearing aids. J Acoust Soc Am. 94(4):1930–3.
12. Kompis M, Dillier N (2001) Performance of an adaptive beamforming noise reduction scheme for hearing aid applications. II. Experimental verification of the predictions. J Acoust Soc Am. 109(3):1134–43.
13. Peterson PM, Wei SM, Rabinowitz WM, Zurek PM (1990) Robustness of an adaptive beamforming method for hearing aids. Acta Otolaryngol Suppl. 469: 85–90.
14. Kates JM, Weiss MR (1996) A comparison of hearing-aid array processing techniques. J Acoust Soc Am. 99(5):3138–48.
15. Ricketts T, Henry P (2002) Evaluation of an adaptive, directional-microphone hearing aid. Int J Audiol. 41(2):100–12.
16. Ricketts T, Dhar S (1999) Comparison of performance across three directional hearing aids. J Am Acad Audiol. 10(4):180–9.
17. Ricketts T, Mueller HG (1999) Making sense of directional microphone hearing aids. Am J Audiol. 8(2):117–27.
18. Bentler RA (2005) Effectiveness of directional microphones and noise reduction schemes in hearing aids: a systematic review of the evidence. J Am Acad Audiol. 16(7):473–84.
19. McCreery RW, Venediktov RA, Coleman JJ, Leech HM (2012) An Evidence-Based Systematic Review of Directional Microphones and Digital Noise Reduction Hearing Aids in School-Age Children with Hearing Loss. Am J Audiol. 21(2):295–312.
20. Mackenzie E, Lutman ME (2005) Speech recognition and comfort using hearing instruments with adaptive directional characteristics in asymmetric listening conditions. Ear Hear. 26(6):669–79.
21. Kokkinakis K, Azimi B, Hu Y, Friedland DR (2012) Single and Multiple Microphone Noise Reduction Strategies in Cochlear Implants. Trends Amplif. 16(2):102–16.
22. Latzel M (2012) Binaural VoiceStream Technology. Intelligent binaural algorithms to improve speech understanding. Phonak Insight, Phonak AG, Switzerland.
23. Hamacher V, Doering WH, Mauer G, Fleischmann H, Hennecke J (1997) Evaluation of noise reduction systems for cochlear implant users in different acoustic environment. Am J Otol. 18(6 Suppl):S46–9.
24. van Hoesel RJ, Clark GM (1995) Evaluation of a portable two-microphone adaptive beamforming speech processor with cochlear implant patients. J Acoust Soc Am. 97(4):2498–503.
25. Nyffeler M (2010) StereoZoom, Improvements with directional microphones. Field study news, Phonak AG, Switzerland.
26. Elko G, Pong A (1995) Simple adaptive first order differential microphone. Proceedings of IEEE workshop on Applications of Signal Processing to Audio and Acoustics, New Paltz, NY, USA. pp. 169–72.
27. Nogueira W, Litvak L, Edler B, Ostermann J, Buechner A (2009) Signal Processing Strategies for Cochlear Implants Using Current Steering, EURASIP Journal on Applied Signal Processing. 10.1155/2009/531213.
28. Kollmeier B, Wesselkamp M (1997) Development and evaluation of a German sentence test for objective and subjective speech intelligibility assessment. J Acoust Soc Am. 1997; 102(4):2412–21.
29. Wagener KC, Brand T (2005) Sentence intelligibility in noise for listeners with normal hearing and hearing impairment: influence of measurement procedure and masking parameters. Int J Audiol. 44(3):144–56.
30. Dawes P, Munro KJ, Kalluri S, Edwards B (2013) Unilateral and bilateral hearing aids, spatial release from masking and auditory acclimatization. J Acoust Soc Am. 134(1):596–606. doi: 10.1121/1.4807783.
31. Chung K, Zeng FG, Acker KN (2006) Effects of directional microphone and adaptive multichannel noise reduction algorithm on cochlear implant performance. J Acoust Soc Am. 120: 2216–27.
32. Wouters J, Van den Berghe J (2001) Speech recognition in noise for cochlear implantees with a two microphone monaural adaptive noise reduction system. Ear Hear. 22: 420–30.
33. Brockmeyer AM, Potts LG (2011) Evaluation of different signal processing options in unilateral and bilateral cochlear freedom implant recipients using R-Space background noise. J Am Acad Audiol. 22(2):65–80.
34. Gifford RH, Revit LJ (2010) Speech perception for adult cochlear implant recipients in a realistic background noise: effectiveness of preprocessing strategies and external options for improving speech recognition in noise. J Am Acad Audiol. 21(7):441–51.
35. Ricketts T (2000) Directivity quantification in hearing aids: fitting and measurement effects. Ear Hear. 21(1):45–58.
36. Hamacher V, Chalupper J, Eggers J, Fischer E, Kornagel U, et al. (2005) Signal Processing in High-End Hearing Aids: State of the Art, Challenges, and Future Trends, EURASIP Journal on Applied Signal Processing. (18), 2915–2929.

# Targeting of *Slc25a21* Is Associated with Orofacial Defects and Otitis Media Due to Disrupted Expression of a Neighbouring Gene

**Simon Maguire[1], Jeanne Estabel[1], Neil Ingham[1¤a], Selina Pearson[1], Edward Ryder[1], Damian M. Carragher[1¤b], Nicolas Walker[1,2], Sanger MGP Slc25a21 Project Team[1¶], James Bussell[1], Wai-In Chan[3¤c], Thomas M. Keane[1], David J. Adams[1], Cheryl L. Scudamore[4¤d], Christopher J. Lelliott[1], Ramiro Ramírez-Solis[1], Natasha A. Karp[1], Karen P. Steel[1¤a], Jacqueline K. White[1]*, Anna-Karin Gerdin[1]**

**1** Wellcome Trust Sanger Institute, Wellcome Trust Genome Campus, Hinxton, Cambridgeshire, United Kingdom, **2** Department of Physiology, Development and Neuroscience, University of Cambridge, Cambridge, Cambridgeshire, United Kingdom, **3** Department of Haematology, Cambridge Institute for Medical Research, Cambridge, Cambridgeshire, United Kingdom, **4** Department of Pathology and Infectious Diseases, Royal Veterinary College, Hatfield, Hertfordshire, United Kingdom

## Abstract

Homozygosity for *Slc25a21*$^{tm1a(KOMP)Wtsi}$ results in mice exhibiting orofacial abnormalities, alterations in carpal and rugae structures, hearing impairment and inflammation in the middle ear. In humans it has been hypothesised that the 2-oxoadipate mitochondrial carrier coded by *SLC25A21* may be involved in the disease 2-oxoadipate acidaemia. Unexpectedly, no 2-oxoadipate acidaemia-like symptoms were observed in animals homozygous for *Slc25a21*$^{tm1a(KOMP)Wtsi}$ despite confirmation that this allele reduces *Slc25a21* expression by 71.3%. To study the complete knockout, an allelic series was generated using the *loxP* and *FRT* sites typical of a Knockout Mouse Project allele. After removal of the critical exon and neomycin selection cassette, *Slc25a21* knockout mice homozygous for the *Slc25a21*$^{tm1b(KOMP)Wtsi}$ and *Slc25a21*$^{tm1d(KOMP)Wtsi}$ alleles were phenotypically indistinguishable from wild-type. This led us to explore the genomic environment of *Slc25a21* and to discover that expression of *Pax9*, located 3′ of the target gene, was reduced in homozygous *Slc25a21*$^{tm1a(KOMP)Wtsi}$ mice. We hypothesize that the presence of the selection cassette is the cause of the down regulation of *Pax9* observed. The phenotypes we observed in homozygous *Slc25a21*$^{tm1a(KOMP)Wtsi}$ mice were broadly consistent with a hypomorphic *Pax9* allele with the exception of otitis media and hearing impairment which may be a novel consequence of *Pax9* down regulation. We explore the ramifications associated with this particular targeted mutation and emphasise the need to interpret phenotypes taking into consideration all potential underlying genetic mechanisms.

**Editor:** Vladimir N. Uversky, University of South Florida College of Medicine, United States of America

**Funding:** This work was supported by the Wellcome Trust (grant no 098051 to WTSI) (http://www.wellcome.ac.uk/) and the European Union's Seventh Framework program under grant agreement number 282510 - BLUEPRINT (NW) (www.blueprint-epigenome.eu/). The funders had no role in study design, data collection and analysis, decision to publish, or preparation of the manuscript.

**Competing Interests:** The authors have declared that no competing interests exist.

* E-mail: jkw@sanger.ac.uk

¤a Current address: Wolfson Centre for Age-Related Diseases, King's College London, Guy's Campus, London, United Kingdom
¤b Current address: Medical Research Council National Institute for Medical Research, Mill Hill, London, United Kingdom
¤c Current address: State Key Laboratory of Quality Research in Chinese Medicine, Macau University of Science and Technology, Taipa, Macau
¤d Current address: Medical Research Council Harwell, Harwell Science and Innovation Campus, Oxford, Oxfordshire, United Kingdom

¶ Membership of the Sanger MGP Slc25a21 Project Team is provided in the Acknowledgments.

## Introduction

Knockout mice are invaluable tools for studying the function of genes both during embryonic development and in the adult. Classically, gene disruption in mice is achieved by replacing a part of the target gene with a selectable marker, e.g. a *neo* cassette, leading to constitutive ablation of the targeted gene. More contemporary approaches include the creation of conditional alleles and targeted gene traps, as well as small hairpin RNA (shRNA) and the use of lentiviral transgenesis, reviewed in [1]. The Sanger Institute Mouse Genetics Project [2] is contributing to an international effort to conduct systematic, large-scale gene function analysis in a mammalian system, through the generation of mice using targeted ES cells available from the EUCOMM and KOMP resources [3]. The typical EUCOMM and KOMP knockout first conditional ready targeted trap [tm1a(EUCOMM) and tm1a(KOMP)] is a powerful allele configured with the potential to convert to a conditional allele or a *lacZ* tagged null allele [3]. This tm1a allele was selected for pragmatic reasons, including there being no requirement for additional breeding to modify the allele, as targeted traps typically disrupt expression of the targeted gene [3,4], and the major advantage that the allele, with full potential for conversion, would be cryopreserved for subsequent community use. However, it has previously been reported that the presence of selectable markers used for gene targeting, such as the *neo* cassette in the EUCOMM and KOMP tm1a allele, can interfere with the expression of neighbouring genes [5,6,7,8,9]. It is, therefore, important that phenotypes discovered in mice carrying the knockout first conditional ready allele, are verified using the derived deletion allele.

*SLC25A21* has previously been reported to be ubiquitously expressed in all tissues tested [10], and codes for the 2-oxoadipate mitochondrial carrier (ODC) that catalyses the movement of several substrates, primarily 2-oxoadipate and 2-oxoglutarate, across inner mitochondrial membranes [10,11,12]. It is suspected that ODC functions by a counter exchange mechanism, catalysing the uptake of 2-oxoadipate into the mitochondrial matrix, in exchange for internal 2-oxoglutarate [10]. The physiological role of the ODC suggests that it may be involved in the human disease 2-oxoadipate acidaemia (OMIM 204750), characterised by an accumulation of 2-oxoadipate and associated metabolites in urine [11]. This inborn error of metabolism shows clinical symptoms of intellectual disability varying from mild to severe, hypotonia, seizures, motor and developmental delay, and cerebellar ataxia [13,14,15,16].

Here we report characterization of the allelic series derived from the KOMP targeted allele of *Slc25a21*. From this, three distinct observations were made. Firstly, ablation of *Slc25a21* was not found to cause symptoms of 2-oxoadipate acidaemia in mice; animals homozygous for *Slc25a21*$^{tm1b(KOMP)Wtsi}$ and *Slc25a21*$^{tm1d(KOMP)Wtsi}$ null alleles were normal for all parameters tested. Secondly, we report that *Slc25a21*$^{tm1a(KOMP)Wtsi}$ homozygous mice present with profound dental, orofacial and hearing/middle ear phenotypes caused by off-target effects on the expression of the neighbouring gene *Pax9*. Finally, the resulting novel, hypomorphic allele of *Pax9* opens the door to further studies into how *Pax9* is involved in the patterning of the palatal rugae and may represent a novel model of otitis media in the mouse. With the growing resource of knockout first conditional ready targeted ES cells created by the EUCOMM and KOMP initiatives, these results represent a timely reminder that the phenotype observed in the knockout first conditional ready mice should be verified by creating and analysing the deletion allele.

## Materials and Methods

### Ethics Statement

The care and use of all mice in this study were in accordance with UK Home Office regulations, UK Animals (Scientific Procedures) Act of 1986, and were approved by the Wellcome Trust Sanger Institute Ethical Review Committee. All efforts were made to minimize suffering including housing mice in a specific pathogen-free unit at a density of 3–5 animals per cage in polysulfone individually ventilated cages [Tecniplast Seal Safe 1284L (overall dimensions of caging: (L×W×H): 365×207×140 mm, floor area = 530 $cm^2$)]. Sterilised Aspen bedding substrate and standard environmental enrichment of nestlet, cardboard tunnel, and three wooden chew blocks were provided. The light cycle was maintained at 12 h light/12 h dark with lights off at 19:30 hours and no twilight period. Room temperature was 21±2°C and humidity was regulated at 55±10%. Mice were given food and water *ad libitum* unless otherwise stated [2]. Animal welfare is our primary consideration and was assessed routinely for all mice involved in this study. Adult mice were killed by terminal anaesthesia followed by exsanguination and either cervical dislocation or removal of the heart. Embryos were killed by decapitation or cooling followed by immersion in cold tissue fixative. Experimental work was performed in accordance with the Arrive guidelines [17].

### Animals

The *Slc25a21*$^{tm1a(KOMP)Wtsi}$ mice were created by blastocyst injection of targeted ES-cell clone EPD0085_1_D04 from the NIH-funded Knockout Mouse Project (KOMP) [3,18,19]. Generation of mice carrying the *Slc25a21*$^{tm1b(KOMP)Wtsi}$, *Slc25a21*$^{tm1c(KOMP)Wtsi}$ and *Slc25a21*$^{tm1d(KOMP)Wtsi}$ alleles was achieved by breeding to mice expressing *Cre* (*Hprt1*$^{Tg(CMV-Cre)Brd}$) and/or *Flp* (*ROSA26*$^{Fki}$) recombinases. For brevity, the allelic series will be referred to hereafter in figures as tm1a, tm1b, tm1c or tm1d. The *Slc25a21*$^{tm1a(KOMP)Wtsi}$, *Slc25a21*$^{tm1b(KOMP)Wtsi}$, *Slc25a21*$^{tm1c(KOMP)Wtsi}$ and *Slc25a21*$^{tm1d(KOMP)Wtsi}$ colonies were maintained on a C57BL/6N;C57BL/6-*Tyr*$^{c-Brd}$ genetic background.

Mice were fed Mouse Breeders Diet (Lab Diets 5021-3, Richmond, Indiana, USA) unless otherwise specified, including *Slc25a21*$^{tm1d(KOMP)Wtsi}$ mice processed through the Mouse Genetics Project screening protocol [2]. *Slc25a21*$^{tm1a(KOMP)Wtsi}$, *Slc25a21*$^{tm1b(KOMP)Wtsi}$ and *Slc25a21*$^{tm1c(KOMP)Wtsi}$ mice which went through the Mouse Genetics Project screening protocol were transferred to a high-fat (21.4% fat by crude content) dietary challenge (Special Diet Services Western RD-829100, Witham, UK) at 4 weeks of age. Cages were processed randomly and different genotypes could be housed together, hence there was no pattern to the order in which animals were processed. The experimental unit throughout the study was a single mouse.

Viability at postnatal day 14 was assessed from heterozygous (het) intercross matings. Furthermore, viability and embryo morphology for *Slc25a21*$^{tm1a(KOMP)Wtsi}$ mutant mice was assessed at E14.5 and E18.5.

### Validation of targeting event

To confirm the integrity and validity of each allele studied, detailed molecular characterisation was performed using short-range, long-range and quantitative PCR strategies, as described previously [20] and detailed in File S1 and Table S1.

Genotyping for *Slc25a21*$^{tm1a(KOMP)Wtsi}$ animals was performed using a combination of three short range assays (Table S1) and the *neo* count qPCR assay (0 = wt, 1 = het, 2 = hom). Conversion to *Slc25a21*$^{tm1b(KOMP)Wtsi}$, *Slc25a21*$^{tm1c(KOMP)Wtsi}$ and *Slc25a21*$^{tm1d(KOMP)Wtsi}$ was detected using short range PCR assays (Table S1).

Work by Santagati [21] indicated the presence of a regulatory element, named conserved non-coding sequence +6 (CNS+6), for *Pax9* within the allele design for *Slc25a21*$^{tm1a(KOMP)Wtsi}$. A PCR assay was designed (Table S1) to amplify *Slc25a21*$^{tm1a(KOMP)Wtsi}$ samples and the resulting products sequenced to determine if the CNS+6 element was disrupted.

### Expression analysis by quantitative PCR and RNA sequencing

E13.5 embryo heads [*Slc25a21*$^{tm1a(KOMP)Wtsi}$ (wt, n = 4; hom, n = 4), *Slc25a21*$^{tm1b(KOMP)Wtsi}$ (wt, n = 4; hom, n = 3), *Slc25a21*$^{tm1c(KOMP)Wtsi}$ (wt, n = 4; hom, n = 3), and *Slc25a21*$^{tm1d(KOMP)Wtsi}$ (wt, n = 4; hom, n = 3)] were processed for expression analysis by qPCR. For *Slc25a21* a custom FAM-labelled TaqMan assay (Applied Biosystems) spanning the junction of exons 8–9, 3′ to the floxed exon (Slc25a21_E8-9_F: CTGCTTCAAAACAATGGA-GATGAT, Slc25a21_E8-9_R: GGGACCAGGCCTTTGTA-TAAGG, Slc25a21_E8-9_M: CGGGAAGAAGGGATTT) was used. For *Pax9* a pre-designed TaqMan assay was used (Mm00440629_m1, Applied Biosystems). Details of the assays and methods used are described in File S1.

RNA sequencing was performed using 5 μg of total RNA from a subset of the above E13.5 embryo head samples [3 homozygotes and 2 wild-types for each allele (12 mutant and 8 control samples in total)] as detailed in File S1.

## Physical assessment, body composition, radiography and clinical chemistry

Homozygous mice (7M and 7F) from each of the alleles (*Slc25a21*$^{tm1a(KOMP)Wtsi}$, *Slc25a21*$^{tm1b(KOMP)Wtsi}$, *Slc25a21*$^{tm1c(KOMP)Wtsi}$ and *Slc25a21*$^{tm1d(KOMP)Wtsi}$), as well as age, sex and genetic background matched controls, were analysed using the standard Sanger Institute Mouse Genetics Project phenotyping screen [2]. Assays of particular relevance are described in File S1, whilst those not part of the standard phenotyping screen are described below.

At necropsy, skulls were collected and the teeth (both upper and lower jaw) and palate were reviewed and imaged (MZ16A dissecting microscope, Leica, Wetzlar, Germany; DFC490 digital camera, Canon Powershot G5, Japan). A range of 42 additional tissues and organs from homozygous *Slc25a21*$^{tm1a(KOMP)Wtsi}$ mice (2M and 2F), and age, sex and genetic background matched controls, were fixed in 10% neutral buffered formalin (Leica Biosystems, Peterborough, UK) for 15–20 hrs and processed to wax. 5 μm sections were stained with haematoxylin and eosin then reviewed by an experienced pathologist.

Micro-CT (computed tomography) images of skulls from *Slc25a21*$^{tm1a(KOMP)Wtsi}$ mice (wt, n = 2; hom, n = 2) were collected at 18 μm resolution (SkyScan 1176, SkyScan, Kontich, Belgium).

## Auditory Brainstem Response (ABR) recordings

ABRs were recorded in *Slc25a21*$^{tm1a(KOMP)Wtsi}$ mice aged 4 weeks (wt, n = 17; het, n = 27; hom, n = 7), 8 weeks (wt, n = 20; het, n = 33; hom, n = 8), 14 weeks (wt, n = 11; hom, n = 14), and 26 weeks (wt, n = 17; hom, n = 10), using the methods described in detail in Ingham et al. [22]. In addition, mice from the *Slc25a21*$^{tm1b(KOMP)Wtsi}$ colony (hom, n = 8), *Slc25a21*$^{tm1c(KOMP)Wtsi}$ colony (hom, n = 5) and *Slc25a21*$^{tm1d\ (KOMP)Wtsi}$ colony (hom, n = 8) were tested at 14 weeks of age.

Anaesthetised mice were placed on a heating blanket inside a sound attenuating booth and recording electrodes inserted in the skin to record responses of the left ear. For ABR threshold determination, click (0.01 ms duration) and tone pip (6, 12, 18, 24, and 30 kHz of 5 ms duration, 1 ms rise/fall time) stimuli over a range of intensity levels from 10–95 dB sound pressure level (SPL) in 5 dB steps were presented in free-field. Averaged responses to 256 stimuli, presented at 42.2/s, were analysed and thresholds established as the lowest sound intensity giving a visually-detectable ABR response.

## Middle ear analysis

Following ABR testing, *Slc25a21*$^{tm1a(KOMP)Wtsi}$ mice aged 9 weeks (wt, n = 8; het, n = 11; hom, n = 8) were killed by cervical dislocation and the right external and middle ears were examined in detail using a dissecting microscope for any signs of malformation or inflammation, including: appearance of excess cerumen in the external ear canal; thickening, whitening, sponginess or excess vascularisation of the bulla wall; clarity and vascularisation of the tympanic membrane; presence of fluid or white inflammatory material in the middle ear cavity; and solid masses or bony outgrowths of the middle ear wall or ossicles. In addition, the left side of the head of these mice was fixed in 10% formalin for 48 hours, and decalcified in 10% EDTA diluted in phosphate buffered saline (PBS) for 10 days, dehydrated, embedded in paraffin wax, sectioned at 8 μm and stained with haematoxylin and eosin.

## Reporter gene analysis

*LacZ* reporter gene wholemount expression analysis was performed on *Slc25a21*$^{tm1a(KOMP)Wtsi}$ adults [aged 15–18 weeks (wt, n = 2; het, n = 3; hom, n = 9)] as described previously [23] and detailed in File S1.

## Bone and cartilage staining

Bone and cartilage staining of *Slc25a21*$^{tm1a(KOMP)Wtsi}$ E18.5 embryos (wt, n = 10; het, n = 27; hom, n = 12) was performed using a protocol based on the Cold Spring Harbour method for Alcian blue/Alizarin Red staining [24], and detailed in File S1.

## Data analysis and statistics

A reference range approach was used to assess continuous data, including time course. For categorical data, a Fisher's exact test was used to identify phenotypic variants. More details of both approaches are presented in File S1. Since both of the above approaches to automatically identify significant calls are known to be conservative and assess each parameter in isolation, they were complemented by a manual assessment made by a biological expert who used knowledge of events on the day, or across sexes, or between related variables, to highlight additional potentially abnormal phenotypes (Table S2).

To assess the ABR data, a one-way Kruskall-Wallis ANOVA on Ranks was used where three genotypes were assessed and Mann-Whitney rank sum test where only homozygote and wild-type animals were assessed. The qPCR gene expression results for mutant mice were compared to littermate wild-type mice using a Student's t-Test assuming two-sample unequal variance. P-values for the RNA sequencing were adjusted for multiple testing with the Benjamini-Hochberg procedure. Pre-weaning lethality was assessed using the Test for One Proportion.

# Results

## Characterisation of *Slc25a21*$^{tm1a(KOMP)Wtsi}$ homozygous mice

*Slc25a21*$^{tm1a(KOMP)Wtsi}$ mice were generated and characterised on a C57BL/6N;C57BL/6-*Tyr*$^{c-Brd}$ background by the Sanger Mouse Genetics Project. Homozygous *Slc25a21*$^{tm1a(KOMP)Wtsi}$ mice were under-represented at post natal day 14 (P14), as a result of pre-weaning lethality, with 25 homozygous mutants detected among 304 progeny from heterozygous intercrosses (Table 1. Test for one proportion; $\chi^2 = 44.74$, df = 1, p = 1.124e-11).

Those homozygous animals surviving to weaning, presented with decreased body weight (Fig. 1A–B), fat mass (Fig. 1C–D) and fat percentage estimate (data not shown), in both sexes, compared to wild-type controls. Furthermore, a range of dental abnormalities were observed in *Slc25a21*$^{tm1a(KOMP)Wtsi}$ homozygous mice. At 10 weeks of age 13 out of 14 homozygous *Slc25a21*$^{tm1a(KOMP)Wtsi}$ mice were found to have an abnormally shortened snout (data not shown). At 16 weeks of age all fourteen homozygous *Slc25a21*$^{tm1a(KOMP)Wtsi}$ mice were found to have macroscopically visible dental abnormalities ranging from white or translucent to severely hypoplastic lower incisors (Fig. 2A–B) compared to wild-type (Fig. 2C). The molars of homozygous *Slc25a21*$^{tm1a(KOMP)Wtsi}$ adult mice (Fig. 2D), in particular of the lower jaw, were found to be strongly stained with X-gal (requiring β-galactosidase activity) compared to heterozygous and wild-type (Fig. 2E–F). Microscopic examination of sections from representative animals confirmed that in unaffected areas, the molars were fully developed with normal odontoblast morphology. In affected areas of the molars, there was focal fracturing of the surface dentine and necrosis of the pulp with associated inflammation and bacterial colonies (Fig. 2G).

**Table 1.** Genotype distribution for *Slc25a21*$^{tm1a(KOMP)Wtsi}$ mice.

| Allele and Stage | Number of Progeny | Number of Wild-types | Number of Heterozygotes | Number of Homozygotes | Percentage Homozygote Viability |
|---|---|---|---|---|---|
| **tm1a E14.5** | 35 | 3 | 22 | 8 | 23% |
| **tm1a E18.5** | 44 | 10 | 27 | 7 | 16% |
| **tm1a P14** | 304 | 111 | 168 | 25 | 8% |
| **tm1b P14** | 130 | 24 | 68 | 38 | 29% |
| **tm1c P14** | 145 | 26 | 84 | 35 | 24% |
| **tm1d P14** | 193 | 44 | 113 | 36 | 19% |

From heterozygous inter-crossing, homozygous progeny for *Slc25a21*$^{tm1a(KOMP)Wtsi}$ were recorded at a sub-Mendelian ratio at post natal day 14 (P14), but a normal ratio at two embryonic time points (E14.5 and E18.5). *Slc25a21*$^{tm1b(KOMP)Wtsi}$, *Slc25a21*$^{tm1c(KOMP)Wtsi}$ and *Slc25a21*$^{tm1d(KOMP)Wtsi}$ homozygotes were detected at the expected ratio.

Micro-CT scanning revealed that the lower incisor root area in homozygous *Slc25a21*$^{tm1a(KOMP)Wtsi}$ mice was severely under-developed and that the lower incisors appeared to be lacking the enamel coating (Fig. 2H–I) compared to wild-type (Fig. 2J). Furthermore, two dimensional X-ray images revealed several changes of the manidibular morphology including pronounced pogonion, pronounced anterior tuberosity, under-developed incisor process and alveolus (data not shown), potentially indicating a change in the developmental dynamics of the mandible in homozygous *Slc25a21*$^{tm1a(KOMP)Wtsi}$ mice. Taken together, the 2D X-ray images, micro-CT and X-gal staining in tooth cavities suggests feeding might be uncomfortable for homozygous *Slc25a21*$^{tm1a(KOMP)Wtsi}$ mice which may explain their reduced body weight and fat mass.

Further characterisation uncovered craniofacial abnormalities in adult homozygous *Slc25a21*$^{tm1a(KOMP)Wtsi}$ mice. Specifically, they presented with abnormal development of palatal rugae number 3 (Fig. 3A–C) compared to wild-type (Fig. 3D). Micro-CT scanning revealed that the anterior part of the vomer bone was completely absent in homozygous *Slc25a21*$^{tm1a(KOMP)Wtsi}$ mice (Fig. 3E–F) compared to wild-type (Fig. 3G), this was confirmed by macroscopic observations (Fig. 3H). The vomeronasal organ (VNO) appeared to be intact. Morphological examination of E18.5 embryo heads from homozygous *Slc25a21*$^{tm1a(KOMP)Wtsi}$ mice did not reveal any further craniofacial abnormalities.

Finally, 14 week old *Slc25a21*$^{tm1a(KOMP)Wtsi}$ homozygous mice were found to have a hearing impairment as they presented with elevated auditory brainstem response thresholds across all frequencies, with severity of impairment increasing with age (Fig. 4A–D). *Slc25a21*$^{tm1a(KOMP)Wtsi}$ homozygous mice displayed an approximately parallel pattern of threshold elevation across the range of frequency stimuli used, a profile which is typical of conductive hearing loss. Fig. 4E shows that click threshold in wild-types was stable with increasing age, at least up to 26 weeks of age, whereas a progressive deterioration was seen in *Slc25a21*$^{tm1a(KOMP)Wtsi}$ homozygous mice over the same age range. At 26 weeks of age, some wild-type mice showed age-related high-frequency hearing loss (indicated by larger standard deviations at 24–30 kHz). The thresholds recorded in the *Slc25a21*$^{tm1a(KOMP)Wtsi}$ homozygous mice at all ages were significantly elevated above age-matched wild-types ($p<0.001$) (Fig. 4F).

To investigate the morphology of the middle ear, the right temporal bone, containing the entire ear, was dissected from *Slc25a21*$^{tm1a(KOMP)Wtsi}$ homozygous mice at 9 weeks of age (n = 8) along with wild-type (n = 8) and heterozygous (n = 11) littermates. Compared to wild-types (Fig. 5A), most of the homozygotes (7/8) showed opaque fluid or white debris in the middle ear cavity indicating otitis media (Fig. 5B). Other features of otitis media were more variable, including excessive vascularisation (n = 3) or whitening of the bulla (n = 4) or tympanic membrane (n = 1). The one homozygous *Slc25a21*$^{tm1a(KOMP)Wtsi}$ mouse in which exudate was not observed in the middle ear also had ABR thresholds only slightly above those seen in wild-type mice. Heterozygotes had normal middle ears.

The left side temporal bones from the same eight *Slc25a21*$^{tm1a(KOMP)Wtsi}$ homozygous mice and wild-type controls were sectioned through the middle ear, stained with haemotoxylin and eosin, and examined microscopically. Inflammatory changes and accumulation of exudate consistent with otitis media were observed in six of the eight homozygotes (Fig. 5D, F).

The middle ear cavity of the six affected *Slc25a21*$^{tm1a(KOMP)Wtsi}$ homozygous mice contained variable amounts of an amorphous eosinophilic exudate containing cholesterol crystals, foamy macrophages and neutrophils, indicating an active inflammatory response. In these mice, the lining epithelium of the middle ear cavity was variably hyperplastic and the underlying lamina propria was oedematous with congestion of blood vessels (Fig. 5D, F). None of the littermate controls showed evidence of inflammation (Fig. 5A, C, E).

Of the two *Slc25a21*$^{tm1a(KOMP)Wtsi}$ homozygous mice showing little or no effusion one had comparatively normal ABR thresholds, whilst the other had raised ABR thresholds.

The tympanic ring size was normal in *Slc25a21*$^{tm1a(KOMP)Wtsi}$ homozygous mice; assessment of micro-CT images revealed no change in adults whilst alizarin red/alcian blue stained embryos revealed no changes at E18.5 (data not shown).

Systematic histopathology assessment of a range of tissues from homozygous *Slc25a21*$^{tm1a(KOMP)Wtsi}$ mice did not reveal any further abnormalities, and in particular, no indication of any inflammation other than in the middle ear was found.

## Ablation of *Slc25a21* does not cause signs of 2-oxoadipate acidaemia in mice

It has been proposed that loss of function of ODC, the protein encoded by *SLC25A21*, causes the human disease 2-oxoadipate acidaemia which is clinically characterised by hypotonia, seizures, motor and developmental delay, cerebellar ataxia and varying severities of intellectual disability [13,14,15,16]. Unexpectedly, homozygous *Slc25a21*$^{tm1a(KOMP)Wtsi}$ mice did not phenocopy this human disease. In particular, lean mass, grip strength and gait, correlates of the human disease manifestation, were all normal for these mice (data not shown), and no seizures were detected.

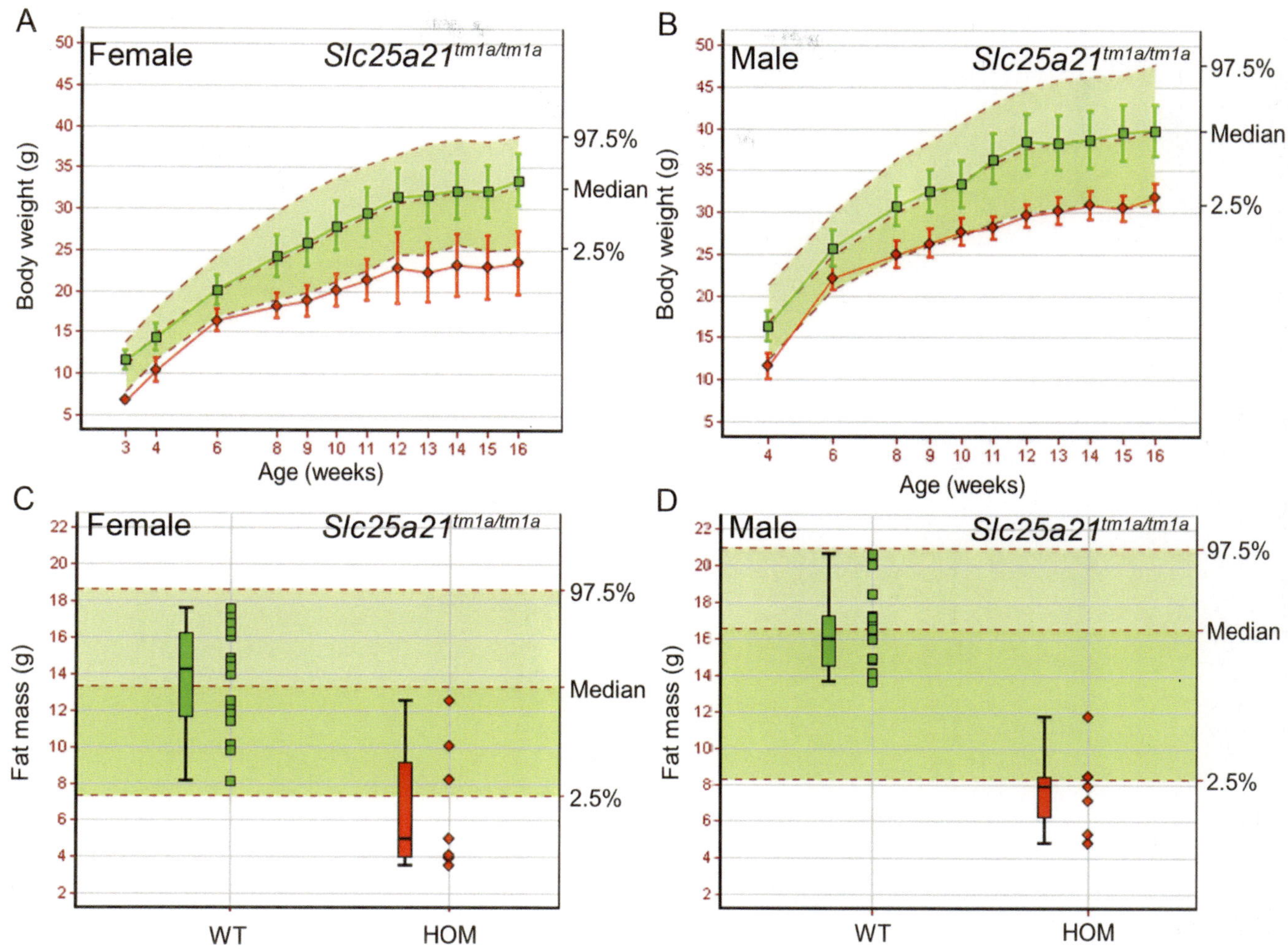


**Figure 1. Body weight and fat mass were reduced in homozygous *Slc25a21*$^{tm1a(KOMP)Wtsi}$ mice.** Homozygous (red symbols) *Slc25a21*$^{tm1a(KOMP)Wtsi}$ female (A,C) (n = 7) and male (B,D) (n = 7) mice showed decreased body weight and fat mass compared to local wild-type controls run on the same week (green symbols) (female, n = 22; male, n = 15). Mean (± SD) body weight is plotted against age (A,B). Fat mass is presented as a boxplot, with median, 25$^{th}$ and 75$^{th}$ percentile (box), and the lowest and highest data point within 1.5× inter quartile range (whiskers) shown (C,D). The median and 95% reference range (2.5–97.5$^{th}$ percentiles, dotted lines) for all wild-type mice of the same genetic background and sex (n>750) are displayed on the pale green background.

To ascertain the molecular consequence of the targeting event, expression analysis of *Slc25a21*$^{tm1a(KOMP)Wtsi}$ was performed on RNA extracted from embryo heads (E13.5). When using the *Slc25a21* TaqMan assay which spanned exons 8–9, 3′ of the cassette insertion, expression was found to be reduced in homozygous *Slc25a21*$^{tm1a(KOMP)Wtsi}$ samples (28.7% of wild-type expression, p = 2.0e-05) but not completely ablated (Fig. 6A). The hypomorphic nature of this allele may have explained the absence of the predicted phenotypes, therefore an allelic series was created (Fig. 6B–E) where tm1b was a *lacZ* reporter tagged deletion with the critical exon (exon 4) removed, tm1c a conditional allele with wild-type function restored, and tm1d the deletion allele where both exon 4 and the *lacZ* reporter were removed. Expression analysis of each of these *Slc25a21* alleles was performed on RNA extracted from embryo heads (E13.5). *Slc25a21* RNA expression was found to be ablated in homozygous *Slc25a21*$^{tm1b(KOMP)Wtsi}$ (0% of wild-type expression, expression was below the limit of detection) and greatly reduced in *Slc25a21*$^{tm1d(KOMP)Wtsi}$ homozygotes (12.9% of wild-type expression, p = 0.043) (Fig. 6A). As expected, expression levels of *Slc25a21* in embryos homozygous for *Slc25a21*$^{tm1c(KOMP)Wtsi}$ were not significantly different from wild-type expression (Fig. 6A).

We proceeded by phenotyping animals homozygous for the *Slc25a21*$^{tm1b(KOMP)Wtsi}$, *Slc25a21*$^{tm1c(KOMP)Wtsi}$ and *Slc25a21*$^{tm1d(KOMP)Wtsi}$ alleles. Following heterozygous intercrossing, homozygous animals for all three alleles were detected at the expected Mendelian ratio. Furthermore, body weight, fat mass and auditory brainstem response thresholds (Mann-Whitney Rank Sum Tests; tm1b, p = 0.12; tm1c, p = 0.48; tm1d, p = 0.59) (Fig. 7A–I) were all found to be normal compared with wild-types, as were the teeth and palatal rugae (data not shown). Full data from the phenotyping pipeline can be viewed online (www.sanger.ac.uk/mouseportal).

These results led us to conclude that the phenotypes observed in mice homozygous for the *Slc25a21*$^{tm1a(KOMP)Wtsi}$ targeted allele were not due to ablation of Slc25a21 function, and speculate that off-target effects due to the selection cassette present in the tm1a allele affected expression of neighbouring genes.

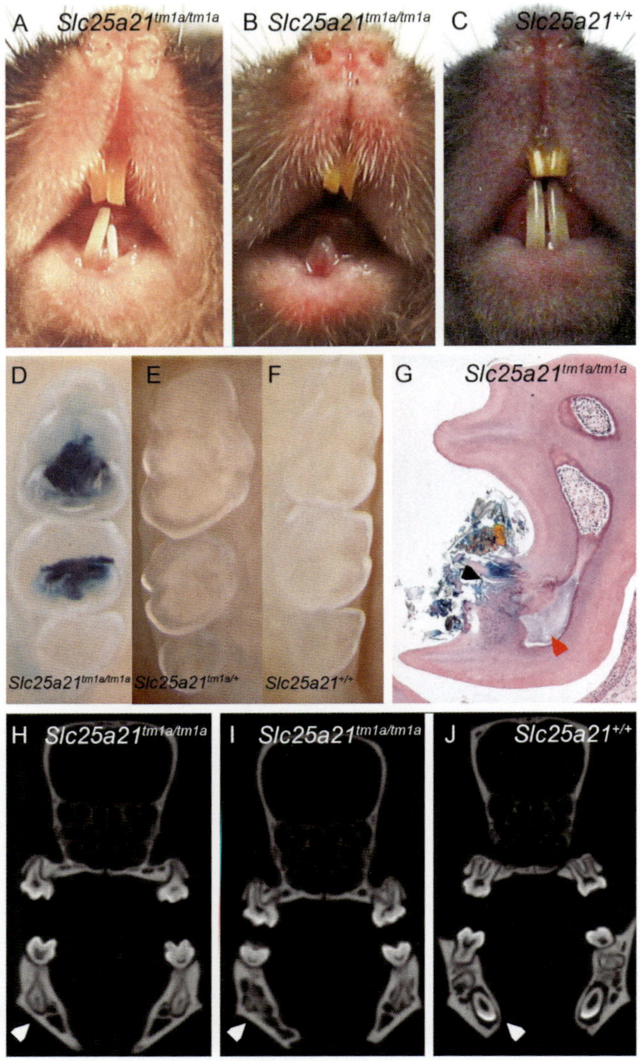


**Figure 2. Dental abnormalities observed in homozygous *$Slc25a21^{tm1a(KOMP)Wtsi}$* mice.** Dysmorphology analysis revealed under-developed, white incisors (A–B) in *$Slc25a21^{tm1a(KOMP)Wtsi}$* homozygous mice as compared to wild-type (C). Wholemount (D–F) and subsequent histological sections (G) demonstrated bacterial *lacZ* activity in cavities within lower jaw molars of *$Slc25a21^{tm1a(KOMP)Wtsi}$* homozygous (D,G) mice compared to heterozygous (E) and wild-type (F) mice. Focal fracturing of the surface dentine is indicated with a black arrow and necrosis of the pulp indicated with a red arrow (G). Micro-CT imaging demonstrated that the root aspect of lower jaw incisors was severely under developed (white arrow) and lacked enamel coating in homozygous *$Slc25a21^{tm1a(KOMP)Wtsi}$* mice (H–I) compared to wild-type (J).

### Hypomorphic expression of *Pax9* may account for observed phenotypes

The 1 Mb genomic interval containing *Slc25a21* (500 kb flanking the target gene) is predicted to contain seven known protein coding genes, one non coding RNA, one novel antisense and one putative processed transcript (Fig. S1). Of particular interest is *Pax9*, located at the 3′ end of *Slc25a21* and orientated on the opposite strand. The 3′UTR regions of *Slc25a21* and *Pax9* overlap by 188 bp. Consistent with the phenotypes observed in *$Slc25a21^{tm1a(KOMP)Wtsi}$* homozygous animals, mice carrying a hypomorphic *Pax9* allele had previously been reported as causing reduced viability at weaning [25], and presented with a range of dental and craniofacial abnormalities [25,26] similar to those described herein.

RNA expression analysis of *Pax9* was performed on embryo heads (E13.5) for all four alleles in the *Slc25a21* series. *Pax9* expression was found to be down regulated [approximately 34% of wild-type *Pax9* levels ($p = 1.1E\text{-}06$)] in homozygous *$Slc25a21^{tm1a(KOMP)Wtsi}$* samples (Fig. 8) confirming our hypothesis that we had inadvertently created a *Pax9* hypomorphic allele. *Pax9* levels were found to be unaffected in homozygous *$Slc25a21^{tm1b(KOMP)Wtsi}$*, *$Slc25a21^{tm1c(KOMP)Wtsi}$* and *$Slc25a21^{tm1d(KOMP)Wtsi}$* samples (Fig. 8). A known *Pax9* regulatory element (CNS+6) was located within the targeting construct used to create the *$Slc25a21^{tm1a(KOMP)Wtsi}$* allele [21]. PCR and sequence analysis was used to demonstrate that this sequence was not disrupted during the vector construction or at the homologous recombination stage (Table S1; data not shown). Consequently, we hypothesise that the presence of the promoter driven neomycin cassette in the homozygous *$Slc25a21^{tm1a(KOMP)Wtsi}$* mice caused the reduction of *Pax9* expression.

RNA sequencing was performed to further explore the impact of the targeting event on the genomic environment around *Slc25a21*. Comparing RNA from wild-type and homozygous *$Slc25a21^{tm1a(KOMP)Wtsi}$* E13.5 embryo heads, the only gene in the 1 Mb interval surrounding *Slc25a21* that had significantly altered expression levels was *Pax9* [q (adjusted p value) = 7.10E-06 (data not shown)]. *Pax9* was not found to be differentially expressed in homozygous *$Slc25a21^{tm1b(KOMP)Wtsi}$*, *$Slc25a21^{tm1c(KOMP)Wtsi}$* and *$Slc25a21^{tm1d(KOMP)Wtsi}$* embryo heads. The low endogenous expression level of *Slc25a21* in wild-type mice was below the threshold where significant changes could be detected.

The phenotypes we observed in homozygous *$Slc25a21^{tm1a(KOMP)Wtsi}$* mice were broadly consistent with those reported previously in mice carrying hypomorphic *Pax9* alleles [26] with the exception that the otitis media and hearing impairment reported in this study have not been assessed previously in *Pax9* mutant mice and may represent a novel consequence of *Pax9* suppression.

## Discussion

### Characteristics of 2-oxoadipate acidaemia are absent in mice ablated for *Slc25a21* expression

We report the generation and phenotypic characterisation of the *Slc25a21* allelic series derived from a typical KOMP-CSD allele [3]. Subject to the sensitivity and scope of the phenotyping performed, ablation of *Slc25a21* expression was not found to phenocopy the human disease 2-oxoadipate acidaemia (OMIM 204750) for which it is a candidate gene [11]. There are several possible explanations for this. Whilst no hypotonia, ataxia or seizures were detected in *Slc25a21* null mice [homozygous for the tm1b (KOMP)Wtsi or tm1d (KOMP)Wtsi alleles], a subset of other clinical symptoms associated with 2-oxoadipate acidaemia, including intellectual disability and urine metabolites, were not assessed by the standard Mouse Genetics Project primary phenotyping pipeline with which these animals were screened [2]. Therefore it cannot be ruled out that additional tests, or analysis performed with increased sensitivity, may reveal subtle disease similarities. Alternatively, mitochondrial transport of metabolites is a complex process involving many carrier proteins. Unknown compensatory mechanisms may be at play in *Slc25a21* null mice that prevent the cytoplasmic build-up of oxoadipate and the associated disruption in the catabolism of key amino acids such as lysine [11]. For example, it is known that the substrate specificity of Slc25a21 itself varies between species [11]. Finally,

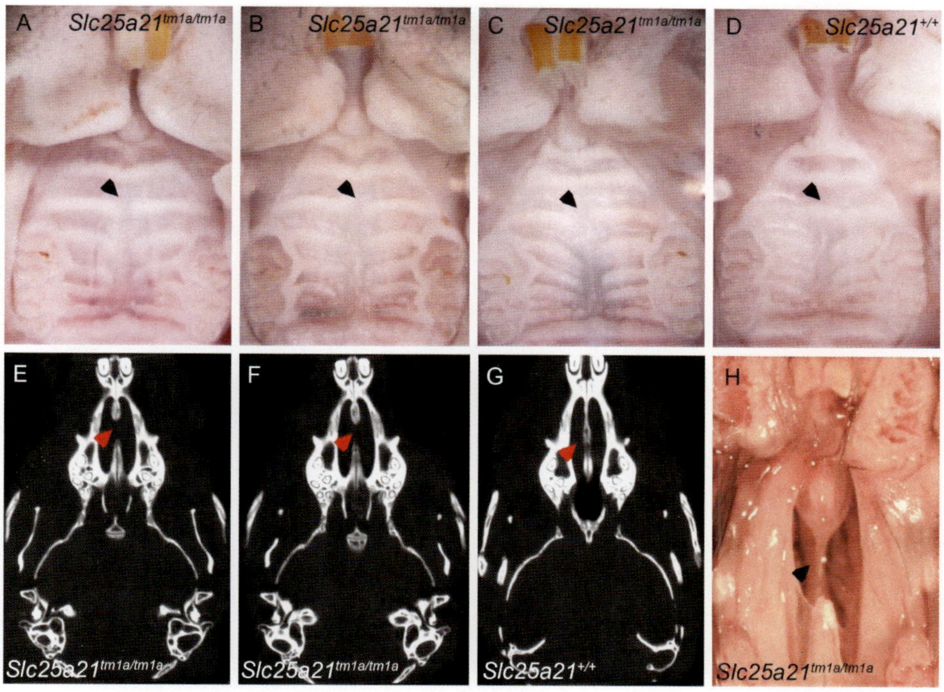


**Figure 3. Rugae and vomer abnormalities observed in homozygous *Slc25a21*$^{tm1a(KOMP)Wtsi}$ mice.** Abnormalities in rugae (in particular number 3) were observed in homozygous *Slc25a21*$^{tm1a(KOMP)Wtsi}$ mice (A–C) compared to wild-type (D), indicated with arrows (wt, n = 11; hom, n = 11). Micro-CT analysis revealed that the anterior part of the vomer bone was absent in *Slc25a21*$^{tm1a(KOMP)Wtsi}$ homozygous mice (E–F) compared to wild-type (G) (wt, n = 2; hom, n = 12). This was confirmed by dissection of the palate of *Slc25a21*$^{tm1a(KOMP)Wtsi}$ mice (H).

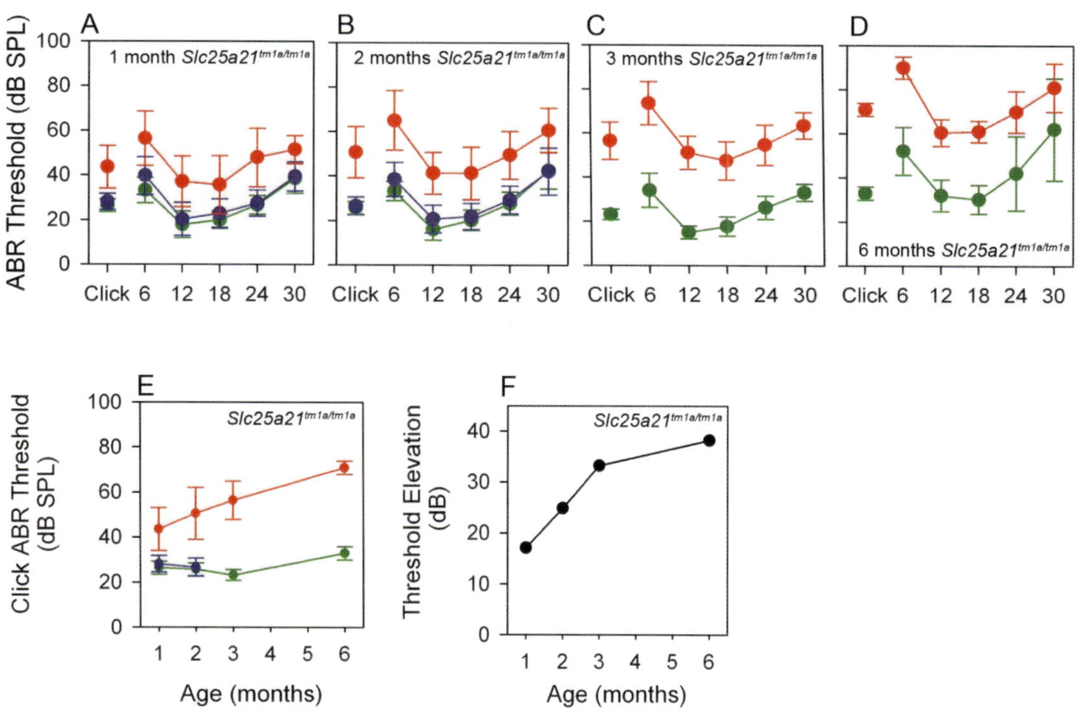


**Figure 4. Auditory brainstem response threshold was elevated in *Slc25a21*$^{tm1a(KOMP)Wtsi}$ mice.** Auditory brainstem response threshold was elevated across all frequencies in homozygous *Slc25a21*$^{tm1a(KOMP)Wtsi}$ mice aged 1, 2, 3 and 6 months respectively. Mean ABR thresholds (± SD) are shown for wild-type (green symbols), heterozygote (blue symbols) and homozygote (red symbols) *Slc25a21*$^{tm1a(KOMP)Wtsi}$ mice (A–D). The click-evoked ABR thresholds (mean ± SD) plotted as a function of age (months) demonstrated a progressive deterioration in *Slc25a21*$^{tm1a(KOMP)Wtsi}$ mice (E); an observation clearly demonstrated by plotting the mean click-evoked ABR threshold elevation of mutants above wild-types as a function of age (months) (F).

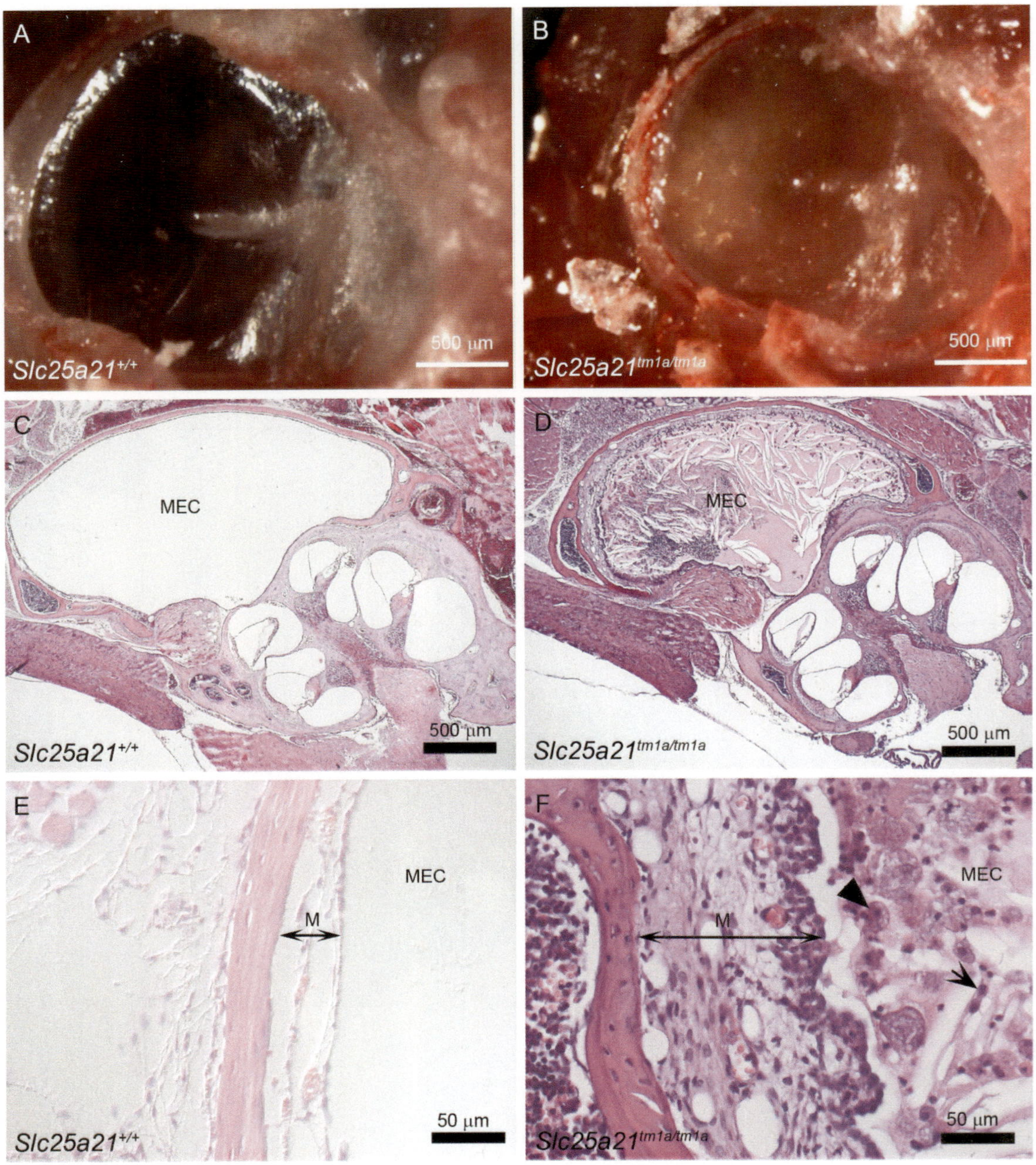


**Figure 5. Signs of otitis media in *Slc25a21$^{tm1a(KOMP)Wtsi}$* mice.** The tympanic membrane viewed from the external ear canal showed an opaque fluid present in *Slc25a21$^{tm1a(KOMP)Wtsi}$* homozygous mice (B) that was not present in wild-type controls (A). The opaque exudate was clearly visible on haematoxylin and eosin stained histology sections through the middle ear of *Slc25a21$^{tm1a(KOMP)Wtsi}$* homozygous mice (D) compared to wild-types (C). Examination at higher magnification revealed that the exudate containing inflammatory cells including foamy macrophages (solid arrow head), and neutrophils (short arrow) in the middle ear cavity (MEC), and a thickened mucosa (M, double headed arrow) in *Slc25a21$^{tm1a(KOMP)Wtsi}$* homozygous mice due to epithelial hyperplasia, oedema and congestion (F). Wild-type mice appeared normal (E).

definitive proof of the candidacy of *Slc25a21* for 2-oxoadipate acidaemia is not published and it has been speculated that the disease may be due to defective 2-oxoadipate dehydrogenase, an alternative gene in the same metabolic pathway [11].

## *Slc25a21$^{tm1a(KOMP)Wtsi}$* allele affects expression of a neighbouring gene

The *Slc25a21$^{tm1a(KOMP)Wtsi}$* homozygous mice investigated in this study were found to be sub-viable. Those homozygous animals surviving to weaning presented with growth retardation, orofacial abnormalities, brittle, white incisors and hearing impairment. Given the absence of any detectable phenotype in mice homozygous for the *Slc25a21* tm1b (KOMP)Wtsi, tm1c (KOMP)Wtsi or tm1d (KOMP)Wtsi derived alleles, we conclude that the phenotypes observed in mice homozygous for *Slc25a21$^{t-m1a(KOMP)Wtsi}$* were not due to ablation of *Slc25a21* function, and propose that off-target effects of the tm1a allele affected expression of a neighbouring gene. The spatial, temporal and quantitatively correct activity of a gene requires the presence of not only intact coding sequence but also properly functioning regulatory control.

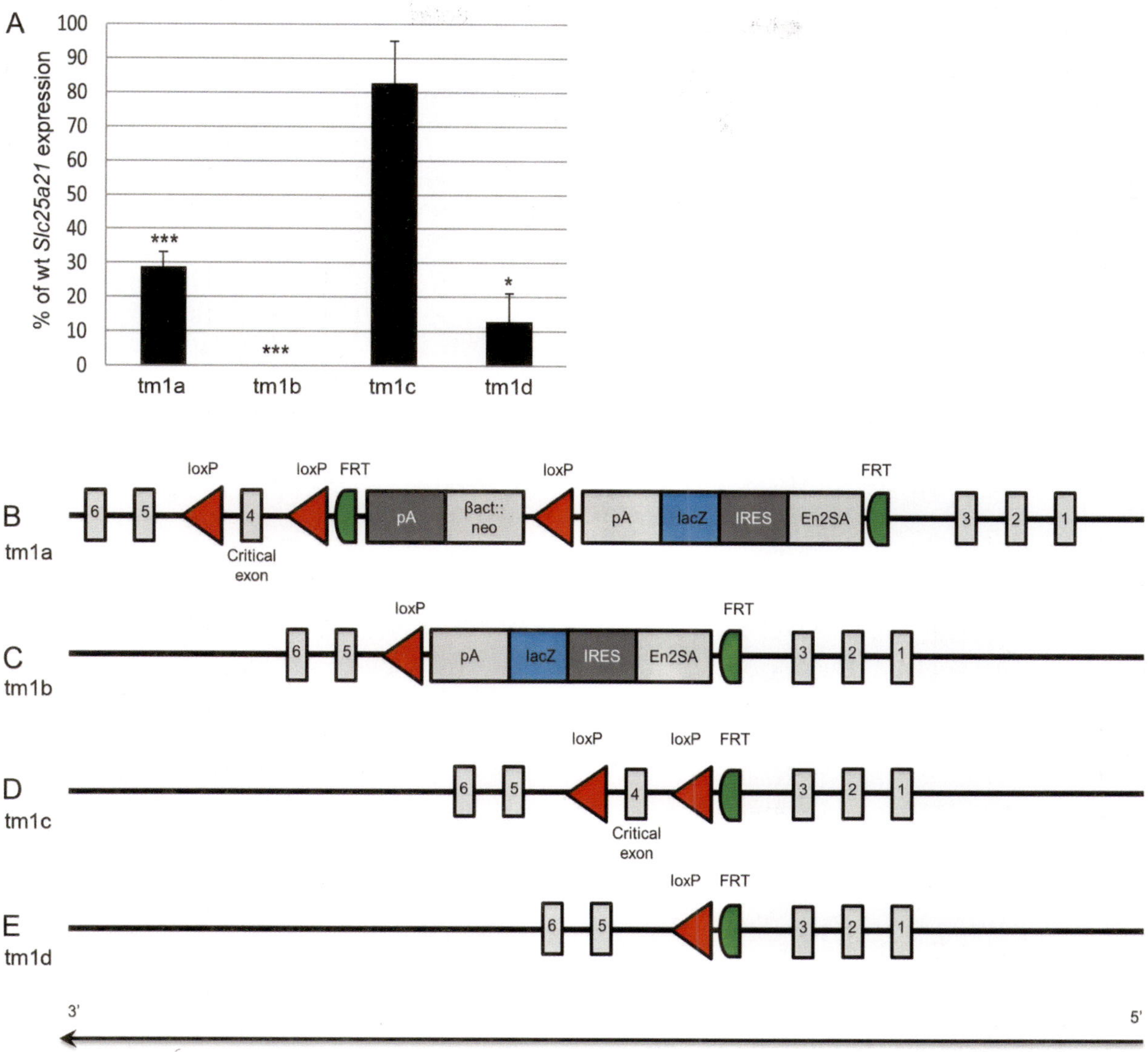


**Figure 6. Schematic of the *Slc25a21*$^{tm1(KOMP)Wtsi}$ allelic series and the associated RNA expression levels.** Quantitative PCR on RNA from E13.5 embryo heads demonstrated that *Slc25a21* RNA expression was significantly reduced in *Slc25a21*$^{tm1a(KOMP)Wtsi}$, *Slc25a21*$^{tm1b(KOMP)Wtsi}$ and *Slc25a21*$^{tm1d(KOMP)Wtsi}$ homozygotes (* $p<0.05$; *** $p<0.001$), but equivalent to wild-type levels in *Slc25a21*$^{tm1c(KOMP)Wtsi}$ homozygotes (A). A schematic of the *Slc25a21*$^{tm1(KOMP)Wtsi}$ allelic series is presented, consisting of: (B) *Slc25a21*$^{tm1a(KOMP)Wtsi}$, the knockout first reporter (*lacZ*) tagged insertion allele; (C) *Slc25a21*$^{tm1b(KOMP)Wtsi}$, the *lacZ* tagged deletion allele generated by breeding with mice ubiquitously expressing Cre recombinase; (D) *Slc25a21*$^{tm1c(KOMP)Wtsi}$, the conditional allele generated by breeding mice carrying the *Slc25a21*$^{tm1a(KOMP)Wtsi}$ allele with mice ubiquitously expressing Flp recombinase; and (E) *Slc25a21*$^{tm1d(KOMP)Wtsi}$, the deletion allele arising after breeding mice carrying the *Slc25a21*$^{tm1c(KOMP)Wtsi}$ allele with mice ubiquitously expressing Cre recombinase (E).

Interference of the expression of neighbouring genes by the presence of selectable marker cassettes or short DNA sequences [5,6,7,8,9] has been reported for genes in close vicinity to the target gene and as far as >100 kb from the targeted gene [6]. Transcriptional silencing of neighbouring genes due to CpG rich sequences within the standard, non-codon optimised, *lacZ* reporter gene used in this KOMP-CSD allele has also been reported [27]. Furthermore, disruption of *cis*-regulatory elements has been linked with abnormal phenotypes in both mice [5] and humans [28,29]. In addition, a wide variety of mechanisms which cause disruption of gene expression by a change in its chromosomal environment, while leaving the transcription unit intact, have been identified [29].

At E13.5, RNA sequencing revealed that the only gene within the 1 Mb genomic interval surrounding *Slc25a21* that was differentially expressed, compared to wild-type, in homozygous *Slc25a21*$^{tm1a(KOMP)Wtsi}$ embryos was *Pax9*, an observation confirmed by quantitative PCR. *Pax9* is located in a 21.06 kb genomic interval directly 3′ of *Slc25a21* and orientated on the opposite strand. Evolutionarily conserved non-coding sequences are present both up-and down-stream of *Pax9*, some of which have been demonstrated to induce *Pax9* expression [21]. One such conserved region, CNS+6, [21] was located within the homology arm of the *Slc25a21*$^{tm1a(KOMP)Wtsi}$ targeting construct, and therefore a candidate for causing altered *Pax9* expression. However, sequencing confirmed the integrity of CNS+6 in the *Slc25a21*$^{tm1a(KOMP)Wtsi}$ allele. Since homozygous *Slc25a21*$^{tm1b(KOMP)Wtsi}$ mice, which still

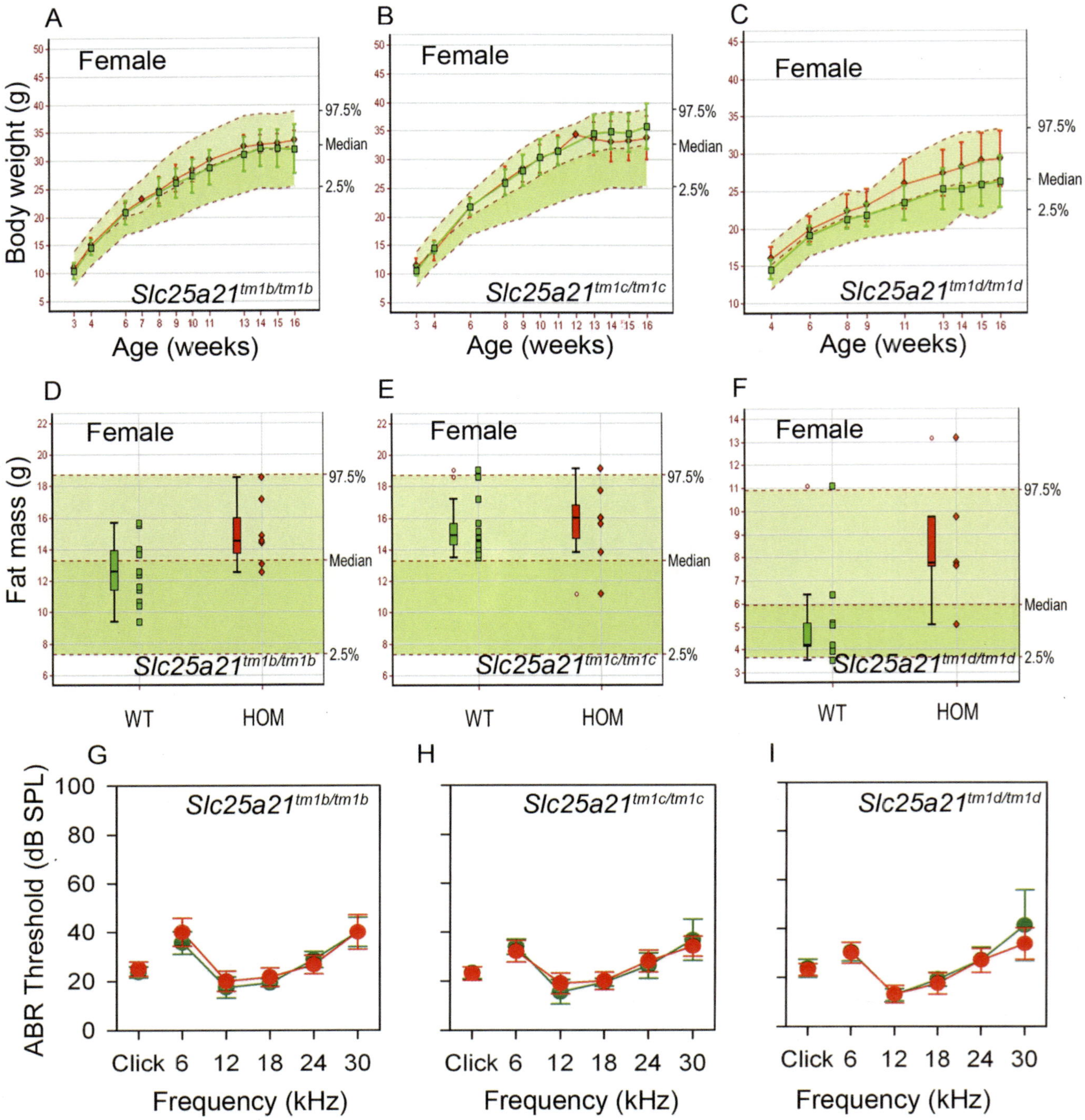


**Figure 7. Normal phenotype observed in *Slc25a21*$^{tm1b(KOMP)Wtsi}$, *Slc25a21*$^{tm1c(KOMP)Wtsi}$ and *Slc25a21*$^{tm1d(KOMP)Wtsi}$ homozygous mice.** Body weight and fat mass were normal in females homozygous (red symbols) for *Slc25a21*$^{tm1b(KOMP)Wtsi}$ (A,D) (n = 7), *Slc25a21*$^{tm1c(KOMP)Wtsi}$ (B,E) (n = 7), and *Slc25a21*$^{tm1d(KOMP)Wtsi}$ mice (C,F) (body weight n = 7, fat mass n = 5) compared to local wild-type controls run on the same week (green symbols) (n≥9). Male homozygotes for each of these three alleles and two parameters were also phenotypically normal (data not shown). Mean (± SD) body weight is plotted against age (A–C). Fat mass is presented as a boxplot, with median, 25th and 75th percentile (box), and the lowest and highest data point within 1.5× inter quartile range (whiskers) shown (D–F). The median and 95% reference range (2.5–97.5th percentiles, dotted lines) for all wild-type mice of the same genetic background and sex (n>80) are displayed on the pale green background. ABR thresholds were normal in homozygous *Slc25a21*$^{tm1b(KOMP)Wtsi}$ (G), *Slc25a21*$^{tm1c(KOMP)Wtsi}$ (H) and *Slc25a21*$^{tm1d(KOMP)Wtsi}$ mice (I) (red symbols) compared to wild-type controls (green symbols).

have part of the targeting cassette present (Fig. 6C), were found to be phenotypically normal, interference by the polyA-*β-actin::neo* cassette is the most likely cause of the reduction of *Pax9* expression seen in homozygous *Slc25a21*$^{tm1a(KOMP)Wtsi}$ mice. The findings in this study highlight the need to confirm phenotypes found in animals carrying the knockout first conditional ready [tm1a (KOMP)Wtsi or tm1a (EUCOMM)Wtsi] allele by creating and analysing the derived deletion allele. This is a timely reminder, with direct implications on the 3Rs, given the growing resource of

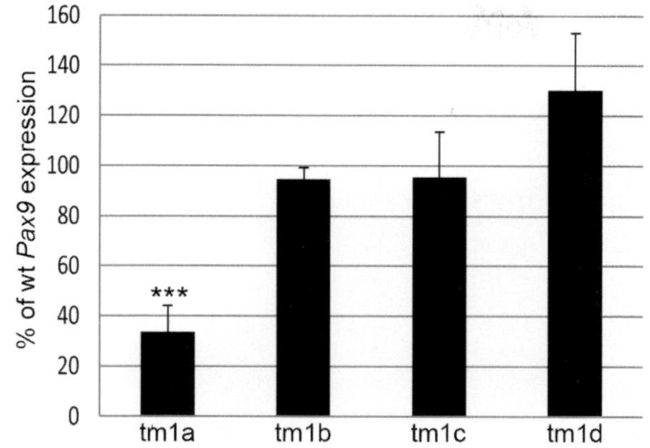


**Figure 8. RNA expression of *Pax9* was reduced in *Slc25a21*$^{tm1a(-KOMP)Wtsi}$ mice.** Quantitative PCR on RNA from E13.5 embryo heads demonstrated that *Pax9* RNA expression was significantly reduced in *Slc25a21*$^{tm1a(KOMP)Wtsi}$ (*** p = 1.1E-06) homozygotes, but equivalent to wild-type levels in *Slc25a21*$^{tm1b(KOMP)Wtsi}$, *Slc25a21*$^{tm1c(KOMP)Wtsi}$ and *Slc25a21*$^{tm1d(KOMP)Wtsi}$ homozygotes.

knockout first conditional ready targeted ES cells created by the EUCOMM and KOMP initiatives.

## Hypomorphic expression of *Pax9* may account for orofacial abnormalities

The *Pax* family of transcription factors plays a pivotal role in embryonic patterning and disease. The expression of each *Pax* gene is highly regulated in a temporal and spatial manner [30]. During mouse embryogenesis, *Pax9* is expressed mainly in the sclerotome of somites, the pharyngeal pouch endoderm and its derivatives, developing limb buds, and in facial mesenchyme of neural-crest cell origin, including nasal and jaw processes and tooth buds [26,31]. There is strong expression of *Pax9* in the medial edge epithelium during the critical time points of palate fusion [32]. In adult mice, *Pax9* is expressed in oesophagus and tongue [33]. Looking at published models of *Pax9* deficiency, homozygous *Pax9* knockout mice die shortly after birth and exhibit a wide range of developmental defects [26] including the absence of teeth. Death has been attributed to cleft palate, affecting the maxillary and palatine shelves, resulting in an inability to suckle and respiratory issues [26]. Two hypomorphic alleles of *Pax9* have been published previously [25]. The first, which expressed wild-type *Pax9* mRNA at 7% of control levels, presented with hypoplastic upper incisors lacking enamel, missing lower incisors, unilateral or bilateral absence of the third molar in the upper jaw and the second and third molar in the lower jaw, and the lower molars that were present showed severe attrition. In comparison, the hypomorphic allele with 20% of wild-type *Pax9* mRNA expression relative to controls presented with less severely affected dentition including relatively normal upper incisors, hypoplastic lower incisors lacking enamel and unilateral or bilateral absence of the upper and lower third molar. We now report homozygous *Slc25a21*$^{tm1a(KOMP)Wtsi}$ mice which express wild-type *Pax9* mRNA at 34% of control levels and present with an even milder dental phenotype including upper incisors that were commonly maloccluded, which may be due to abnormal snout morphology or the fact that the incisors do not wear against each other. We found fragile, damaged or missing lower incisors which were white or translucent; normally incisors in mice are brownish/yellow due to incorporation of iron-containing pigment in the enamel [34]. The lower incisor root area was severely under-developed. Lower jaw molars showed focal fracturing of the surface dentine and necrosis of the pulp with associated inflammation and bacterial accumulation. The presence of *lacZ* activity within the cavities of the lower molars of homozygous *Slc25a21*$^{tm1a(KOMP)Wtsi}$ mice but not heterozygous mice, confirms that bacterial β-galactosidase is the cause of the staining, not expression of the lacZ reporter gene within the targeted allele. Molars in the upper jaw were less affected. The more severe findings in the lower jaw are consistent with findings in the other *Pax9* hypomorphic alleles [25].

Only limited assessment of the palate has been published for the previous *Pax9* hypomorphic lines and no abnormalities were reported [25]. In this study, more extensive analysis was performed and whilst the phenotype was significantly less severe than that reported in *Pax9* null mice [26], abnormalities were identified, characterised largely by discordance of rugae 3 and an incomplete fusion of the vomer bone to the maxilla.

This gradated allelic series of *Pax9* expression levels, extended by the data reported herein, clearly demonstrates that dosage of this gene affects orofacial development and that lower jaw dentition in the mouse is more susceptible to reduced *Pax9* expression [25]. This is consistent with humans where dentition is not uniformly affected by a reduced Pax9 expression [35,36,37] and the observation that the minimal *Pax9* gene dosage required for the formation of individual teeth varies, the posterior tooth in each tooth family being the most sensitive to a reduction in *Pax9* levels.

## Otitis media and hearing impairment in mice may be due to disrupted *Pax9* expression

A reduction in the size of the tympanic ring has previously been described in Pax9 mutant mice [26], however the effect on hearing has not previously been assessed. The homozygous *Slc25a21*$^{tm1a(-KOMP)Wtsi}$ mice have a normal sized tympanic ring but display a clear hearing impairment with increased thresholds at all frequencies tested. The moderate hearing impairment seen in homozygous *Slc25a21*$^{tm1a(KOMP)Wtsi}$ mice is robust and reproducible across different cohorts of mice, tested at ages from 4 to 26 weeks of age. The degree of impairment in mutant mice is progressive from 4–14 weeks old, with slower progression to 26 weeks of age. The parallel shifts in audiometric profiles across frequencies at the different ages (Fig. 4) are consistent with an underlying conductive hearing loss. Middle ears of the majority of homozygous *Slc25a21*$^{tm1a(KOMP)Wtsi}$ mice were filled with fluid of varying viscosity at all ages examined and sections revealed inflammation of the lining of the middle ear. The presence of eosinophilic exudate and the thickening of the mucosa are evident in the homozygous *Slc25a21*$^{tm1a(KOMP)Wtsi}$ mice, indicating an on-going inflammatory process. Whilst the aetiology of otitis media is complex [38] and was beyond the scope of this study, the correlation between signs of otitis media and elevated ABR thresholds supports our suggestion that the otitis media is a major contributor to the hearing impairment observed in the young adult homozygous *Slc25a21*$^{tm1a(KOMP)Wtsi}$ mice. However, cochlear dysfunction cannot be ruled out especially in the 26 week-old group of both mutants and controls. ABR data from *Slc25a21*$^{tm1b(KOMP)Wtsi}$, *Slc25a21*$^{tm1c(KOMP)Wtsi}$ and *Slc25a21*$^{tm1d(KOMP)Wtsi}$ homozygotes indicate that hearing thresholds are normal.

## Conclusion

In conclusion, ablation of *Slc25a21* expression was not found to phenocopy the human disease 2-oxoadipate acidaemia (OMIM 204750) for which it is a candidate gene. The phenotypes observed in mice homozygous for *Slc25a21*$^{tm1a(KOMP)Wtsi}$ were not due to ablation of *Slc25a21* function, but instead the presence of the selection cassette affected expression of the neighbouring gene, *Pax9*. The resulting mutant line confirmed and extended the existing knowledge of *Pax9* gene dosage effect on orofacial development and represents a novel model of otitis media that may be due to reduced *Pax9* expression.

## Supporting Information

**Figure S1 Ensembl view of 1 Mb genomic interval encompassing *Pax9* and *Slc25a21*.** Ensembl view of the 500 kb of genomic DNA flanking the 5′ and 3′ end of *Slc25a21*. The *Slc25a21*$^{tm1a(KOMP)Wtsi}$ targeting construct (shown in blue) designates exon 4 as the critical exon.

**File S1 Supplementary materials.**

**Table S1 The sequence of primers used for molecular characterisation.** Molecular characterisation of the targeting event was performed using a combination of PCR assays. The 5′ to 3′ primer sequence along with the expected product size (bp) is presented.

**Table S2 Comparison of the outcomes from automatic data evaluation and manual assessment.** Comparison of the outcomes from automatic data evaluation and manual assessment for each parameter included in the dataset is presented. Discrepancies between these two methods of assessment are highlighted, and the rationale behind the manual assessment is provided in each instance there was a discrepancy.

## Acknowledgments

We thank the staff from the Sanger Institute's Research Support Facility and Mouse Informatics Group for their excellent support and Darren Logan for useful discussions. We thank Skyscan for use of the SkyScan1176 micro-CT machine. We thank the Illumina Bespoke Team for the RNA-seq data.

**The Sanger MGP Slc25a21 Project Team was led by:** Hannah Wardle Jones and included Caroline Barnes, Ryan Beveridge, Emma Cambridge, Diane Gleeson, Ozama Ismail, Lee Mulderrig, Hayley J. Protheroe, Laura-Anne Roberson, Grace Salsbury, Mark Sanderson, Daniel Sanger, Agnes Swiatkowska, David Tino Lafont and Valerie E. Vancollie. All members of the Sanger MGP Slc25a21 Project Team were affiliated with the Wellcome Trust Sanger Institute at the time the work was performed.

## Author Contributions

Conceived and designed the experiments: AKG JKW KPS DJA SM. Performed the experiments: SM JB RRS ER CLS WIC NI SP JE DMC Sanger MGP Slc25a21 Project Team. Analyzed the data: AKG JKW SM NAK NW TMK NI SP JE CJL. Wrote the paper: AKG JKW SM KPS DJA CJL.

## References

1. van der Weyden L, White JK, Adams DJ, Logan DW (2011) The mouse genetics toolkit: revealing function and mechanism. Genome Biol 12: 224.
2. White JK, Gerdin AK, Karp NA, Ryder E, Buljan M, et al. (2013) Genome-wide Generation and Systematic Phenotyping of Knockout Mice Reveals New Roles for Many Genes. Cell 154: 452–464.
3. Skarnes WC, Rosen B, West AP, Koutsourakis M, Bushell W, et al. (2011) A conditional knockout resource for the genome-wide study of mouse gene function. Nature 474: 337–342.
4. Mitchell KJ, Pinson KI, Kelly OG, Brennan J, Zupicich J, et al. (2001) Functional analysis of secreted and transmembrane proteins critical to mouse development. Nat Genet 28: 241–249.
5. Meier ID, Bernreuther C, Tilling T, Neidhardt J, Wong YW, et al. (2010) Short DNA sequences inserted for gene targeting can accidentally interfere with off-target gene expression. FASEB J 24: 1714–1724.
6. Pham CT, MacIvor DM, Hug BA, Heusel JW, Ley TJ (1996) Long-range disruption of gene expression by a selectable marker cassette. Proc Natl Acad Sci U S A 93: 13090–13095.
7. Hug BA, Wesselschmidt RL, Fiering S, Bender MA, Epner E, et al. (1996) Analysis of mice containing a targeted deletion of beta-globin locus control region 5′ hypersensitive site 3. Mol Cell Biol 16: 2906–2912.
8. Fiering S, Kim CG, Epner EM, Groudine M (1993) An "in-out" strategy using gene targeting and FLP recombinase for the functional dissection of complex DNA regulatory elements: analysis of the beta-globin locus control region. Proc Natl Acad Sci U S A 90: 8469–8473.
9. Olson EN, Arnold HH, Rigby PW, Wold BJ (1996) Know your neighbors: three phenotypes in null mutants of the myogenic bHLH gene MRF4. Cell 85: 1–4.
10. Fiermonte G, Dolce V, Palmieri L, Ventura M, Runswick MJ, et al. (2001) Identification of the human mitochondrial oxodicarboxylate carrier. Bacterial expression, reconstitution, functional characterization, tissue distribution, and chromosomal location. J Biol Chem 276: 8225–8230.
11. Palmieri F (2004) The mitochondrial transporter family (SLC25): physiological and pathological implications. Pflugers Arch 447: 689–709.
12. Palmieri F (2013) The mitochondrial transporter family SLC25: Identification, properties and physiopathology. Molecular Aspects of Medicine 34: 465–484.
13. Duran M, Beemer FA, Wadman SK, Wendel U, Janssen B (1984) A patient with α-ketoadipic and α-aminoadipic aciduria. Journal of Inherited Metabolic Disease 7: 61–61.
14. Fischer MH, Brown RR (1980) Tryptophan and lysine metabolism in alpha-aminoadipic aciduria. Am J Med Genet 5: 35–41.
15. Przyrembel H, Wendel U, Becker K, Bremer HJ, Bruinvis L, et al. (1976) Glutaric aciduria type II: Report on a previously undescribed metabolic disorder. Clinica Chimica Acta 66: 227–239.
16. Wilson RW, Wilson CM, Gates SC, Higgins JV (1975) Alpha-ketoadipic aciduria: a description of a new metabolic error in lysine-tryptophan degradation. Pediatr Res 9: 522–526.
17. Kilkenny C, Browne WJ, Cuthill IC, Emerson M, Altman DG (2010) Improving Bioscience Research Reporting: The ARRIVE Guidelines for Reporting Animal Research. PLoS Biol 8: e1000412.
18. Collins FS, Rossant J, Wurst W (2007) A mouse for all reasons. Cell 128: 9–13.
19. Pettitt SJ, Liang Q, Rairdan XY, Moran JL, Prosser HM, et al. (2009) Agouti C57BL/6N embryonic stem cells for mouse genetic resources. Nat Methods 6: 493–495.
20. Ryder E, Gleeson D, Sethi D, Vyas S, Miklejewska E, et al. (2013) Molecular Characterization of Mutant Mouse Strains Generated from the EUCOMM/KOMP-CSD ES Cell Resource. Mamm Genome 24: 286–294.
21. Santagati F, Abe K, Schmidt V, Schmitt-John T, Suzuki M, et al. (2003) Identification of Cis-regulatory elements in the mouse Pax9/Nkx2-9 genomic region: implication for evolutionary conserved synteny. Genetics 165: 235–242.
22. Ingham NJ, Pearson S, Steel KP (2011) Using the Auditory Brainstem Response (ABR) to Determine Sensitivity of Hearing in Mutant Mice. Curr Protoc Mouse Biol 1: 279–287.
23. Adams DJ, van der Weyden L (2008) Contemporary approaches for modifying the mouse genome. Physiol Genomics 34: 225–238.
24. Ovchinnikov D (2009) Alcian blue/alizarin red staining of cartilage and bone in mouse. Cold Spring Harb Protoc 2009: pdb prot5170.
25. Kist R (2005) Reduction of Pax9 gene dosage in an allelic series of mouse mutants causes hypodontia and oligodontia. Human Molecular Genetics 14: 3605–3617.
26. Peters H, Neubuser A, Kratochwil K, Balling R (1998) Pax9-deficient mice lack pharyngeal pouch derivatives and teeth and exhibit craniofacial and limb abnormalities. Genes & Development 12: 2735–2747.
27. Chevalier-Mariette C, Henry I, Montfort L, Capgras S, Forlani S, et al. (2003) CpG content affects gene silencing in mice: evidence from novel transgenes. Genome Biology 4: R53.
28. Kleinjan DJ, Coutinho P (2009) Cis-ruption mechanisms: disruption of cis-regulatory control as a cause of human genetic disease. Brief Funct Genomic Proteomic 8: 317–332.
29. Kleinjan DA, Lettice LA (2008) Long-range gene control and genetic disease. Adv Genet 61: 339–388.
30. Lang D, Powell S, Plummer R, Young K, Ruggeri B (2007) PAX genes: Roles in development, pathophysiology, and cancer. Biochemical Pharmacology 73: 1–14.
31. Neubuser A, Koseki H, Balling R (1995) Characterization and developmental expression of Pax9, a paired-box-containing gene related to Pax1. Dev Biol 170: 701–716.

32. Sasaki Y, Okane S, Dixon J, Dixon M, Ferguson M (2007) Temporal and spatial expression of Pax9 and Sonic hedgehog during development of normal mouse palates and cleft palates in TGF-β3 null embryos. Archives of Oral Biology 52: 260–267.
33. Peters H, Schuster G, Neubuser A, Richter T, Hofler H, et al. (1997) Isolation of the Pax9 cDNA from adult human esophagus. Mamm Genome 8: 62–64.
34. Mataki S (1991) Studies on the transport mechanism of iron in rat incisor enamel. In: Ohya K, Ino M, Ogura H, editors. Tokyo: Springer-Verlag. pp. 298–301
35. Das P, Hai M, Elcock C, Leal SM, Brown DT, et al. (2003) Novel missense mutations and a 288-bp exonic insertion in Pax9 in families with autosomal dominant hypodontia. American Journal of Medical Genetics 118A: 35–42.
36. Frazier-Bowers SA, Guo DC, Cavender A, Xue L, Evans B, et al. (2002) A Novel Mutation in Human Pax9 Causes Molar Oligodontia. Journal of Dental Research 81: 129–133.
37. Nieminen P, Arte S, Tanner D, Paulin L, Alaluusua S, et al. (2001) Identification of a nonsense mutation in the Pax9 gene in molar oligodontia. Eur J Hum Genet 9: 743–746.
38. Tyrer HE, Crompton M, Bhutta MF (2013) What have we learned from murine models of otitis media? Curr Allergy Asthma Rep 13: 501–511.

# 13

# Audio-Tactile Integration in Congenitally and Late Deaf Cochlear Implant Users

**Elena Nava[1]*, Davide Bottari[1], Agnes Villwock[1], Ineke Fengler[1], Andreas Büchner[2], Thomas Lenarz[2], Brigitte Röder[1]**

**1** University of Hamburg, Biological Psychology and Neuropsychology, Hamburg, Germany, **2** German Hearing Centre, Medical Clinic Hannover, Hannover, Germany

## Abstract

Several studies conducted in mammals and humans have shown that multisensory processing may be impaired following congenital sensory loss and in particular if no experience is achieved within specific early developmental time windows known as sensitive periods. In this study we investigated whether basic multisensory abilities are impaired in hearing-restored individuals with deafness acquired at different stages of development. To this aim, we tested congenitally and late deaf cochlear implant (CI) recipients, age-matched with two groups of hearing controls, on an audio-tactile redundancy paradigm, in which reaction times to unimodal and crossmodal redundant signals were measured. Our results showed that both congenitally and late deaf CI recipients were able to integrate audio-tactile stimuli, suggesting that congenital and acquired deafness does not prevent the development and recovery of basic multisensory processing. However, we found that congenitally deaf CI recipients had a lower multisensory gain compared to their matched controls, which may be explained by their faster responses to tactile stimuli. We discuss this finding in the context of reorganisation of the sensory systems following sensory loss and the possibility that these changes cannot be "rewired" through auditory reafferentation.

**Editor:** Maurice Ptito, University of Montreal, Canada

**Funding:** The study was supported by the European Research Council (ERC-2009-AdG 249425-CriticalBrainChanges) to BR. The funder had no role in study design, data collection and analysis, decision to publish, or preparation of the manuscript.

**Competing Interests:** The authors have declared that no competing interests exist.

* E-mail: elena.nava@uni-hamburg.de

## Introduction

Neurophysiological studies conducted in mammals have shown that multisensory neurons and the ability to integrate crossmodal information require an extensive time of sensory experience during early development in order to fully mature [1,2]. This predicts that sensory deprivation may impair multisensory processing, as has been extensively documented in visually deprived animals [3,4] and in blind humans too [5,8]. In particular, [5] have suggested that there may be a sensitive period for the development of multisensory integration, after which – if adequate experience has not been made - multisensory processing will remain impaired.

The closing of these sensitive periods is in line with a regressive notion of a developmental process known as "perceptual narrowing" [6]. One of the prevailing theories of brain development is that human infants are born with the ability to sense a broader variety of stimuli than later in life [28]. Special experience available in the environment results in the functional tuning of neural systems and the emergence of expert systems. In parallel, the ability to discriminate and perceive unexplored stimuli within the same domain is lost. For example, [29] showed that within the first year of life, there is an increase in performance for the native language and a decline in non-native perception over the same period of time. The same pattern has been observed for multisensory perception too [7]. Indeed, [7] presented 4-, 6-, 8- and 10-month old infants with two side-by-side faces of a monkey producing two different species-specific calls (i.e., "coo" and "grunt"). The faces were presented either alone or concurrently with the matching call. Four- and 6-month-old infants were found to look longer at the matching audio-visual stimulus compared to the presentation of the face alone. On the contrary, older infants did not show any looking preference, suggesting the inability to match non-native faces and calls.

Both experiments suggest that perceptual narrowing shapes our perceptual expertise and that the time window for building up such expertise seems to close early in development constraining multisensory learning in adulthood.

Furthermore, it has been shown that broadly tuned basic multisensory abilities, such as intersensory synchrony, is present at birth and puts the basis for the development of other basic features of multimodal temporal experience (e.g., temporal synchrony, duration, temporal rate, and rhythm, see [31] for a review) as development progresses [6]. This suggests that atypical sensory experience may result in altered multisensory processes that require functional tuning (multisensory perceptual narrowing) and thus altered multisensory functions [23]. Indeed, a study [9] on individuals with a history of congenital cataracts which were removed between six weeks and three years employed a simple detection task for crossmodal stimuli, including combinations of audio-visual, audio-tactile and visuo-tactile stimuli. Results showed that cataract patients benefitted from redundant stimulation over unimodal stimulation (e.g., audio-visual together vs. visual alone) comparably to normally sighted and visually impaired controls, suggesting that basic multisensory processing, such as simultaneity detection, is not disrupted following congenital visual loss. In contrast, for functions, which seem to rely on multisensory,

experience based tuning (i.e., higher level perceptual abilities), [5] found that congenital cataract patients did not show any multisensory gain. Indeed, these individuals were not able to improve auditory speech comprehension by reading congruent lip movements, although they were able to lipread.

The consequences of auditory deprivation have started receiving larger attention in the past twenty years (for a review see [13]), newly triggered by to the possibility of partially restoring auditory functions through a cochlear implant (CI). A CI is a surgically implanted electronic device that allows deaf individuals to perceive auditory input to some degree. Similarly as cataract patients, these individuals allow us to investigate the developmental consequences of an early or late sensory deprivation on multisensory functions (depending on age at deafness onset and age at CI implantation).

Most of the research interested in multisensory processing in CI recipients has focused on audio-visual interactions for speech comprehension, likely because the main aim of the CI is allowing recipients to communicate with other people. For example, [10] investigated the ability of late deaf CI recipients to fuse audio-visual information in the McGurk task, a classical demonstration of how visual speech can modify audition when presented with an incongruent auditory signal (e.g., presenting a spoken syllable/ba/ matched with synchronous lips pronouncing the syllable/ga/, is often perceived as a third syllable:/da/). The authors found that adult CI recipients were able to fuse the incongruent crossmodal information to the same degree as controls did, in line with results of [11], who tested a group of congenitally deaf CI children on the same task. However, [11] documented audio-visual fusion only in children, who had received a CI before age 2.5 years but not in children who had received their implants later. This result suggests the existence of a sensitive period for the acquisition of audio-visual speech integration. Similarly, [12] investigated audio-visual integration for simple stimuli in early deaf CI children (i.e., who became deaf within their first year of life) who were fitted with their CI either early (between 1 and 4 years of age) or late (between 5 and 10 years of age). They employed a simple detection task, in which reaction times to auditory and visual stimuli were measured when presented alone or concurrently. The authors found that while early implanted CI children gained from cross-modal redundant stimulation similarly to hearing controls, late implanted CI children did not. These results suggest, in line with [11] that typical auditory experience within a sensitive period during the first years of life is necessary in order to develop unimpaired multisensory functions. Thus, it might be assumed that the tuning of crossmodal simultaneity detection depends on experience within the first years of life as well (note that the participants of [5] were mostly deprived for a few months only).

Overall, it appears that most studies in deaf CI recipients have investigated audio-visual integration, possibly because audio-visual integration is crucial in the context of speech perception. However, audio-tactile integration is important in many everyday situations as well, for example in the context of temporal perception, action control and object recognition [27,30]. Furthermore, audio-tactile interactions represent another case to observe possible plastic reorganisation in the deaf brain. As has been previously shown for visually deprived individuals [3,4], it might be that multisensory areas reorganise following auditory deprivation for the processing of visual and tactile stimuli. In other words, auditory input reaching multisensory areas after the closing of sensitive phases in development might not be able to establish contacts with neither the visual nor the tactile inputs, thus explaining the presence of impaired crossmodal interactions. For CI recipients, this would translate into showing impaired cross-modal interactions if CI implantation does not take place before the closing of sensitive phases.

To our knowledge, there is only one study that has addressed audio-tactile integration in CI recipients [15]. In this study, the authors employed an audio-tactile illusion, in which participants commonly perceive additional tactile stimuli when one touch is accompanied multiple successive sounds (see [16]). Results revealed that whereas hearing controls perceived the illusion, CI recipients did not; that is, the latter group did not show any sign of integration capability. Furthermore, the authors suggested that temporary auditory deprivation impairs multisensory integration even if deafness had not occurred at birth, since no difference was found between congenitally and late deaf CI recipients.

The findings of [15] overall suggest that prolonged deafness, irrespective of age at onset, impairs integration of audio-tactile stimuli. This is in contrast with other results showing that CI recipients with congenital onset and early surgery or late deafness are able to fuse incongruent audio-visual information ([11,10] or are even better integrators of auditory and visual speech signals, respectively [17].

In the present study we investigated whether multisensory abilities relying on simultaneity detection develop typically or are impaired following temporary deafness acquired at different stages of development. To this aim, we tested congenitally and late deaf CI recipients, age-matched with a group of hearing controls, on an audio-tactile redundancy paradigm, in which reaction times for unisensory and crossmodal redundant signals were measured. Commonly, healthy adults show faster reaction times for redundant targets compared to unimodal stimuli [18], and this has been generally explained by coactivation models [18]. These models assume that faster reaction times for redundant signals result from an integration of the two sensory channels at some processing stage, and not by one sensory channel "winning the race" over the other (race model, [19]). [18] has proposed a race model inequality test, in which reaction times to bimodal stimulation can be assessed as deriving from integration or mere statistical facilitation (i.e., violation or non-violation of the race model, respectively).

Because the redundant target effect makes use of synchronous stimuli only, we assumed it to be the ideal paradigm to document whether CI recipients are able to integrate audio-tactile information. If experience is necessary to further shape at birth broadly tuned multisensory integration processes, we would expect only - or at least higher - redundancy gains in late deaf CI recipients with respect to congenitally deaf CI recipients.

## Method

### Participants

Ten congenitally (5 female; mean age: 25 years, range: 20–37) and ten late deaf CI recipients (4 female; mean age: 48 years, range: 23–59) participated in this study. The ten age-matched controls for the congenitally deaf CI recipients (MCCD from now on) comprised 7 females and 3 males (mean age: 24 years, range: 20–38), while the ten age-matched controls for the late deaf CI recipients (MCLD from now on) comprised 5 females and 5 males (mean age: 41, range: 20–57).

The CI recipients were recruited through local advertising and some of the late deaf CI recipients were recruited at the Medical School in Hannover (Germany). All CI recipients were profoundly deaf (>90 dB) in both ears before receiving their CI. While the congenitally deaf CI recipients became deaf at birth or immediately after, the late deaf CI recipients became deaf at different ages during development, ranging between 7 and 42 years of age. For

**Table 1.** Description of CI recipients.

| ID | age | gender | etiology | age at deafness onset | years of deafness | age at first implant | years of CI use | type of CI | implanted ear (side) |
|---|---|---|---|---|---|---|---|---|---|
| 1 | 23 | male | unknown | 0 | 2 | 2 | 21 | Cochlear | right |
| 2 | 20 | female | unknown | 0 | 10 | 10 | 10 | Advanced Bionics | bilateral |
| 3 | 37 | female | unknown | 0 | 33 | 33 | 4 | Cochlear | right |
| 4 | 23 | male | unknown | 0 | 11 | 11 | 12 | Cochlear | right |
| 5 | 23 | male | unknown | 0 | 9 | 9 | 14 | Advanced Bionics | right |
| 6 | 23 | female | unknown | 0 | 18 | 18 | 5 | Cochlear | right |
| 7 | 23 | male | unknown | 0 | 14 | 14 | 9 | Cochlear | right |
| 8 | 23 | female | unknown | 0 | 8 | 8 | 15 | Cochlear | bilateral |
| 9 | 23 | female | unknown | 0 | 4 | 4 | 19 | Cochlear | left |
| *mean* | **24** (SD: 4.6) | | | **0** | **12** (SD: 8.7) | **12** (SD: 8.7) | **12** (SD: 5.5) | | |
| 10 | 47 | female | unknown | 23 | 1 | 24 | 23 | Cochlear | bilateral |
| 11 | 58 | male | unknown | 32 | 21 | 53 | 5 | Advanced Bionics | bilateral |
| 12 | 56 | female | unknown | 7 | 43 | 50 | 6 | Advanced Bionics | bilateral |
| 13 | 59 | female | tumor | 42 | 12 | 54 | 5 | Cochlear | bilateral |
| 14 | 56 | female | unknown | 17 | 29 | 46 | 10 | Clarion | bilateral |
| 15 | 51 | male | unknown | 30 | 16 | 46 | 5 | Med El | bilateral |
| 16 | 38 | female | Scarlet fever | 20 | 13 | 33 | 5 | Advanced Bionics | right |
| 17 | 42 | male | German measles | 40 | 1 | 41 | 1 | Cochlear | bilateral |
| 18 | 23 | female | unknown | 18 | 1 | 19 | 4 | Cochlear | right |
| 19 | 45 | male | unknown | 31 | 1 | 32 | 13 | Advanced Bionics | bilateral |
| *mean* | **48** (SD: 10.6) | | | **26** (SD: 10.4) | **14** (SD: 13.4) | **40** (SD: 11.6) | **8** (SD: 6) | | |

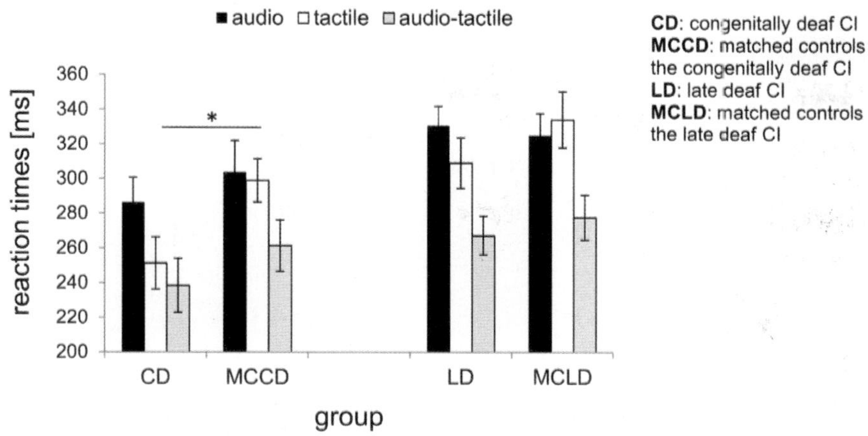


**Figure 1. RT for unimodal auditory, unimodal tactile and bimodal.** Mean reaction times (in ms, with error bars indicating the standard error) for each condition (unimodal auditory, unimodal tactile and audio-tactile), separately for the group of congenitally deaf CI recipients and their age-matched controls (left panel), and late deaf CI recipients and their age-matched controls (right panel). Note that despite all participants being faster for bimodal compared to unimodal stimuli, congenitally deaf CI recipients were faster for unimodal tactile stimuli compared their matched controls.

the congenitally deaf CI recipients, implantation occurred at different ages during development, ranging between 2 and 33 years of age. For the late deaf CI recipients, age at implantation occurred in adulthood only, ranging between 19 and 54 years of age. The CI recipients had had on average 10 years of experience with their implant prior to testing (range: 1–23 years). Although the cause of deafness was unknown for most CI participants, we only recruited participants for which possibilities of cognitive impairment could be excluded (e.g., as a consequence of meningitis).

Further details about the participants, including aetiology of deafness, type of device implanted, ear implanted, age at first CI implant (i.e., in case of bilateral sequential CI, we refer to the age at which the first CI was implanted; no CI recipients was implanted simultaneously), years of experience with the CI and years of CI use are reported in Table 1.

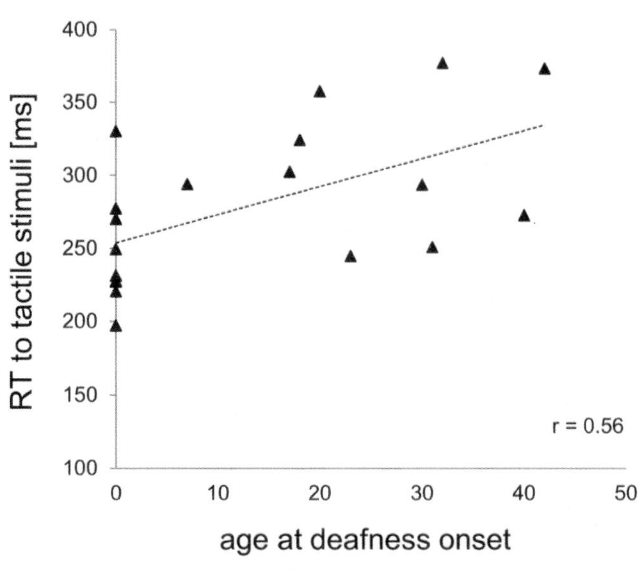


**Figure 2. Correlation between unisensory tactile stimuli and age at deafness onset.** Reaction times (in ms) to unisensory tactile stimuli as a function of age at deafness onset (in years).

All participants had normal or corrected-to-normal vision, reported normal sensitivity to their fingertips and had no neurological impairment.

All participants provided written informed consent before being tested and received a reimbursement for their time and expenses associated with the testing, which took place in a room of the laboratory at the University of Hamburg or in one of the rooms of the Medical School of Hannover.

The study was approved by the ethical commission of the German Society of Psychology and the Medical School of Hannover. The study was conducted according to the principles expressed in the Declaration of Helsinki.

## Stimuli and Procedure

The auditory stimulus consisted of a 50 ms burst of white noise at 80 dB and was presented from two loudspeakers (Bose, Multimedia Speaker System) positioned side-by-side 60 cm in front of the participant.

Tactile stimuli were 50 ms vibrations of plastic cubes at the left index finger controlled by cell phone motors with a direct current, with a tuning frequency of 200 Hz. To ensure spatial proximity of the stimuli, participants were asked to keep their left hand close to the loudspeakers throughout the experiment. To mask the faint noise generated by the tactile stimulators, all participants wore closed headphones throughout the experiment. For CI participants, the sound pressure of the auditory stimulus was adjusted to a comfortable level.

During the experiment, participants were presented with 180 unimodal auditory, 180 unimodal tactile and 180 audio-tactile stimuli divided in two blocks and presented in random order at 1000 or 2000 ms intervals. In addition, 36 catch trials (i.e., no stimulus presented) were included to prevent participants from guessing the onset of the upcoming stimulus. The task for all participants simply consisted of pressing the space bar of the computer keyboard each time a stimulus was perceived. Trials with a stimulus, in which no response was provided, were considered as "miss". Trials without a stimulus but with a response were counted as "false alarm". Participants were allowed to take breaks between the two blocks. The experiment took approximately 20 minutes to complete and before the start participants were familiarized with the experiment by training them on a set of 36 trials.

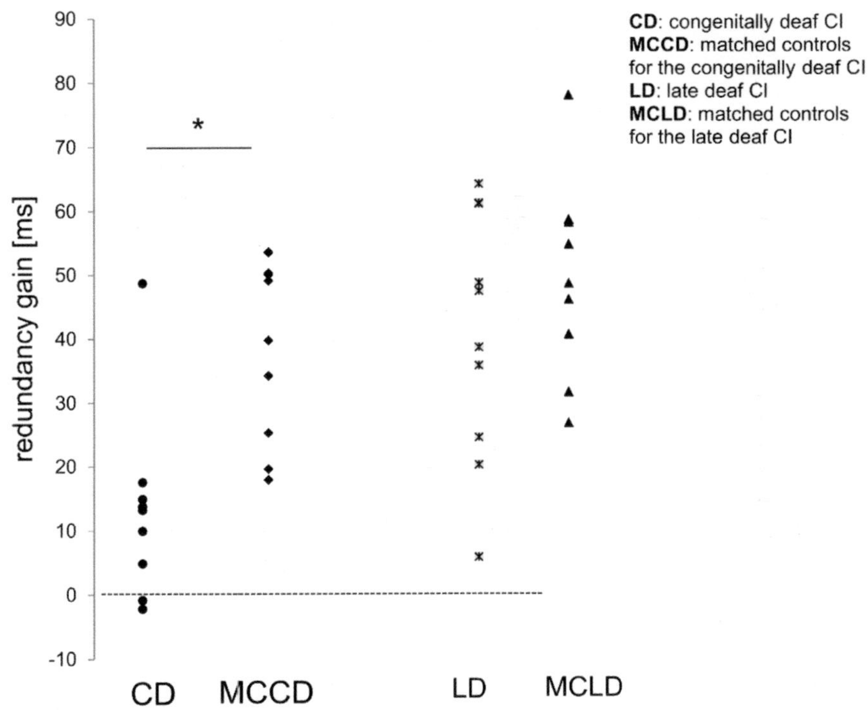


**Figure 3. Redundancy gains (in ms).** Redundancy gains for each participant (in ms), computed as the difference between the mean reaction times of bimodal stimuli and the fastest unimodal stimuli. Note that congenitally but not late deaf CI recipients showed lower redundancy gains compared to their matched controls.

## Data Analysis

We measured reaction times for all conditions (unimodal auditory, unimodal tactile and audio-tactile) for each participant. For all controls, the number of "misses" and "false alarms" was negligible (maximum of 2 for each condition). For CI participants, "misses" were on average below 3% and were not further analysed. "False alarms" were negligible (maximum 3 for each condition).

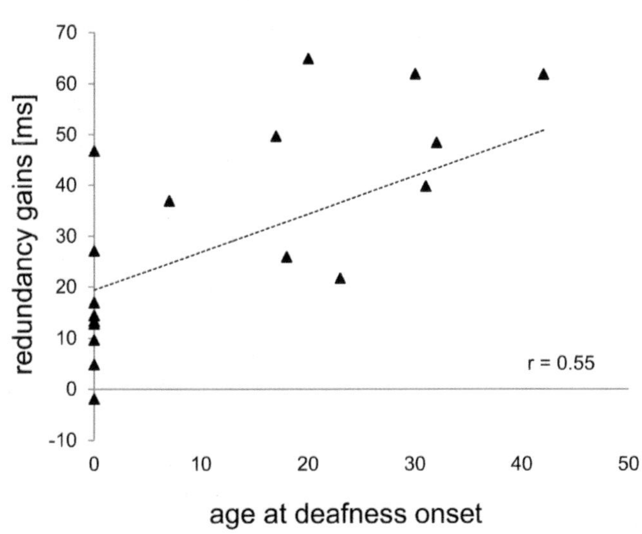


**Figure 4. Correlation between redundancy gain and age at deafness onset.** Redundancy gains (in ms) plotted as a function of age at deafness onset (in years).

For each group, we calculated a repeated-measures ANOVA with Condition (single auditory, single tactile and bimodal stimuli) as the within-participants factor and reaction times as dependent variable. To assess the redundant target effect and reaction time differences in the different conditions we used Helmert contrasts [26].

To compare the two groups (congenitally and late deaf CI users) we ran two separate repeated-measures ANOVAS for congenitally deaf CI recipients and their matched controls, and for late deaf CI recipients and their matched controls, with Condition as the within-participants factor, Group as the between-participants factor and reaction times as the dependent variable. Furthermore, we ran independent samples t-tests to compare performance of congenitally and late deaf CI recipients to their matched controls for each condition. To assess whether the redundancy gain differed between groups, we calculated the difference between the mean reaction times in the bimodal condition and the fastest reaction time of the two unimodal stimuli with independent-samples t-test. Finally, we correlated the redundancy gain with age at deafness onset, years of deafness, age at CI implantation and years of CI use. While for the factor "age at deafness onset" the performance of all CI recipients was included, for the other factors we conducted separate correlations for each group of CI recipients.

To assess whether faster responses in bimodal trials can be explained by integration of redundant input, we used the RMITest (http://psy.otago.ac.nz/miller/Software.htm#RMITest), which tests for violations of the race model inequality described by [15] by implementing the algorithm described in [20]. More precisely, it estimates the cumulative probability distributions of the reaction times for each condition and tests whether the bimodal condition is significantly faster than the race model predicts.

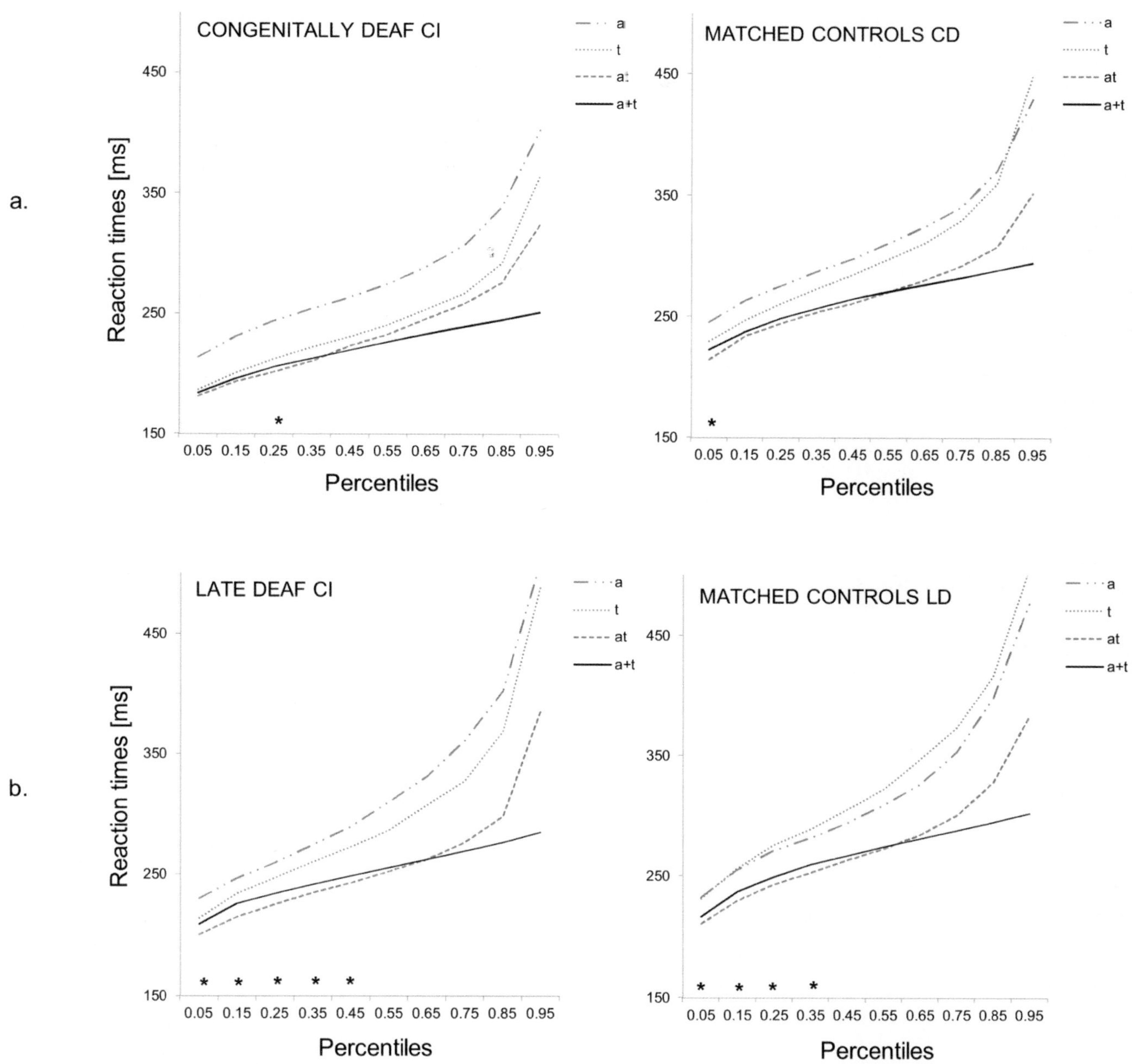


**Figure 5. Multisensory facilitation indexed by violation of the race model.** Cumulative distribution functions for response time to unisensory auditory and tactile stimuli and crossmodal stimuli for a. congenital deaf CI recipients and their age-matched controls and b. late deaf CI recipients and their age-matched controls. The filled black line indicates the summed proportions to unimodal stimuli (*a+t*, race model), *at* the violation of the race model, and *a* and *t* the responses to single auditory and tactile stimuli, respectively.

In 1962, [19] proposed the well-known race model to explain why redundant targets speed up the response of most healthy participants with respect to responses to unimodal stimuli. According to this model, each signal activates a separate process that will lead one of the two to "win the race", so that faster reaction times for bimodal stimulation end up being the expression of one of the two unimodal signals, hence to what it's called a "statistical facilitation".

However, [18] proposed the race model inequality (RMI), by which a violation of the inequality between redundant stimuli and the sum of unimodal stimuli should be interpreted as integration of the sensory information by neural summation (also called "co-activation mechanism").

Therefore, for each group we tested whether the race model was violated at 10 different points (percentiles) on the cumulative distribution of their reaction times. Additionally, we compared distributions of the fastest unisensory signal and redundant targets between groups for each percentile.

Finally, to compare the amount of RMI violations between groups, we calculated the amount of violation area for each participant (computed as the difference between the minima obtained from the two unisensory signals using the method of antithetic variates and the mean reaction time in the redundant signals; see [21]), and compared the groups by means of independent samples t-tests. A negative or zero value of the violation area indicates that the amount of observed facilitation (in terms of reaction times) is likely explained by the race model; on the contrary, positive values cannot be explained by the race model. The amount of violation was also correlated to the aforementioned factors (age at deafness onset, age at implant, years of deafness and years of CI use).

## Results

One congenitally deaf CI recipient had to be discarded from the analyses because her reaction times were three standard deviations above mean. The number of MCCD was not modified because the matching participant had an age that was compatible with the mean age of the group.

Figure 1 shows mean reaction times for each group in the unimodal and bimodal conditions. For each group, mean reaction times significantly differed between conditions (*congenitally deaf CI recipients*: $F(1.4, 10.8) = 26.5$, $p<0.001$, effect size $\eta_p^2 = 0.8$; *late deaf CI recipients*: $F(1.6, 14.4) = 33.6$, $p<0.001$, effect size $\eta_p^2 = 0.8$; *MCCD*: $F(1.4, 12.2) = 25.7$, $p<0.001$, effect size $\eta_p^2 = 0.7$; *MCLD*: $F(1.3, 11.8) = 22.0$, $p<0.001$, effect size $\eta_p^2 = 0.7$), and for each group reaction times to bimodal stimuli were faster compared to unimodal stimuli (*congenitally deaf CI recipients*: $F(1, 8) = 32.9$, $p< 0.001$, effect size $\eta_p^2 = 0.8$; *late deaf CI recipients*: $F(1, 9) = 27.4$, $p = 0.001$, effect size $\eta_p^2 = 0.7$; *MCCD*: $F(1, 9) = 10.4$, $p = 0.01$, effect size $\eta_p^2 = 0.5$; *MCLD*: $F(1, 9) = 6.2$, $p = 0.03$, effect size $\eta_p^2 = 0.4$).

In particular, for the MCCD the bimodal condition was faster compared to the tactile ($t(9) = 8.9$, $p<0.001$, $d = 5.6$) and the auditory condition ($t(9) = 6.7$, $p<0.001$, $d = 4.2$) while the two unimodal conditions did not differ ($p = 0.7$). Similarly, for the MCLD the bimodal condition was faster compared to the tactile ($t(9) = 6.0$, $p<0.001$, effect size $d = 3.8$) and the auditory condition ($t(9) = 8.8$, $p<0.001$, effect size $d = 5.6$) while the two unimodal conditions did not differ ($p = 0.4$).

On the contrary, for the congenitally deaf CI recipients, not only was the bimodal condition faster compared to the tactile ($t(8) = 2.6$, $p = 0.03$, effect size $d = 1.7$) and auditory condition ($t(8) = 7.7$, $p<0.001$, effect size $d = 5.1$), but also the two unimodal conditions differed ($t(8) = 4.0$, $p = 0.004$, effect size $d = 2.7$), in that this group responded faster to tactile than to auditory stimuli (251 ms (SE = 15) vs. 286 ms (SE = 14), respectively). Similarly, late deaf CI recipients showed faster reaction times for bimodal compared to the tactile ($t(9) = 7.0$, $p<0.001$, effect size $d = 4.4$) and auditory condition ($t(9) = 8.1$, $p<0.001$, effect size $d = 5.1$) and faster reaction times for tactile than auditory stimuli (309 ms (SE = 14) vs. 331 ms (SE = 11), respectively; $t(9) = 2.3$, $p = 0.05$, effect size $d = 1.5$).

In order to compare the two groups (congenitally and late deaf CI recipients), we ran two separate ANOVAS for each group matched with its control group (congenitally deaf CI vs. MCCD and late deaf CI vs. MCLD). The comparison between congenitally deaf CI recipients and MCCD revealed a main effect of condition ($F(1.4, 23.1) = 45.7$, $p<0.001$, effect size $\eta_p^2 = 0.7$) and a significant interaction between condition and group ($F(1.4, 23.1) = 6.4$, $p = 0.01$, effect size $\eta_p^2 = 0.3$) but no significant group effect ($p = 0.2$). Independent-samples t-tests showed that congenitally deaf CI were faster for unimodal tactile stimuli only compared to their matched controls ($t(17) = 2.3$, $p = 0.03$, effect size $d = 1.1$).

On the contrary, the comparison between late deaf CI recipients and their matched controls revealed a significant main effect of Condition ($F(1.5, 27.8) = 50.6$, $p<0.001$, effect size $\eta_p^2 = 0.3$) but only a marginally significant interaction between Condition and Group ($F(1.5, 27.8) = 3.3$, $p = 0.06$, effect size $\eta_p^2 = 0.2$). Moreover, independent samples t-tests showed no difference for any condition between groups.

To document whether faster responses to tactile stimuli are influenced by age at deafness onset, years of deafness, age at implantation or years of CI use, we correlated these factors with the mean response to unimodal tactile stimuli. To avoid confounds (i.e., our congenital and late deaf CI recipients have different characteristics, such as age, and age at implantation is statistically different between groups) only for age at deafness onset the correlation was made between both groups and their reaction times. For the other factors, analyses were kept separate. Note, that age at implantation and years of deafness have the same numerical value for congenitally deaf CI, so that disambiguating the role of these two factors is rather difficult.

Figure 2 shows that only age at deafness onset ($r = 0.56$, $n = 19$, $p = 0.01$) was a significant factor, while all others did not explain our results. However, it is worth noting that years of CI use showed a trend towards significance for the late deaf CI recipients ($r = -0.57$, $n = 10$, $p = 0.09$), in that reaction times to tactile stimuli tend to get faster the longer the CI recipients has worn his implant.

Figure 3 shows redundancy gains for each participant, separately for group. Between groups analyses (congenitally deaf CI vs. MCCD and late deaf CI vs. MCLD) showed redundancy gains differences, specifically between congenitally deaf CI recipients and their matched controls ($t(17) = 3.8$, $p = 0.001$, effect size $d = 1.8$), caused by lower redundancy gains in congenitally deaf CI recipients compared to their matched controls (mean: 13 ms (SE = 4.5), vs. 38 ms (SE = 4.1), respectively). On the contrary, we found no difference between late deaf CI recipients and their matched controls. Furthermore, the correlations (see Fig. 4) proved significant for age at deafness onset only ($r = 0.55$, $n = 19$, $p = 0.02$).

To document whether there is a trade-off between redundancy gain and reaction times to unimodal tactile stimuli (i.e., shorter reaction times to tactile stimuli parallel lower multisensory gains), we correlated these two factors separately for congenitally and late deaf CI recipients. We found a significant correlation for the congenitally ($r = 0.7$, $n = 9$, $p = 0.05$) but not for the late deaf CI recipients ($r = 0.6$, $n = 10$, $p = 0.07$).

The race model inequality test revealed a significant violation of the race model assumption in all three groups (see Fig. 5). It is worth noting that the violation of the race model occurred in the third percentile for the MCCD, in the first 4 percentiles for the MCLD, in the first percentile for the congenitally deaf CI recipients and in the first five percentiles for the late deaf CI recipients. However, we found no difference in the amount of violation between groups. Moreover, the correlations between amount of violation and the factors of interest did not prove significant.

## Discussion

The present study examined whether congenitally and late deaf CI recipients are able to integrate simple audio-tactile stimuli as measured in a redundant target paradigm.

We found reliable redundancy gains for audio-tactile stimuli compared to unimodal stimuli and a violation of the race model for both congenitally and late deaf CI recipients. A violation of the race model is commonly accepted evidence for a true coactivation and thus crossmodal integration. The finding that not only late but congenitally deaf CI recipients were able to integrate audio-tactile stimuli as well suggests that, congenital sensory deprivation does not prevent the development of multisensory integration of simple synchronous stimuli, which is in line with [9], who tested congenital cataract individuals on the same paradigm as used in the present study. The similar results obtained in the two studies allow us speculating on the fact that crossmodal integration might build on broadly tuned innate abilities (i.e., detection of simultaneously presented multimodal information). However, it is worth discussing the differences between our results and [9]. Indeed, cataract patients [9] showed more similar multisensory gains with respect to their matched controls compared to our CI recipients (particularly the congenitally CI recipients), suggesting a more fully recovery in the cataract patients compared to our CI recipients. This may be due to the earlier sensory restoration performed in the cataract patients compared to our congenitally CI recipients, who received their CI on average in adulthood. Indeed, the earliest surgery in the deaf CI recipients was performed at a higher age (>2 years) than the latest cataract surgery in most of the patients studied in [9]. If the critical period for multisensory processes exists within the first about 2.5 years [11], it is not surprising that we did not find a statistically significant correlation between age at implant or years of CI experience and reaction times or redundancy gains.

It is worth considering why our results appear in conflict with [15], who used simple audio-tactile stimuli too and found no integration abilities for both congenitally and late deaf CI recipients, thus concluding that years of deafness, and not age at deafness onset, influence multisensory processing capabilities. First, it should be noted that the authors adopted a paradigm that tests the ability to fuse crossmodal incongruent information, while our task made use of congruent, synchronous stimuli. The lack of fusion of incongruent audio-tactile information could be explained by the enhanced tactile abilities of CI recipients as reported earlier for deaf individuals [14] and confirmed in the present study by showing shorter reaction times to tactile stimuli in the congenitally deaf CI recipients. Based on an optimal integration rule [22], higher tactile performance could result in higher reliance upon tactile information and thus less interference when incongruent auditory input is presented (see [16] for an analogous reasoning for lower audio-tactile fusion in the blind). Recently, it has been speculated as well that enhanced skills in the intact modality after sensory deprivation might originate from a reorganisation at the level of multisensory brain structures as a consequence of sensory deprivation and that these neural changes in turn would interfere with functional recovery [23,24]. Our data do not allow disambiguating between these two alternatives. Both accounts are able to explain the positive correlation between redundancy gain and reaction times to unimodal tactile stimuli in congenitally deaf CI recipients only, namely participants who were faster at detecting unimodal tactile stimuli also had a lower multisensory gain. This leads to the discussion as to why congenitally deaf CI recipients showed lower redundancy gains compared to their matched controls. While it could be argued that this difference stems from less multisensory integrating abilities, it might similarly emerge as a consequence of congenitally deaf CI recipients responding faster to unimodal tactile stimuli compared to their matched controls (the redundancy gain was computed as a difference between bimodal stimuli and the faster of the two unisensory stimuli). The advantage in reaction times for unimodal tactile stimuli in the congenitally deaf CI recipients, as discussed above could be explained in terms of a reorganisation of the sensory systems, by which the remaining senses improve to compensate the sensory loss [25,14]. Our results showed that faster responses to tactile stimuli are only significantly influenced by one factor, namely age at deafness onset, which suggests that this cross-modal reorganisation may decrease the later deafness is acquired in development. Furthermore, because for our congenitally deaf CI recipients other factors such as age at implantation and years of CI use were not found significant, it could be speculated that once cross-modal changes have taken place, they cannot be "re-wired" through auditory reafferentation, at least not after the age of 2 years. In support to this claim, several studies [32,33,34] have provided evidence that particularly deafened individuals with massive crossmodal take-over of auditory regions by visual input are less likely to benefit from implantation, thus questioning, for some specific cases, the potential of restoring hearing. Recently, [35] examined the relationship between crossmodal plasticity and speech perception in prelingually and postlingually deafened CI recipients by correlating the amplitude of visual evoked potential (VEP) over the right temporal lobe with the word perception scores of each CI recipient. The authors found that the amplitude of the VEP increased while the word perception scores decreased. Most importantly, this was observed in prelingually but not postlingually CI recipients, suggesting that, in accord with our findings, the influence of crossmodal plasticity on speech perception abilities depends upon deafness onset.

In conclusion, the present study provides evidence that basic audio-tactile stimuli can be integrated following congenital and late deafness after sensory restoration. We provide evidence for compensatory plasticity early in life, leading to an improvement in the tactile modality accompanied by lower multisensory gains following auditory loss.

## Acknowledgments

We thank all the CI recipients for participating in the study, and the Medical School in Hannover, in particular Dr. Angelika Illg, for supporting the study and allowing recruiting a part of the CI participants. Additionally, we thank Sarah Kolb and Gerhild Klein for helping recruiting and testing the participants.

## Author Contributions

Conceived and designed the experiments: EN BR. Performed the experiments: EN AV IF. Analyzed the data: EN DB. Contributed reagents/materials/analysis tools: AB TL. Wrote the paper: EN BR.

## References

1. Wallace MT, Stein BE (2007) Early experience determines how the senses will interact. J Neurophysiol 97: 921–926.
2. Yu L, Rowland BA, Stein BE (2010) Initiating the development of multisensory integration by manipulating sensory experience. J Neurosci 30: 4904–4913.
3. Carriere BN, Royal DW, Perrault TJ, Morrison SP, William Vaughan J, et al. (2007) Visual deprivation alters the development of cortical multisensory integration. J Neurophysiol 98: 2858–2867.
4. Wallace MT, Perrault TJ, David Hairston P, Stein BE (2004) Visual experience is necessary for the development of multisensory integration. J Neurosci 24: 9580–9584.
5. Putzar L, Goerendt I, Lange K, Rösler F, Röder B (2007) Early visual deprivation impairs multisensory interactions in humans. Nat Neurosci 10: 1243–1245.
6. Lewkowicz DJ, Ghazanfar AA (2009) The emergency of multisensory systems through perceptual narrowing. Trends Cogn Sci 13: 470–478.
7. Lewkowicz DJ, Ghazanfar AA (2006) The decline of cross-species intersensory perception in human infants. P Natl Acad Sci U S A 103: 6771–6774.
8. Putzar L, Hötting K, Röder B (2010) Early visual deprivation affects the development of face recognition and of audio-visual speech perception. Restor Neurol Neurosci 28: 251–257.

9. Putzar L, Gondan M, Röder B (2012) Basic multisensory functions can be acquired after congenital visual pattern deprivation in humans. Dev Neuropsychol 37: 697–711.
10. Tremblay C, Champoux F, Lepore F, Théoret H (2010) Audiovisual fusion and cochlear implant proficiency. Restor Neurol Neurosci 28: 283–291.
11. Schorr E, Fox NA, van Wassenhove V, Knudsen E (2005) Auditory-visual fusion in speech perception in children with cochlear implants. P Natl Acad Sci U S A 102: 18748–18750.
12. Gilley PM, Sharma A, Mitchell TV, Dorman MF (2010) The influence of a sensitive period for auditory-visual integration in children with cochlear implants. Restor Neurol Neurosci 28: 207–218.
13. Pavani F, Röder B (2012) Crossmodal plasticity as a consequence of sensory loss: insights from blindness and deafness. In: Stein B, editor. The New Handbook of Multisensory Processes. Cambridge, MIT Press. 737–760.
14. Levänen S, Hamdorf D (2001) Feeling vibrations: enhanced tactile sensitivity in congenitally deaf humans. Neurosci Lett 301: 75–77.
15. Landry SP, Guillemot JP, Champoux F (2013) Temporary deafness can impair multisensory integration. A study of cochlear implant users. Psychol Sci 24: 1260–1268.
16. Hötting K, Röder B (2004) Hearing cheats touch, but less in congenitally blind than in sighted individuals. Psychol Sci 15: 60–64.
17. Rouger J, Lagleyre S, Fraysse B, Deguine O, Barone P (2007) Evidence that cochlear-implanted deaf patients are better multisensory integrators. P Natl Acad Sci U S A 105: 7295–7300.
18. Miller J (1982) Divided attention: evidence for coactivation with redundant targets. Cognitive Psychol 14: 247–279.
19. Raab DH (1962) Statistical facilitation of simple reaction times. T New York Acad Sci 24: 574–590.
20. Ulrich R, Miller J, Schröter H (2007) Testing the race model inequality: an algorithm and computer programs. Behav Res Methods 39: 291–302.
21. Colonius H, Diederich A (2006) The race model inequality: a geometric measure of the amount of violation. Psychol Rev 113: 148–154.
22. Ernst MO, Banks MS (2002) Humans integrate visual and haptic information in a statistically optimal fashion. Nature: 415, 429–433.
23. Lewkowicz D, Röder B (2011) Development of multisensory processes and the role of early experience. In: Stein B, editor. The New Handbook of Multisensory Processes. MIT Press, Cambridge/MA, USA.
24. Lomber SG, Meredith MA, Kral A (2012) Cross-modal plasticity in specific auditory cortices underlies visual compensations in the deaf. Nat Neurosci 13: 1421–1427.
25. Levänen S, Jousmäki V, Hari R (1998) Vibration-induced auditory-cortex activation in a congenitally deaf adult. Curr Biol 8: 869–872.
26. Gondan M, Lange K, Röder B (2004) The redundant target effect is affected by modality switch costs. Psychon B Rev 11: 307–313.
27. Occelli V, Spence C, Zampini M (2011) Audiotactile interactions in temporal perception. Psychon B Rev 18: 429–454.
28. Slater A, Kirby R (1998) Innate and learned perceptual abilities in the newborn infant. Exp Brain Res 123: 90–94.
29. Kuhl PK, Stevens E, Hayashi A, Deguchi T, Kiritani S, et al. (2006) Infants show a facilitation effect for native language phonetic perception between 6 and 12 months. Dev Sci 9: F13-F21.
30. Amedi A, Von Kriegstein K, Van Atteveldt NM, Beauchamp MS, Naumer MJ (2005) Functional imaging of human crossmodal identification and object recognition. Exp Brain Res, 166: 559–571.
31. Lewkowicz DJ (2000) The development of intersensory temporal perception: an epigenetic systems/limitations view. Psychol Bull, 126: 281.
32. Sandmann P, Dillier N, Eichele T, Meyer M, Kegel A, et al. (2011) Visual activation of auditory cortex reflects maladaptive plasticity in cochlear implant users. Brain 135: 555–568.
33. Lee DS, Lee JS, Oh SH, Kim SK, Kim JW, et al. (2001) Cross-modal plasticity and cochlear implants. Nature 409: 149–150.
34. Lee HJ, Giraud AL, Kang E, Oh SH, Kang H, et al. (2007) Cortical activity at rest predicts cochlear implantation outcome. Cereb Cortex 17: 909–917.
35. Buckley KA, Tobey EA (2011) Cross-modal plasticity and speech perception in pre- and postlingually deaf cochlear implant users. Ear Hearing 32: 2–15.

# Altered Regional and Circuit Resting-State Activity Associated with Unilateral Hearing Loss

**Xingchao Wang[1]**, **Yang Fan[2]**, **Fu Zhao[3]**, **Zhenmin Wang[1]**, **Jianqiao Ge[2]**, **Kai Zhang[1]**, **Zhixian Gao[1]**, **Jia-Hong Gao[2,4]**, **Yihong Yang[5]**, **Jin Fan[6,7,8,9]**, **Qihong Zou[2*]**, **Pinan Liu[1,3*]**

**1** Department of Neurosurgery, Beijing Tiantan Hospital, Capital Medical University, Beijing, China, **2** MRI Research Center and Beijing City Key Lab for Medical Physics and Engineering, Peking University, Beijing, China, **3** Department of Neural reconstruction, Beijing Neurosurgery Institute, Capital Medical University, Beijing, China, **4** McGovern Institute for Brain Research, Peking University, Beijing, China, **5** Neuroimaging Research Branch, National Institute on Drug Abuse, National Institutes of Health, Baltimore, Maryland, United States of America, **6** Department of Psychology, Queens College, The City University of New York, Flushing, New York, United States of America, **7** Department of Psychiatry, Mount Sinai School of Medicine, New York, New York, United States of America, **8** Friedman Brain Institute, Mount Sinai School of Medicine, New York, New York, United States of America, **9** Fishberg Department of Neuroscience, Mount Sinai School of Medicine, New York, New York, United States of America

## Abstract

The deprivation of sensory input after hearing damage results in functional reorganization of the brain including cross-modal plasticity in the sensory cortex and changes in cognitive processing. However, it remains unclear whether partial deprivation from unilateral auditory loss (UHL) would similarly affect the neural circuitry of cognitive processes in addition to the functional organization of sensory cortex. Here, we used resting-state functional magnetic resonance imaging to investigate intrinsic activity in 34 participants with UHL from acoustic neuroma in comparison with 22 matched normal controls. In sensory regions, we found decreased regional homogeneity (ReHo) in the bilateral calcarine cortices in UHL. However, there was an increase of ReHo in the right anterior insular cortex (rAI), the key node of cognitive control network (CCN) and multimodal sensory integration, as well as in the left parahippocampal cortex (lPHC), a key node in the default mode network (DMN). Moreover, seed-based resting-state functional connectivity analysis showed an enhanced relationship between rAI and several key regions of the DMN. Meanwhile, lPHC showed more negative relationship with components in the CCN and greater positive relationship in the DMN. Such reorganizations of functional connectivity within the DMN and between the DMN and CCN were confirmed by a graph theory analysis. These results suggest that unilateral sensory input damage not only alters the activity of the sensory areas but also reshapes the regional and circuit functional organization of the cognitive control network.

**Editor:** Yu-Feng Zang, Hangzhou Normal University, China

**Funding:** This work was supported by National Science and Technology Support Program of the 12th Five-Year of China (grant number: 2012BAI12B03), Natural Science Foundation of Beijing (grant number: 7112049), China's National Strategic Basic Research Program (973) (grant number: 2012CB720700), and Natural Science Foundation of China (grant numbers: 81201142 and 31200761). The funders had no role in study design, data collection and analysis, decision to publish, or preparation of the manuscript.

**Competing Interests:** The authors have declared that no competing interests exist.

* E-mail: pinanliu@ccmu.edu.cn (PL); zouqihong@pku.edu.cn (QZ)

These authors contributed equally to this work.

## Introduction

The functional organization of brain continues to change after prenatal development and can undergo remodeling throughout a person's life to adapt to changing sensory experiences [1,2]. Previous research has demonstrated that non-auditory sensory stimulation could activate the regions responsible for auditory processing in deaf people [3–5], which implies the existence of cross-modal plasticity in the sensory cortex of those who are completely deaf [6]. In addition, studies on the aging and cochlear implant populations [7–10] have demonstrated that hearing loss can alter different aspects of human cognitive functions in both pre- and post-lingual deafness [11–13], such as enhanced peripheral visual attention across time or space [14–17], behavioral inhibition defects [9,18], distributed short-term memory [19] and compromised executive function [20–22]. Thus, there are at least two important forms of remodeling of the brain during hearing damage: the cross-modal plasticity implies that functional reorganization in sensory regions compensate for the compromised hearing input by optimizing multi-sensory perception [6] and changes in cognitive function suggest that more cognitive resources must be engaged during auditory processing to compensate for hearing impairment [11,19].

Unlike those with bilateral deafness, unilateral hearing loss (UHL) individuals preserve much of the ability to capture auditory information, and the changes in auditory processing are more complicated [23–26]. Moreover, the brain is organized into intrinsic networks, which work cooperatively to facilitate an individual's responses to stimuli [27], and these networks instantiate the maintenance of information for interpreting, responding to and even predicting environmental demands [28]. When one of the sensory perceptions is compromised, such as the asymmetrical auditory processing in UHL, it may affect not only the integral auditory perception [29] but also the auditory processing for higher-order representations [30–32]. It is therefore reasonable to predicate that the internal connectivity within sensory and high-order control networks as well as integration between these networks might be reorganized in UHL patients functionally. Previous research has addressed the issue of how UHL affects the plasticity in central auditory pathway, however, most of these studies are confined to the auditory cortex by examining task-related brain activation [33–36]. No study to date has investigated the functional changes associated with asymmetrical hearing damage and considered the reorganizations related to both sensation and cognitive functions. It remains unclear whether the deprivation of unilateral auditory input would affect the neural circuitry of the cognitive control network in addition to sensory cortex.

Resting-state fMRI is a promising noninvasive technique for mapping whole brain functional activity. Previous studies have demonstrated that regional homogeneity (ReHo) [37], a robust index with high test-retest reliability [38] can be used to map the synchronization of time courses between neighboring regions, as well as resting state functional connectivity (RSFC) [39] with excellent test-retest reliability [40] for measuring the temporal relationship among spatially distant regions, were quite informative for investigating the neural basis of individual differences in sensory deprivation [41–43] [32,44,45]. Moreover, resting-state fMRI is especially useful in clinical populations which have difficulty in task performances [27] such as patients with UHL, and it could provide functional information for simultaneously investigating the mechanisms of auditory and non-auditory higher order functional changes underlying UHL.

We hypothesized that the sensory cortex as well as regions subserving the higher order control network would be the primary regions affected by reduced hearing in UHL. We collected resting-state fMRI data from participants with UHL that resulted from acoustic neuroma and compared them to healthy controls to examine the plastic changes in regional homogeneity and functional connectivity in UHL. We predict that UHL patients would show abnormal resting activity not only in primary sensory regions, but also in the networks involving in cognitive control.

## Materials and Methods

### Participants

All participants were right-handed and reported no previous or current psychiatric disorders (see Table 1 for all participants' demographic and clinical characteristics). Informed consent was obtained from all subjects prior to their participation, and all participants provided their written informed consent to participate in this study. The study was approved by the Institutional Review Board of Beijing Tiantan Hospital, Capital Medical University.

Thirty-six untreated UHL patients with primary ipsilateral acoustic neuroma (AN) and 24 normal controls (NCs) participated in the study. Two UHL participants (One left UHL and one right UHL) and 2 NCs were excluded due to excessive head motion (please refer to Data Preprocessing). Finally, 34 UHL patients and 22 NCs were included in the study. Among the patients, 17 had hearing loss in the left ear and 17 had hearing loss in the right ear. NC were recruited from local communities in Beijing.

### Cognitive and Clinical Assessments

The cognition of all participants was evaluated by the Mini-Mental State Examination (MMSE) [46], which has been widely used clinically for screening cognitive impairment. It includes 11 items that assess eight categories of cognition: orientation to time, orientation to place, registration, attention and calculation, recall, language, repetition, and complex commands. The full score is 30 points and a low score indicates cognitive impairment. MMSE evaluation was performed to provide a brief and accurate report of the neurological status including mental status, cranial nerves, motor, sensory, coordination, and reflex functions of all patients.

Pure tone audiometry (PTA) is a gold standard for the assessment of hearing loss. We used the standard Hughson-Westlake PTA procedure to identify hearing threshold level of both ears for all participants in the study. The air-conduction pure-tone audiogram was assessed by a clinical audiologist under standard conditions. Audiometric measurements were performed using a GSI-61 audiometer, including TDH39 headphones. Audiologic equipment was calibrated on a regular basis. Pure tone audiometry was conducted at frequencies of 0.25, 0.5, 1, 2, 4, and 8 kHz. Acoustic thresholds of the affected ears were compared with those of the contralateral (unaffected) ears at each frequency level. The mean acoustic thresholds in speech frequency ([0.5 kHz +1 kHz +2 kHz +4 kHz]/4) were calculated to estimate the level of hearing loss.

### Demographic and Auditory Profile

Based on the evaluations of MMSE and standard neurological examinations, all the participants did not show cognitive, language, or somatosensory deficit besides hearing loss. As shown in Table 1, there was no significant group difference in age ($F=0.338$, $p=0.715$), gender ($\chi^2=1.945$, $p=0.378$), education ($F=1.565$, $p=0.219$) or MMSE ($F=2.033$, $p=0.141$) among three groups of subject. Most of the UHL participants had severe-to-profound hearing loss in the impaired ear (eleven left UHL with PTA $\geq 50$ dB and the other six $50>\text{PTA}\geq 20$ dB; twelve right UHL with PTA $\geq 50$ dB and the other five $50>\text{PTA}\geq 20$ dB). UHL patients showed higher PTA levels of the impaired ear than those of the same side of ears in NCs ($t=-5.9$, $p<0.001$ for left UHLs; $t=-7.2$, $p<0.001$ for right UHLs). Meanwhile, no significant difference was found between PTA levels of unaffected ears in UHL patients and those of the same side of ears in normal controls ($t=1.272$, $p=0.211$ for left UHL; $t=1.925$, $p=0.062$ for right UHL). There was no significant differences in the duration of hearing loss ($t=0.437$, $p=0.665$), PTA between the left and right ears that were compromised ($t=0.034$, $p=0.973$), or the contralateral ears with intact hearing ($t=-0.257$, $p=0.799$) between these two patient groups.

### Imaging Acquisition

All functional and structural images were acquired on a 3.0 Tesla scanner (Siemens Trio, Erlangen, Germany) using 12-channel head coil. Head movement was minimized using foam pads, and earplugs were used to attenuate acoustic noise during scanning. For the ten-minute resting-state fMRI scan, participants were instructed to hold still and keep their eyes closed, but not to fall asleep nor think of anything in particular. Resting-state fMRI data were acquired using an echo-planar image pulse sequence (41 axial slices, slice thickness/gap = 3.5/0.7 mm, repetition time = 2500 ms, echo time = 30 ms, flip angle = 90°, and field of view (FOV) = $256\times256$ mm$^2$ with in-plane resolution of $3.75\times3.75$ mm$^2$). A T1-weighted sagittal anatomical image was also obtained using a gradient echo sequence (176 slices, slice thickness/gap = 1/0 mm, inversion time = 900 ms, repetition time = 2300 ms, echo time = 3 ms, flip angle = 7°, number of excitations = 1, FOV = $256\times256$ mm$^2$ with in-plane resolution of $0.9375\times0.9375$ mm$^2$).

**Table 1.** Demographic and auditory characteristics of the participant groups.

| | Left UHL | Right UHL | NC | *F* value | *p* value |
|---|---|---|---|---|---|
| Age (years) | 45.7±6.5 | 43.0±5.4 | 46.0±4.8 | 0.337 | 0.715 |
| Gender | 12f/5m | 8f/9m | 13f/9m | 1.945* | 0.378 |
| Handness | R | R | R | NA | NA |
| Education (years) | 12.4±1.9 | 11.5±2.3 | 13.7±1.2 | 1.565 | 0.219 |
| MMSE | 26.8±1.2 | 27.5±1.1 | 28.1±0.6 | 2.033 | 0.141 |
| Left ears PTA (dB) | 67.2±19.2 | 18.5±3.8 | 16.0±2.2 | 1.925a | 0.062 |
| | | | | −5.9[b] | 0.000 |
| Right ears PTA (dB) | 19.1±2.3 | 66.8±15.6 | 15.6±2.4 | 1.272[c] | 0.211 |
| | | | | −7.2[d] | 0.000 |
| | | | | 0.034[e] | 0.973 |
| Duration of UHL (months) | 26.1±10.9 | 22.5±11.7 | NA | 0.437** | 0.665 |

Abbreviations: UHL = unilateral hearing loss patients, MMSE = Mini-Mental Status Examination, f = female, m = male, R = right, NC = normal controls. Left and Right PTA = pure tone audiometry results of [0.5 kHz +1 kHz +2 kHz +4 kHz]/4 of the left and right ears,
*: $\chi^2$ value of Chi-square test,
**: *t* value of t-test between duration of left and right UHL,
[a]: t value of t-test between PTA in left ears of right UHL and NC,
[b]: t value of t-test between PTA in left ears of left UHL and NC,
[c]: t value of t-test between PTA in right ears of left UHL and NC,
[d]: t value of t-test between PTA in right ears of right UHL of NC,
[e]: t value of t-test between PTA in impaired ears of left and right UHL,

## Data Preprocessing

The resting-state fMRI data were preprocessed using SPM8 (http://www.fil.ion.ucl.ac.uk/spm ) and a pipeline analysis toolbox, DPARSF [47] http://www.restfmri.net/). To avoid transient signal changes before the longitudinal magnetization reached a steady state, the first ten volumes were discarded. The remaining images were preprocessed using a procedure, which included slice timing correction, head motion correction, T1-weighted image based spatial normalization to the Montreal Neurological Institute (MNI) space, linear trend removal, and band-pass filtering (0.01–0.08 Hz). All of the participants' head motion parameters were less than 3 mm in translation and less than 3 degrees in rotation. To further reduce the effects of head motion on estimates of resting-state activity, we censored volumes within each participant's fMRI time series that were associated with sudden head motion [48,49]. For each participant, fMRI volumes were censored if framewise displacement (FD) of head position, calculated as the sum of the absolute values of the derivatives of the realignment estimates, was above 0.5. As a result, four participants (one left UHL, one right UHL and two NCs) with less than five minutes of data after "scrubbing" were excluded from the further analysis.

## Data Length and Mean FD after "scrubbing"

The mean numbers of volumes of left UHLs, right UHLs and NCs after scrubbing were 229.9, 224.5 and 226.2, respectively. There waere no significant differences in the number of volumes between the three groups of subjects ($p = 0.77$). Mean FD of the three groups after scrubbing were 0.11 mm, 0.12 mm and 0.13 mm, respectively. No significant statistical difference was found between mean FD of the three groups of subjects ($p = 0.68$).

## ReHo Analysis

ReHo [37] was used to measure local synchronization of spontaneous BOLD fluctuations within a given cluster (e.g. 27 nearest neighboring voxels). Kendall's coefficient of concordance (ranged from 0 to 1) was used as a measurement of ReHo for each voxel, an indication of similarity between the time series of that voxel and its nearest neighboring voxels. It was measured in a voxel-wise way for each participant within a whole brain mask provided by REST [50]. To reduce nuisance sources of variation [51], individual ReHo maps were divided by the global mean value within the whole brain mask for normalization. Then, all normalized ReHo maps were spatially smoothed with a 6-mm full width at half-maximum (FWHM) Gaussian isotropic kernel.

To detect differences in ReHo amongst the three groups of participants, a one-way analysis of covariance (ANCOVA) was conducted based on the ReHo maps within the whole brain mask with age and gender information as covariates. The Gaussian Random Field theory, which has been implemented in REST, was used to correct for multiple comparisons. The corrected $p<0.05$ (uncorrected $p<0.001$ and minimum 21 voxels in a cluster) was used as threshold. To determine which pairs of groups contributed to the significant group difference, post hoc Tukey pairwise comparison was conducted between each pair of groups for each cluster, with a significance threshold set at 0.05.

## Seed-based Resting-state Functional Connectivity Analysis

Significant clusters were extracted from ANCOVA of ReHo maps and served as seeds in resting-state functional connectivity analysis. First, non-neuronal-related covariates, including six parameters of head motion correction, the average time courses of the whole brain (global mean signal), the average time courses within the white matter mask, and the average time courses within the CSF mask, were removed from the preprocessed data by linear regression analysis. Then, the images were spatially smoothed with a 6-mm FWHM Gaussian kernel. We computed the functional connectivity between each seed region and every voxel within the whole brain mask. The individual functional connectivity maps were transformed to $z$-maps using Fisher's $z$-transformation to improve data normality. A series of one-sample $t$-tests were conducted to detect cortical areas functionally connected with each seed region in each group of participants (Figs. S2–S3). A group connectivity mask was generated with an "OR" operation of the corrected functional connectivity maps of the three groups for each seed. For each seed region, one-way ANCOVA, with age and gender as covariates, was used to identify brain regions within the mask, with significant differences in connectivity to the seed region among the three groups. Multiple comparison correction was performed according to the Gaussian Random Field theory with a corrected $p<0.05$ (uncorrected $p<0.001$ and minimum 21 voxels in a cluster) within the whole brain mask. Similar to ReHo analysis, post hoc Tukey pairwise comparisons were conducted between each pair of groups for each significant cluster identified by the ANCOVA of seed-based functional connectivity.

Further, to examine more directly the potential reorganization of brain activity in the default mode network (DMN) and cognitive control networks (CCN) subserving higher-order cognitive functions, we performed ROI-based functional connectivity analysis using previously defined ROIs (Table S1) of the DMN and cinguloopercular network, a representative networks that compose the CCN involving rAI.

### Correlation between Intrinsic Resting-state Activity and Degree and Duration of Hearing Loss

To investigate the relationship between brain plasticity and PTA as well as hearing loss duration in participants with UHL, we calculated the correlation between the above computed resting-state activity indices (i.e. ReHo/RSFC) and PTA and hearing loss duration. Corrected $p<0.05$ was used as threshold for multiple comparisons correction (uncorrected $p<0.01$, corrections for ReHo and for RSFC analyses were performed using the whole brain mask and the Group connectivity mask, respectively).

## Results

### Abnormal Regional Activity of UHL Patients in ReHo

The ANOVA of ReHo showed significant group differences in cortical regions, including left parahippocampal cortex (lPHC), right anterior insular cortex (rAI), and bilateral calcarine cortices (see Fig. 1), indicating that the neural synchronization of local brain areas during resting state were reshaped by auditory deprivation in UHL. Further post hoc comparisons amongst the lPHC, rAI and bilateral calcarine cortices (Fig. 1, see Table 2 for details, $p<0.05$) showed that left UHL and right UHL participants had higher ReHo values in the rAI compared to NCs (post-hoc $p<0.001$) (Fig. 1A). Right UHL participants showed higher ReHo values than NC and left UHL participants (post-hoc $p<0.001$) in the left PHC (Fig. 1B). Meanwhile, left and right UHL participants had lower ReHo in bilateral calcarine cortices compared to NCs (post-hoc $p<0.001$) (Fig. 1C–1D).

### Abnormal Circuit Activity of UHL Patients within and Beyond the Auditory System

Four regions identified from ReHo analyses were used as seeds for RSFC analysis, including lPHC, rAI and bilateral calcarine cortices, respectively. ANCOVA on the functional connectivity of the rAI seed region showed significant group differences in the medial prefrontal cortex (rMPFC), right pregenual anterior cingulate cortex (pACC) and right postcentral gyrus (rPCG) (post-hoc $p<0.05$, see Fig. 2). Using lPHC as a seed, DMN regions (i.e. right angular gyrus, right precuneus, left cuneus) showed the stronger connectivity among UHL patients compared with NC (post-hoc $p<0.05$, see Fig. 3). There was no significant difference among three groups in RSFC with bilateral calcarine cortices as the seeds. Post-hoc pairwise comparisons (see Table 3 for details, $p<0.05$) showed increased strength of functional connectivity in UHL patients compared to normal controls by using lPHC and rAI as seeds, while no findings of decreased RSFC strength in UHL. Importantly, most of these regions showing altered RSFC were associated with higher-order brain structures including those of the DMN (lPHC, left cuneus, right precuneus and MPFC) and CCN (rAI, rACC), and these results were confirmed by a graph theory analysis (see Text S1, Fig. S6 and Fig. S7).

To note, neither ReHo nor RSFC showed a significant correlation with hearing loss duration or auditory ratings.

## Discussion

Exploring intrinsic brain activity is important for the understanding of brain organization and it may best capture the essence of brain function [55]. In current study, we found decreased ReHo in bilateral calcarine cortices in UHL patients. Moreover, ReHo was increased in the rAI, the key node of CCN, and in the lPHC, a key node of DMN, while the reorganization of RSFC within DMN and between DMN and CCN was confirmed by graph theory analysis. These findings support the notion that adaptive sensory-driven plasticity is involved in widespread brain areas during unilateral hearing processing. The UHL not only reshapes the activity of the sensory cortex but also alters the regional and circuit functional organization of the higher order control networks.

### Plasticity of Sensory Cortices

As ReHo during resting state might be the foundation of the activity change during task-state [56], the decreased ReHo of bilateral calcarine cortices in UHL compared with controls may present the baseline abnormality of sensory cortices in UHL during resting state. The calcarine cortex processes visual information and is considered to be the primary visual cortex. Decreased ReHo of the bilateral calcarine cortices in UHL groups compared with controls may represent an adaptation to engage other sensory systems to compensate for the partial loss of hearing [57]. It has been suggested that sensory deprivation in one modality (auditory) could affect the functions of the remaining modalities (visual) [6,58] [59]. Previous research of auditory brain plasticity on congenitally deaf individuals suggested that early deafness is associated with activation and hyper-functionality in the visual cortex when having auditory stimulation [58,60], which implies cross-modal plasticity. In the current study, all the hearing damage participants were post-lingual UHL adults, and they were not in the critical onset of age for cortical development. Therefore, the progressive UHL caused by AN may influence the calcarine cortex and induce reorganization of visual processing. The reduced ReHo in calcarine cortex may suggest the local reorganization in visual areas. The progressive UHL disrupted the integrity of sensory perceptions, and the visual cortex might not able to reorganize promptly but be in the process of remodeling showing as the reduced functional coherences. We inferred that the decreased ReHo may reflect the functional differentiation for better visual perception in order to cover the hearing deficits. To not, however, this does not mean a causal relationship between decreased ReHo and dysfunction of the visual region. Moreover, we did not find a significant difference in RSFC of bilateral calcarine cortex amongst three groups in current study. We propose that this may be due to the fact that UHL participants largely preserve the ability to capture auditory information in the unaffected ear. UHL may only cause local functional changes in visual areas, rather than long distance reorganization related to cross-model plasticity.

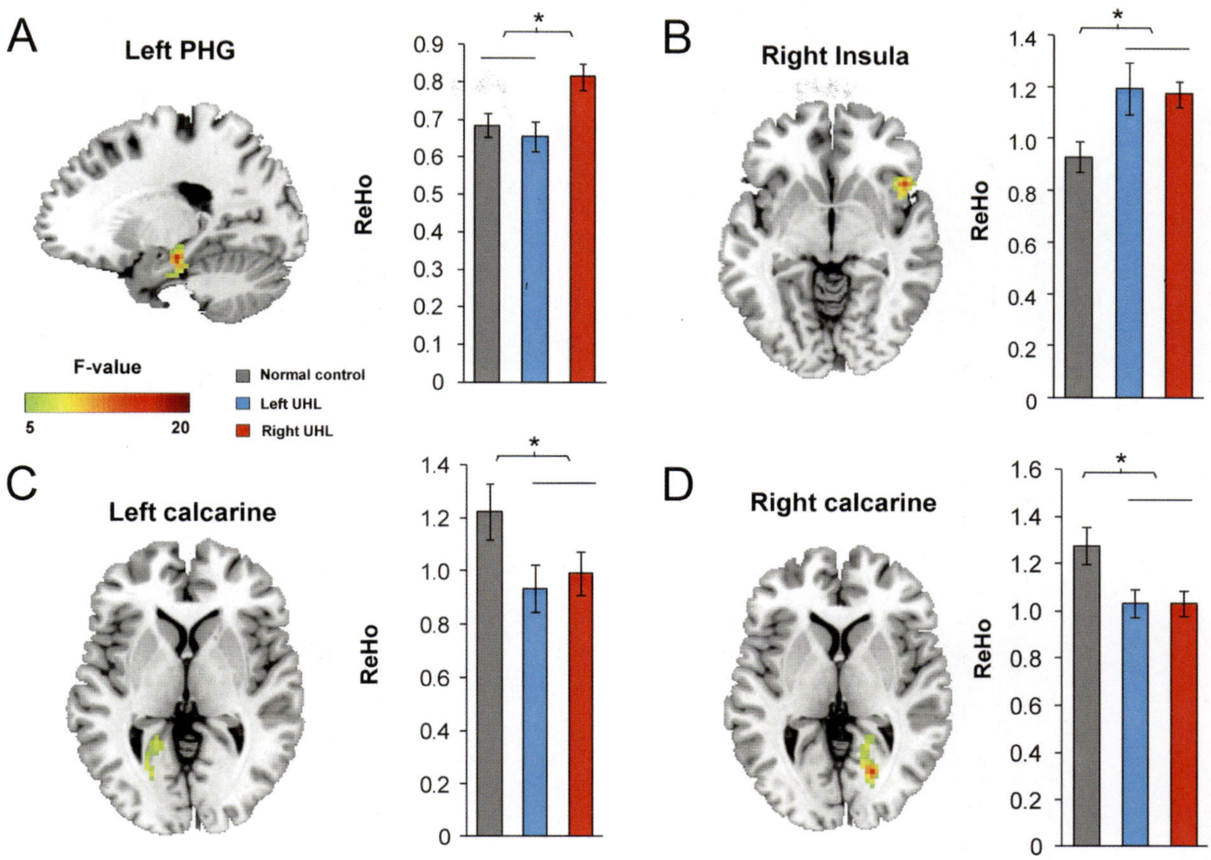


**Figure 1. Group difference in ReHo revealed by ANCOVA.** Significant differences, location and ReHo values of each group in right anterior insular cortex (rAI) (A), left parahippocampal cortex (lPHC) (B), left calcarine cortex (C) and right calcarine cortex (D). The bar and error bar represent the mean value and SD, respectively, of the ReHo values in the region. * $p<0.05$, corrected. UHL, unilateral hearing loss, NC, normal controls.

It is worth noting that, the auditory cortex is expected to be reorganized during UHL intuitively. In current study, attenuation of hearing input leads to a functional in-coordination between auditory perception and goal-directed attention as long as we assess the RSFC for auditory areas particularly (see Text S1,Table S2, Fig, S4 and Fig. S5). However, The UHL patients in current study were all postlingual deaf and their hearing loss started after the critical onset for cortical development. In addition, the UHL individuals did not suffer from totally deafness for a long enough duration. Previous study proved that the age of the onset of deafness is critical to plasticity of deaf brain[41]. Therefore, we could only find the impact on the auditory areas of UHL showing as a trend of alteration of ReHo and RSFC in regions related to auditory function such as temporal cortex (Fig. S1, Fig. S2 and Fig. S3). Nevertheless, the plastic changes in auditory cortex is too mild to pass the strict multiple-comparisons correction of ANOVA. The intrinsic activity changes within auditory cortex of UHL may be little but complex which needs to investigated by further studies.

## Functional Reorganization in the Higher Order Control Network

In this study, key nodes in the functional networks of CCN and DMN, such as rAI, lPHC, rather than primary sensory areas demonstrated both abnormal regional and circuit activity/connectivity in UHL, supporting our hypothesis that compensa-

**Table 2.** Group difference in ReHo among the three groups of participants.

| Location | Peak F-value | MNI coordinate (mm) x | y | z | Volume (mm³) | Post hoc analysis (Tukey $p<0.05$) |
|---|---|---|---|---|---|---|
| right AI | 15.41 | 48 | 18 | −6 | 39 | Left UHL and Right UHL>NC |
| left PHC | 17.22 | −21 | −21 | −18 | 46 | Right UHL>Left UHL and NC |
| left calcarine cortex | 11.87 | −21 | −48 | −3 | 43 | Left UHL and Right UHL<NC |
| Right calcarine cortex | 16.00 | 21 | −69 | 3 | 77 | Left UHL and Right UHL<NC |

Abbreviations: AI = anterior insular cortex, PHC = parahippocampal cortex, UHL = unilateral hearing loss, NC = normal controls.

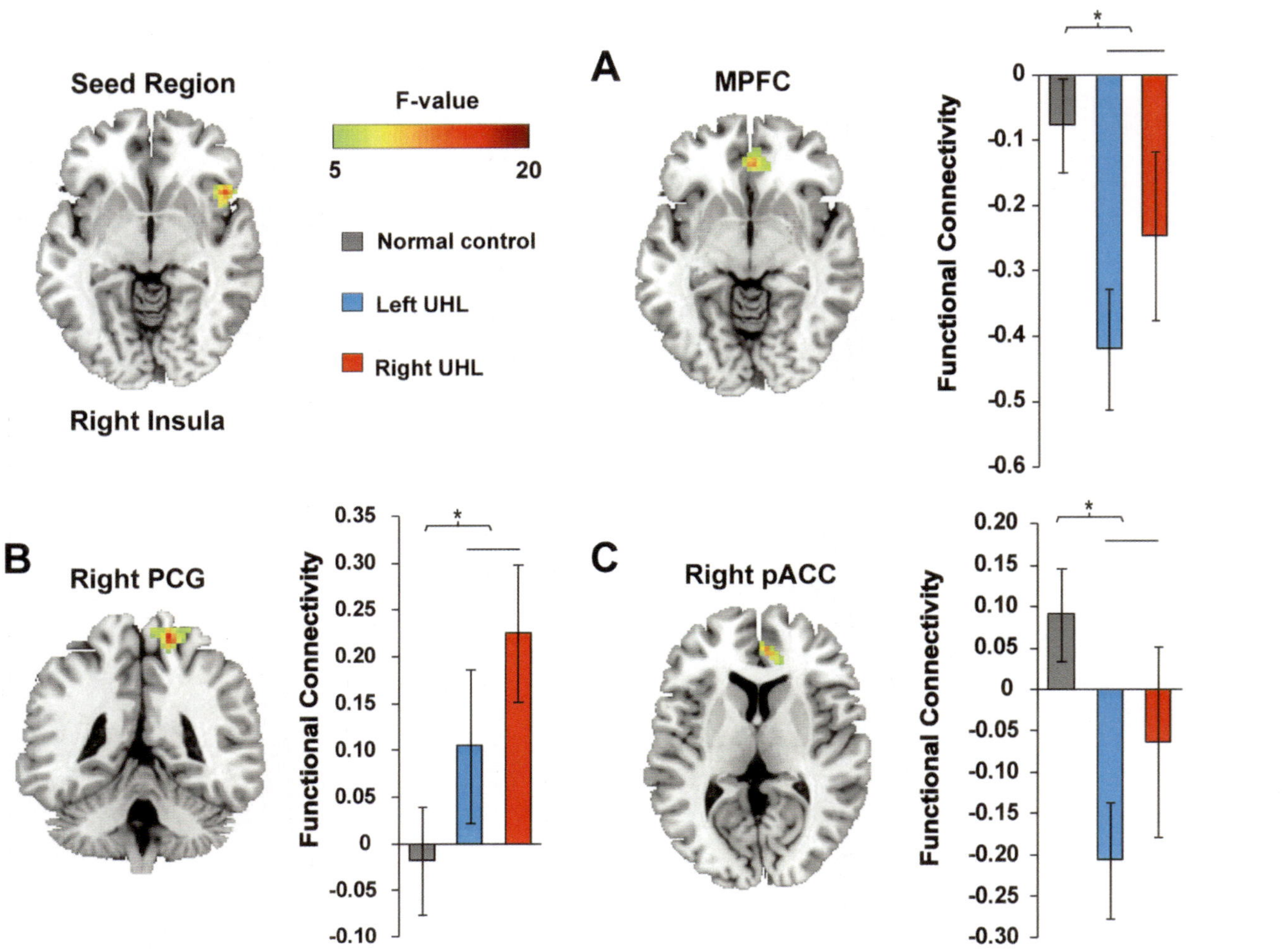


**Figure 2. Group difference in resting state functional connectivity with rAI (the seed region) revealed by ANCOVA.** The significant differences were shown in right medial prefrontal cortex (rMPFC) (A), right postcentral gyrus (rPCG) (B) and pregenual anterior cingulate cortex (pACC) (C). The bar and error bar represent the mean value and SD, respectively, of the functional connectivity values in the region. * $p<0.05$, corrected.

tory remodeling of higher order cognitive processes was involved in asymmetric auditory impairment.

**Remodeling of the CCN.** In the current study, rAI was demonstrated to show increased ReHo, increased strength of negative RSFC with pACC and MPFC in UHL participants compared to control subjects, supporting the notion that UHL lead to hyperactivity of rAI with local and long-distance plastic changes, which may suggest remodeling in cognitive control regions necessary for auditory processing of unilateral hearing damage.

It is recognized that complex auditory information processing may be hindered by UHL, such as phonological processing, musical perception, vocal communication sounds, and spatial and temporal auditory processing [23–26]. Virtually, all these high-level auditory processes rely on the cognitive control and conditioning of cognitive process [61,62]. The AI plays an important role in several independent but interrelated CCN simultaneously [53,63,64]. For instance, AI serves in the cinguloopercular network which contribute to flexible control of human goal-directed behavior [54,65,66], as well as in salience networks which are required for detecting and orienting to salient external stimuli and internal events [31,67,68]. These networks have been proposed to exhibit altered intrinsic activity or connectivity in the AI due to compromised cognitive control in a number of pathological situations [69,70] [71] [68,72,73]. These features serve as the theoretical basis for the speculation that alterations of spontaneous fMRI BOLD signals in rAI might due to the harder cognitive control as a compensation to the partial hearing loss in UHL.

In addition, the insula is also a critical region for the integration of information from diverse functional systems. It connects functional networks together to make perceptual decisions and support complex behavior [67,74–76]. The AI integrates bottom-up signaling with top-down predictions to generate current awareness state [77–81]. Moreover, the AI is also believed to be novelty-sensitive region for involuntary attention to events in the sensory environment [82,83]. For UHL individuals, the asymmetrical auditory deficits is aberrant from the vast and continuous stream of normal bilateral auditory stimuli, which might engage the rAI mediating cognitive control as well as engage different cognitive processes to compensate the perceptional deficits.

Taken together, in line with the hypothesis that altered functional connectivity reflects the brain characteristic in hearing loss [11,19,84], we speculated that the hyperactivity of the rAI and its abnormal RSFC in UHL as an indication of the alteration in cognitive control, namely, that reorganization in UHL individuals

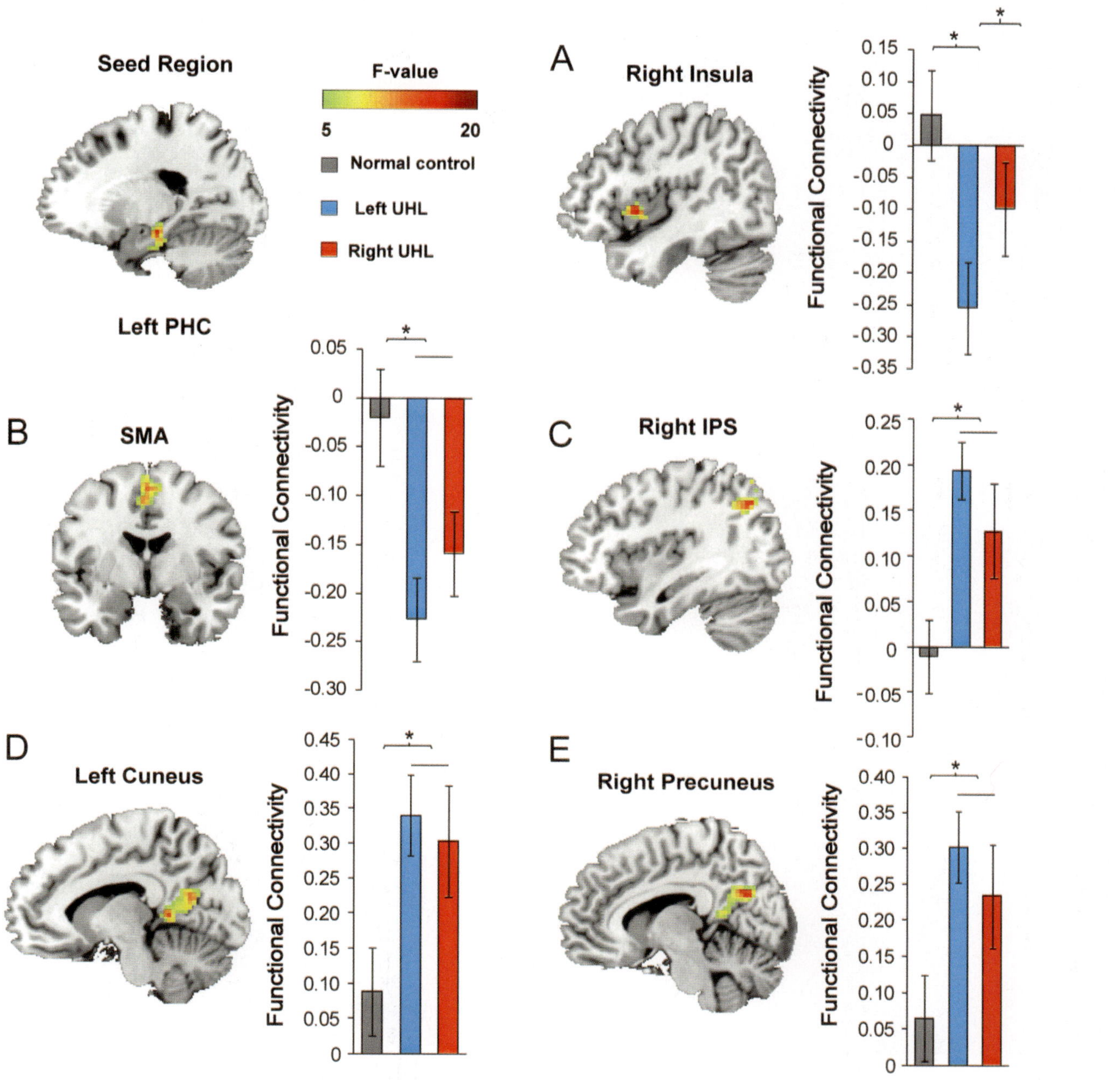


**Figure 3. Group difference in resting state functional connectivity with lPHC (seed region) revealed by ANCOVA.** The significant differences are shown in (A) right insula, (B) supplementary motor area (SMA), (C) right angular gyrus (rAG), (D) left cuneus and (E) right precuneus. The bar and error bar represent the mean value and SD, respectively, of the functional connectivity values in the region. * $p<0.05$, corrected.

tend to favor efforts to resume the effective perception by remodeling the cognitive processing. However, future fMRI studies employing cognitive tasks are needed to further clarify the specific modalities of such cognitive reorganization.

**Alteration of regional and circuit resting-state activity in DMN.** Further, we found increased ReHo in the lPHC as well as enhanced positive RSFC between the lPHC and right angular gyrus, right precuneus and left cuneus in UHL compared to control subjects, suggesting reorganization within the DMN. The DMN, with all the above described regions as important nodes [52], is a task-negative, cross- spatial and intrinsically organized network in the brain. Numerous studies have found that the DMN remains stable amongst healthy individuals [85,86] and can be affected by neurological and psychiatric diseases [87,88]. In healthy subjects, the DMN involved in the integration of self-monitoring, autobiographical, and related social cognitive functions [86,89]. The anti-correlated interactions between cognitive-demanding regions and the DMN are intrinsic through the human brain, occurring naturally and spontaneously [86], and it is correlated to a more consistent behavioral performance [90] as well as exact control of efficient goal-directed behavior and focused attention [91]. Viewed from this context, the increased positive RSFC between core nodes in DMN, which consistent with the enhanced correlation among key nodes within DMN in ROI-based functional connectivity analysis, indicated hyperfunction of

**Table 3.** Group difference in functional connectivity with seed regions selected from ReHo analysis.

| Seed | Location | Peak | MNI coordinate (mm) | | | Volume | Post hoc analysis |
|---|---|---|---|---|---|---|---|
| | | F-value | x | y | z | (mm$^3$) | (Tukey $p$<0.05) |
| | MPFC | 13.46 | 3 | 39 | −6 | 48 | Right UHL and Left UHL< NC <0 |
| Right AI | right pACC | 13.30 | 6 | 45 | 9 | 39 | Right UHL and Left UHL <0< NC |
| | right PCG | 17.94 | 15 | −45 | 69 | 89 | Right UHL and Left UHL >0> NC |
| | right AI | 17.26 | 48 | 9 | −3 | 76 | Left UHL< Right UHL<NC <0 |
| | SMA | 15.02 | 0 | 9 | 51 | 121 | Right UHL and Left UHL< NC <0 |
| Left PHC | Right AG | 18.77 | 36 | −69 | 39 | 227 | Right UHL and Left UHL >0> NC |
| | Left cuneus | 14.95 | −9 | −48 | 3 | 139 | Right UHL and Left UHL>NC >0 |
| | Right precuneus | 16.27 | 9 | −66 | 24 | 123 | Right UHL and Left UHL>NC >0 |

Abbreviations: AI = anterior insular cortex, PHC = parahippocampal cortex, MPFC = medial prefrontal cortex, pACC = pregenual anterior cingulate cortex, PCG = postcentral gyrus, SMA = supplementary motor area, AG = angular gyrus, UHL = unilateral hearing loss, NC = normal controls.

DMN in UHL participants, suggesting that UHL induced an alteration in the intrinsic circuit for DMN in UHL.

**Reorganization of the connectivity between CCN and DMN.** In addition, we found increased strength of negative RSFC between the important nodes of DMN (MPFC, rAG and lPHC) and rAI in UHL participants compared to their control counterparts. Enhanced connectivity between CCN and the DMN was also demonstrated by the graph theory analysis. The alteration in RSFC has been demonstrated due to changes in the different sensory experience [32,44,45], such as blindness. In this study, the enhanced RSFC between nodes of CCN and DMN may indicate the more rapid and intensive coordination between these two networks for assisting the detection of dynamic environment and compensating the perceptional deficit resulting from UHL [90]. Moreover, the rAI plays a critical and causal role in switching between activation and deactivation of large-scale brain networks involving the central-executive network and the DMN [92]. The enhanced synchronization between lPHC and rAI in UHL may also indicate a prompt switching from resting state to an activated state in order to facilitate the cognitive process to adapt to attenuation of hearing information input. It would be in line with the notion that neural synchrony between spatially distinct regions helps to coordinate information processing in those regions [93]. Thus, changes within and between functional networks during resting-state might be an indicator of abnormal task activation and deactivation patterns and task performances, which encourages further investigations using task-based fMRI.

## No Correlation between Intrinsic Resting-state Activity and Degree and Duration of Hearing Loss

Neither ReHo nor RSFC showed a significant correlation with hearing loss duration or auditory ratings. The null findings might be due to some possible reasons. Firstly, a previous study has suggested that the influence of plasticity may be more so influenced by the onset of (pre- or post-lingually) the patients acquires a profound hearing impairment rather than the duration of auditory deprivation [94]. Secondly, duration of hearing loss in the current study was reported by the patients potentially be with subjective bias, and the unit for duration of hearing loss (months) may not offer enough temporal resolution to detect correlations between hearing loss duration and resting-state brain activity. It is also possible that the correlations between resting-state activity and degree or duration of hearing loss may not be linear.

## The Lateralization of UHL

For most of the result, the UHL groups showed significant differences compared to normal control groups with non significant differences between left and right UHL groups. However, most reorganizations of ReHo and RSFC found in the current study were more pronounced in left UHL patients than right UHL ones, although not significant statistically. This may have resulted from the fact that greater resilience against reduced hearing damage in right ear [95]. The left ear pathway demonstrates a stronger contralateral effect during monaural acoustic stimulation [96,97]. In other words, the right ear delivers information to both hemispheres more evenly, while the left ear delivers information more lateralized. Accordingly, once the normal pattern was interfered by UHL, the dysfunction of left ear interrupt the brain more significantly. Meanwhile, the right UHL participants show more stabilization in cortex.

## Conclusion

The present study confirms and extends the previous findings of reorganizations in the brain associated with auditory damage. The reduced regional homogeneity in calcarine cortex suggested a dysfunctional reorganization for post-lingual UHL patients in sensory cortex. Furthermore, both regional and circuit plastic changes in rAI and lPHC which involving in high-order cognitive networks may indicate the adapted cognitive process for attenuation of hearing information input. Taken together, abnormal resting-state brain activity in UHL participants suggests that brain areas involved in cognitive control as well as the sensory cortices, are modulated by asymmetric auditory function preservation.

## Supporting Information

**Figure S1** One-sample t-maps of ReHo in the whole brain for each of the three groups ($p<0.05$, corrected). L and R represent the left and right hemispheres, respectively. The results were mapped onto the cortical surfaces using in-house developed BrainNet viewer software (www.nitrc.org/projects/bnv/). UHL, unilateral hearing loss, NC, normal controls.

**Figure S2** One-sample t-maps of resting-state functional connectivity of the right anterior insular cortex in the whole brain for each of the three groups ($p<0.05$, corrected). L and R represent the left and right hemispheres, respectively. The results were mapped onto the cortical surfaces using in-house developed BrainNet viewer software (www.nitrc.org/projects/bnv/).

**Figure S3** One-sample t-maps of resting-state functional connectivity of the left parahippocampal cortex in the whole brain for each of the three groups ($p<0.05$, corrected). L and R represent the left and right hemispheres, respectively. The results were mapped onto the cortical surfaces using in-house developed BrainNet viewer software (www.nitrc.org/projects/bnv/).

**Figure S4** Group difference in resting state functional connectivity with left HG(the seed region) revealed by ANCOVA. The significant differences were shown in left medial frontal gyrus (MPG) (A) and right superior parietal lobule (SPL) (B). The bar and error bar represent the mean value and SD, respectively, of the functional connectivity values in the region. * $p<0.05$, corrected.

**Figure S5** Group difference in resting state functional connectivity with right HG (the seed region) revealed by ANCOVA. The significant differences were shown in left medial frontal gyrus (MFG) (A). The bar and error bar represent the mean value and SD, respectively, of the functional connectivity values in the region. * $p<0.05$, corrected.

**Figure S6** The distribution of connections with significant group effects in the functional connectivity strength among the three groups at $p<0.01$ (uncorrected). The thicknesss of connections indicate the significance of between-group differences. ROIs in purple belong to DMN while ROIs in blue belong to CCN. Connections in gray indicate those connections were between DMN and CCN (A–C), while connections in purple indicate those connections were within DMN [ipsilateral connetions (D–E), contralateral connections (F–J)]. For each connection, the bar and error bar represent the mean value and SD, respectively, of the functional connectivity strength in each group. Post hoc tests showed that all the ROIs have increased functional connectivity strength in the left UHL patients versus the controls. Three of these six ROI, including the rIPL, rTPJ and rAI/fO showed reduced functional connectivity strength in the right UHL patients compared with the left ones. Only one region (lHF) showed increased functional connectivity strength in right UHL patients compared to normal controls. * $p<0.05$. The connecitons were mapped onto the cortical surfaces using in-house BrainNet viewer software (www.nitrc.org/projects/bnv/).

**Figure S7** The distribution of brain regions with significant group effects in the functional connectivity strength among the three groups at $p<0.05$ (uncorrected). The sizes of ROIs indicate the significance of between-group differences. ROIs in purple belong to DMN while ROIs in blue belong to CCN. For each ROI, the bar and error bar represent the mean value and SD, respectively, of the functional connectivity strength in each group. Post hoc tests showed that all the ROIs have increased functional connectivity strength in the left UHL patients versus the controls. Three of these six ROI, including the rIPL, rTPJ and rAI/fO showed reduced functional connectivity strength in the right UHL patients compared with the left ones. Only one region (lHF) showed increased functional connectivity strength in right UHL patients compared to normal controls. * $p<0.05$. The ROIs were mapped onto the cortical surfaces using in-house BrainNet viewer software (www.nitrc.org/projects/bnv/). For the abbreviations of the ROIs, see Table S1.

**Table S1** Regions of interest in graph analysis.

**Table S2** Group difference in functional connectivity with seed regions at primary auditory cortex.

**Text S1**

## Acknowledgments

We wish to thank M.D. Shujie Ma who helped with the data collection and Tuyen Nguyen who helped with the English language editing.

## Author Contributions

Conceived and designed the experiments: XW YF FZ JG KZ ZG QZ PL. Performed the experiments: XW ZW YF QZ ZG KZ. Analyzed the data: XW YF QZ PL JHG JG. Contributed reagents/materials/analysis tools: XW FZ KZ ZG PL ZW. Wrote the paper: XW YF QZ JF YY.

## References

1. King AJ, Moore DR (1991) Plasticity of auditory maps in the brain. Trends Neurosci 14: 31–37.
2. Eggermont JJ (2008) The role of sound in adult and developmental auditory cortical plasticity. Ear Hear 29: 819–829.
3. Bavelier D, Tomann A, Hutton C, Mitchell T, Corina D, et al. (2000) Visual attention to the periphery is enhanced in congenitally deaf individuals. J Neurosci 20: RC93.
4. Finney EM, Fine I, Dobkins KR (2001) Visual stimuli activate auditory cortex in the deaf. Nat Neurosci 4: 1171–1173.

5. Auer ET Jr, Bernstein LE, Sungkarat W, Singh M (2007) Vibrotactile activation of the auditory cortices in deaf versus hearing adults. Neuroreport 18: 645–648.
6. Bavelier D, Neville HJ (2002) Cross-modal plasticity: where and how? Nat Rev Neurosci 3: 443–452.
7. Humes LE, Busey TA, Craig J, Kewley-Port D (2013) Are age-related changes in cognitive function driven by age-related changes in sensory processing? Atten Percept Psychophys 75: 508–524.
8. Lin FR, Yaffe K, Xia J, Xue QL, Harris TB, et al. (2013) Hearing loss and cognitive decline in older adults. JAMA Intern Med 173: 293–299.
9. Horn DL, Davisa RA, Pisoni DB, Miyamoto RT (2004) Visual attention, behavioral inhibition and speech/language outcomes in deaf children with cochlear implants. Int Congr Ser 1273: 332–335.
10. Shin MS, Kim SK, Kim SS, Park MH, Kim CS, et al. (2007) Comparison of cognitive function in deaf children between before and after cochlear implant. Ear Hear 28: 22S–28S.
11. Dye MW, Bavelier D (2010) Attentional enhancements and deficits in deaf populations: an integrative review. Restor Neurol Neurosci 28: 181–192.
12. Parasnis I, Samar VJ, Berent GP (2003) Deaf adults without attention deficit hyperactivity disorder display reduced perceptual sensitivity and elevated impulsivity on the Test of Variables of Attention (T.O.V.A.). J Speech Lang Hear Res 46: 1166–1183.
13. Lazard DS, Lee HJ, Truy E, Giraud AL (2012) Bilateral reorganization of posterior temporal cortices in post-lingual deafness and its relation to cochlear implant outcome. Hum Brain Mapp 4: 1208–19
14. Dye MW, Baril DE, Bavelier D (2007) Which aspects of visual attention are changed by deafness? The case of the Attentional Network Test. Neuropsychologia 45: 1801–1811.
15. Proksch J, Bavelier D (2002) Changes in the spatial distribution of visual attention after early deafness. J Cogn Neurosci 14: 687–701.
16. Weisberg J, Koo DS, Crain KL, Eden GF (2012) Cortical plasticity for visuospatial processing and object recognition in deaf and hearing signers. Neuroimage 60: 661–672.
17. Daza MT, Phillips-Silver J (2013) Development of attention networks in deaf children: Support for the integrative hypothesis. Res Dev Disabil 34: 2661–2668.
18. Quittner AL, Leibach P, Marciel K (2004) The impact of cochlear implants on young deaf children: new methods to assess cognitive and behavioral development. Arch Otolaryngol Head Neck Surg 130: 547–554.
19. Husain FT, Pajor NM, Smith JF, Kim HJ, Rudy S, et al. (2011) Discrimination task reveals differences in neural bases of tinnitus and hearing impairment. PLoS One 6: e26639.
20. Oberg E, Lukomski J (2011) Executive functioning and the impact of a hearing loss: performance-based measures and the Behavior Rating Inventory of Executive Function (BRIEF). Child Neuropsychol 17: 521–545.
21. Figueras B, Edwards L, Langdon D (2008) Executive function and language in deaf children. J Deaf Stud Deaf Educ 13: 362–377.
22. Kronenberger WG, Pisoni DB, Henning SC, Colson BG (2013) Executive functioning skills in long-term users of cochlear implants: a case control study. J Pediatr Psychol 38: 902–914.
23. Vasama JP, Makela JP (1995) Auditory pathway plasticity in adult humans after unilateral idiopathic sudden sensorineural hearing loss. Hear Res 87: 132–140.
24. Schmithorst VJ, Holland SK, Ret J, Duggins A, Arjmand E, et al. (2005) Cortical reorganization in children with unilateral sensorineural hearing loss. Neuroreport 16: 463–467.
25. Wu CM, Ng SH, Wang JJ, Liu TC (2009) Diffusion tensor imaging of the subcortical auditory tract in subjects with congenital cochlear nerve deficiency. AJNR Am J Neuroradiol 30: 1773–1777.
26. Araujo PG, Mondelli MF, Lauris JR, Richieri-Costa A, Feniman MR (2010) Assessment of the auditory handicap in adults with unilateral hearing loss. Braz J Otorhinolaryngol 76: 378–383.
27. Zhang D, Raichle ME (2010) Disease and the brain's dark energy. Nat Rev Neurol 6: 15–28.
28. Raichle ME (2006) Neuroscience. The brain's dark energy. Science 314: 1249–1250.
29. Salvador KK, Pereira TC, Moraes TF, Cruz MS, Feniman MR (2011) Auditory processing in unilateral hearing loss: case report. J Soc Bras Fonoaudiol 23: 381–384.
30. Kral A, Eggermont JJ (2007) What's to lose and what's to learn: development under auditory deprivation, cochlear implants and limits of cortical plasticity. Brain Res Rev 56: 259–269.
31. Seeley WW, Menon V, Schatzberg AF, Keller J, Glover GH, et al. (2007) Dissociable intrinsic connectivity networks for salience processing and executive control. J Neurosci 27: 2349–2356.
32. Bengoetxea H, Ortuzar N, Bulnes S, Rico-Barrio I, Lafuente JV, et al. (2012) Enriched and deprived sensory experience induces structural changes and rewires connectivity during the postnatal development of the brain. Neural Plast 2012: 305693.
33. Suzuki M, Kouzaki H, Nishida Y, Shiino A, Ito R, et al. (2002) Cortical representation of hearing restoration in patients with sudden deafness. Neuroreport 13: 1829–1832.
34. Bilecen D, Seifritz E, Radu EW, Schmid N, Wetzel S, et al. (2000) Cortical reorganization after acute unilateral hearing loss traced by fMRI. Neurology 54: 765–767.
35. Welsh LW, Welsh JJ, Rosen LF, Dragonette JE (2004) Functional impairments due to unilateral deafness. Ann Otol Rhinol Laryngol 113: 987–993.
36. Hutson KA, Durham D, Imig T, Tucci DL (2008) Consequences of unilateral hearing loss: cortical adjustment to unilateral deprivation. Hear Res 237: 19–31.
37. Zang Y, Jiang T, Lu Y, He Y, Tian L (2004) Regional homogeneity approach to fMRI data analysis. Neuroimage 22: 394–400.
38. Zuo XN, Xu T, Jiang L, Yang Z, Cao XY, et al. (2013) Toward reliable characterization of functional homogeneity in the human brain: preprocessing, scan duration, imaging resolution and computational space. Neuroimage 65: 374–386.
39. Biswal B, Yetkin FZ, Haughton VM, Hyde JS (1995) Functional connectivity in the motor cortex of resting human brain using echo-planar MRI. Magn Reson Med 34: 537–541.
40. Shehzad Z, Kelly AM, Reiss PT, Gee DG, Gotimer K, et al. (2009) The resting brain: unconstrained yet reliable. Cereb Cortex 19: 2209–2229.
41. Li Y, Booth JR, Peng D, Zang Y, Li J, et al. (2012) Altered Intra- and Inter-Regional Synchronization of Superior Temporal Cortex in Deaf People. Cereb Cortex 23: 1988–96
42. Tibbetts K, Ead B, Umansky A, Coalson R, Schlaggar BL, et al. (2011) Interregional brain interactions in children with unilateral hearing loss. Otolaryngol Head Neck Surg 144: 602–611.
43. Liu C, Liu Y, Li W, Wang D, Jiang T, et al. (2011) Increased regional homogeneity of blood oxygen level-dependent signals in occipital cortex of early blind individuals. Neuroreport 22: 190–194.
44. Liu Y, Yu C, Liang M, Li J, Tian L, et al. (2007) Whole brain functional connectivity in the early blind. Brain 130: 2085–2096.
45. Yu C, Liu Y, Li J, Zhou Y, Wang K, et al. (2008) Altered functional connectivity of primary visual cortex in early blindness. Hum Brain Mapp 29: 533–543.
46. Folstein MF, Folstein SE, McHugh PR (1975) "Mini-mental state". A practical method for grading the cognitive state of patients for the clinician. J Psychiatr Res 12: 189–198.
47. Chao-Gan Y, Yu-Feng Z (2010) DPARSF: A MATLAB Toolbox for "Pipeline" Data Analysis of Resting-State fMRI. Front Syst Neurosci 4: 13.
48. Power JD, Barnes KA, Snyder AZ, Schlaggar BL, Petersen SE (2012) Spurious but systematic correlations in functional connectivity MRI networks arise from subject motion. Neuroimage 59: 2142–2154.
49. Liang X, Zou Q, He Y, Yang Y (2013) Coupling of functional connectivity and regional cerebral blood flow reveals a physiological basis for network hubs of the human brain. Proc Natl Acad Sci U S A 110: 1929–1934.
50. Song XW, Dong ZY, Long XY, Li SF, Zuo XN, et al. (2011) REST: a toolkit for resting-state functional magnetic resonance imaging data processing. PLoS One 6: e25031.
51. Yan CG, Craddock RC, Zuo XN, Zang YF, Milham MP (2013) Standardizing the intrinsic brain: towards robust measurement of inter-individual variation in 1000 functional connectomes. Neuroimage 80: 246–262.
52. Andrews-Hanna JR, Reidler JS, Sepulcre J, Poulin R, Buckner RL (2010) Functional-anatomic fractionation of the brain's default network. Neuron 65: 550–562.
53. Fan J, Van Dam NT, Gu X, Liu X, Wang H, et al. (2013) Quantitative Characterization of Functional Anatomical Contributions to Cognitive Control under Uncertainty. Journal of Cognitive Neuroscience Jan 6. Epub ahead of print
54. Dosenbach NU, Fair DA, Miezin FM, Cohen AL, Wenger KK, et al. (2007) Distinct brain networks for adaptive and stable task control in humans. Proc Natl Acad Sci U S A 104: 11073–11078.
55. Raichle ME (2010) Two views of brain function. Trends Cogn Sci 14: 180–190.
56. Tian L, Ren J, Zang Y (2012) Regional homogeneity of resting state fMRI signals predicts Stop signal task performance. Neuroimage 60: 539–544.
57. Driver J, Spence C (2000) Multisensory perception: beyond modularity and convergence. Curr Biol 10: R731–735.
58. Bavelier D, Dye MW, Hauser PC (2006) Do deaf individuals see better? Trends Cogn Sci 10: 512–518.
59. Dieterich M, Bauermann T, Best C, Stoeter P, Schlindwein P (2007) Evidence for cortical visual substitution of chronic bilateral vestibular failure (an fMRI study). Brain 130: 2108–2116.
60. Sladen DP, Tharpe AM, Ashmead DH, Wesley Grantham D, Chun MM (2005) Visual attention in deaf and normal hearing adults: effects of stimulus compatibility. J Speech Lang Hear Res 48: 1529–1537.
61. Leaver AM, Rauschecker JP (2010) Cortical representation of natural complex sounds: effects of acoustic features and auditory object category. J Neurosci 30: 7604–7612.
62. Sharda M, Singh NC (2012) Auditory perception of natural sound categories–an fMRI study. Neuroscience 214: 49–58.
63. Cauda F, Costa T, Torta DM, Sacco K, D'Agata F, et al. (2012) Meta-analytic clustering of the insular cortex: characterizing the meta-analytic connectivity of the insula when involved in active tasks. Neuroimage 62: 343–355.
64. Taylor KS, Seminowicz DA, Davis KD (2009) Two systems of resting state connectivity between the insula and cingulate cortex. Hum Brain Mapp 30: 2731–2745.
65. Morecraft RJ, Geula C, Mesulam MM (1993) Architecture of connectivity within a cingulo-fronto-parietal neurocognitive network for directed attention. Arch Neurol 50: 279–284.
66. Dosenbach NU, Fair DA, Cohen AL, Schlaggar BL, Petersen SE (2008) A dual-networks architecture of top-down control. Trends Cogn Sci 12: 99–105.
67. Menon V, Uddin LQ (2010) Saliency, switching, attention and control: a network model of insula function. Brain Struct Funct 214: 655–667.

68. Menon V (2011) Large-scale brain networks and psychopathology: a unifying triple network model. Trends Cogn Sci 15: 483–506.
69. Repovs G, Csernansky JG, Barch DM (2011) Brain network connectivity in individuals with schizophrenia and their siblings. Biol Psychiatry 69: 967–973.
70. Tu PC, Hsieh JC, Li CT, Bai YM, Su TP (2012) Cortico-striatal disconnection within the cingulo-opercular network in schizophrenia revealed by intrinsic functional connectivity analysis: a resting fMRI study. Neuroimage 59: 238–247.
71. Sylvester CM, Corbetta M, Raichle ME, Rodebaugh TL, Schlaggar BL, et al. (2012) Functional network dysfunction in anxiety and anxiety disorders. Trends Neurosci 35: 527–535.
72. Palaniyappan L, Liddle PF (2012) Does the salience network play a cardinal role in psychosis? An emerging hypothesis of insular dysfunction. J Psychiatry Neurosci 37: 17–27.
73. Sullivan EV, Muller-Oehring E, Pitel AL, Chanraud S, Shankaranarayanan A, et al. (2013) A Selective Insular Perfusion Deficit Contributes to Compromised Salience Network Connectivity in Recovering Alcoholic Men. Biol Psychiatry 74: 547–55
74. Wiech K, Lin CS, Brodersen KH, Bingel U, Ploner M, et al. (2010) Anterior insula integrates information about salience into perceptual decisions about pain. J Neurosci 30: 16324–16331.
75. Manoliu A, Riedl V, Zherdin A, Muhlau M, Schwerthoffer D, et al. (2013) Aberrant Dependence of Default Mode/Central Executive Network Interactions on Anterior Insular Salience Network Activity in Schizophrenia. Schizophr Bull 40: 428–37
76. Stephani C, Fernandez-Baca Vaca G, Maciunas R, Koubeissi M, Luders HO (2011) Functional neuroanatomy of the insular lobe. Brain Struct Funct 216: 137–149.
77. Nagai M, Kishi K, Kato S (2007) Insular cortex and neuropsychiatric disorders: a review of recent literature. Eur Psychiatry 22: 387–394.
78. Craig AD (2010) The sentient self. Brain Struct Funct 214: 563–577.
79. Craig AD, Chen K, Bandy D, Reiman EM (2000) Thermosensory activation of insular cortex. Nat Neurosci 3: 184–190.
80. Gu X, Hof PR, Friston KJ, Fan J (2013) Anterior Insular Cortex and Emotional Awareness. The Journal of Comparative Neurology 521: 3371–88
81. Gu X, Hof PR, Friston KJ, Fan J (2013) Anterior insular cortex and emotional awareness. J Comp Neurol 521: 3371–3388.
82. Downar J, Crawley AP, Mikulis DJ, Davis KD (2002) A cortical network sensitive to stimulus salience in a neutral behavioral context across multiple sensory modalities. J Neurophysiol 87: 615–620.
83. Downar J, Crawley AP, Mikulis DJ, Davis KD (2000) A multimodal cortical network for the detection of changes in the sensory environment. Nat Neurosci 3: 277–283.
84. Moussa MN, Vechlekar CD, Burdette JH, Steen MR, Hugenschmidt CE, et al. (2011) Changes in cognitive state alter human functional brain networks. Front Hum Neurosci 5: 83.
85. Harrison BJ, Pujol J, Lopez-Sola M, Hernandez-Ribas R, Deus J, et al. (2008) Consistency and functional specialization in the default mode brain network. Proc Natl Acad Sci U S A 105: 9781–9786.
86. Fox MD, Snyder AZ, Vincent JL, Corbetta M, Van Essen DC, et al. (2005) The human brain is intrinsically organized into dynamic, anticorrelated functional networks. Proc Natl Acad Sci U S A 102: 9673–9678.
87. Bonnelle V, Ham TE, Leech R, Kinnunen KM, Mehta MA, et al. (2012) Salience network integrity predicts default mode network function after traumatic brain injury. Proc Natl Acad Sci U S A 109: 4690–4695.
88. Whitfield-Gabrieli S, Ford JM (2012) Default mode network activity and connectivity in psychopathology. Annu Rev Clin Psychol 8: 49–76.
89. Spreng RN, Mar RA, Kim AS (2009) The common neural basis of autobiographical memory, prospection, navigation, theory of mind, and the default mode: a quantitative meta-analysis. J Cogn Neurosci 21: 489–510.
90. Kelly AM, Uddin LQ, Biswal BB, Castellanos FX, Milham MP (2008) Competition between functional brain networks mediates behavioral variability. Neuroimage 39: 527–537.
91. Leech R, Kamourieh S, Beckmann CF, Sharp DJ (2011) Fractionating the default mode network: distinct contributions of the ventral and dorsal posterior cingulate cortex to cognitive control. J Neurosci 31: 3217–3224.
92. Sridharan D, Levitin DJ, Menon V (2008) A critical role for the right fronto-insular cortex in switching between central-executive and default-mode networks. Proc Natl Acad Sci U S A 105: 12569–12574.
93. Buzsaki G, Draguhn A (2004) Neuronal oscillations in cortical networks. Science 304: 1926–1929.
94. Buckley KA, Tobey EA (2011) Cross-modal plasticity and speech perception in pre- and postlingually deaf cochlear implant users. Ear Hear 32: 2–15.
95. Burton H, Firszt JB, Holden T, Agato A, Uchanski RM (2012) Activation lateralization in human core, belt, and parabelt auditory fields with unilateral deafness compared to normal hearing. Brain Res 1454: 33–47.
96. Scheffler K, Bilecen D, Schmid N, Tschopp K, Seelig J (1998) Auditory cortical responses in hearing subjects and unilateral deaf patients as detected by functional magnetic resonance imaging. Cereb Cortex 8: 156–163.
97. Jancke L, Wustenberg T, Schulze K, Heinze HJ (2002) Asymmetric hemodynamic responses of the human auditory cortex to monaural and binaural stimulation. Hear Res 170: 166–178.

# Deficiency of Transcription Factor Brn4 Disrupts Cochlear Gap Junction Plaques in a Model of DFN3 Non-Syndromic Deafness

**Yoshinobu Kidokoro[1], Keiko Karasawa[1], Osamu Minowa[2], Yoshinobu Sugitani[3], Tetsuo Noda[2,3], Katsuhisa Ikeda[1], Kazusaku Kamiya[1]***

**1** Juntendo University Faculty of Medicine, Department of Otorhinolaryngology, Tokyo, Japan, **2** BioResource Center, Institute of Physical and Chemical Research (RIKEN), Tsukuba, Japan, **3** Department of Cell Biology, Japanese Foundation for Cancer Research, Cancer Institute, Tokyo, Japan

## Abstract

*Brn4*, which encodes a POU transcription factor, is the gene responsible for DFN3, an X chromosome–linked, non-syndromic type of hearing loss. Brn4-deficient mice have a low endocochlear potential (EP), hearing loss, and ultrastructural alterations in spiral ligament fibrocytes, however the molecular pathology through which Brn4 deficiency causes low EP is still unclear. Mutations in the Gjb2 and Gjb6 genes encoding the gap junction proteins connexin26 (Cx26) and connexin30 (Cx30) genes, respectively, which encode gap junction proteins and are expressed in cochlear fibrocytes and non-sensory epithelial cells (i.e., cochlear supporting cells) to maintain the proper EP, are responsible for hereditary sensorineural deafness. It has been hypothesized that the gap junction in the cochlea provides an intercellular passage by which $K^+$ is transported to maintain the EP at the high level necessary for sensory hair cell excitation. Here we analyzed the formation of gap junction plaques in cochlear supporting cells of Brn4-deficient mice at different stages by confocal microscopy and three-dimensional graphic reconstructions. Gap junctions from control mice, which are composed mainly of Cx26 and Cx30, formed linear plaques along the cell-cell junction sites with adjacent cells. These plaques formed pentagonal or hexagonal outlines of the normal inner sulcus cells and border cells. Gap junction plaques in Brn4-deficient mice did not, however, show the normal linear structure but instead formed small spots around the cell-cell junction sites. Gap junction lengths were significantly shorter, and the level of Cx26 and Cx30 was significantly reduced in Brn4-deficient mice compared with littermate controls. Thus the Brn4 mutation affected the assembly and localization of gap junction proteins at the cell borders of cochlear supporting cells, suggesting that Brn4 substantially contributes to cochlear gap junction properties to maintain the proper EP in cochleae, similar to connexin-related deafness.

**Editor:** Eliana Scemes, Albert Einstein College of Medicine, United States of America

**Funding:** This work was supported in part by a research grant from the Ministry of Education, Science and Culture (to K. K.), Ministry of Health, Labor and Welfare of Japan (to K. K.), Takeda Science Foundation (to K. K.), MEXT-support program for the Strategic Research Foundation at Private Universities, 2011–2013 (to K. I.). The funders had no role in study design, data collection and analysis, decision to publish, or preparation of the manuscript.

**Competing Interests:** The authors have declared that no competing interests exist.

* Email: kkamiya@juntendo.ac.jp

## Introduction

Congenital sensorineural hearing loss occurs in 1 out of every 1000 births and is one of the most common congenital diseases. Deafness type 3 (DFN3) is the most common type of in X chromosome–linked, non-syndromic hearing loss. DFN3 is caused by mutations in Brn4, which is the gene that encodes the POU domain, class 3, transcription factor 4 (POU3F4) [1]. During embryogenesis, Brn4 is expressed in mesenchymal cells of the inner ear [2]. Brn4 is also associated with neuronal development, as radial bundle fasciculation and synapse formation are disrupted when POU3F4 is deleted from the otic mesenchyme [3]. This neuronal defect does not, however, explain the pathophysiology of the severe hearing loss that is present in Brn4-deficient mice and that is caused by the decreased EP [4].

To investigate the function of Brn4 in the cochlea, we developed Brn4-deficient mice as a model of DFN3 non-syndromic deafness [4]. Although, these mice show no gross morphological changes in their cochleae, there are severe ultrastructural alterations in the cochlear spiral ligament fibrocytes, which might have caused the decrease in EP that resulted in severe hearing loss [4]. This suggests that the initial pathology of Brn4 deficiency may be related to an impairment of intercellular junctions including gap junctions.

Cochlear fibrocytes of the mesenchymal non-sensory regions express gap junction proteins such as Cx26 and Cx30 and have important roles in the cochlear physiology of hearing, including the transport of potassium ions to generate an endocochlear potential in the endolymph, which is essential for the transduction of sound by hair cells. Cx26 and Cx30 are the two most abundantly expressed gap junction proteins in the cochlea, and both Cx26 and Cx30 are expressed at high levels in the supporting cells of the organ of Corti and fibrocytes in the spiral ligament [5]. Furthermore, co-immunostaining indicates that Cx26 and Cx30 are expressed in the same gap junction plaques (GJPs), and their co-assembly has been confirmed by co-immunoprecipitation of proteins extracted from cochlear tissues [5].

Mutations in the Cx26 and Cx30 genes are well known to be responsible for hereditary sensorineural deafness [6] [7], as are mutations in POU3F4 [1]. In this study, we analyzed the morphology, structure, or length formation of GJPs, the functional molecular complex of the gap junction, of Brn4-deficient mice at different stages by confocal microscopy and three-dimensional graphic reconstructions to clarify the relationship between the connexins and Brn4.

## Materials and Methods

### Animals and ethics statement

The care, maintenance, and treatment of animals in these studies followed protocols approved by the Institutional Animal Care and Use Committee at Juntendo University (Permit Number: 250192). 2–6 week old male mice were deeply anesthetized with an i.p. injection of Nembutal (50 mg/ml DAINIPPON SUMITOMO PHARMA) 0.5 mg per 10 g body weight before all examinations. POU3F4 mutant mice, in which the coding region was replaced with a pgk-neo (neomycin-resistance gene driven by the phosphoglycerate kinase gene promoter) cassette [4] were maintained in a C57BL/6 background. The absence of Brn4 protein was confirmed by immunohistochemistry with rabbit anti-POU3F4 (SIGMA) in inner ear frozen sections (data not shown). We minimized, to the extent possible, the number of animals used and their suffering.

### Immunohistochemistry

Mice were anesthetized and killed, and the inner-ear tissues were then removed. The cochleae were further dissected and fixed in 4% paraformaldehyde. Immunofluorescence staining with antibodies against Cx26 (mouse IgG; LifeSpan Biosciences) and Cx30 (rabbit IgG; Invitrogen) was performed on whole-mount preparations of the finely dissected organ of Corti, which included inner sulcus cells (ISCs). We incubated the tissues in the antibody solutions for 1 hour at room temperature after blocking (with 2% BSA in 0.01 M PBS). Fluorescence confocal images were obtained with a LSM510-META confocal microscope (Carl Zeiss). Cx30 was immunolabeled by red fluorescence, Cy3 (rabbit IgG; Sigma Aldrich), and observed by confocal laser microscopy using a 543-nm laser. Cx26 was immunolabeled by green fluorescence, Alexa488 (mouse IgG; Life Technologies), and observed by confocal microscopy using a 488-nm laser. Three-dimensional images were constructed with *z*-stacked confocal images by IMARIS (Bitplane). Quantitative analysis of the GJP length (mean ± S.E.M.) was measured with an LSM Image Browser (Zeiss), and data were compared using Student's *t*-test (Microsoft Excel).

### Western blotting

Mouse cochlear proteins were extracted with T-PER Tissue Protein Extraction Reagent (Thermo Scientific) from at least six cochleae, which included the organ of Corti, lateral wall, and stria vascularis. The proteins were resolved by SDS–polyacrylamide gel electrophoresis (PAGE) with 4–20% mini-PROTEAN TGX gels (Bio-Rad Laboratories, Inc.) and then transferred onto a polyvinyl difluoride (PVDF) membrane (Amersham Hybond-P; GE Healthcare). After blocking, membranes were processed through sequential incubations with rabbit anti-Cx26 (1:1000; Invitrogen), rabbit anti-Cx30 (1:1000; Invitrogen) and mouse monoclonal anti–β-actin (1:5000; Sigma) with horseradish peroxidase–conjugated anti–rabbit or anti–mouse IgG (1:20000; GE Healthcare) as the secondary antibody. Amersham ECL Prime Western Blotting Detection Reagent (GE Healthcare) was then used for visualization, and the signal was developed on X-ray film (Amersham Hyperfilm ECL; GE Healthcare). Each experiment was repeated at least three times. The densitometric analysis of band intensities was performed with the NIH ImageJ software, and data were compared using Student's *t*-test (Microsoft Excel).

### Auditory brainstem response (ABR)

All the recordings were performed in the soundproof chamber with electrostatic shield to avoid the electrical noise. Mice ranging in age from 2 weeks to 6 weeks were studied. For the ABR measurement, stainless-steel needle electrodes were placed at the vertex and ventrolateral to the left and right ears. The ABR was measured using the waveform storing and stimulus control of the Scope software from the Power Laboratory system (model PowerLab4/25; AD Instruments), and the electroencephalogram recording was made with an extracellular amplifier AC PreAmplifier (model P-55; Astro-Med). Acoustic stimuli were delivered to the mice through a coupler-type speaker (model ES1spc; Bio Research Center). The threshold was determined for frequencies of 8 and 20 kHz from a set of responses at varying intensities with 5-dB intervals, and the electrical signals were averaged at 512 repetitions. The maximum output level was 93.5 and 83.4 dB at 8 and 20 kHz, respectively, and 5 dB was added to these values when the ABR was not detected in the maximum output for statistical analysis.

### Transmission electron microscopy

Animals were deeply anesthetized and perfused intracardially with 0.01 M PBS, followed by 2% paraformaldehyde and 2% glutaraldehyde in 0.1 M cacodylate buffer. The cochleae were opened and flushed with the fixative for 2 h at room temperature. After washing, the specimens were post-fixed for 1.5 h in 2% osmium tetroxide in 0.1 M phosphate buffer and then were dehydrated through a graded ethanol series and embedded in Epon (Oken Shoji). Ultrathin sections of the cochleae were cut, stained with uranyl acetate and lead citrate, and examined by electron microscopy (HT-7700, Hitachi).

## Results

In this study, we performed a detailed analysis of cochlear GJPs using a mouse model of a major type of DFN3. These mice have severe sensorineural hearing loss together with decreased EP, fewer cytoplasmic extensions, and a reduction in the cytoplasmic volume and the number of mitochondria in the fibrocytes of the spiral ligament, although no abnormalities have been observed in other organs [4].

In littermate controls, gap junctions formed linear GJPs along the cell-cell junction sites with adjacent cells, and these formed pentagonal or hexagonal outlines of normal inner sulcus cells and border cells (Figure 1 A, C, E, G, I, K). The GJPs in 6-week-old Brn4-deficient mice did not show the normal linear structure but instead were present as small spots around the cell-cell junction sites (Figure 1 J, L). The gap junction units of the Brn4-deficient mice were substantially shorter than those in the control mice (Figure 1 I, K). In 2-week-old littermate control and Brn4-deficient mice, GJPs formed linear units around the cells (Figure 1 A–D). In 4-week-old littermate control and Brn4-deficient mice, the linear structure of the GJPs was present, although some plaques were disrupted and scattered in the cochleae of Brn4-deficient mice (Figure 1 E–H). In 6-week-old Brn4-deficient mice, a number of small GJPs that contained Cx30 were scattered around the cell-cell junction sites (Figure 1 J, L). The length of each GJP was notably shorter than those in the littermate controls (Figure 1 I, K).

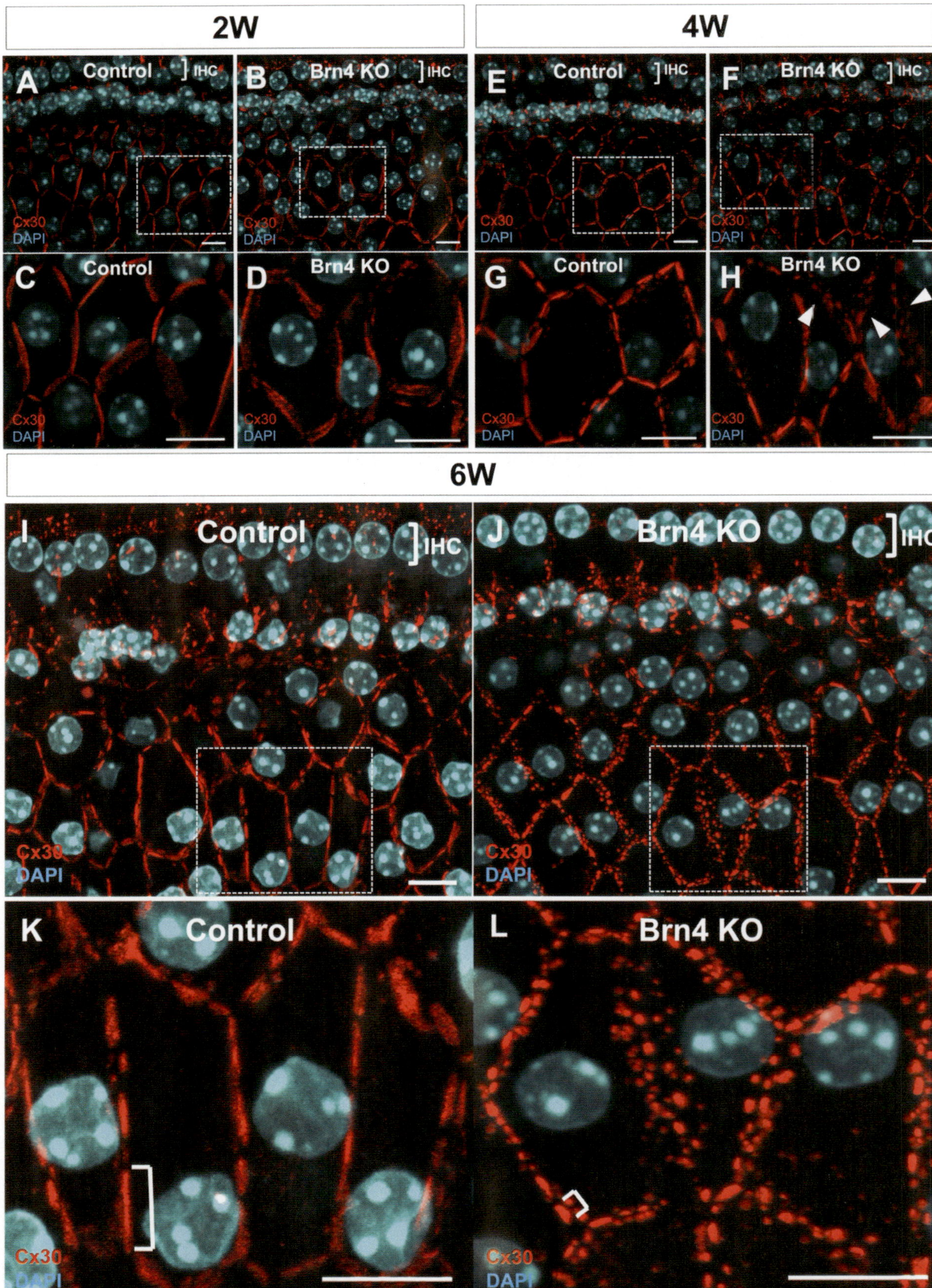


**Figure 1. Brn4-deficient mice show a drastic disruption of GJPs with increasing age.** Z-Stack images of cochlear inner sulcus cells from 2-, 4-, and 6-week-old littermate control and Brn4-deficient mice were obtained by confocal microscopy. GJPs were immunolabeled for Cx30 (red) (A–L). Nuclei were counterstained with DAPI (blue) (A–L). The positions of inner hair cells (IHCs) indicate the orientation of the irages (A, B, E, F, I and J).

High-magnification images of each boxed region in A, B, E, F, I and J are shown in C, D, G, H, K and L. The GJPs in 6-week-old Brn4-deficient mice were present as small spots around the cell-cell junction sites (J, L). In 2-week-old and 4-week-old littermate control and Brn4-deficient mice, the linear structure of the GJPs was present, although some plaques 4-week-old Brn4-deficient mice were disrupted and scattered (H, arrowheads). The lengths of the largest GJPs (brackets in K and L) along a single cell border were analyzed and are shown in Figure 4. Scale bars indicate 10 μm.

In littermate controls, gap junctions were composed mainly of Cx26 and Cx30 (Figure 2 A–C). GJPs co-immunolabeled for Cx26 and Cx30 in inner sulcus cells were also observed in Brn4-deficient mice (Figure 2 D–F). Although there was a possibility that the Connexin-immunostaining might not indicate gap junction but hemichannel, the transmission electron microscopy showed the typical structures for gap junctions with inter-membrane layer also in Brn4-deficient mice as well as littermate controls (Figure S1).

In the detailed analysis with three-dimensional graphic reconstruction of the GJP structure in the inner sulcus cells (ISCs; Figure 1 I, K), cochleae from adult littermate control mice showed large planar GJPs (Figure 3 A) at the cell borders that formed orderly pentagonal or hexagonal outlines around normal ISCs. In contrast, cochleae from Brn4-deficient mice (Figure 1 J, L) showed drastically fragmented small vesicle-like GJPs (Figure 3 B). To compare the size differences of the GJPs between Brn4-deficient mice and their littermate controls, the lengths of the largest GJPs with Cx30 (e.g., brackets in Figure 1 K, L) along a single cell border were analyzed in four Brn4-deficient mice and four control littermates. In 6-week-old Brn4-deficient mice, the average length of the GJPs was significantly shorter than that in the littermate controls (Figure 4).

In addition to GJP disruptions by the confocal analysis, 3D construction and their size analysis (Figure 1, 3 and 4), the significantly reduced levels of Cx26 and Cx30 in the Brn4-deficient mice (Figure 5) suggested that the gap junction macromolecular complex had degraded. Recently, we reported that assembly of the cochlear gap junction macromolecular complex requires connexin 26 [8]. In this paper, we demonstrated that

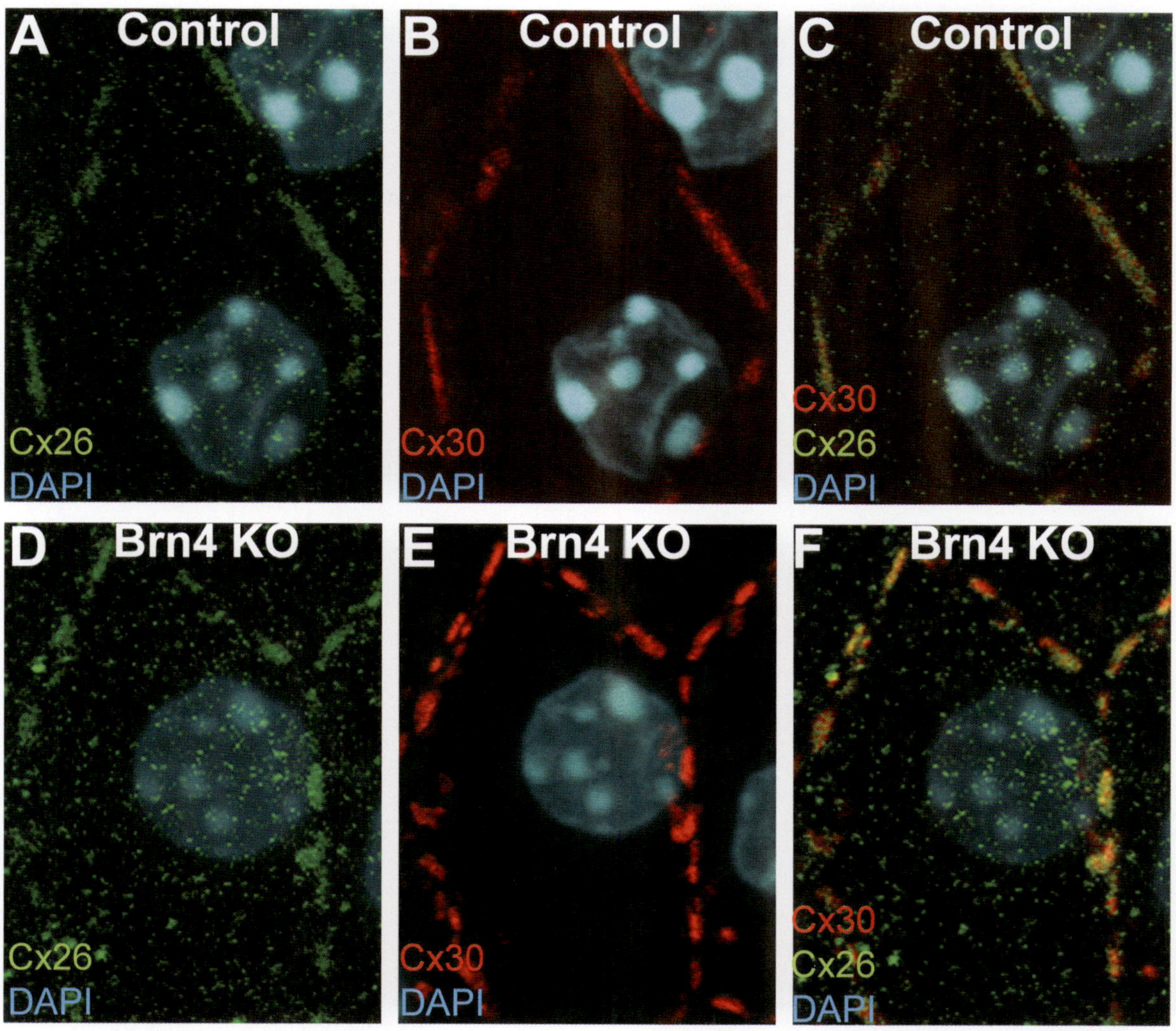


**Figure 2. GJPs in Brn4-deficient cochleae are composed of Cx26 and Cx30 as in control littermates.** Inner sulcus cells in cochlear whole-mount sections from a 6-week-old littermate control (A–C) and Brn4-deficient (knockout, KO) mouse (D–F). Images were obtained by confocal microscopy and z-stacking after immunolabeling for Cx26 (green) (A, D) and Cx30 (red) (B, E). Merged images are also shown (C, F). Nuclei were counterstained with DAPI (blue) (A–F). Bars indicate 10 μm.

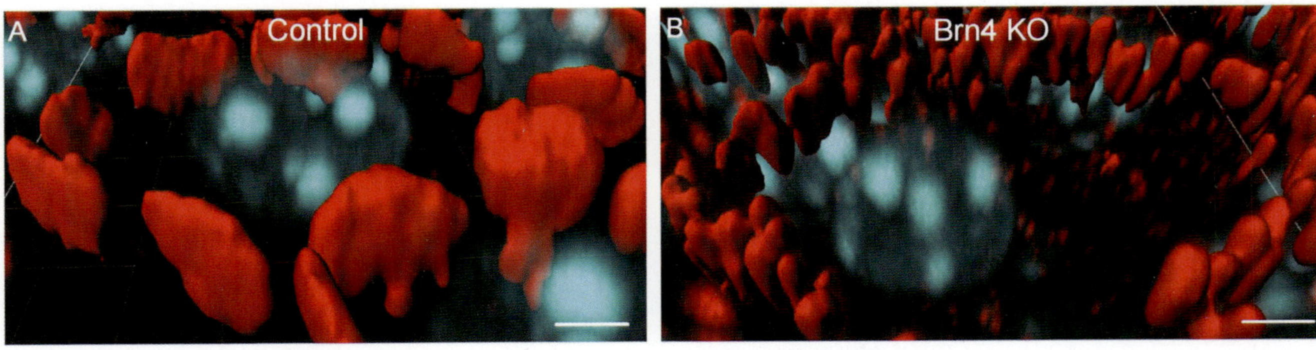


**Figure 3. Three-dimensional reconstruction shows disrupted GJPs in Brn4-deficient mice.** Three-dimensional images were reconstructed to show the detailed structure of GJPs from the *z*-stack images shown in Figure 1 I, J. GJP formation in adult (6w) cochleae from a littermate control (A) and a Brn4-deficient mouse (B). GJPs were immunolabeled for Cx30 (red), and nuclei were counterstained with DAPI (blue) (A, B). Scale bars indicate 5 μm.

cochlear gap junction plaque, macromolecular complex were mainly composed of Connexin 26 and Connexin 30, and this molecular complex were degraded together with the activation of endocytosis with upregulation of Caveolin proteins, in case of the Cx26-deficiency. It has also been reported in the other papers that the gap junction molecular complex were degraded via some proteasome pathways such as ubiquitination, autophagy, or endocytosis [9–11]. To assess the change in hearing function, ABR analyses were performed for 2- and 6-week-old male Brn4-deficient mice. ABR thresholds were significantly higher in the 6-week-old mice than in the 2-week-old Brn4-deficient mice (Figure 6, Figure S2). On the other hand, wild type mice in 2 and 6-week old showed normal ABR threshold (9.4±2.9 dB SPL, $n=5$ for 2-week-old and 4.8±2.6 dB SPL, $n=7$ for 6-week-old wild type mice).

## Discussion

In the present study, we examined the novel molecular pathology of hereditary deafness caused by Brn4 gene deficiency in a mouse model of DFN3. An abnormal morphology of the cell-to-cell adhesion of fibrocytes has been observed in 11-week-old Brn4-deficient mice [4]. At the spiral ligament, type IV and V otic fibrocytes are absent in these Brn4-deficient mice [4]. Cx26 expression is lost in type I and V fibrocyte regions of the spiral ligament [4]. In postnatal day 12 mice, Cx26 expression in type I and V fibrocyte regions is present in wild-type mice but not in Brn4-deficient mice [4]. In contrast to the spiral ligament, the cellular and molecular pathology of cochlear supporting cells has not been reported. In our previous study [4,12], we have not identified any changes in connexin expression of the lateral wall fibrocytes in younger stage than 11-week old. However in the present study, we analyzed the subcellular expression of connexins with the 3D structure of GJP acquired from the z-scan confocal images of whole mount cochlea together with quantitative western blotting, and found the significant change in connexin expressions in postnatal development of Brn4-deficient mouse. Here we showed that Brn4 substantially contributes to cochlear gap junction properties to maintain the proper EP in cochleae, similar

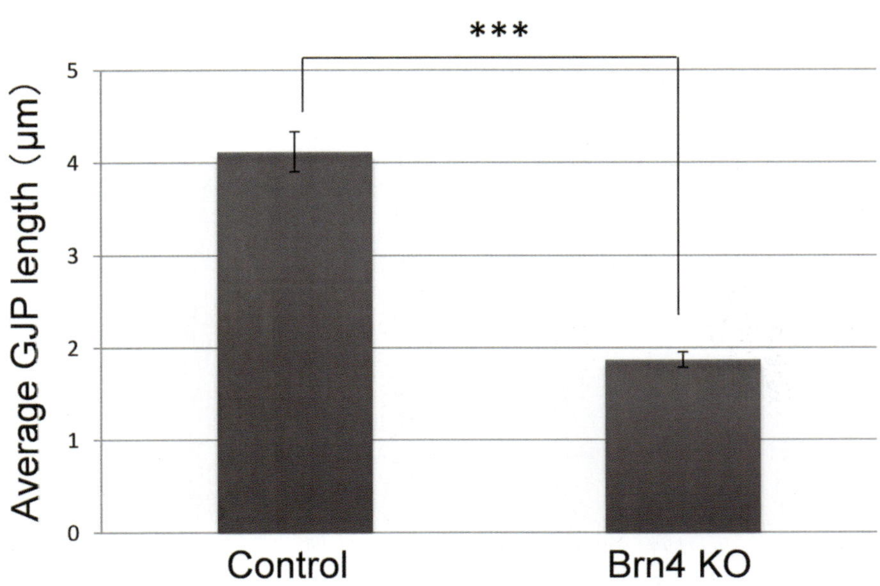


**Figure 4. GJPs were significantly shorter in Brn4-deficient mice as compared with littermate controls at 6 weeks.** The lengths of the largest GJPs (e.g., brackets in Figure 1 K and L) along a single cell border were measured in the *z*-stack confocal images and are expressed as the mean ± Standard Error (SE) ($n=81$ GJPs per mouse type). ***$P=6.49\times10^{-16}$ (Student's *t*-test).

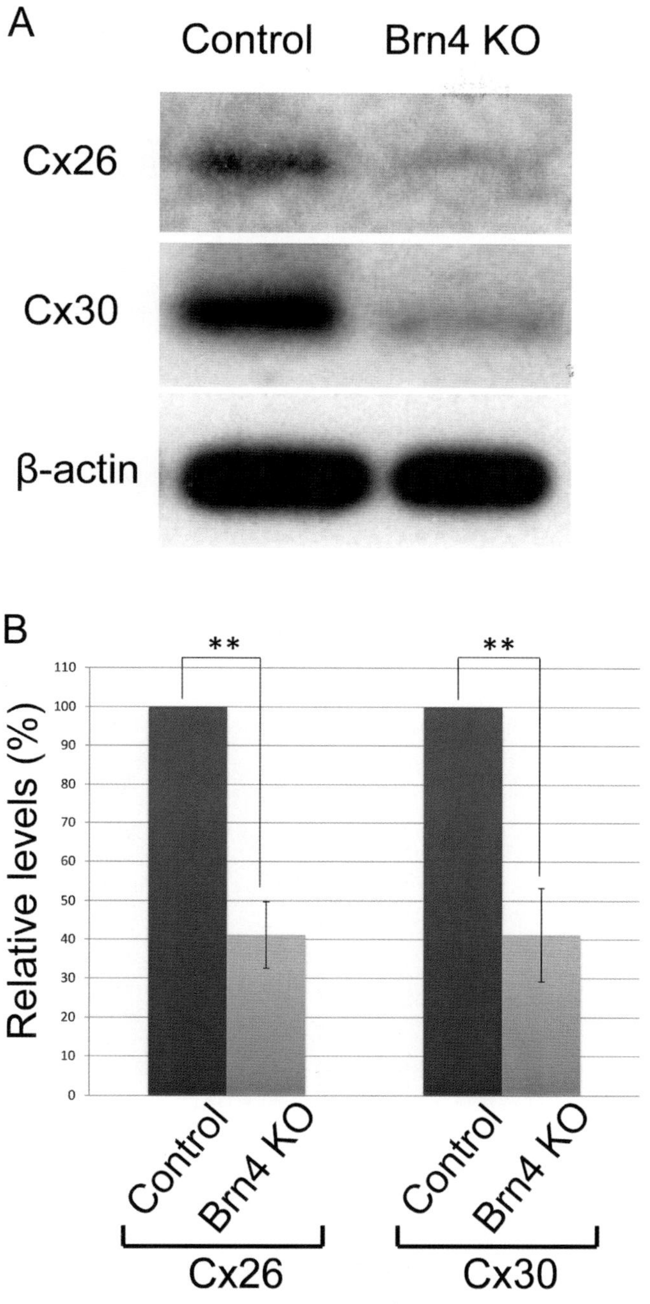


**Figure 5. Gap junction protein levels were reduced in Brn4-deficient mice at 6 weeks.** Western blot analysis of Cx26 and Cx30 was performed in 6-week-old Brn4-deficient mice and littermate controls. The level of Cx26 and Cx30 was normalized to the corresponding β-actin levels and expressed relative to the amount present in each of the littermate controls. Values represent the mean ± SE ($n = 3$ mice). $^{***}P = 7.943 \times 10^{-3}$ for Cx26 and $^{***}P = 8.137 \times 10^{-3}$ for Cx30, Student's *t*-test.

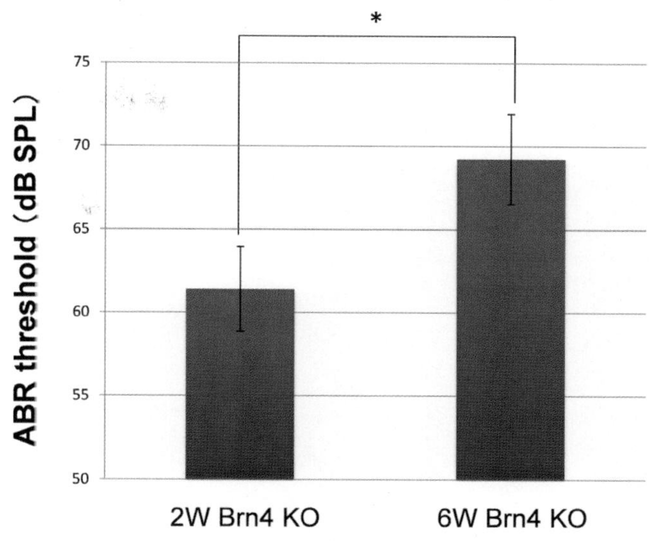


**Figure 6. ABR thresholds were higher in Brn4-deficient mice at 6 weeks as compared with 2 weeks.** ABR thresholds were analyzed in 2- and 6-week-old Brn4-deficient mice. In 2-week-old mice, the ABR threshold was 61.4±2.5 dB SPL ($n = 5$ mice), and in 6-week-old mice the ABR threshold was 69.2±2.7 dB SPL ($n = 6$ mice). Values represent the mean ± SE. $^{*}P = 3.40 \times 10^{-2}$ (Student's *t*-test).

to connexin-related deafness. This finding suggests that the hearing loss was caused by an effect on connexins such as Cx26 and Cx30, which represent the proteins that are most frequently mutated in hereditary deafness. The disruption of GJPs observed after 4 weeks in the Brn4-deficient mice was also observed in our two Cx26 mutant mice [8]. This suggests that Brn4 expression is directly or indirectly involved in gap junction formation in ISCs. The reduction in the GJP area may then abolish the proper biophysical potential needed for intercellular communication in the cochlea, resulting in a significant elevation of the ABR threshold (Figure 6). This may explain why Brn4-deficient mice showed significantly decreased EPs in our previous study [4]. In that study, EP was not absent but reduced from 85 mV (wild-type mice) to 38 mV in 11-week-old male Brn4 deficient mice. Although we have not measured EP before 11 weeks old and the biochemical or structural changes of GJP have not been detected around 2-week-old mice, there is a possibility that the EP was not absent but already lower than the control level (~+80 mV) in 2-week-old, and then progressively reduced to around 38 mV or maintained low EP level by 11 weeks old, because the ABR data in the present study (Figure 6) indicated the hearing loss already in 2-week-old Brn4-KO mice. Currently, the downstream targets of POU3F4, including gap junction genes and their proposed transcription factors in the cochlear supporting cells, are unknown. Only a few genes have been reported to be involved in fibrocyte differentiation including Otospiralin (Otos) [13] and Tbx18 [14], although Song et al. reported that neither Otos nor Tbx18 expression was affected in the spiral ligament of Brn4-deficient mice [15]. Although the entire molecular pathway between Brn4 and the cochlear gap junction has not yet been worked out, our data clearly demonstrated that POU3F4 affects the expression and assembly of the gap junction proteins Cx30 (GJB6) and Cx26 (GJB2) in cochlear supporting cells. GJP degradation along with a decrease in the component connexins may explain the decrease in the EP and the severe hearing loss in Brn4-deficient mice and DFN3 patients. Furthermore, gene therapy targeting cochlear gap junction proteins, such as Cx26 gene transfer, may also be effective for DFN3 patients.

## Supporting Information

**Figure S1 Ultrastructures of gap junctions in Brn4 deficient mice by Transmission Electron Microscopy (TEM).** Ultrathin sections of ISCs showed the gap junctions in 6-week-old Brn4 deficient mice (B) with an inter-membrane layer

between both clearly visible plasma membranes that maintains the same distance (2–4 nm) in both mutant mice and control littermates (A). There were no obvious differences between Brn4 deficient mice (B) and control mice (A). Inset shows high-magnification image of boxed area, which contains a gap junction. Bars indicate 100 nm.
(DOCX)

**Figure S2 ABR waveforms of control (+/Y) and Brn4 deficient (−/Y) males at 6 weeks old of age, measured at 60-, 70- and 80-dB SPL.**

## Acknowledgments

We thank M. Yoshida for help with transmission electron microscopy, K. Kobayashi, Y. Yokoyama and B. Kuerban for experimental assistance.

## Author Contributions

Conceived and designed the experiments: K. Kamiya. Performed the experiments: YK K. Karasawa. Analyzed the data: YK KI. Contributed reagents/materials/analysis tools: OM YS TN. Wrote the paper: K. Kamiya.

## References

1. de Kok YJ, Merkx GF, van der Maarel SM, Huber I, Malcolm S, et al. (1995) A duplication/paracentric inversion associated with familial X-linked deafness (DFN3) suggests the presence of a regulatory element more than 400 kb upstream of the POU3F4 gene. Hum Mol Genet 4: 2145–2150.
2. Phippard D, Heydemann A, Lechner M, Lu L, Lee D, et al. (1998) Changes in the subcellular localization of the Brn4 gene product precede mesenchymal remodeling of the otic capsule. Hear Res 120: 77–85.
3. Coate TM, Raft S, Zhao X, Ryan AK, Crenshaw EB 3rd, et al. (2012) Otic mesenchyme cells regulate spiral ganglion axon fasciculation through a Pou3f4/EphA4 signaling pathway. Neuron 73: 49–63.
4. Minowa O, Ikeda K, Sugitani Y, Oshima T, Nakai S, et al. (1999) Altered cochlear fibrocytes in a mouse model of DFN3 nonsyndromic deafness. Science 285: 1408–1411.
5. Ahmad S, Chen S, Sun J, Lin X (2003) Connexins 26 and 30 are co-assembled to form gap junctions in the cochlea of mice. Biochem Biophys Res Commun 307: 362–368.
6. Kelsell DP, Dunlop J, Stevens HP, Lench NJ, Liang JN, et al. (1997) Connexin 26 mutations in hereditary non-syndromic sensorineural deafness. Nature 387: 80–83.
7. del Castillo I, Villamar M, Moreno-Pelayo MA, del Castillo FJ, Alvarez A, et al. (2002) A deletion involving the connexin 30 gene in nonsyndromic hearing impairment. N Engl J Med 346: 243–249.
8. Kamiya K, Yum SW, Kurebayashi N, Muraki M, Ogawa K, et al. (2014) Assembly of the cochlear gap junction macromolecular complex requires connexin 26. J Clin Invest 124: 1598–1607.
9. Bejarano E, Yuste A, Patel B, Stout RF Jr, Spray DC, et al. (2014) Connexins modulate autophagosome biogenesis. Nat Cell Biol 16: 401–414.
10. Falk MM, Kells RM, Berthoud VM (2014) Degradation of connexins and gap junctions. FEBS Lett 588: 1221–1229.
11. Gilleron J, Fiorini C, Carette D, Avondet C, Falk MM, et al. (2008) Molecular reorganization of Cx43, Zo-1 and Src complexes during the endocytosis of gap junction plaques in response to a non-genomic carcinogen. J Cell Sci 121: 4069–4078.
12. Xia AP, Kikuchi T, Minowa O, Katori Y, Oshima T, et al. (2002) Late-onset hearing loss in a mouse model of DFN3 non-syndromic deafness: morphologic and immunohistochemical analyses. Hear Res 166: 150–158.
13. Delprat B, Ruel J, Guitton MJ, Hamard G, Lenoir M, et al. (2005) Deafness and cochlear fibrocyte alterations in mice deficient for the inner ear protein otospiralin. Mol Cell Biol 25: 847–853.
14. Trowe MO, Maier H, Schweizer M, Kispert A (2008) Deafness in mice lacking the T-box transcription factor Tbx18 in otic fibrocytes. Development 135: 1725–1734.
15. Song MH, Choi SY, Wu L, Oh SK, Lee HK, et al. (2011) Pou3f4 deficiency causes defects in otic fibrocytes and stria vascularis by different mechanisms. Biochem Biophys Res Commun 404: 528–533.

# Activated Notch Causes Deafness by Promoting a Supporting Cell Phenotype in Developing Auditory Hair Cells

**Grace Savoy-Burke[1], Felicia A. Gilels[3], Wei Pan[1,2], Diana Pratt[1], Jianwen Que[2], Lin Gan[1,3], Patricia M. White[3], Amy E. Kiernan[1,2]***

**1** Department of Ophthalmology, University of Rochester Medical Center, Rochester, New York, United States of America, **2** Department of Biomedical Genetics, University of Rochester Medical Center, Rochester, New York, United States of America, **3** Department of Neurobiology and Anatomy, University of Rochester Medical Center, Rochester, New York, United States of America

## Abstract

***Purpose:*** To determine whether activated Notch can promote a supporting cell fate during sensory cell differentiation in the inner ear.

***Methods:*** An activated form of the Notch1 receptor (NICD) was expressed in early differentiating hair cells using a Gfi1-Cre mouse allele. To determine the effects of activated Notch on developing hair cells, Gfi1-NICD animals and their littermate controls were assessed at 5 weeks for hearing by measuring auditory brainstem responses (ABRs) and distortion product otoacoustic emissions (DPOAEs). The differentiation of NICD-expressing hair cells was assessed at postnatal day (P) 6, 11 and 20, using histological and molecular markers for hair cells, as well as supporting cells/progenitor cells. We also examined whether the effects of Notch were mediated by SOX2, a gene expressed in supporting cells and a likely downstream target of Notch, by crossing an inducible form of SOX2 to the Gfi1-Cre.

***Results:*** Activation of Notch1 in developing auditory hair cells causes profound deafness. The NICD-expressing hair cells switch off a number of hair cell markers and lose their characteristic morphology. Instead, NICD-expressing hair cells adopt a morphology resembling supporting cells and upregulate a number of supporting cell markers. These effects do not appear to be mediated by SOX2, because although expression of SOX2 caused some hearing impairment, the SOX2-expressing hair cells did not downregulate hair cell markers nor exhibit a supporting cell-like phenotype.

***Conclusions:*** Our data show that Notch signaling inhibits hair cell differentiation and promotes a supporting cell-like phenotype, and that these effects are unlikely to be mediated by SOX2.

**Editor:** Domingos Henrique, Instituto de Medicina Molecular, Portugal

**Funding:** Support was provided by the National Institutes of Health www.nih.gov; DC009250 (AK), DC008856 (LG), DK082650 (JQ), Research to Prevent Blindness, http://www.rpbusa.org/rpb/; Research to Prevent Blindness unrestricted grant to the Department of Ophthalmology at the University of Rochester Medical Center, the Schmitt Program on Integrative Brain Research (AK and PW) (http://www.urmc.rochester.edu/neurobiology-anatomy/schmitt/). The funders had no role in study design, data collection and analysis, decision to publish, or preparation of the manuscript.

**Competing Interests:** The authors have declared that no competing interests exist.

* Email: amy_kiernan@urmc.rochester.edu

## Introduction

The vertebrate inner ear is a complex structure that includes a variety of sensory regions that transduce both sound and vestibular information. Each sensory region is composed of two major cell types, the sensory hair cell and associated supporting cells, which arise from a common progenitor [1]. The mosaic arrangement of the sensory cells, in which each hair cell is surrounded by supporting cells, led investigators to suggest that the pattern was produced through the process of lateral inhibition mediated by the Notch signaling pathway [2,3]. Notch signaling is an evolutionarily conserved pathway in which interactions between the cell-bound ligands (Jagged1–2, and Delta-like1,3–4) and receptors (NOTCH1-4) trigger the release of the activated form of the receptor (the intracellular domain or NICD) to the nucleus where it interacts with the nuclear effector RBPJ (also known as RBPjκ or CSL) and causes changes in transcription (reviewed in [4]).

Disruptions in Notch signaling in a variety of different vertebrate models have been shown to cause alterations in sensory patterning, supporting the lateral inhibitory model in the ear [5–9]. Based on studies from Drosophila [10], a model of lateral inhibition in the ear mediated by Notch signaling has emerged in which cells developing as the primary cell type (the hair cell) express a Notch ligand and activate Notch in the surrounding cells, thereby inhibiting them from adopting the same cell fate. These surrounding cells will instead adopt the secondary cell fate, in this case the supporting cell fate [11,12]. This traditional model of lateral inhibition supports a role for Notch in inhibiting the primary cell fate, but indicates no instructive role in the secondary cell fate. This idea was challenged a number of years ago in the vertebrate central nervous system, in which it was shown that Notch can play an instructive role in the glial cell fate [13–16]. For example, expression of an activated form of Notch in the retina leads to an increase in cells expressing Müller glial markers [13]. Similarly in the forebrain Notch promotes the acquisition of a radial glial phenotype [14]; while in the cerebellum, loss of a novel Notch ligand (DNER) or Jagged1 leads to defects in Bergmann glial differentiation [15,16]. However, whether Notch can play an instructive role in non-glial cell fates, such as the supporting cells of the inner ear, is not known.

Here, to test the role of Notch activation in supporting cell differentiation, we expressed an activated form of the receptor (NICD) in early differentiating hair cells to determine whether Notch signaling can (1) prevent the adoption of the hair cell fate and (2) promote the adoption of the supporting cell fate. Our results show that activation of Notch in differentiating hair cells leads to profound deafness. Histologically, the auditory hair cells shut off a number of different hair cell markers and the inner hair cells lose their characteristic morphology. Specifically, the NICD-expressing inner hair cells gradually adopt a more supporting cell-like morphology and express several supporting cell markers. In addition, our data demonstrates that these effects are not mediated by SOX2, a gene expressed in supporting cells that is upregulated by activating Notch. These results show that Notch actively promotes the supporting cell phenotype in addition to suppressing sensory hair cell marker expression, and that these effects are not dependent upon SOX2 expression.

## Materials and Methods

### Mice

The mouse strains used were as follows: *Gfi1-Cre* [17], *ROSA26-NICD* [18], *ROSA26-LacZ* [19], *ROSA26-SOX2* [20]. The day of birth was considered postnatal day (P)0. This study was carried out in strict accordance with the recommendations in the Guide for the Care and Use of Laboratory Animals of the National Institutes of Health. The animal protocol was approved by the University Committee of Animal Resources (UCAR Protocol No. 101414) at the University of Rochester.

### Histology

**Paraffin sections.** The inner ear was dissected from postnatal mice, fixed in 4% paraformaldehyde overnight and washed in PBS. Ears were then decalcified in 0.2M EDTA (pH 7.3) for 14 days. The tissue was dehydrated through serial EtOH washes from 70% to 100%, cleared in xylene, embedded in paraffin and then sectioned at a thickness of 10 µm.

**Frozen sections.** Heads of P6 mice were bisected, fixed in 4% paraformaldehyde overnight and embedded in Tissue Freezing Medium. Half heads were then cryosectioned at 20 µm.

### Immunohistochemistry

Antigen retrieval was performed on all paraffin sections prior to staining by incubating in 10 mM Sodium Citrate Buffer (pH 6, 0.05% Tween 20) for 20 minutes at 98°C. Sections were incubated in primary antibodies overnight at 4°C, secondary antibodies for 2 hours at room temperature and DAPI nucleic acid stain (1:24,000) for 8 minutes. The primary antibodies used were as follows: rabbit anti-MYO6 (Proteus Biosciences), rabbit anti-calretinin (Millipore), mouse anti-parvalbumin (Sigma), goat anti-prestin (Santa Cruz), goat anti-SOX2 (Santa Cruz) anti-P27KIP1 (Lab Vision), anti-PROX1 (Chemicon), anti-Na-K-ATPase α1 (Millipore), and anti-β-galactosidase (Abcam).

### Quantification of inner hair cell marker expression

Images of P20 paraffin sections were captured through the mid-modiolar region of the cochlea (ranging between 24 and 36 sections for each mutant or control including roughly equal numbers of basal and apical regions) and relative expression levels of each marker were assessed exclusively in the inner hair cells. Three controls and three mutants were analyzed for each of the hair cell markers (calretinin, parvalbumin and myosinVI). When inner hair cells were brightly and fully stained by the hair cell marker a score of 2 was given (strong), and cells in which hair cell markers were completely negative were assigned a score of 0 (absent). In cases where only a portion of the cell demonstrated signal, or the signal was very low compared to average control expression, these images received a score of 1 (weak).

### Auditory testing

Auditory testing was conducted using a Smart EP Universal Smart Box (Intelligent Hearing Systems). 5 week old mice were anesthetized with an intraperitoneal injection of ketamine (80 mg/kg) in a sterile acepromazine/saline mixture (3 mg/kg). A 10B+ (high frequency transducer/stimulator) probe was placed at the opening to the external auditory meatus. ABR stimuli were 5-ms clicks, or 5-ms tone pips presented at 5 frequencies between 8 and 32 kHz. Stimuli began at 75 dB amplitude and decreased by 5 dB steps to 15–25 dB. 512 sweeps were averaged for each frequency and amplitude. Electrical responses were measured with three subdermal needle electrodes (Grass): one inserted beneath each pinna, and a third, the ground electrode, placed at the vertex. ABR thresholds for a particular frequency were determined by the last visible trace where waves one and two were seen for each stimulus (dB). Wave amplitudes and latencies were determined using IHS software computing capabilities.

To measure DPOAEs, we measured the amplitude of evoked otoacoustic emissions to paired pure tones of frequencies f1 and f2, where $f1/f2 = 1.2$ and the f1 level was 10 dB above f2. 32 sweeps were made in 5 dB steps starting with f1 at 65 dB and ending at 40 dB. For our equipment, the threshold of DPOAE detection is 3 dB. To calculate the threshold, we used linear regression to fit a line to the points closest to the threshold and calculated the level of f2 necessary for an output of 3 dB.

## Results

### Activation of Notch in early developing hair cells causes deafness

To test the role of Notch during sensory cell differentiation, we generated a mouse model in which activated Notch is expressed in early developing hair cells, allowing us to examine the effects of activated Notch on both hair cell and supporting cell differentiation. To generate this model, we crossed mice expressing Cre under the Gfi1 promoter [17] to mice expressing an activated form of the Notch receptor, NICD (Notch Intracellular Domain) under the ubiquitous ROSA26 promoter [18] (Fig. 1A). Gfi1 is a transcription factor expressed soon after hair cells begin differentiating in the ear, approximately embryonic (E)13–14 in the vestibular system and E15–16 in the cochlea [17,21,22]. The ROSA26-NICD allele contains an intervening floxed-stop cassette, preventing NICD expression unless Cre is present. Offspring containing both a Cre allele and an NICD allele (hereafter referred to as Gfi1-NICD mutants) were born and survived until adulthood. In addition, a ROSA26-lacZ allele [19] was also bred into the cross, so that hair cells expressing NICD would be marked by ß-galactosidase. Upon weaning it was apparent that some of the Gfi1-NICD offspring lacked a Preyer reflex, the ear flick response to sound, indicating a hearing impairment. To investigate this further, we measured auditory brainstem responses (ABRs) and distortion product otoacoustic emissions (DPOAEs) in Gfi1-NICD mutants (n = 8) and their littermate controls (n = 8). Results of the ABRs showed that the Gfi1-NICD mutants showed no responses to even the highest levels of sound (80 dB SPL), indicating profound deafness (Fig. 1B). In addition, measurements of outer hair cell function, DPOAEs, also demonstrated raised thresholds when compared to controls at most frequencies, indicating that outer hair cell function is compromised (Fig. 1C). These results show that expression of activated Notch in early differentiating hair cells affects the function of the organ of Corti.

## Hair cell markers are downregulated in NICD-expressing hair cells and SOX2 is upregulated

To examine the effects of activated Notch on the molecular and histological differentiation of cochlear hair cells, we sectioned postnatal day (P)20 Gfi1-NICD cochleae and littermate controls and examined the expression of several hair cell markers by immunohistochemistry. Results of these studies showed that a number of established hair cell markers, including calretinin, parvalbumin, and myosin VI, were either not expressed in the hair cells or were severely downregulated when compared to controls (Fig. 2). In the case of calretinin and parvalbumin, the majority of both inner and outer hair cells did not express these markers (Fig. 2A–F). In the case of myosin VI, while the majority of inner hair cells downregulated this marker, the outer hair cells largely maintained expression of myosin VI (Fig. 2G–I). The absence of hair cell markers was not due to cell loss, as the cells still expressed ß-galactosidase (Fig. 2C,F,I). Inner hair cell marker expression was quantified for each marker (myosin VI, calretinin, and

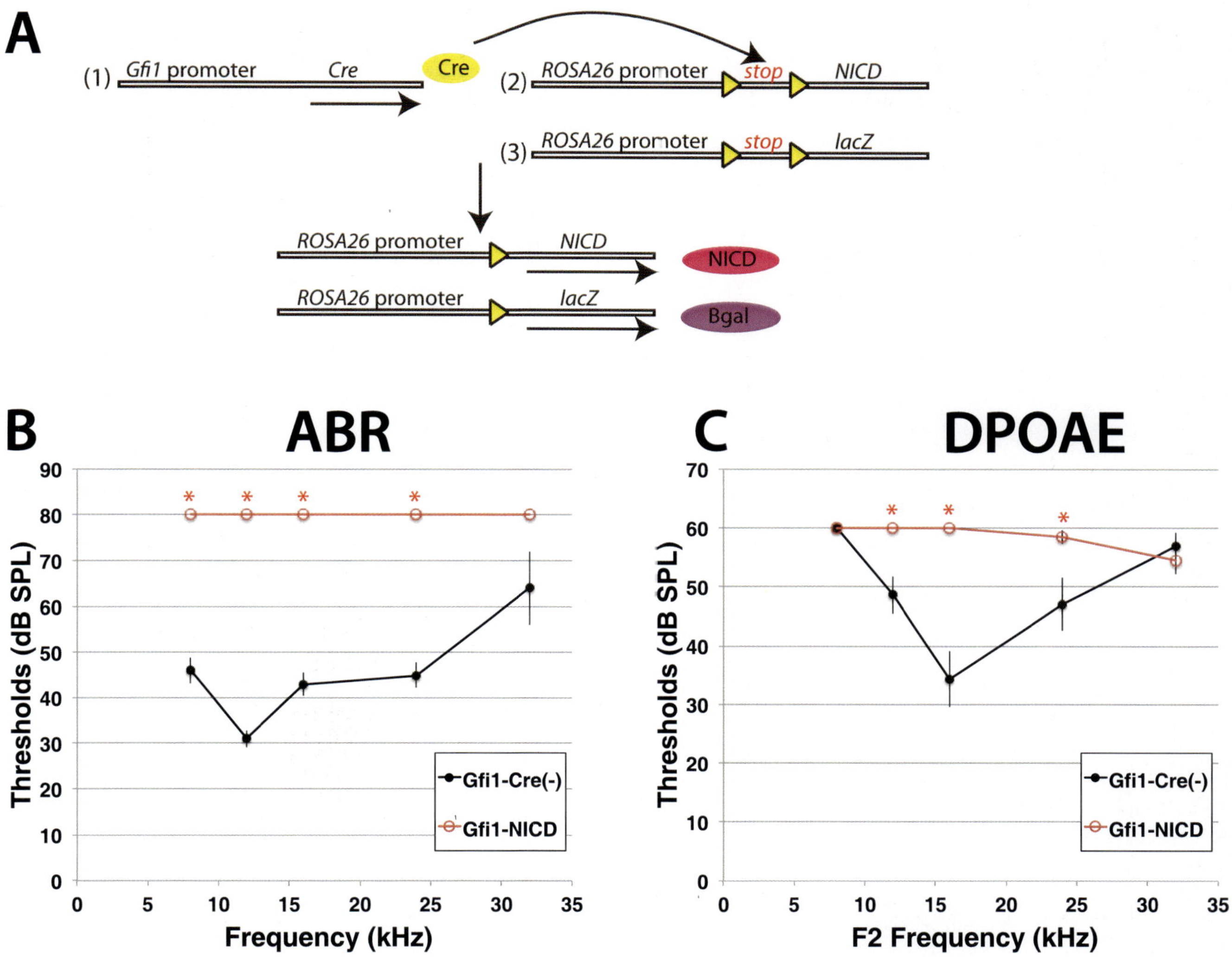


**Figure 1. Activation of Notch in differentiating hair cells causes profound deafness.** A. Schematic diagram demonstrating constructs for NICD expression in hair cells. (1) Cre is expressed in early developing hair cells under the Gfi1 promoter, causing recombination of a floxed-stop cassette and expression of NICD (2). The cross also contains a ROSA26-lacZ allele, which is similarly recombined upon expression of Cre and marks by lineage the cells expressing NICD (3). B–C. Hearing assessments of Gfi1-NICD mutants and their littermate Cre-negative controls at 5weeks of age. B. Auditory brainstem recordings (ABRs) show that Gfi1-NICD mutants have no responses to the highest sounds levels (80 dB SPL). C. Measurements of distortion product otoacoustic emissions (DPOAEs) also show raised thresholds, but have some responses to sound. To determine significance, a 2-way ANOVA was performed, with pairwise comparisons to determine significance for each frequency, * = $p<0.001$.

parvalbumin) in three Gfi1-NICD mutant cochleae and controls (Fig. 2J). Sections through the mid-modiolar regions of the cochlea were scored for presence (black regions of bars) or absence of the marker signal (white). If the marker was only partially expressed within the cell, or was very weak, those inner hair cells were scored as weak (gray area of bars). As expected, the control sections showed greater than 95% strong expression, with only a few inner hair cells exhibiting weak expression, and no control sections showing absent expression. In contrast, at least 50% of the mutant sections showed no expression of the marker in the inner hair cells (for parvalbumin it was greater than 80%). Even when the marker wasn't completely absent, weak expression was observed in 15–40% of the inner hair cells in the mutant cochlea, whereas weak expression constituted only 3–4% of the control inner hair cells. These results show that greater than 80% of the hair cells expressing NICD have either downregulated or completely shut off hair cell-specific markers by P20.

In addition to the downregulation of the hair cell markers, the NICD-expressing hair cells upregulated the HMG transcription factor SOX2 (Fig. 2), a progenitor and supporting cell marker that is normally downregulated in auditory hair cells early postnatally. As expected SOX2 was not detectable in control hair cells at P20 (Fig. 2A,D,G), but was apparent in the Gfi1-NICD inner and outer hair cells (Fig. 2B,E,H). Interestingly, as SOX2 is a transcription factor localized to the nucleus, it was apparent that the nuclei of the NICD-expressing inner hair cells were more basally positioned than in control inner hair cells (Fig. 2B,E,H, arrows; insets in C,F, and I). This nuclear position is consistent with the position of the nucleus in supporting cells rather than hair cells, where it is more apically situated.

To determine how early these markers were shut off, we examined Gfi1-NICD cochleae and littermate controls at P6. Results of these experiments showed that many inner hair cells did not express either calretinin or parvalbumin, similar to results at P20, whereas the outer hair cells largely still expressed these markers (Fig. 3A–F). Interestingly, the majority of both inner and outer hair cells continued to express myosin VI (Fig. 3G–I), indicating that not all hair cell markers were downregulated at the same time. As at P20, the hair cells also expressed SOX2, although unlike P20, the NICD-expressing inner hair cell nuclei were normally positioned at this time. To get a better idea of how many hair cells had begun downregulating hair cell markers and had upregulated SOX2, we examined Gfi1-NICD cochleae and their littermate controls in wholemount (Fig. 3J–O). These results showed that a majority of the Gfi1-NICD inner hair cells had downregulated parvalbumin and upregulated SOX2, whereas the majority of the outer hair cells still expressed parvalbumin, although there were variations in the levels of expression (Fig. 3M).

## NICD-expressing hair cells demonstrate an abnormal morphology resembling supporting cells, and upregulate supporting cell markers

To further investigate the morphological and molecular changes taking place in the cochlear hair cells, we examined Gfi1-NICD cochlea and controls at P11, using both myosin VI and P27KIP1, a nuclear cell cycle inhibitor expressed in postnatal supporting cells. Results of these studies showed that although most of the inner hair cells appeared to have a normal morphology and maintained expression of myosin VI, some of the inner hair cells had begun downregulating myosin VI and displayed an abnormal hair cell morphology (Fig. 4). Specifically, some of the NICD-expressing inner hair cells had lost their flask-like shape, displayed a more basally-positioned nucleus, and demonstrated processes that contacted the basement membrane (Fig. 4A′–D′). These features are consistent with a supporting cell morphology.

As many of the supporting cell markers examined were also progenitor cell markers that eventually were downregulated in the supporting cells, we were interested in whether the NICD-expressing hair cells expressed any mature supporting cell markers. Since the inner hair cells showed the most dramatic cell morphological and molecular changes in response to NICD expression, we reasoned that these cells may be converting to inner phalangeal cells, the supporting cells that surround the inner hair cells. We therefore examined expression of the Na-K-ATPase $\alpha$1 subunit (NKA$\alpha$1) [23,24], an inner phalangeal cell marker, in P20 cochlea from Gfi1-NICD mutants and their littermate controls (Fig. 5). Results showed that NKA$\alpha$1 was upregulated dramatically not only in the NICD-expressing inner hair cells (Fig. 5D–F), but also more mildly in the outer hair cells (Fig. 5E; arrowhead and arrows). These results demonstrate that the NICD-expressing hair cells express mature supporting cell markers in the adult cochlea, indicating that Notch promotes a supporting cell phenotype, and not simply a progenitor cell phenotype.

Interestingly, although the Gfi1-NICD mutants were profoundly deaf, the mice did not demonstrate any classic behaviors indicative of a vestibular defect, including circling or head-shaking behavior. To investigate this further, we examined the utricular and saccular maculae in Gfi1-NICD mutants to determine whether there were any histological or molecular changes taking place. These studies showed no downregulation of hair cell markers, or changes in cell morphology (Fig. 6), indicating that surprisingly, Notch does not have the same effects on vestibular hair cells that it has on the auditory hair cells.

## Activation of SOX2 in developing hair cells does not recapitulate the effects of NICD overexpression

Given that activation of Notch led to an upregulation of SOX2, and SOX2 is expressed in supporting cell of the inner ear, we were interested in determining whether SOX2 was mediating any of the changes observed in the NICD-expressing hair cells. To accomplish this, we used an experimental paradigm similar to the Notch activation and crossed Gfi1-Cre to mice expressing SOX2 under the ubiquitous ROSA26 promoter [20]. We tested whether expression of SOX2 has any effects on hearing using ABR and DPOAE analysis. Results of these tests showed that Gfi1-SOX2 mutants ($n = 14$) were hearing impaired when compared to littermate controls ($n = 9$), although they were not as profoundly deaf as the Gfi1-NICD mutants (Fig. 7). Specifically, whereas Gfi1-NICD mutants showed no responses at even the highest levels of sound tested, Gfi1-SOX2 mutants demonstrated some responses, although at most frequencies their thresholds were significantly raised (Fig. 7A). Similarly DPOAE responses were also detected in Gfi1-SOX2 animals, although again these responses showed increased thresholds when compared to controls (Fig. 7B), although at most frequencies these increases were not significantly different. These data indicate that both inner and outer hair cells are functionally compromised by SOX2 overexpression, but the effects are not as severe as those produced by NICD overexpression.

To determine the effects of ectopic SOX2 expression on the molecular and histological aspects of sensory cell differentiation, we examined hair cell and supporting cell markers by immunohistochemistry. Surprisingly, these results showed that hair cell markers were maintained normally in SOX2-expressing cells (Fig. 8). No differences were detected in expression of myosin VI or calretinin at P6 (Fig. 8 A–D). Even at P20, no downregulation of either calretinin or parvalbumin was observed in the inner hair

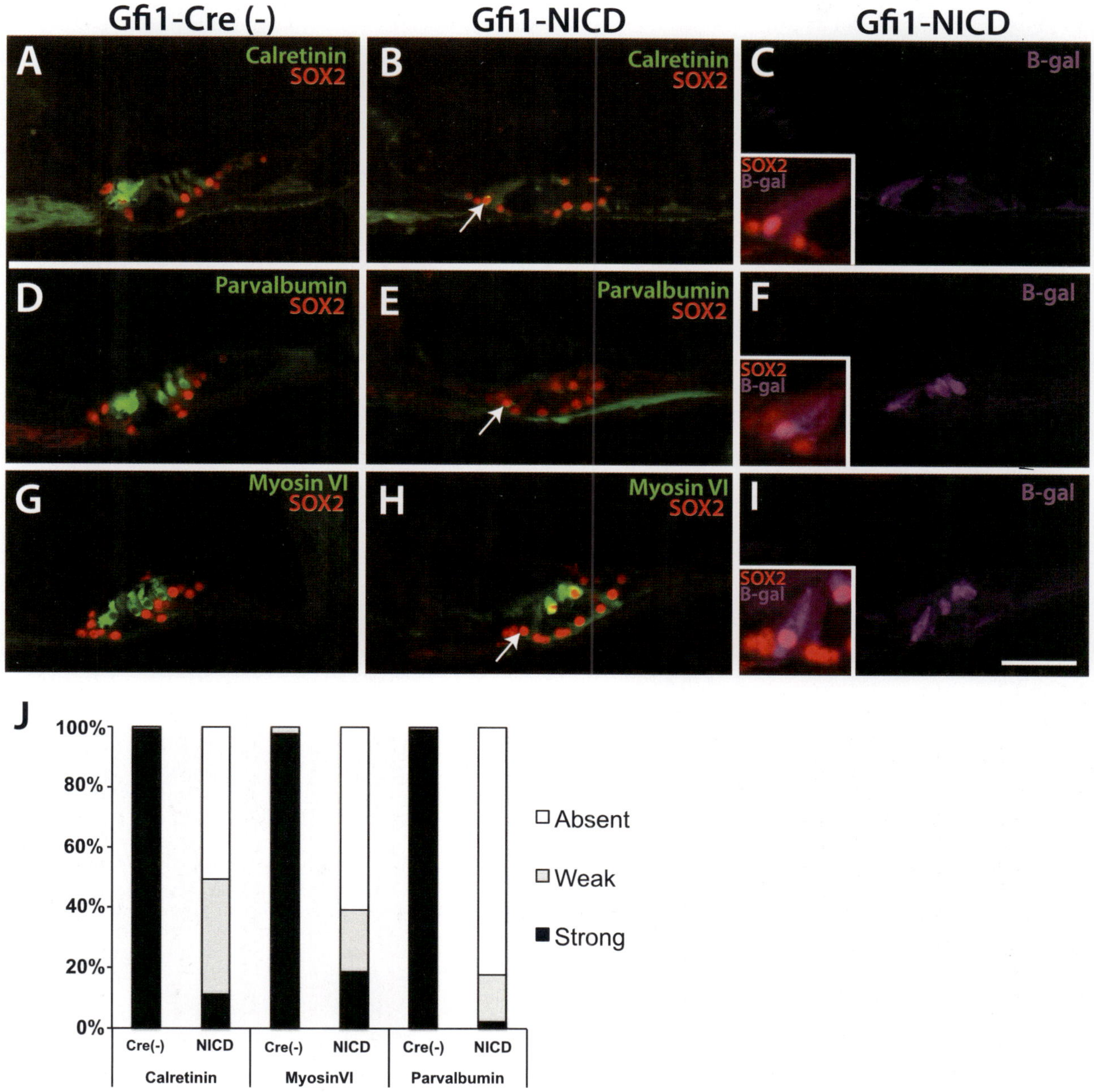


**Figure 2. At P20, NICD-expressing hair cells in the cochlea have downregulated hair cell markers.** A–I Paraffin sections through the P20 cochlea stained for hair cell markers, SOX2, and ß-galactosidase. A, D, G. Calretinin, parvalbumin, and myosin VI all show expression in the inner and outer hair cells at P20 (although calretinin expression is weak in outer hair cells at P20). B, E, H. Both calretinin and parvalbumin are shut off in the Gfi1-NICD inner and outer hair cells, whereas myosin VI is generally still expressed in the outer hair cells in the mutant (H). Gfi1-NICD inner and outer hair cells express SOX2 and the inner hair cells have a more basally-located nucleus than in controls (B,E,H, arrows and insets in C,F,I showing higher power images of inner hair cells expressing ß-galactosidase and SOX2). J. Quantification of relative expression levels of indicated markers in the Gfi1-NICD (NICD) inner hair cells and littermate controls [Cre(-)]. Scale bar in I = 100 microns (= 50 microns for inset panels).

cells (Fig. 8E–H), although in most cases neither marker was detectable at this time in Gfi1-NICD expressing hair cells (Fig. 2). Moreover, no differences were detected in the morphology of the SOX2-expressing hair cells. Specifically, we did not observe any hair cells in contact with the basement membrane, and the hair cell nuclei retained their normal apical position. These data show that while SOX2 expression may have some effects on the function of the hair cell, SOX2 expression does not interfere with hair cell gene expression or morphology, indicating that SOX2 does not mediate the effects of Notch in repressing the hair cell phenotype while promoting a supporting cell phenotype.

## Discussion

Our results indicate that Notch plays an important role in suppressing hair cell gene expression in differentiating supporting cells. In addition, we have shown that Notch actively promotes the expression of a number of supporting cell markers. This change in gene expression is accompanied by changes in cell morphology, particularly in the inner hair cells, in which cells lose their

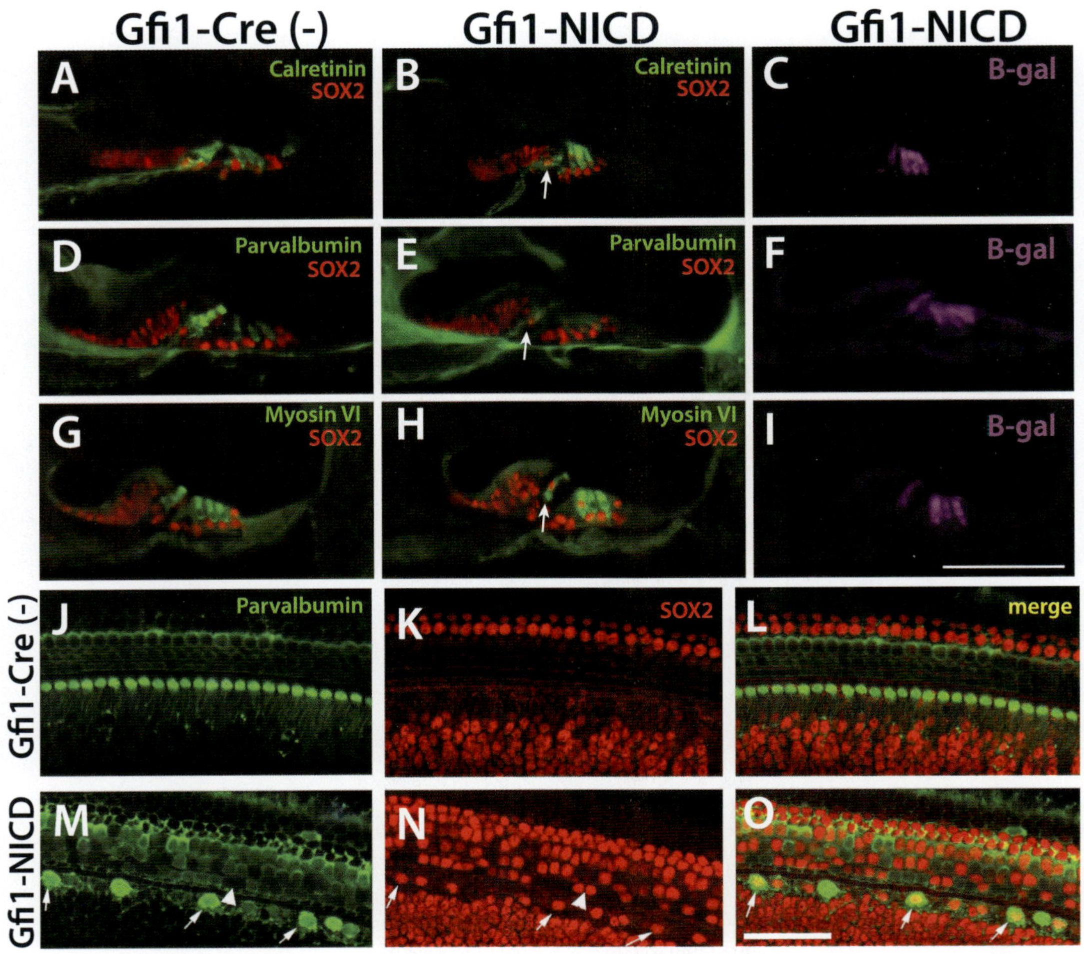


**Figure 3. At P6, Some hair cell markers are downregulated in the inner hair cells.** A–I. Frozen sections through the P6 cochlea stained for hair cell markers, SOX2, and ß-galactosidase. A, D, G. Calretinin, parvalbumin, and myosin VI all show expression in the inner and outer hair cells at P6 (although parvalbumin expression is weaker in outer hair cells at P6). B, E, H. Both calretinin and parvalbumin are downregulated in the Gfi-NICD inner hair cells, although outer hair cell expression is largely maintained. Interestingly, myosin VI (G–I) is generally indistinguishable from the controls at this time point. Scale bar in I = 100microns. J–O. Wholemount cochlea stained for hair cell (parvalbumin) and supporting cell (SOX2) markers. Many of the inner hair cells have shut off parvalbumin and upregulated SOX2 by this time point (M–O, arrows). A few outer hair cells have downregulated parvalbumin (M–O, arrowhead), but most have upregulated SOX2.

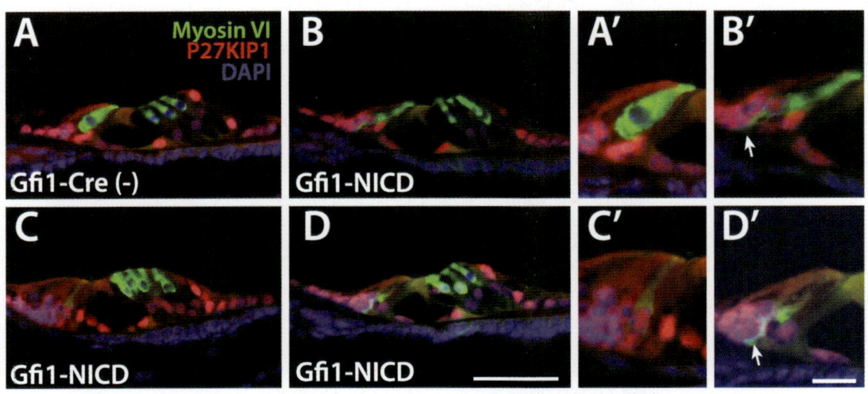


**Figure 4. NICD-expressing inner hair cells show morphology changes and abnormal P27KIP1 expression at P11.** A–D. Paraffin sections from Gfi1-NICD cochlea and littermate controls at P11. A′-D′ show higher power views of the inner hair cells, which demonstrate morphological and molecular changes due to Notch activation. The changes in the inner hair cells in the Gfi1-NICD mutants (B,C,D and B′C′,D,) include weaker MYO6 expression, lack of the normal flask-like shape, more basally positioned nulcei, and nuclear P27KIP1 expression normally only observed in supporting cells at this time. Scale bar in D = 100 microns for A–D, and in D′ = 25 microns for A′–D′.

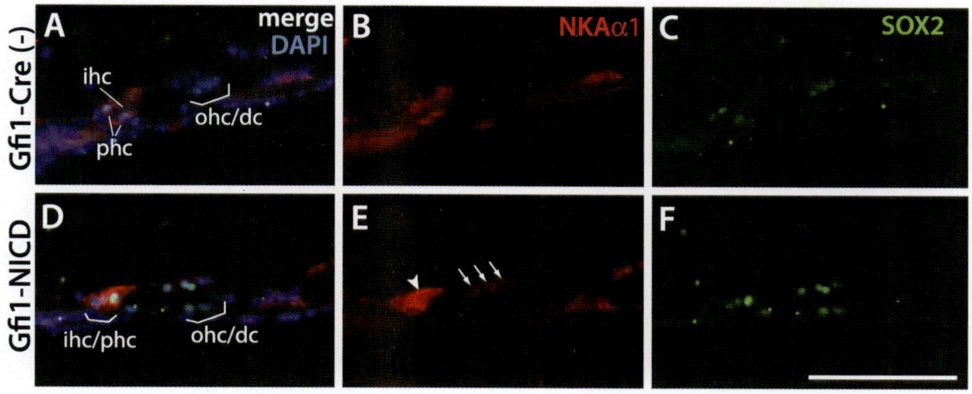


**Figure 5. The mature supporting cell marker NKAα1 is upregulated in NICD-expressing inner and outer hair cells.** A–F. Paraffin sections from Gfi1-NICD and Cre-negative control cochleae at P20. A–C. Control sections showing the normal expression of NKAα1 in the phalangeal cells (phc) surrounding the inner hair cells (ihc), which are also coexpressed with SOX2. Deiter's cells also show expression of SOX2, although not NKAα1. D–F. Gfi1-NICD expressing inner hair cell has upregulated NKAα1 (arrowhead). Surprisingly, the NICD-expressing outer hair cells (ohc) have also upregulated NKAα1, although much more weakly than in the inner hair cells. Both inner and outer hair cells also show upregulation of SOX2. Scale bar = 100 microns.

characteristic flask-like shape, show contact with the basement membrane, and have a more basally-positioned nucleus, features consistent with a supporting cell fate. This instructive role in the supporting cell differentiation is similar to the role that Notch plays in the CNS in promoting the glial cell fate [13–16]. Not surprisingly, this switch in gene expression leads to severe consequences for hair cell function, as the Gfi1-NICD mutants were profoundly deaf. We also examined whether these effects were mediated by SOX2, a likely downstream target of Notch signaling [25–28] expressed in developing and mature supporting cells [29,30]. Interestingly, although SOX2 expression interferes with hair cell function to some degree, we did not observe the same molecular and cell morphology changes in the Gfi1-SOX2 mutants that were seen in the NICD-expressing mutants.

The protracted and gradual nature of the expression and morphology changes in the cochlear hair cells after NICD expression was unexpected. Although we began to express NICD during early hair cell differentiation (E15–E16.5 in the cochlea [17]), widespread changes in gene expression and morphology were not observed until P20, although some downregulation of hair cell markers could be observed at P6. A possible reason for this slow change in phenotype is that although NICD may inhibit expression of hair cell markers immediately through suppression of transcription, ultimately loss of the hair cell markers may depend on the half-life of the protein. Indeed, this may explain why some markers are downregulated more quickly than others (Fig. 2J). Myosin VI, for example, seemed particularly resistant to downregulation compared to calretinin or parvalbumin, as expression was frequently observed at P6 while the other two markers were largely absent (Fig. 3). It also appeared that in some cases, downregulation of hair cell-specific marker expression was required before the cells could express supporting cell markers, or show changes in morphology. For example at P11, upregulation of P27KIP1 and contact with the basement membrane was only observed in a subset of inner hair cells that had significantly downregulated myosin VI (Fig. 4). Thus, suppression of hair cell genes may be a required step for the proper expression of supporting cell genes.

Another surprising result was the differential effects of Notch activation depending on the type of hair cell. For example, while we saw dramatic changes in gene expression, morphology and function in inner hair cells and milder changes in outer hair cells,

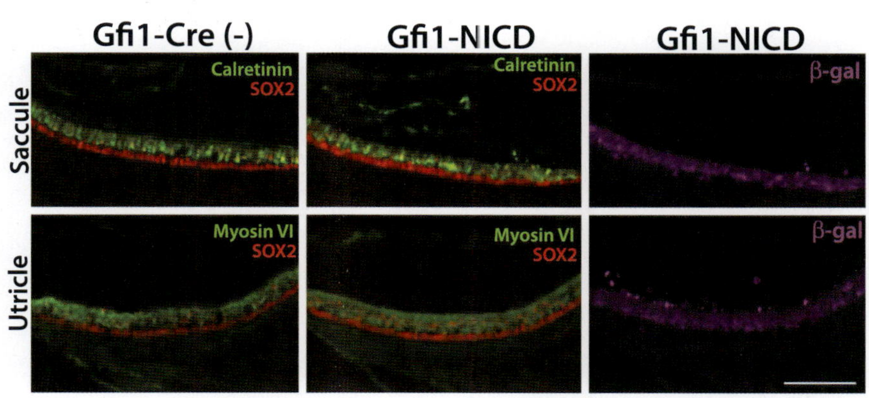


**Figure 6. NICD-expressing hair cells exhibit expected markers in the vestibular regions. A–F**. Frozen sections through the vestibular regions of P6 inner ears. Hair cell markers (calretinin and Myosin VI; B and E) are expressed similarly to controls (A and D) in the indicated regions of the vestibular system. Sections were co-labeled with ß-galactosidase expression, which is shown in a different panel (C, F) to better show the expression. Scale bar in F = 100 microns.

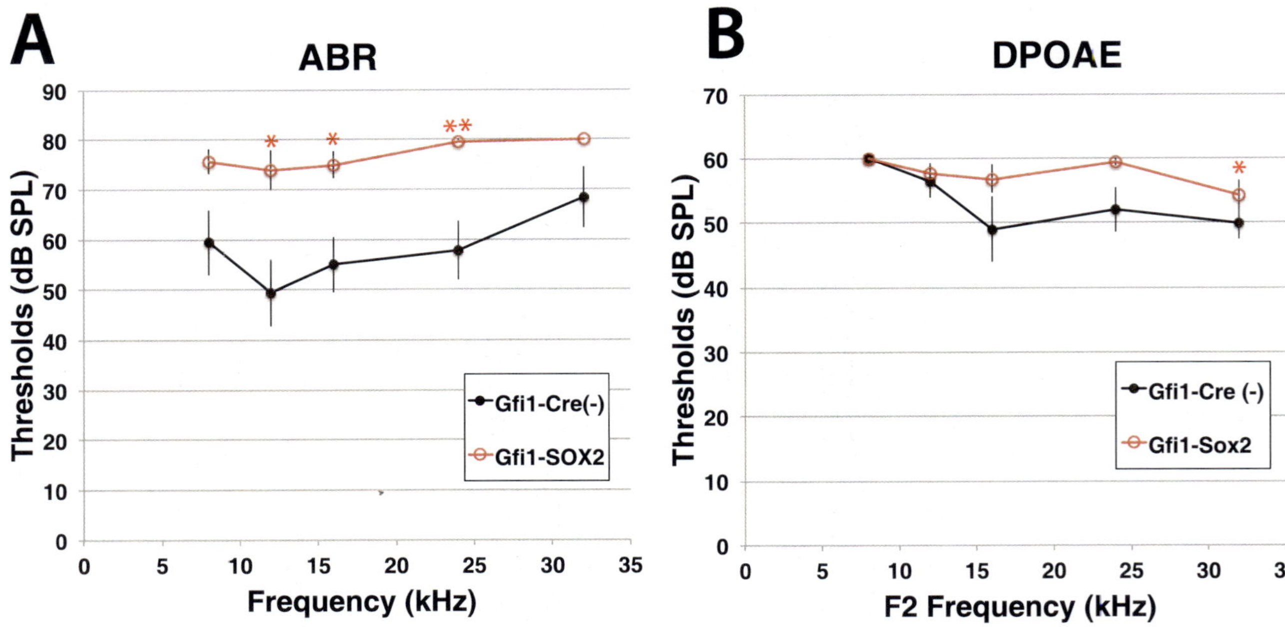


**Figure 7. Auditory testing of Gfi1-SOX2 mutants demonstrates that SOX2 expression causes hearing impairment.** A. Auditory brainstem recordings (ABRs, left) of Gfi1-SOX2 mutants and littermate controls at 5 weeks of age show that SOX2-expressing mice have significantly raised thresholds compared to controls. B. Measurements of distortion product otoacoustic emissions (DPOAEs) of the same mice tested for ABR, also show raised thresholds at 5 weeks. To determine significance, a 2-way ANOVA was performed, with pairwise comparisons to determine significance for each frequency: ** = $p<0.001$, * = $p<0.05$.

there were no apparent effects on the vestibular hair cells. The reasons for this are currently unclear, although it suggests that Notch or its targets are regulated differentially depending on the type of hair cell. In this context, it is interesting to note that some adult vestibular hair cells (likely type II) continue to express SOX2, which is exclusively restricted to supporting cells in the cochlea [30,31]. However, control of SOX2 function may be regulated by aspects other than transcriptional control, including potentially other SoxB members such as SOX21. It is interesting to note that SOX21 is also differentially expressed between the cochlear and vestibular regions in the chicken, and overexpression of SOX21 results in a bias towards the hair cell fate in vestibular regions but not in the cochlea (basilar papilla) [32]. It is also possible that the timing of Gfi1-Cre expression is slightly different in different types of hair cells, and this may account for the differential effects. Our results indicate that activated Notch and SOX2 must be shut off in the hair cells of the cochlea for normal hair cell function, but similar downregulation may not be required for vestibular hair cells.

Our results are in contrast to those of Liu et al., [33], who used the *Atoh1*$^{CreER}$ to express NICD in developing hair cells, and found no changes in hair cell gene expression, hair cell function or morphology, despite upregulation of SOX2. Although these two Cre alleles have slightly different times of induction, with *Atoh1*$^{CreER}$ being slightly earlier than the Gfi1-Cre used in our study [22], we consider it more likely that these differing outcomes are due to the different endpoints examined in each study. For example Lui et al., [33] looked at changes in hair cell gene expression at E19, whereas our study looked at later postnatal ages. Indeed, as discussed above, we demonstrated that there are only mild gene expression changes beginning around P6, which do not become pronounced until P20, along with morphological changes. In addition to the earlier induction, Lui et al., [33] also induced Cre at later time periods, including P0 and P1, to look at the effects of later NICD re-activation in developing and adult hair cells. Similar to their results at the earlier time points, they observed no changes in hair cell gene expression, morphology, or function (as assessed by FM 4–64FX dye) even at adult stages. However, it appeared that very little ectopic SOX2 expression was detected in the inner hair cells, indicating that significant NICD activation was not achieved in this cell type, since in our experience SOX2 expression is an excellent readout for NICD activation [25,34]. Thus, since the major effects that we observed were in the inner hair cells, it is possible that they saw few effects on the cochlea due to the low recombination rates of the NICD allele in the inner hair cell population. However, it is also possible that NICD overexpression at P0–P1 is too late to induce cell fate changes in the hair cells [33]. Therefore, it remains an open question as to whether Notch can induce supporting cell-like changes in postnatal and adult inner hair cells.

Our results show that Notch activation leads to suppression of hair cell markers and an upregulation of supporting cell markers in cells that have begun differentiating as hair cells. These results indicate that Notch not only prevents the hair cell fate, but can promote a supporting cell fate, similar to its role in promoting certain glial cell phenotypes in the central nervous system [13–16]. It is interesting to note that the glial cell types in which Notch has been shown to play an instructive role (including radial glia and particular radial glial subtypes including Bergman and Müller glia) can also act as progenitors [35,36]. It will be interesting to determine if there are further similarities between supporting cells and radial glia subtypes. Our data also shows that, in contrast to a previous study [33], auditory hair cells are not irreversibly specified at embryonic time points, and have the capability of acquiring aspects of the supporting cell phenotype. Our results have important implications for those interested in regenerating sensory region cell types in the inner ear. Specifically, our data indicates that activation of Notch is an important step in the

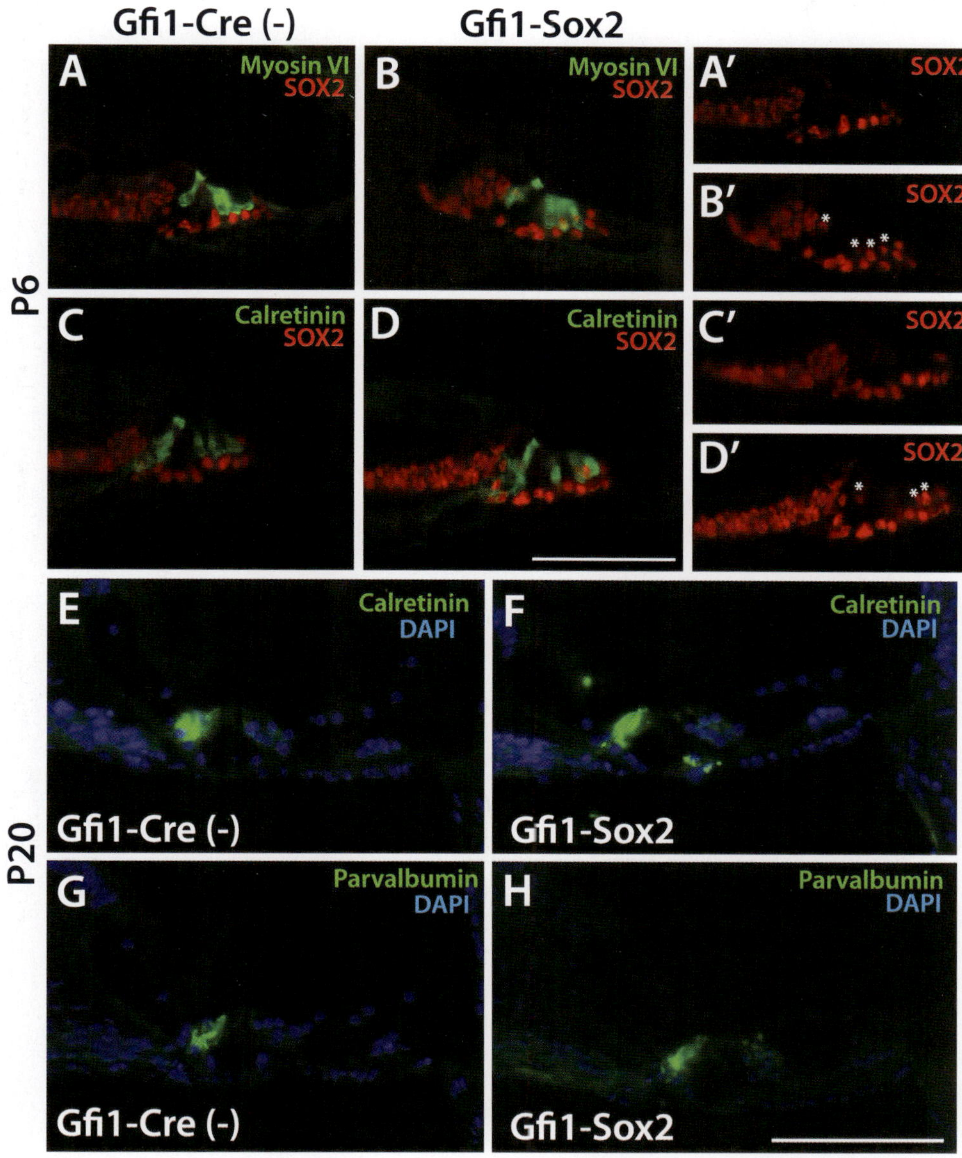


**Figure 8. Histological assessment of SOX2-expressing hair cells shows no morphological changes or downregulation of hair cell markers over time.** A–D. Both calretinin and myosin VI are expressed normally in Gfi1-SOX2 mutants (B,D) at P6 when compared to controls (A,C). A′–D′. Expression of SOX2 alone (shown also in A–D) demonstrates the upregulation of SOX2 in the inner and outer hair cells in Gfi1-SOX2 mutants (asterisks indicate hair cell nuclei expressing SOX2 in B′–D′). Scale bar in D = 100 microns for A–D. E–H. Expression of indicated hair cells markers in Gfi1-SOX2 mutants (F,H) is maintained normally at P20 when compared to controls (E,G). Scale bar in H = 100 microns for E–H.

specification of supporting cells, whereas suppression of Notch activation appears to be a required step in the differentiation of auditory hair cells.

## Acknowledgments

We thank Richard Libby for careful reading of the manuscript, and also thank members of the Kiernan, Libby, Gan, and White laboratories for their input on the project.

## Author Contributions

Conceived and designed the experiments: WP AK. Performed the experiments: GS FG WP DP. Analyzed the data: GS FG WP DP JQ LG PW AK. Contributed reagents/materials/analysis tools: JQ LG PW. Wrote the paper: PM AK.

## References

1. Fekete DM, Muthukumar S, Karagogeos D (1998) Hair cells and supporting cells share a common progenitor in the avian inner ear. J Neurosci 18: 7811–7821.
2. Lewis J (1991) Rules for the production of sensory cells. Ciba Found Symp 160: 25–39; discussion 40–53.
3. Adam J, Myat A, Le Roux I, Eddison M, Henrique D, et al. (1998) Cell fate choices and the expression of Notch, Delta and Serrate homologues in the chick inner ear: parallels with Drosophila sense-organ development. Development 125: 4645–4654.

4. Hori K, Sen A, Artavanis-Tsakonas S (2013) Notch signaling at a glance. J Cell Sci 126: 2135–2140.
5. Haddon C, Jiang YJ, Smithers L, Lewis J (1998) Delta-Notch signalling and the patterning of sensory cell differentiation in the zebrafish ear: evidence from the mind bomb mutant. Development 125: 4637–4644.
6. Brooker R, Hozumi K, Lewis J (2006) Notch ligands with contrasting functions: Jagged1 and Delta1 in the mouse inner ear. Development 133: 1277–1286.
7. Lanford PJ, Lan Y, Jiang R, Lindsell C, Weinmaster G, et al. (1999) Notch signalling pathway mediates hair cell development in mammalian cochlea. Nat Genet 21: 289–292.
8. Riley BB, Chiang M, Farmer L, Heck R (1999) The deltaA gene of zebrafish mediates lateral inhibition of hair cells in the inner ear and is regulated by pax2.1. Development 126: 5669–5678.
9. Kiernan AE, Cordes R, Kopan R, Gossler A, Gridley T (2005) The Notch ligands DLL1 and JAG2 act synergistically to regulate hair cell development in the mammalian inner ear. Development 132: 4353–4362.
10. Bray SJ (2006) Notch signalling: a simple pathway becomes complex. Nat Rev Mol Cell Biol 7: 678–689.
11. Eddison M, Le Roux I, Lewis J (2000) Notch signaling in the development of the inner ear: lessons from Drosophila. Proc Natl Acad Sci U S A 97: 11692–11699.
12. Kiernan AE (2013) Notch signaling during cell fate determination in the inner ear. Semin Cell Dev Biol 24: 470–479.
13. Furukawa T, Mukherjee S, Bao ZZ, Morrow EM, Cepko CL (2000) rax, Hes1, and notch1 promote the formation of Muller glia by postnatal retinal progenitor cells. Neuron 26: 383–394.
14. Gaiano N, Nye JS, Fishell G (2000) Radial glial identity is promoted by Notch1 signaling in the murine forebrain. Neuron 26: 395–404.
15. Eiraku M, Tohgo A, Ono K, Kaneko M, Fujishima K, et al. (2005) DNER acts as a neuron-specific Notch ligand during Bergmann glial development. Nat Neurosci 8: 873–880.
16. Weller M, Krautler N, Mantei N, Suter U, Taylor V (2006) Jagged1 ablation results in cerebellar granule cell migration defects and depletion of Bergmann glia. Dev Neurosci 28: 70–80.
17. Yang H, Gan J, Xie X, Deng M, Feng L, et al. (2010) Gfi1-Cre knock-in mouse line: A tool for inner ear hair cell-specific gene deletion. Genesis 48: 400–406.
18. Murtaugh LC, Stanger BZ, Kwan KM, Melton DA (2003) Notch signaling controls multiple steps of pancreatic differentiation. Proc Natl Acad Sci U S A 100: 14920–14925.
19. Soriano P (1999) Generalized lacZ expression with the ROSA26 Cre reporter strain. Nat Genet 21: 70–71.
20. Lu Y, Futtner C, Rock JR, Xu X, Whitworth W, et al. (2010) Evidence that SOX2 overexpression is oncogenic in the lung. PLoS One 5: e11022.
21. Wallis D, Hamblen M, Zhou Y, Venken KJ, Schumacher A, et al. (2003) The zinc finger transcription factor Gfi1, implicated in lymphomagenesis, is required for inner ear hair cell differentiation and survival. Development 130: 221–232.
22. Hertzano R, Montcouquiol M, Rashi-Elkeles S, Elkon R, Yucel R, et al. (2004) Transcription profiling of inner ears from Pou4f3(ddl/ddl) identifies Gfi1 as a target of the Pou4f3 deafness gene. Hum Mol Genet 13: 2143–2153.
23. McLean WJ, Smith KA, Glowatzki E, Pyott SJ (2009) Distribution of the Na,K-ATPase alpha subunit in the rat spiral ganglion and organ of corti. J Assoc Res Otolaryngol 10: 37–49.
24. Peters TA, Kuijpers W, Curfs JH (2001) Occurrence of NaK-ATPase isoforms during rat inner ear development and functional implications. Eur Arch Otorhinolaryngol 258: 67–73.
25. Pan W, Jin Y, Stanger B, Kiernan AE (2010) Notch signaling is required for the generation of hair cells and supporting cells in the mammalian inner ear. Proc Natl Acad Sci U S A 107: 15798–15803.
26. Jeon SJ, Fujioka M, Kim SC, Edge AS (2011) Notch signaling alters sensory or neuronal cell fate specification of inner ear stem cells. J Neurosci 31: 8351–8358.
27. Ehm O, Goritz C, Covic M, Schaffner I, Schwarz TJ, et al. (2010) RBPJkappa-dependent signaling is essential for long-term maintenance of neural stem cells in the adult hippocampus. J Neurosci 30: 13794–13807.
28. Liu Z, Owen T, Fang J, Zuo J (2012) Overactivation of Notch1 signaling induces ectopic hair cells in the mouse inner ear in an age-dependent manner. PLoS One 7: e34123.
29. Kiernan AE, Pelling AL, Leung KK, Tang AS, Bell DM, et al. (2005) Sox2 is required for sensory organ development in the mammalian inner ear. Nature 434: 1031–1035.
30. Hume CR, Bratt DL, Oesterle EC (2007) Expression of LHX3 and SOX2 during mouse inner ear development. Gene Expr Patterns 7: 798–807.
31. Oesterle EC, Campbell S, Taylor RR, Forge A, Hume CR (2007) Sox2 and Jagged1 Expression in Normal and Drug-Damaged Adult Mouse Inner Ear. J Assoc Res Otolaryngol.
32. Freeman SD, Daudet N (2012) Artificial induction of Sox21 regulates sensory cell formation in the embryonic chicken inner ear. PLoS One 7: e46387.
33. Liu Z, Owen T, Fang J, Srinivasan RS, Zuo J (2012) In vivo Notch reactivation in differentiating cochlear hair cells induces Sox2 and Prox1 expression but does not disrupt hair cell maturation. Dev Dyn 241: 684–696.
34. Pan W, Jin Y, Chen J, Rottier RJ, Steel KP, et al. (2013) Ectopic Expression of Activated Notch or SOX2 Reveals Similar and Unique Roles in the Development of the Sensory Cell Progenitors in the Mammalian Inner Ear. J Neurosci 33: 16146–16157.
35. Goldman D (2014) Muller glial cell reprogramming and retina regeneration. Nat Rev Neurosci 15: 431–442.
36. Barry DS, Pakan JM, McDermott KW (2014) Radial glial cells: key organisers in CNS development. Int J Biochem Cell Biol 46: 76–79.

# 17

# Targeted High-Throughput Sequencing Identifies Pathogenic Mutations in KCNQ4 in Two Large Chinese Families with Autosomal Dominant Hearing Loss

**Hongyang Wang[1]ⓐ, Yali Zhao[1]ⓐ¤, Yuting Yi[2]ⓐ, Yun Gao[1], Qiong Liu[1], Dayong Wang[1], Qian Li[1], Lan Lan[1], Na Li[1], Jing Guan[1], Zifang Yin[1], Bing Han[1], Feifan Zhao[1], Liang Zong[1], Wenping Xiong[1], Lan Yu[1], Lijie Song[2], Xin Yi[2], Ling Yang[2], Christine Petit[3,4,5,6], Qiuju Wang[1]***

**1** Institute of Otolaryngology, Chinese PLA General Hospital, Medical School of Chinese PLA, Beijing, China, **2** BGI-Tianjin, Tianjin, China, **3** Unité de Génétique et Physiologie de l'Audition, Institut Pasteur, Paris, France, **4** UMRS 1120, Institut National de la Santé et de la Recherche Médicale (INSERM), Paris, France, **5** Université Pierre et Marie Curie (Paris VI), Paris, France, **6** Collège de France, Paris, France

## Abstract

Autosomal dominant non-syndromic hearing loss (ADNSHL) is highly heterogeneous, among them, *KCNQ4* is one of the most frequent disease-causing genes. More than twenty *KCNQ4* mutations have been reported, but none of them were detected in Chinese mainland families. In this study, we identified a novel *KCNQ4* mutation in a five generation Chinese family with 84 members and a known *KCNQ4* mutation in a six generation Chinese family with 66 members. Mutation screening of 30 genes for ADNSHL was performed in the probands from thirty large Chinese families with ADNSHL by targeted region capture and high-throughput sequencing. The candidate variants and the co-segregation of the phenotype were verified by polymerase chain reaction (PCR) amplification and Sanger sequencing in all ascertained family members. Then we identified a novel *KCNQ4* mutation p.W275R in exon 5 and a known *KCNQ4* mutation p.G285S in exon 6 in two large Chinese ADNSHL families segregating with post-lingual high frequency-involved and progressive sensorineural hearing loss. This is the first report of *KCNQ4* mutation in Chinese mainland families. *KCNQ4*, a member of voltage-gated potassium channel family, is likely to be a common gene in Chinese patients with ADNSHL. The results also support that the combination of targeted enrichment and high-throughput sequencing is a valuable molecular diagnostic tool for autosomal dominant hereditary deafness.

**Editor:** You-Qiang Song, The University of Hong Kong, Hong Kong

**Funding:** This work was supported by the grants of the National Key Basic Research Program of China, No. 2014CB943001, the National Natural Science Foundation of China, Major Project, No. 81120108009. The funders had no role in study design, data collection and analysis, decision to publish, or preparation of the manuscript.

**Competing Interests:** The authors have declared that no competing interests exist.

* Email: wqcr@263.net

ⓐ These authors contributed equally to this work.

¤ Current address: Department of Otolaryngology, Beijing Tongren Hospital, Beijing, China

## Introduction

Hereditary hearing loss can be inherited in many patterns, such as autosomal dominant audosomal recessive, X-linked dominant, X-linked recessive, Y-linked pattern, among which ADNSHL has strikingly genetic heterogeneity. To date, more than 60 loci for ADNSHL have been mapped and only 30 corresponding genes have been identified (http://hereditaryhearingloss.org). During the past twenty years, linkage analysis and candidate gene sequencing has been proved to be a powerful tool to identify responsible genes for ADNSHL. However, limited number of samples in the clinical part, the large number of genes in the mapped region, and the large size of many genes restrained the application of this method. Recently, high-throughput sequencing, also known as next-generation sequencing (NGS) has been proved to be an ideal tool to decipher the genetic heterogeneity of deafness. More than ten deafness genes have been identified using NGS including *TPRN*, *GPSM2*, *HSD17B4*, *MASP1*, *CACAM1*, *HARS2*, *SMPX*, *DNMT1*, *ABHD12*, *TSPEAR*, *TNC* and *P2RX2* [1,2,3].

Among ADNSHL genes, *KCNQ4* (MIM*600101), one of the most frequent genes [4], was firstly identified as the causal gene for ADNSHL at DFNA2 by Kubisch and colleagues [5]. As a member of voltage-gated potassium channel family, *KCNQ4* plays a crucial role in potassium recycling in the inner ear. *KCNQ4* has six predicted transmembrane domains encoded by six exons (exon 2 to 7) and a P-loop between transmembrane domains S5 and S6. The P-loop domain forms a channel pore, containing a potassium ion-selective filter, whose function is eliminated by mutations in the pore region [5]. To date, 20 mutations in *KCNQ4* have been reported (Table 1) and it is identified as a common gene with a frequency up to 6.62% in ADNSHL in Japan, predicted to be the most prevalent gene responsible for Japanese ADNSHL patients [6]. However, these mutations have not been found in Chinese mainland populations before this study. Almost all reported cases showed a similar phenotype characterized by post-lingual, progressive, high-frequency hearing impairment (one mid-frequency predominant hearing loss caused by the p.V230E mutation was reported) [6].

Recently, we performed targeted capture and NGS to analyze a cohort of 30 hearing loss probands from Chinese families with ADNSHL (data not shown). Among these families, we identified a novel *KCNQ4* mutation p.W275R in exon 5 in family 025 and a known *KCNQ4* mutation p.G285S in exon 6 in family 727.

## Materials and Methods

### Ethics Statement

The study was approved by the Committee of Medical Ethics of Chinese People's Liberation Army (PLA) General Hospital. We obtained written informed consents from all the participants in this study. Written informed consents were obtained from the next of kin on the behalf of the minors/children participants involved in this study.

### Family Recruitment and Clinical Evaluations

A six-generation family (025) with 66 members segregating ADNSHL and a five-generation family (727) with 84 members segregating ADNSHL were ascertained from the Department of Otolaryngology, Head and Neck Surgery, at the Institute of Otolaryngology of PLA, Chinese PLA General Hospital (Figure 1A, 1B). Either personal or family medical evidence of hearing loss, tinnitus, vestibular symptoms, use of aminoglycosides, and other clinical abnormalities of the participants were identified by a team of experienced doctors and audiologists. Audiometric evaluations included pure tone audiometry, auditory brainstem responses (ABR) and distortion product otoacoustic emissions (DPOAE). High resolution computed tomography (HRCT) was also performed on some subjects to verify whether the family members had other complications other than hearing disorders.

### Targeted capture and NGS

Genomic DNA (gDNA) was extracted from the whole blood samples using the Blood DNA kit (TIANGEN BIOTECH, Beijing, China), and 1 ug of purified gDNA fragmented to 200–300 base pairs using an ultrasonoscope (Covaris S2, Massachusetts, USA). End-repair, adenylation and adapter ligation were performed for library preparation following the Illumina's protocol. The same amount of library were pooled then hybridized to the customized capture array (NimbleGen, Roche) including exons, splicing sites and immediate flanking intron sequences of 29 genes for non-syndromic autosomal dominant hearing loss and TNC, a novel causative gene for ADNSHL identified in our previous research (Table S1). Sequencing was carried out on Illumina HiSeq2000 to generate paired end reads (90 bps at each end) [7].

Raw image files were processed by Illumina Pipeline (version 1.3.4) for base-calling with default parameters. Reads were aligned

**Table 1.** Overview of all *KCNQ4* mutations identified to date.

| Mutation DNA | Protein | Exon | Origin | reference |
|---|---|---|---|---|
| c.211_223del13 | p.Q71fs | 1 | Belguim | Coucke et al. (1999) |
| c.211delC | p.Q71fs | 1 | Japan | Kamada et al. (2006) |
| c.229_230insGC | P.H77fs | 1 | Japan | Naito, et al. (2013) |
| c.546C>G | p.F182L | 4 | Taiwan, | Su, et al. (2007); |
| | | | Japan | Naito, et al. (2013) |
| c.664_681del18 | p.G215_220del6 | 4 | Korea | Beak, et al. (2010) |
| c.689T>A | p.V230E | 4 | Japan | Naito, et al. (2013) |
| c.725G>A | p.W241X | 5 | USA | Hildebrand, et al. (2008) |
| c.778G>A | p.E260K | 5 | USA | Hildebrand, et al. (2008) |
| c.785A>T | p.D262V | 5 | USA | Hildebrand, et al. (2008) |
| c.821T>A | p.L274H | 5 | Neth | Van Hauwe, et al. (2000); De Heer, et al. (2011) |
| **c.823T>C** | **p.W275S** | **5** | **China** | **Present study** |
| c.827G>C | p.W276S | 5 | Neth, Japan | Coucke et al. (1999), Akita et al. (2001), Camp, et al. (2002), Topsakal, et al. (2005) |
| c.842T>C | p.L281S | 6 | USA | Talebizadeh, ea al. (1999) |
| c.853G>T | p.G285C | 6 | USA | Coucke et al. (1999) |
| **c.853G>A** | **p.G285S** | **6** | France, | Kubisch, et al. (1999) |
| | | | **China** | **Present study** |
| c.859G>C | p.G287R | 6 | USA | Arnett, et al. (2011) |
| c.871C>T | p.P291S | 6 | Japan | Naito, et al. (2013) |
| c.872C>T | p.P291L | 6 | Japan | Naito, et al. (2013) |
| c.886G>A | p.G296S | 6 | Spain | Mencia, et al. (2008) |
| c.891G>T | p.R297S | 6 | Japan | Naito, et al. (2013) |
| c.961G>A | p.G321S | 7 | Neth | Coucke et al. (1999) |

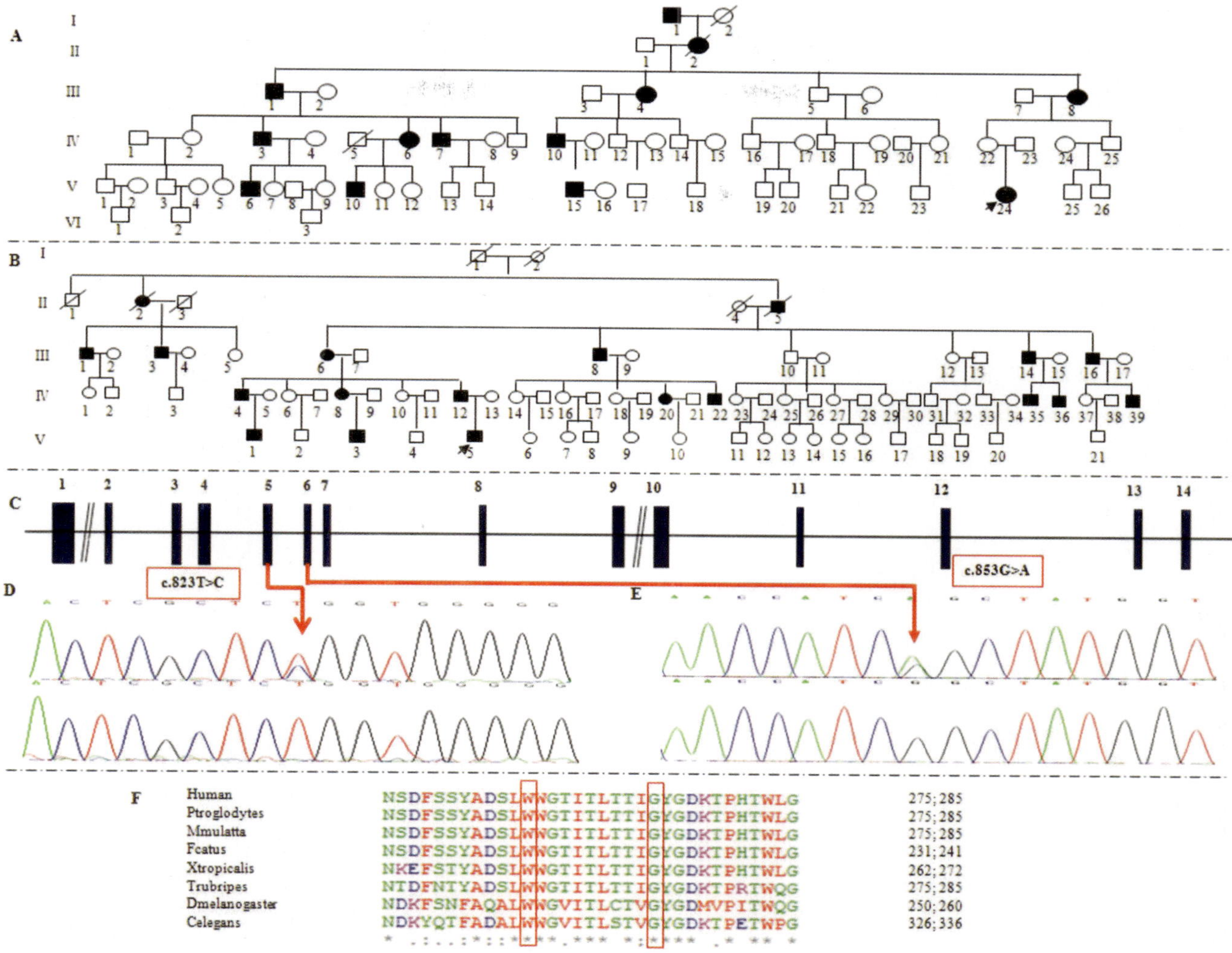


**Figure 1. Pedigrees and mutation analysis of the two large Chinese families.** (A) & (B) Pedigrees of family 025 and 727. Filled symbols for males (squares) and female (circles) represent affected individuals, and empty, unaffected individuals. (C) Structure of *KCNQ4* gene. *KCNQ4* gene has 14 exons. Mutations of c.823T>C (p.W275R) and c.853G>A (p.G285S) identified in *KCNQ4* are located in exon5 and exon6 respectively. (D) DNA sequence chromatograms showing the two heterozygous missense mutations c.823T>C and c.853G>A in affected individuals (upper panel) compared with the wild type controls (lower panel). (F) Conservation analysis shows that the Trp residue at 275 and the Gly residue at 285 in *KCNQ4* is conserved across human, Ptroglodytes, Mmulatta, Fcatus, Trubripes, Dmelanogaster, Celegans, Xtropicalis.

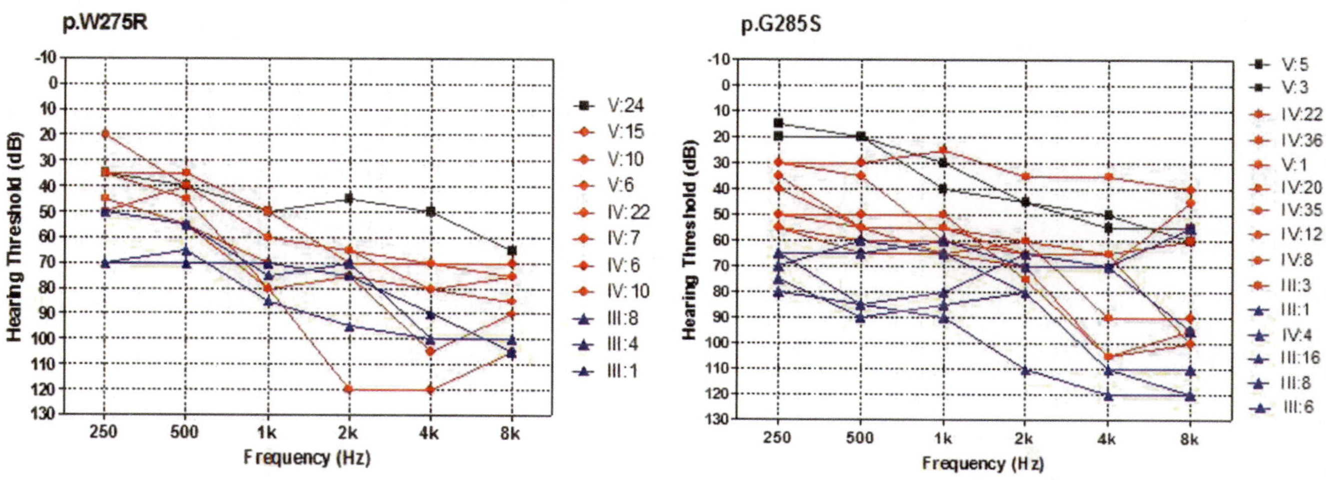


**Figure 2. Overlapping audiograms from the better ear for each genotype.** In the two cases of p.W275R and p.G285S, black colored audiograms were from the patients aged less than 20 years old, red colored audiograms were from individuals aged 20–49 years old and the blue audiograms were from the patients in their 50 s and over.

**Table 2.** Summary of clinical data for hearing impaired members in family 727.

| Subject | Gender[a] | Age of test (year) | Age of onset (year) | PTA (dB HL)[b] | Hearing impairment[c] | Audiogram | Tinnitus |
|---|---|---|---|---|---|---|---|
| III:1 | M | 50 | 6 | 78.75 | severe | downslope | + |
| III:3 | M | 44 | 10 | 72.50 | severe | downslope | − |
| III:6 | F | 68 | N/A | 91.25 | profound | flat | + |
| III:8 | M | 67 | 20 | 100.00 | profound | downslope | + |
| III:16 | M | 54 | 15 | 66.25 | moderately severe | flat | − |
| IV:4 | M | 50 | 30 | 75.00 | severe | flat | + |
| IV:8 | F | 41 | 24 | 58.75 | moderately severe | downslope | + |
| IV:12 | M | 34 | 17 | 57.50 | moderately severe | flat | + |
| IV:20 | F | 25 | 5 | 70.00 | moderately severe | flat | − |
| IV:22 | M | 21 | 6 | 61.25 | moderately severe | flat | + |
| IV:35 | M | 25 | 10 | 73.75 | severe | downslope | − |
| IV:36 | M | 22 | 10 | 62.50 | moderately severe | flat | − |
| V:1 | M | 23 | N/A | 31.25 | mild | downslope | N/A |
| V:3 | M | 13 | 11 | 38.75 | mild | downslope | + |
| V:5 | F | 8 | 6 | 37.50 | mild | downslope | + |

[a]M, male; F, female.
[b]PTA, pure-tone air-conduction averages (0.5, 1, 2 and 4 kHz) for the better-hearing ear of affected subjects in family 727.
[c]Diagnosed at the time of test. The severity of hearing impairment was defined as mild (26–40 dB HL), moderate (41–55 dB HL), moderately severe (56–70 dB HL), severe (71–90 dB HL) and profound (>90 dB HL).
N/A, not available; +, positive finding; −, negative finding.

**Table 3.** Summary of clinical data for hearing impaired members in family 025.

| Subject | Gender[a] | Age of test (year) | Age of onset (year) | PTA (dB HL)[b] | Hearing impairment[c] | Audiogram | Tinnitus[d] |
|---|---|---|---|---|---|---|---|
| III:1 | M | 76 | 15 | 76.25 | severe | flat | + |
| III:4 | F | 72 | 20 | 86.25 | severe | downslope | − |
| III:8 | F | 57 | 20 | 75 | severe | downslope | + |
| IV:3 | M | 52 | 16 | 70 | moderately severe | flat | + |
| IV:6 | F | 46 | 30 | 70 | moderately severe | downslope | + |
| IV:7 | M | 39 | 25 | 66.25 | moderately severe | downslope | − |
| IV:10 | M | 49 | 20 | 56.25 | moderately severe | flat | − |
| V:6 | M | 25 | 17 | 61.25 | moderately severe | downslope | − |
| V:10 | M | 25 | 15 | 56.25 | moderately severe | downslope | − |
| V:15 | M | 24 | 10 | 58.75 | moderately severe | flat | N/A |
| V:24 | F | 9 | 2 | 46.25 | moderate | downslope | N/A |

[a]M, male; F, female.
[b]PTA, pure-tone air-conduction averages (0.5, 1, 2 and 4 kHz) for the better-hearing ear of affected subjects in family 727.
[c]Diagnosed at the time of test. The severity of hearing impairment was defined as mild (26–40 dB HL), moderate (41–55 dB HL), moderately severe (56–70 dB HL), severe (71–90 dB HL) and profound (>90 dB HL).
[d]N/A, not available; +, positive finding; −, negative finding.

**Table 4.** Target region capture sequencing results.

| Proband | Length of target region (bp) | Target Region Map Bases (Mbp) | Coverage (%) | Coverage at least 20× (%) | Mean Depth |
|---|---|---|---|---|---|
| 025 | 132,789 | 54.21 | 99.71 | 99.49 | 408.23 |
| 727 | 132,789 | 56.11 | 99.71 | 99.38 | 422.59 |
| **Average** | **132,789** | **55.16** | **99.71** | **99.44** | **415.41** |

to NCBI37/hg19 assembly using the BWA (Burrows Wheeler Aligner). SNPs and indels (inserts and deletions) were detected using the GATK software [8].

## Sanger sequencing

After filtering against multiple databases, sanger sequencing was used in all available members from family 025 and 727 to determine whether the potential mutations in causative genes co-segregated with the disease phenotype in these families or not. Direct PCR products were sequenced using Bigdye terminator v3.1 cycle sequencing kits (Applied Biosystems. Foster City, CA) and analyzed using a ABI 3700XL Genetic Analyzer.

# Results

## Clinical description

For family 727, a total of 41 family members, composed of 15 clinical affected and 26 unaffected individuals were ascertained in this study. While in family 025, 11 patients and 26 control individuals were ascertained. Age of onset in family 727 ranged from 5 to 30 years old, with average onset age 13.08 years old, while in 025 the onset age ranged from 2 to 30 years old, with average onset age 16.45 years old. For both two autosomal families, affected members showed a post-lingual, symmetrical, and bilateral non-syndromic sensorineural hearing loss. The hearing loss was initially presented as high frequencies with subsequent gradual progression to severe level involving all frequencies at later ages. Some patients had associated tinnitus, but no vestibular symptoms or signs were reported (Table 2, Table 3, Figure 1A, 1B, Figure 2). High resolution computed tomography (HRCT) of the temporal bone in the probands showed normal middle ears structure, including normal vestibular aqueduct and internal auditory canal. None of the affected members had a history of exposure to aminoglycosides, noise, or other causes that may account for the hearing impairment.

## Targeted high-throughput sequencing

Approximately 133K bp of exons and adjacent intronic regions of the 30 genes known to be responsible for ADNSHL were captured and sequenced. The average sequencing depth for target region is about 415×, and 99.44% of the average coverage for targeted region is more than 20×, which is satisfied with the requirements for calling SNPs and InDels (Table 4). For the proband of family 025, a total of 484 variants were identified, 47 of which were nonsynonymous variants, splice acceptor and donor site mutations and coding indels that were more likely to be pathogenic mutations; only 3 of the 47 variants were with the allele frequency which were less than 0.01 in dbSNP137, HapMap, 1000 human genome and local dataset; and a missense variant, c.823T>C (p.W275R) in exon5 of *KCNQ4* (NM_004700), predicted to be "Damaging", "Probably Damaging", "Deleterious", "Disease_causing", "Conserved" and "Conserved" by SIFT, Polyphen2, LRT, Mutation Taster, GERP++, and PhyloP respectively (Tables 5 and 6). For this site, 45% (114/254) reads supported for C vs. 55% (140/254) reads supported for T, which means it is a heterozygote (Het) (Figure S1). This indicated that this novel mutation may be the cause of the hearing loss in this Chinese family. In the proband of family 727, another missense mutation, c.853G>A (p.G285S) in *KCNQ4*, a previously reported mutation (rs28937588) was identified (Figure S2).

## Mutation detection and analysis

Sanger sequencing confirmed the co-segregation of p.W275R and p.G285S with the disease phenotype in Family 025 and 727 respectively (Figure 1C and D and E). The two mutations were not detected in other 28 probands from Chinese families with ADNSHL. Both of the mutations occurred at highly conserved amino acids (Figure 1F), and are predicted to be deleterious by the SIFT, Polyphen2, LRT, Mutation Taster, GERP++, and PhyloP programs (IS IT NOT IDENTICAL TO WHAT HAVE MENTIONNED JUST ABOVE (Table 6). Based on these results and the phenotypes of these two families, we concluded that these

**Table 5.** Candidate genetic variants identified for the proband of family 025.

| Filter process | NO. of Variants |
|---|---|
| All SNPs/InDels | 484 |
| Functional_variations | 47 |
| Genotype frequency in dbSNP137, HapMap, 1000 human genome dataset ≤0.01 | 8 |
| Genotype frequency in local dataset≤0.01 | 3 |
| Predicted to be deleterious by SIFT, Polyphen2, LRT and MutationTaster | 1 |

**Table 6.** A novel variant in the proband of family 025.

| Gene | NM No. | Nucleotide | Amino Acid | Zygosity | Prediction information | | | | | |
|---|---|---|---|---|---|---|---|---|---|---|
| | | | | | SIFT | Polyphen2 | LRT | MutationTaster | GERP++ | PhyloP |
| *KCNQ4* | NM_004700 | c.823T>C | p.W275R | Het | Damaging | Probably Damaging | Deleterious | Disease_causing | Conserved | Conserved |

two mutations in the *KCNQ4* are responsible for the hearing loss in the family 025 and 727.

## Discussion

As is known, mutations in gene *KCNQ4* have been associated with ADNSHL, recognized as one of the most frequent causes of ADNSHL, is characterized by post-lingual autosomal dominant non-syndromic progressive sensorineural hearing loss, first affected the high frequencies according to GeneReviews. In this present study, we identified a known mutation and a novel mutation in the P-loop region of the *KCNQ4* potassium channel which yielded dominant non-syndromic hearing loss by high-throughput sequencing as well as conventional genetic testing. It is noteworthy that this is the first report of heterozygous mutations in the *KCNQ4* genes as a cause of ADNSHL in Chinese mainland families. In family 727, the G285S mutation in exon6 affects the first glycine in the GYG signature sequence of K+ channel pores, which has been identified in three affected members of a small French family with DFNA2. This mutation exert a strong dominant-negative effect on the wild type and render heteromeric channels nonfunctional [5]. By using adenoviral delivery of *KCNQ4* channels carrying G285S, Holt JR and colleagues demonstrated that *KCNQ4* channels contributed to the M-like conductances: $G_{K,n}$ of the cochlear outer hair cells and $G_{K,L}$ of the vestibular type I hair cells [9]. As far as we know, this is the second report about this mutation. Recurrent mutations in *KCNQ4* also include c.211delC (p.Q71fs), c.821T>A (p.L274H), c.827G>C (p.W276S), having been reported in more than one family. Among these recurrent mutations, mutation W276S is a hot spot mutation in Belgian, Dutch and Japanese families [10]. Together with specific audiogram configuration, recurrent mutations may promote genetic testing for ADNSHL with a particular phenotype [6]. In family 025, we found a novel missense mutation W275R in exon 5 of KCNQ4. The mutation c.823T>C (W275R) is immediately adjacent to the previously reported mutation c.827G>C (W276S). These two adjacent tryptophan residues, located with the pore helix, are highly conserved across different potassium channel families and play a important role in $K^+$ channel function, presumably holding the pore open at a correct diameter [11]. Mutations in these conserved tryptophan residues result in a complete loss of function of $K^+$ channel [12]. Previous studies have demonstrated that the W276S mutation lead to a dramatic decrease in *KCNQ4* surface expression with strong dominant-negative effects on the wild type (WT) *KCNQ4* subunit. We presume that the W275R mutation may have the similar functional mechanism [13,14].

It is noteworthy that this is the first report of *KCNQ4* mutation in Chinese mainland families. Before this report, there was a report of *KCNQ4* missense mutation P182L in a Taiwan family. The mutation locates in the S3 domain of *KCNQ4*. However, it is not conserved in all KCNQ family and unlikely to be pathogenic according to some prediction program, such as SIFT, Polyphen Phylop, LRT, etc. In this study, we found a P182L mutation in one of the 30 probands from ADNSHL families which did not co-segregate with the disease phenotype in the family members. It was also found in a Japanese control sample with normal hearing [4,15].

To date, 16 missense mutations and 4 indels in *KCNQ4* have been reported (Table 1). Phenotype-genotype correlation of *KCNQ4* has been summarized, most of the patients with missense mutation are younger-onset and pure all-frequency hearing loss, while patients with deletion mutations are later-onset and pure high-frequency hearing loss, so the two families in this study are

[16,17]. *KCNQ4* is also predicted to be a candidate gene for age-related hearing loss (ARHI) since *KCNQ4* mutation families have similar pattern of hearing loss with ARHI, especially a unique pattern of hearing loss with striking resemblance to ARHI, in which only the high frequencies were progressively affected while the lower frequencies remained intact until an older age [18]. To investigate the association of *KCNQ4* with ARHI, Van Eyken et al. examined *KCNQ4* and detected a significant association between *KCNQ4* and ARHI in two independent Caucasian populations. All SNPs are located in the same 13-kb region in the middle of the *KCNQ4* gene, indicating that the pathogenic variants for ARHI may locate in this region [19].

*KCNQ4* is likely to be a common gene in Chinese ADNSHL: i) *KCNQ4* is one of the more frequent genes in ADNSHL in comparison to the other reported genes [4]; ii) In a large Japanese cohort, *KCNQ4* is found to be the most prevalent gene responsible for Japanese ADNSHL. In their study, 19 families with 7 different mutations were identified in 287 probands from ADNSHL families [6]. Mutations of *KCNQ4* were also found in other east Asian region, such as Korea and other Japanese population (Table 1). iii) Our group found a copy variation of 47 base pairs insertion or deletion in the exon2 and exon3 intron sequence, supposing to be a specific marker for the hearing loss of the pedigree [20]. Then we performed mutation screening of *KCNQ4* in 71 patients with high frequency hearing loss and 40 unaffected individuals of matched geographical ancestry, and found the deletion of the second intron 47 bp in 5 patients as well as 2 males with normal hearing, the insertion of 47 bp in 11 patients [21].

Despite an increasing number of pathogenic *KCNQ4* mutations have been identified, the molecular aetiology of DFNA2 still unknown. The missense mutations are believed to exert a dominant-negative effect by interfering with the normal channel subunit. The two deletions, c.211delC and c.211_223del13, are proposed to exert a pathogenic effect through haploinsufficiency [3]. In the mouse models, loss of *KCNQ4* function leads to progressive sensorineural hearing loss, paralleled by selective degeneration of outer hair cells and spiral ganglion neurons [22]. Among the missense mutations, L274H, W276S, L281S, G285S, G296S and G321S are loss of function mutations and eletrophysiological studies have shown that these mutations lead to loss of *KCNQ4* currents [5,13,22,23,24]. However, the molecular mechanisms about how these mutations lead the loss of *KCNQ4* currents remain unknown. Recently Gao YH et al. reported two mechanisms underlying DFNA2, the decreased cell surface expression detected by immunofluorescent microscopy and Western blot and the impaired conductance of *KCNQ4* demonstrated by electrophysiological studies [14]. Because of the restriction of the lack of the understanding of the molecular aetiology, no therapeutic methods to prevent progressive hearing loss are available for now. Further functional studies regarding mutations in these residues in *KCNQ4* may help clarify the molecular mechanism, which in turn, will facilitate informative genetic counseling, early diagnosis and even treatment of hearing impairment [25]. It is anticipated that future management of these genetic hearing disorders will be more targeted to the cellular processes involved and improve the likelihood of hearing recovery.

In conclusion, we have shown two mutations in Chinese ADNSHL families using targeted high-throughput sequencing. This is the first report of *KCNQ4* mutation in Chinese mainland families, providing more information for discovering the molecular mechanism of KCNQ4 mutation-induced hearing loss. The results also support that the combination of targeted capture and NGS is a valuable molecular diagnostic tool for autosomal dominant hereditary deafness.

## Supporting Information

**Figure S1 Reads of proband from family 025 (chr1 41285133).**

**Figure S2 Reads of proband from family 727 (chr1 41285565).**

**Table S1 The non-syndromic autosomal dominant genes captured.**

**File S1 Data S1–S4.** Data S1. Next generation sequencing results of proband of family 025 (including all SNP and INDEL results). Data S2. Next generation sequencing results of proband of family 727 (including all SNP and INDEL results). Data S3. Sanger sequencing results of family 025. This file shows the sanger sequencing results of 36 members ascertained in this study. Data S4. Sanger sequencing results of family 727. This file shows the sanger sequencing results of 41 members ascertained in this study.

## Acknowledgments

We thank the families for their invaluable cooperation and participation in this work.

## Author Contributions

Conceived and designed the experiments: QW HW. Performed the experiments: HW YZ YY. Analyzed the data: HW YZ YY LS YG. Contributed reagents/materials/analysis tools: Q. Liu LL NL ZY WX LY. Contributed to the writing of the manuscript: HW YZ YY. Critical reading and discussion of manuscript: DW Q. Li JG BH FZ LZ XY LY CP QW.

## References


1. Gao X, Su Y, Guan LP, Yuan YY, Huang SS, et al. (2013) Novel compound heterozygous TMC1 mutations associated with autosomal recessive hearing loss in a Chinese family. PLoS One 8: e63026.
2. Yan D, Zhu Y, Walsh T, Xie DH, Yuan HJ, et al. (2013) Mutation of the ATP-gated $P2X_2$ receptor leads to progressive hearing loss and increased susceptibility to noise. Proc Natl Acad Sci 110: 2228–2233.
3. Zhao YL, Zhao FF, Zong L, Zhang P, Guan LP, et al. (2013) Exome sequencing and linkage analysis identified tenascin-C (TNC) as a novel causative gene in nonsyndromic hearing loss. PLoS One 8: e69549.
4. Hilgert N, Smith RJ, Van Camp G (2009) Forty-six genes causing nonsyndromic hearing impairment: which ones should be analyzed in DNA diagnostics? Mutat Res 681: 189–196.
5. Kubisch C, Schroeder BC, Friedrich T, Lutjohann B, El-Amraoui A, et al. (1999) KCNQ4, a novel potassium channel expressed in sensory outer hair cells, is mutated in dominant deafness. Cell 96: 437–446.
6. Naito T, Nishio SY, Iwasa Y, Yano T, Kumakawa K, et al. (2013) Comprehensive genetic screening of KCNQ4 in a large autosomal dominant nonsyndromic hearing loss cohort: genotype-phenotype correlations and a founder mutation. PLoS One 8: e63231.
7. Wei XM, Ju XC, Yi X, Zhu Q, Qu N, et al. (2011) Identification of sequence variants in genetic disease-causing genes using targeted next-generation sequencing. PLoS One 6: e29500.
8. Wei XM, Sun Y, Xie JS, Shi Q, Qu N, et al. (2012) Next-generation sequencing identifies a novel compound heterozygous mutation in MYO7A in a Chinese patient with Usher Syndrome 1B. Clin Chim Acta 413: 1866–1871.
9. Holt JR, Stauffer EA, Abraham D, Geleoc GS (2007) Dominant-negative inhibition of M-like potassium conductances in hair cells of the mouse inner ear. J Neurosci 27: 8940–8951.
10. Van Camp G, Coucke PJ, Akita J, Fransen E, Abe S, et al. (2002) A mutational hot spot in the KCNQ4 gene responsible for autosomal dominant hearing impairment. Hum Mutat 20: 15–19.

11. Doyle DA, Cabral JM, Pfuetzner RA, Kuo A, Gulbis JM, et al. (1998). The Structure of the Potassium Channel: Molecular Basis of K+ Conduction and Selectivity. Science 280: 69–77.
12. Perozo E, MacKinnon R, Bezanilla F, Stefani E (1993) Gating currents from a nonconducting mutant reveal open-closed conformations in Shaker K+ channels. Neuron 11: 353–358.
13. Kim HJ, Lv P, Sihn CR, Yamoah EN (2011) Cellular and molecular mechanisms of autosomal dominant form of progressive hearing loss, DFNA2. J Biol Chem 286: 1517–1527.
14. Gao YH, Yechikov S, Vazquez AE, Chen DY, Nie LP (2013) Impaired surface expression and conductance of the KCNQ4 channel lead to sensorineural hearing loss. J Cell Mol Med 17: 889–900.
15. Su CC, Yang JJ, Shieh JC, Su MC, Li SY (2007) Identification of novel mutations in the KCNQ4 gene of patients with nonsyndromic deafness from Taiwan. Audiol Neurotol 12: 20–26.
16. Topsakal V, Pennings RJ, te Brinke H, Hamel B, Huygen PL, et al. (2005) Phenotype determination guides swift genotyping of a DFNA2/KCNQ4 family with a hot spot mutation (W276S). Otol Neurotol 26: 52–58.
17. Kamada F, Kure S, Kudo T, Suzuki Y, Oshima T, et al. (2006). A novel KCNQ4 one-base deletion in a large pedigree with hearing loss: implication for the genotype-phenotype correlation. J Hum Genet 51: 455–460.
18. Coucke PJ, Van Hauwe P, Kelley PM, Kunst H, Schatteman I, et al. (1999) Mutations in the KCNQ4 gene are responsible for autosomal dominant deafness in four DFNA2 families. Hum Mol Genet 8: 1321–1328.
19. Van Eyken E, Van Laer L, Fransen E, Topsakal V, Lemkens N, et al. (2006) KCNQ4: a gene for age-related hearing impairment? Hum Mutat 27: 1007–1016.
20. Wang QJ, Cao JY, Li N, Yang Y, Wang QG, et al. (2002) KCNQ4 gene mutations affected pedigree with autosomal dominant hereditary hearing loss. Chin J Otorhinolaryngol 37: 343–347.
21. Li LN, Li QZ, Wu WM, Wang QJ (2007). Screening the mutation of KCNQ4 in patients with high frequency hearing impairment. J of audio and speech pathol 15: 25–27.
22. Kharkovets T, Dedek K, Maier H, Schweizer M, Khimich D, et al. (2006). Mice with altered KCNQ4 K+ channels implicate sensory outer hair cells in human progressive deafness. EMBO J 25: 642–652.
23. Baek JI, Park HJ, Park K, Choi SJ, Lee KY, et al. (2011) Pathogenic effects of a novel mutation (c.664_681del) in KCNQ4 channels associated with auditory pathology. Biochim Biophys Acta 1812: 536–543.
24. Mencia A, Gonzalez-Nieto D, Modamio-Hoybjor S, Etxeberria A, Aranguez G, et al. (2008). A novel KCNQ4 pore-region mutation (p.G296S) causes deafness by impairing cell-surface channel expression. Hum Genet 123: 41–53.
25. Trune DR (2010) Ion homeostasis in the ear: mechanisms, maladies, and management. Current Opinion in Otolaryngology & Head and Neck Surgery 18: 413–419.

18

# Whole-Exome Sequencing to Decipher the Genetic Heterogeneity of Hearing Loss in a Chinese Family with Deaf by Deaf Mating

**Jie Qing[1,2], Denise Yan[2], Yuan Zhou[1], Qiong Liu[2], Weijing Wu[1], Zian Xiao[1], Yuyuan Liu[1], Jia Liu[1], Lilin Du[2], Dinghua Xie[1]*, Xue Zhong Liu[1,2]***

**1** Department of Otolaryngology-Head and Neck Surgery, Institute of Otology, the Second Xiangya Hospital, Central South University, Changsha, Hunan, China, **2** Departments of Otolaryngology-Head and Neck Surgery, Leonard M. Miller School of Medicine, University of Miami, Miami, Florida, United States of America

## Abstract

Inherited deafness has been shown to have high genetic heterogeneity. For many decades, linkage analysis and candidate gene approaches have been the main tools to elucidate the genetics of hearing loss. However, this associated study design is costly, time-consuming, and unsuitable for small families. This is mainly due to the inadequate numbers of available affected individuals, locus heterogeneity, and assortative mating. Exome sequencing has now become technically feasible and a cost-effective method for detection of disease variants underlying Mendelian disorders due to the recent advances in next-generation sequencing (NGS) technologies. In the present study, we have combined both the Deafness Gene Mutation Detection Array and exome sequencing to identify deafness causative variants in a large Chinese composite family with deaf by deaf mating. The simultaneous screening of the 9 common deafness mutations using the allele-specific PCR based universal array, resulted in the identification of the 1555A>G in the *mitochondrial DNA (mtDNA) 12S rRNA* in affected individuals in one branch of the family. We then subjected the mutation-negative cases to exome sequencing and identified novel causative variants in the *MYH14* and *WFS1* genes. This report confirms the effective use of a NGS technique to detect pathogenic mutations in affected individuals who were not cand dates for classical genetic studies.

**Editor:** Andreas R. Janecke, Innsbruck Medical University, Austria

**Funding:** This study was supported by grants from the Cochlear Implantation Program of Hunan, China, and National Basic Research Program of China (973) (grants 2012CB967900 and 2012CB967904). This work also was supported by National Institutes of Health (NIH) (grant R01DC005575, R01DC012546 and R01DC012115) to XZL. The funders had no role in study design, data collection and analysis, decision to publish, or preparation of the manuscript.

**Competing Interests:** The authors have declared that no competing interests exist.

* Email: xliu@med.Miami.edu (XZL); dhuaxie@163.com (DX)

## Introduction

Hereditary hearing loss is highly heterogeneous, with hundreds of mutations in more than 60 genes found to disrupt auditory function (http://hereditaryhearingloss.org). Yet it is estimated that for the majority of patients with a presumed genetic deafness the etiology is still undetermined. In many of those unsolved cases, the cause may involve a known or a novel mutation in currently known causative genes. However, because of practical limitations including the large number and size of many genes and the high cost and cumbersomeness of Sanger sequencing, these genes are not routinely screened in a diagnosis setting. Although for many decades, genome wide linkage analysis has been used for disease gene identification, this approach is time consuming and unsuitable for small families with an inadequate number of affected individuals. Moreover, other traditional strategies including candidate gene study, combined linkage study and positional cloning have been very challenging in detecting extremely rare cases or sporadic cases caused by *de novo* mutation. As a result, the causal variant for these hearing-impaired patients has remained elusive and the genes for many human deafness associated loci have not been identified.

Recent developments in high-throughput sequence capture methods and next-generation sequencing (NGS) technologies have now made Whole exome sequencing (WES) technically feasible and more cost-effective to elucidate the genetic basis of Mendelian disorders with hitherto unknown etiology and diseases with genetic and phenotypic heterogeneity [1]. Targeted or WES has proved to be a robust and powerful tool to discover mutations or genes for both nonsyndromic and complex syndromic forms of hearing loss, especially in small families with a distinct and particular phenotypic expression that were once too small to map [2–4].

A typical WES screen will identify between 20,000 and 50,000 exonic variants [5]. A multitude of programs and databases are thus required to handle such a wealth of information. NGS data analysis normally involves applying multiple filters to the data in order to prioritize candidate functional variants from the large pool of candidates. With regard to deafness, because of its extreme genetic heterogeneity, WES analysis of several affected and healthy relatives from one family may be powerful strategy to discover rare causative genes or mutations. In the present study, we applied WES to determine the deafness causative genes and mutations in a large composite Chinese family with assortative mating. Among the mutations detected, we identified the 1555A>G mutation in the *mtDNA 12S rRNA* gene and novel mutations (c.541G>A; p.A181 T and c.449C>T; p.A150 V) in the genes encoding MYH14 and WFS1, respectively.

## Materials and Methods

### Clinical Evaluation

A large Chinese family with nonsyndromic sensorineural hearing loss was identified through the Department of Otolaryngology-Head and Neck Surgery, the Second Xiangya Hospital of Central South University, China. All patients underwent a complete history and physical exam as well as audiogram including air and bone (AC/BC) conduction pure tone thresholds, auditory brainstem response (ABR) thresholds, and auditory steady state response (ASSR). Audiological assessment was performed by measuring the average hearing thresholds level at 500, 1000, and 2000 Hz. High-resolution, thin-section computed tomography (CT) and magnetic resonance imaging (MRI) of the temporal bone were used to detect any congenital malformations in two children (IIIC:2 and IIIC:3) prior to cochlear implant surgery. This study was approved by the Ethics Review Committee of the Second Xiangya Hospital of Central South University. And the written consent form of the study was obtained from the study participants or their guardians.

### Preparation of DNA

Peripheral blood samples were collected from patients and their lineal relatives. Genomic DNA was then extracted from the blood using RelaxGene Blood DNA System (TIAGEN Biotech, Beijing, China).

### Simultaneous deafness gene mutation detection using microarray

Hereditary hearing loss allele-specific PCR based universal array (ASPUA) (CapitalBio, Beijing, China) was used to simultaneously screen 9 mutations causing hereditary hearing loss (*GJB2*: c.35delG, c.176del16, c.235delC, c.299-300delAT; *GJB3*: c.538C>T (R180X); *SLC26A4*: c.IVS7-2A>G, c.2168A>G (p.H723R); *mtDNA 12S rRNA*: 1555A>G, 1494C>T). Multiplex allele-specific PCR was performed and chips were imaged with a LuxScan TMHT 24 Microarray Scanner (CapitalBio, Beijing, China).

### Whole exome sequencing and data analysis

Enrichment of coding exons and flanking intronic regions was performed using a solution hybrid selection method with the SureSelect human all exon 50 Mb kit (Agilent Technologies) following the manufacturer's standard protocol. Adapter sequences for the Illumina Hiseq2000 were ligated and the enriched DNA samples were sequenced on the Hisq2000 instrument (Illumina). The resulting data were processed and annotated with Burrows-Wheeler Aligner (BWA), Genome Analysis Toolkit (GATK), and SeattleSeq. Details of read mapping, variant detection, filtering and annotation have previously been described [6].

### *GJB2, TRMU* genes analysis and candidate variants validation by direct Sanger sequencing

Whole coding region of the *GJB2* gene and the exon 1 of the *TRMU* gene were analyzed using previously reported primers [7]. Positive sequence variants detected in WES were tested for segregation in the family by first performing Sanger sequencing of the DNA of affected members. If all affected members were found to be carriers of the sequence variant, unaffected members of the family were also sequenced.

The primers were designed using Primer3, v.0.4.0 (http://frodo.wi.mit.edu/). Polymerase Chain Reaction (PCR) reactions included 10–40 ng of genomic DNA with Taq DNA polymerase (Roche), were performed using standard methods, and sequenced using the ABI PRISM Big Dye Terminator Cycle Sequencing V3.1 Ready Reaction Kit and the ABI PRISM 3730 DNA Analyzer (Applied Biosystems).

## Results

### Clinical manifestation

Genealogy of the composite family with deaf individuals is shown in Fig. 1. Physical examination of all members did not demonstrate any dysmorphic features suggestive of syndromic disease. A computed tomography (CT) scan and magnetic resonance tomography (MRI) performed in subjects IIIC:2 and IIIC:3 prior to cochlear implant surgery and did not show any abnormalities. Age at onset of hearing impairment in affected individuals varied from congenital to fourth decades of life. They exhibited symmetric progressive sensorineural hearing loss that ranged from moderate to profound in degree with sloping, flat or U-shaped audio profiles. One affected male (IIA:3) had a history of aminoglycoside exposure (Table 1; Fig. 1).

### Allele-specific PCR-based universal array for simultaneous deafness associated genes detection

Among the individuals (IIC:1; IIA:3; IIIC:1; IIIC:2; IIIC:3) tested for hotspot mutations, only one affected subject (IIA:3) was found to carry the *mtDNA 12S rRNA* 1555A>G mutation in homoplasmic state (Table 1 and Fig. 2A). Sanger sequencing analysis of the *mtDNA* of other family members revealed the presence of a homoplasmic c.1555A>G mutation in IA:2; IIA:1; IIA:2; IIA:3; IIA:4; IIIA:3; IIIA:4; IIIA:5 (Table 1; Fig. 2B), but the mutation was absent in other affected individuals (IIB:3; IIIB:1; IIIB:2; IIC:1; IIIC:1; IIIC:2; IIIC:3) and family members with normal hearing (IIA:5; IIIA:1; IIIA:2) (Fig. 1B and 1C). In addition, no pathogenic mutations were identified in either the coding region of the *GJB2* gene or the exon 1 of the *TRMU* gene by Sanger sequencing in any of the affected individuals tested. Individuals IIA:4, IIIA:3, IIIA:4 and IIIA:5 have normal hearing despite harboring the 1555A>G homoplasmic mutation. These individuals had no known history of aminoglycoside exposure. It has become clear that mtDNA mutations can cause nonsyndromic hearing loss (NSHL), both as a primary or as a predisposing factor. In the absence of exposure to aminoglycosides, the age of onset associated with the 1555A>G mutation may differ considerably among members of the same family. The clinical phenotype can also be variable, ranging from normal hearing, progressive moderate hearing loss starting in adult life, to profound congenital deafness [8]. It has been suggested that certain nuclear modifiers such as the 35delG mutation in the *GJB2* gene and the A10 S mutation in the *TRMU* gene as well as certain mitochondrial haplogroups may modulate the phenotypic expression of the hearing loss associated with the 1555A>G mutation [8,9]. In the present study, we have excluded the role of other common variants in the *mtDNA 12SrRNA* gene and *GJB2* gene in the 1555A>G positive individuals using the Deafness Gene Mutation Detection Array and Sanger sequencing. Thus, the observed variable phenotypic expression could be attributed to other modifier genes. IIA:1 and IIA:2 are both deaf and carry the homoplasmic 1555A>G mutation. Hearing loss is more likely caused by aminoglycoside ototoxicity in these cases. So far, the only well

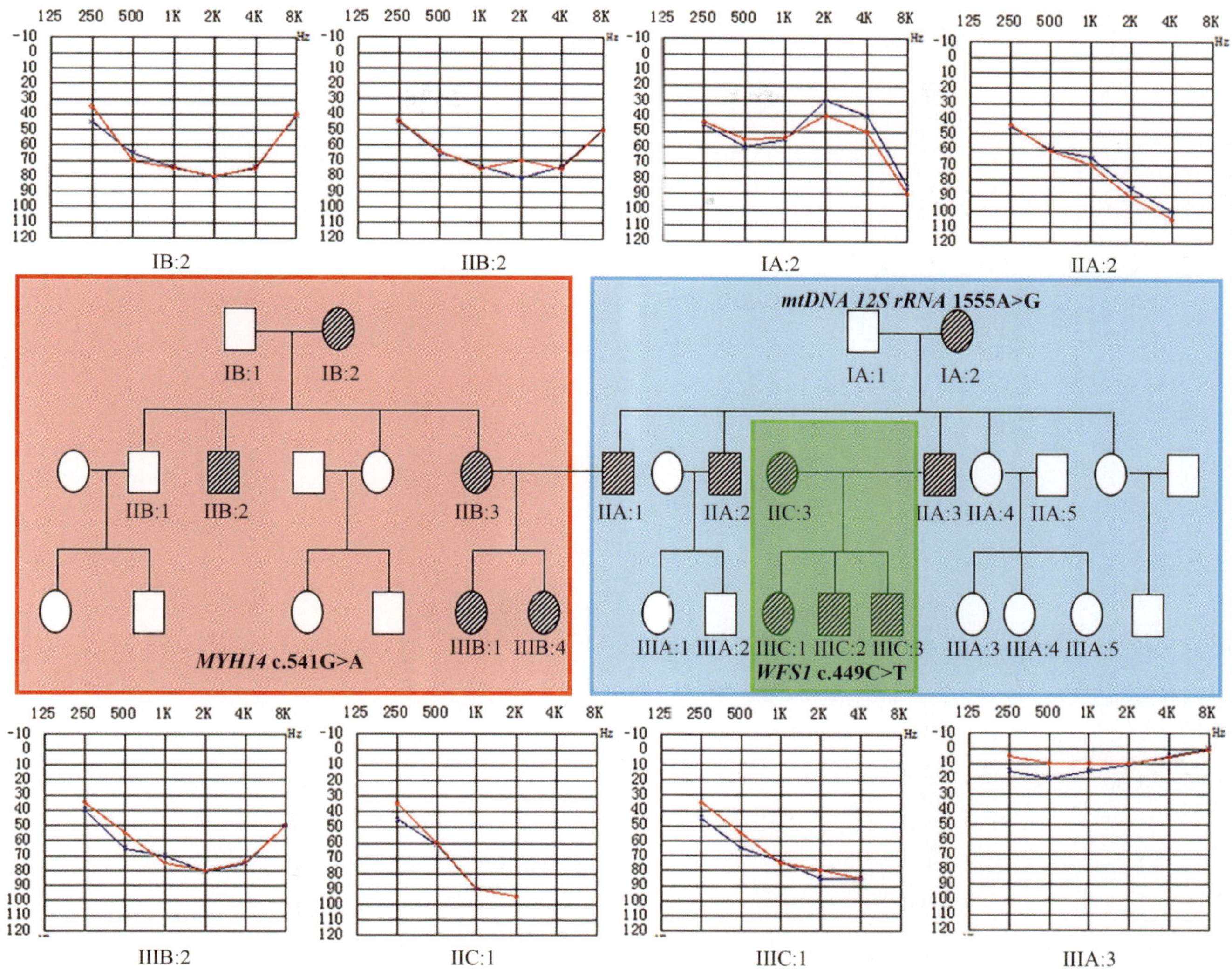


**Figure 1. Pedigrees of the composite family and Audiograms.** Segregation of the *mtDNA 12S rRNA* 1555A>G mutation (A), c.541G>A; p.A181 T in *MYH14* (B) and c.449C>T; p.A150 V in *WSF1* (C). Individuals for whom DNA samples are available and tested are labeled with their identification number. Audiograms of eight individuals exhibiting bilateral, symmetric, sensorineural hearing loss are shown. The blue curves indicate the left ear and red curves indicate the right ear.

documented environmental factor affecting the 1555A>G mutation are the aminoglycosides. This antibiotic class is widely used in developing countries like China, India and South Africa as a first-line treatment against multi-drug resistant tuberculosis due to its broad spectrum activity and cost-effectiveness.

## WES

The DNA samples from 2 distant relatives from the third generation (IIIB:2 and IIIC:2) were used for identification of the causative mutations by WES. Approximately, 94,000 single nucleotide variants and 10,206 INDELS per sample were obtained before variant filtering. Coverage of targeted exons for >10 reads were ranged from 92.3% to 93.5% and >20 reads from 81% to 83.5%. The Genomes Management Application (GEM.app), University of Miami Miller School of Medicine (https://secureforms.med.miami.edu/hihg/gem-app) was applied for data filtering. After analysis and filtering of the data according to the dominant inheritance model, 48 and 35 non-synonymous variants in 21 known deafness genes were detected in affected subject (IIIB:2) and (IIIC:2), respectively. The numbers of variants were further narrowed down by excluding the variants reported in dbSNP137, NHLBI (http://evs.gs.washington.edu/EVS/) or that had a minor allele frequency of more than 0.05% in these databases. Computational functional prediction algorithms (PolyPhen, SIFT, MutationTaster) and conservation scores (PHASTCO, GERP, PHYLOP) were also applied. By this filtering strategy, we have rapidly identified two missense mutations (c.541G>A; p.A181 T and c.2594C>T; p.T865 M) in the *MYH14* gene in IIIB:2 and a missense variant (c.449C>T; p.A150 V) in the *WFS1* gene in IIIC:2.

By filtering the variants according to the inheritance model (autosomal recessive with both homozygous and compound heterozygous), only a homozygous mutation (c.301G>A) in the *C3orf17* gene was found in affected subject IIIC:2. This gene is located on 3q13.2 and code for an uncharacterized single-pass transmembrane protein, consisting of 567 amino acid residues.

**Table 1.** The clinical features and the genetic study of the composite Chinese family with assortative mating.

| Number | Sex | Age at onset | Hearing test (BC[1]/ASSR[2]) | Audiogram profiles | *mtDNA 12S rRNA* 1555A>G | *MYH14* c.541G>A (p.A181 T) | *MYH14* c.2594C>T (p.T865 M) | *WFS1* c.449C>T (p.A150 V) |
|---|---|---|---|---|---|---|---|---|
| IA:1 | Male | - | L[3]:20 dB; R[4]:25 dB | normal | wt | wt[5]/wt | wt/wt | wt/wt |
| IA:2 | Female | The fourth decade | L:51 dB; R:55 dB | sloping | Homoplasmic | wt/wt | wt/wt | wt/wt |
| IIA:1 | Male | The first decade | L:>100 dB; R:>100 dB | sloping | Homoplasmic | wt/wt | wt/wt | wt/wt |
| IIA:2 | Male | The fourth decade | L:70 dB; R:70 dB | sloping | Homoplasmic | wt/wt | wt/wt | wt/wt |
| IIIA:1 | Female | - | L:20 dB; R:20 dB | normal | wt | wt/wt | wt/wt | wt/wt |
| IIIA:2 | Male | - | L:20 dB; R:23 dB | normal | wt | wt/wt | wt/wt | wt/wt |
| IIA:3 | Male | The first decade | L:90 dB; R:98 dB | sloping | Homoplasmic | wt/wt | wt/wt | wt/wt |
| IIA:4 | Female | - | L:25 dB; R:20 dB | normal | Homoplasmic | wt/wt | wt/wt | wt/wt |
| IIA:5 | Male | - | L:20 dB; R:20 dB | normal | wt | wt/wt | wt/wt | wt/wt |
| IIIA:3 | Female | - | L:23 dB; R:20 dB | normal | Homoplasmic | wt/wt | wt/wt | wt/wt |
| IIIA:4 | Female | - | L:25 dB; R:25 dB | normal | Homoplasmic | wt/wt | wt/wt | wt/wt |
| IIIA:5 | Female | - | L:23 dB; R:20 dB | normal | Homoplasmic | wt/wt | wt/wt | wt/wt |
| IB:1 | Male | - | L:25 dB; R:23 dB | normal | wt | wt/wt | wt/wt | wt/wt |
| IB:2 | Female | The first decade | L:70 dB; R:75 dB | U-shape | wt | mt[6]/wt | wt/wt | wt/wt |
| IIB:1 | Male | | L:20 dB; R:20 dB | normal | wt | wt/wt | wt/wt | wt/wt |
| IIB:2 | Male | The first decade | L:85 dB; R:81 dB | U-shape | wt | mt/wt | wt/wt | wt/wt |
| IIB:3 | Female | The first decade | L:85 dB; R:80 dB | U-shape | wt | mt/wt | wt/wt | wt/wt |
| IIIB:1 | Female | The first decade | L:83 dB; R:>100 dB | U-shape | wt | mt/wt | mt/wt | wt/wt |
| IIIB:2 | Female | The first decade | L:80 dB; R:80 dB | U-shape | wt | mt/wt | mt/wt | wt/wt |
| IIC:1 | Female | congenital | L:90 dB; R:90 dB | sloping | wt | wt/wt | wt/wt | mt/wt |
| IIIC:1 | Female | congenital | L:90 dB; R:85 dB | sloping | wt | wt/wt | wt/wt | mt/wt |
| IIIC:2 | Male | congenital | L:>100 dB; R:>100 dB | - | wt | wt/wt | wt/wt | mt/wt |
| IIIC:3 | Male | congenital | L:>100 dB; R:>100 dB | - | wt | wt/wt | wt/wt | mt/wt |

[1]Bone conduction;
[2]Auditory steady state response;
[3]left ear;
[4]Right ear;
[5]wild type;
[6]mutant allele.

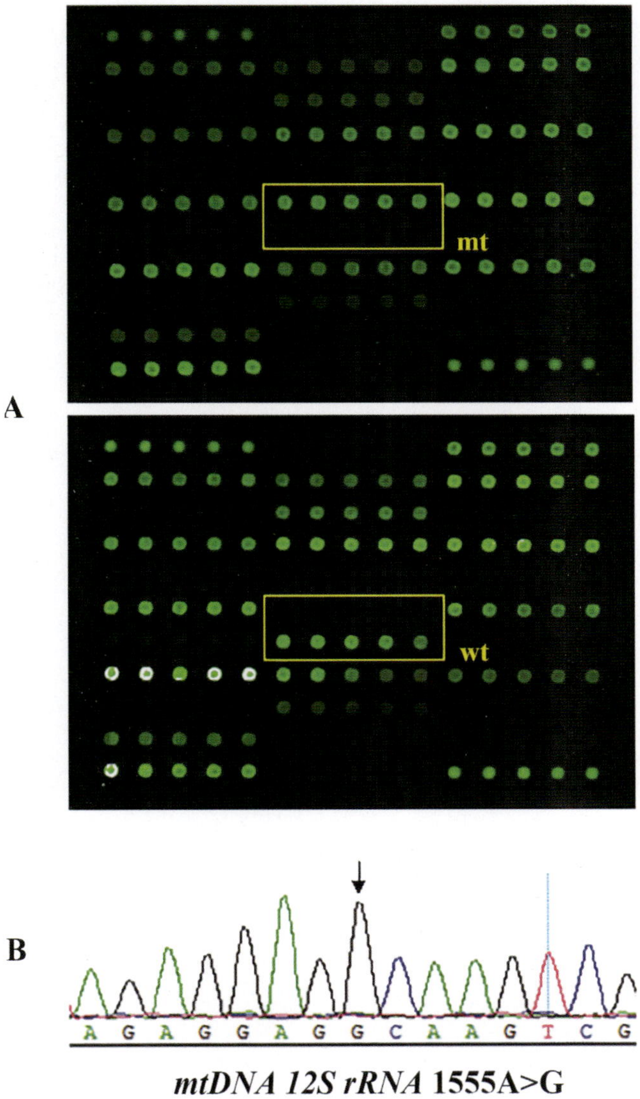


**Figure 2. Deafness genes detection array.** The *mtDNA 12S rRNA* 1555A>G homoplasmic mutation. The box in the scanned image of the microarray chip represents the *mtDNA 12S rRNA* 1555A>G square areas. The upper dark dots indicate the wild-type is absent and the green dots below indicate the 1555A>G homoplasmic mutation (A). Sequence chromatograms showing the homoplasmic 1555A>G mutation as indicated by the arrow (B).

## Expanded familial validation and Sanger sequencing confirmation

To validate the WES results from probands, we performed Sanger sequencing on extended family members. Expanded familial validation revealed that the sequence variation *MYH14* c.541G>A at codon 181 (exon 3) (Fig. 3A) located in the motor domain, near the ATP binding site of the *MYH14* gene (Fig. 3C), co-segregates with the deafness phenotype in all affected individuals (IB:2, IIB:2, IIB:3, IIIB:1 and IIIB:2) in part B of the composite pedigree (Fig. 1B), while the variant c.2594C>T; p.T865 M presents only in subjects IIIB:1 and IIIB:2. This sequence change is neither present in the exome variant server (EVS) database (6448 exomes; http://evs.gs.washington.edu/EVS/) nor in dbSNP (http://www.ncbi.nlm.nih.gov/projects/SNP/). It was absent in the parents and is thus more likely a *de novo* sequence change (Table 1). A number of studies have shown that a significant fraction of single-nucleotide variations (SNVs) occur *de novo*, representing the most extreme form of rare variants [10–12]. One of the superiorities of exome sequencing is the capacity of finding such rare SNVs. Furthermore, Sanger sequencing validated the proband's (IIIC:2) mutation (c.449C>T; p.A150 V) in the *WFS1* gene and demonstrated that the two siblings (IIIC:1 and IIIC:3) and mother (IIC:1) also carry this mutation (Table 1; Fig. 1C). The amino acids A181 in MYH14 and A150 in WFS1 are conserved in all sequenced vertebrates, from zebrafish to mammals (Fig. 3B1). Furthermore, Sequence alignment of the non-muscle class II myosin showed conservation of MYH14 p.A181 (Fig. 3B2). The mutations were predicted to affect protein function, with polyphen 2 score of 0.99 and SIFT score of 0.01 for MYH14 p.A181 T and polyphen 2 score of 0.964 for WFS1 p.A150 V [13]. Neither of these variants was identified in a panel of 320 normal hearing Chinese control subjects. The (c.541G>A; p.A181 T) in the *MYH14* gene was not present in the exome variant server (EVS) database (6448 exomes) or in the dbSNP (http://www.ncbi.nlm.nih.gov/projects/SNP/). The WFS1 (c.449C>T; p.A150 V) is carried by 1 out of 6489 exomes present on the Exome Variant server (MAF = 0.0077%). These observations suggest that the mutations A181 T in MYH14 and A150 V in WFS1 are likely to have a detrimental effect on the protein and its function. Finally, the variant (c.301G>A; pE101 K) in the *C3orf17* gene detected in both subjects with and without hearing loss was excluded as a deafness causative gene.

## Discussion

The simultaneous screening of target genes of interest allows for an efficient and cost-effective method of analyzing panels of genes concurrently, as opposed to testing on a gene-by-gene basis as occurs in Sanger sequencing. This is especially true for a disorder with heterogenic pathology, such as hearing loss (HL). On a larger scale, WES has become a promising tool for detecting novel and known mutations involved in hereditary deafness and for solving many deafness cases, as it screens the exons of all genes in the human genome. In the present study, we first tested the subjects IIA:3, IIC:1, IIIC:2 and IIIC:3 for deafness common mutations, using a targeted microarray, which resulted in the identification of the 1555A>G mutation in the *mtDNA 12S rRNA* gene in individual IIA:3 in a homoplasmic state. To further assess the mutation-negative cases, we performed exome sequencing with DNA from IIIB:2 and IIIC:2. After applying a filtering strategy using GEM.app followed by validation and segregation analysis of the variants in the family, we identified new deafness causative mutations in the *MYH14* and *WFS1* genes in part B and C of the composite family, respectively (Table 1 and Fig. 1). Defects in these genes have previously been described to cause autosomal dominant hearing loss.

The *MYH14* gene encodes nonmuscle myosin heavy chain II-C (NMHCII-C), a member of the NMHCII family of ATP-dependent molecular motor which interacts with cytoskeletal actin and regulates cytokinesis, cell motility, and cell polarity [14]. The *MYH14* encoded a protein that contains a N-terminal myosin domain, a myosin head-like region, two IQ domains, and a C-terminal myosin tail (Fig. 3C). It shares significant similarity with MYH9, MYH10, and MYH11, with highest conservation in the myosin head domain. The amino acid residue at the position 181 is highly conserved between species (Fig. 3B1) and among members of NMHC II, including MYH9, MYH10 and MYH11 (Fig. 3B2). The replacement of the hydrophobic, non-polar

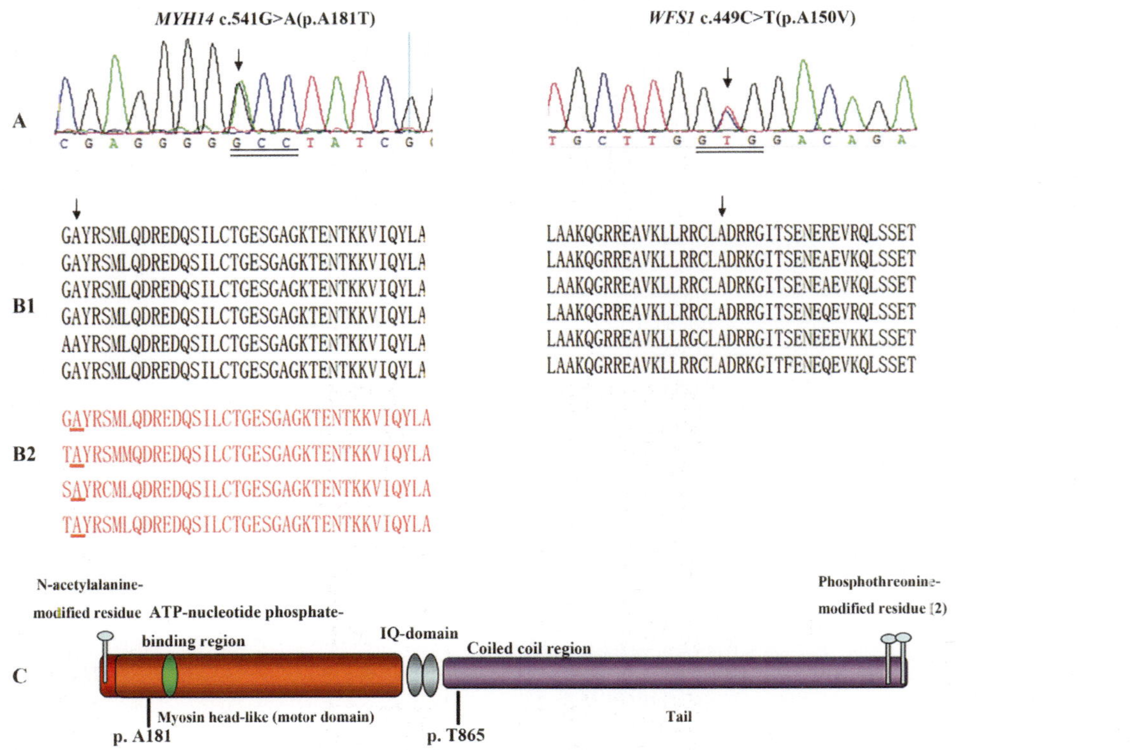


**Figure 3. Mutations analysis and conservations of the identified variants in the *MYH14* and *WFS1* genes.** Chromatogram of exon 3 of the *MYH14* gene showing heterozygous mutation c.541G>A in affected individuals (left panel; arrow) and heterozygous mutation c.449C>T in exon 4 of the *WFS1* gene (right panel; arrow) (A). Protein sequence alignment showing conservation of residues MYH14 A181 (left panel; arrow) and WFS1 A150 (right panel; arrow) across six species. Sequence alignment of the non-muscle class II myosin showing conservation of MYH14 A181 (left panel; red underlined) (B). Diagram of the human MYH14 consisting of a N-terminal myosin domain, a myosin head region, a motor domain, two IQ motifs, a coiled-coil region and a tail domain (C).

residue Alanine by the hydrophilic, polar residue Threonine may change the protein property. Moreover, according to the Chou-Fasman parameters [15,16], Alanine is one of the strongest helix formers whereas Threonine is one of the strongest β-sheet formers, which further supports the "probable" damaging effect of the amino acid change on the structure of protein. Furthermore, because the variant is located between the actin binding region and the ATP-binding (198–205$^{th}$) domain of the myosin head-like domain of MYH14, the mutation is more likely to affect the binding activity of the protein. The identification of this additional novel mutation further confirms the crucial role of MYH14 in auditory function.

The *MYH14* gene was identified as a causal gene of DFNA4 deafness [17]. Until now, only 4 *MYH14* causative mutations have been reported in DFNA4 families [17–19]. In the present study, we identified a new mutation (c.541G>A; p.A181 T) in the *MYH14* gene. The phenotype of this family is different to that of the previously reported DFNA4 families. Affected members have a moderate to profound sensorineural hearing loss with a U-shaped audio profile. We have also identified a novel mutation (c.449C>T; p.A150 V) in the *WFS1* gene in another branch of the pedigree. Hearing loss in this family is nonsyndromic and segregated in an autosomal dominant manner. Hearing impairment is congenital and affected mid and high frequencies. The WFS1 (c.449C>T; p.A150 V) is carried by 1 out of 6489 exomes present on the Exome Variant server (MAF = 0.0077%). The wild-type nucleotide C at cDNA position 449 is also highly conserved, with a PhyloP score of 4.13, phasCons 0.927 and Polyphen-2 predicts this variant as 'probably damaging' with a score of 0.964.

The protein product of WFS1, wolframin, is a membrane glycoprotein that is estimated to have nine helical transmembrane segments. It is primarily localized in the endoplasmic reticulum, with a hydrophilic extracytoplasmic N-terminus and a hydrophobic intracytoplasmic C-terminus [20–22]. Mutations in this gene are reported to be responsible for Wolfram Syndrome (WS), characterized by juvenile onset diabetes mellitus and optic atrophy, with 60% of the patients showing various degrees of hearing impairment by 20 years of age [23]. *WFS1* has also been linked to an autosomal dominant form of low-frequency sensorineural hearing loss (LFSNHL) [24–26], autosomal dominant optic atrophy (ADOA) [26–28], type 2 diabetes [29–31] and psychiatric problems [27,32,33]. Mutation analysis of *WFS1* in families with DFNA6/14 revealed that the identified pathogenic mutations in this disorder tend to be non-inactivating and cluster at the C-terminus or N-terminus of the protein domain [34,35], whereas most of the pathogenic mutations in Wolfram syndrome patients are distributed over the entire coding region and are often inactivating mutations resulting in loss of function of the encoded protein [36]. The WFS1 (c.449C>T; p.A150 V) identified in the present study is located in the extracellular N-terminus domain of the wolframin protein. Three other mutations in the N-terminal cytoplasmic domain of the protein, p.R161Q, p.D171N and p.K193Q, have been associated with LFSNHL [34,37] [45]. Other clinical features including optic atrophy have not been reported as concomitant features in families with LFSNHL. DFNA1, DFNA6/14/38 and DFNA54 are the loci so far reported as being associated with LFSNHL [38]. The progression of hearing impairment caused by a mutation in any of these three loci exhibits different characteristics. Patients carrying a mutation in the DFNA1 locus typically experience a rapidly deteriorating hearing loss progressing from low to involve all higher frequencies [39]. In contrast, those with a mutation in the DFNA54 or DFNA6/14/38 locus experience deafness propagating from low to high frequencies [40] or have no or mild progression beyond presbycusis [25,41,42]. The difference in phenotype across families may reflect influences of a modifier gene similar to DFNB1. The congenital, sharply sloping profound high frequency hearing loss in the individuals (IIC:1, IIIC:1, IIIC:2 and IIIC:3) carrying the WFS1 p.A150 V mutation is thus far unexplained, as we have ruled out involvement of *GJB2* and mitochondrial defect 12S rRNA in the phenotypic expression of the WFS1 p.A150 V mutation in those affected subjects. The fact that the carriers of the *WFS1* mutations associated with WS do not exhibit hearing loss and heterozygosity for other *WFS1* mutations resulting in nonsyndromic autosomal dominant LSFHNL reveals our incomplete knowledge of the function of the WFS1 protein and the impact of the different types of *WFS1* mutations. Another interesting point to be considered is a possible correlation between the location of the mutations within the WFS1 protein and the severity of the phenotype. Chaussenot et al (2011) [43] showed that the presence of at least 1 mutation that affects the carboxy-terminal tail of the protein seems to be more frequent in patients with neurologic symptoms whereas mutation in the N-terminal region was significantly correlated with the absence of neurologic complications. It has also been suggested that homozygosity or compound heterozygosity for missense mutation is more likely to lead to a "mild" phenotype whereas patients with one or more inactivating mutations would have a more severe phenotype. This distinction is rather arbitrary because only functional studies can determine which mutations are really inactivating. Our findings are broadening the mutational and phenotypic spectrum associated with the *WFS1* gene (Table 1).

Exome sequencing is not without limitations. For example, it does not detect mitochondrial disorders and may not capture each exon in every gene and insufficient depth of coverage in some regions can hinder detection of potential disease-causing genetic variants. The total proportion of gene variants that can be missed by current exome sequencing methods may be as high as 15%–20% [44].

In summary, we have combined both the Deafness Gene Mutation Detection Array and exome sequencing to identify deafness causative variants in this composite family with deaf by deaf mating. We first simultaneously screened the deaf patients for the 9 deafness common mutations using the allele-specific PCR based universal array, and then performed exome sequencing to identify the deafness causative gene in the mutation-negative cases. In the WES method, we consecutively filtered the variants by subjecting them to an analytical pipeline for high confidence variant calling and annotation. This simple filtering strategy rapidly led to the identification of causative variants in the *MYH14* and *WFS1* genes, and effectively demonstrates the potential of this combined approach to identify disease causative mutations in both novel and known genes in families with a small number of affected individuals.

## Acknowledgments

We express our deepest thanks and gratitude to this family for the cooperation of the members.

## Author Contributions

Conceived and designed the experiments: JQ DY QL WW ZX DX XZL. Performed the experiments: JQ DY YZ YL LD JL. Analyzed the data: QJ DY DX XZL. Contributed reagents/materials/analysis tools: JQ DY QL WW ZX DX XZL. Contributed to the writing of the manuscript: QJ DY DX XZL. Family contact: JQ YL DX.

## References


1. Ku CS, Naidoo N, Pawitan Y (2011) Revisiting Mendelian disorders through exome sequencing. Hum Genet 129: 351–370.
2. Yan D, Tekin M, Blanton SH, Liu XZ (2013) Next-generation sequencing in genetic hearing loss. Genet Test Mol Biomarkers 17: 581–587.
3. Shearer AE, Hildebrand MS, Sloan CM, Smith RJ (2011) Deafness in the genomics era. Hear Res 282: 1–9.
4. Lin X, Tang W, Ahmad S, Lu J, Colby CC, et al. (2012) Applications of targeted gene capture and next-generation sequencing technologies in studies of human deafness and other genetic disabilities. Hear Res 288: 67–76.
5. Genomes Project C, Abecasis GR, Altshuler D, Auton A, Brooks LD, et al. (2010) A map of human genome variation from population-scale sequencing. Nature 467: 1061–1073.
6. Gonzalez MA, Lebrigio RF, Van Booven D, Ulloa RH, Powell E, et al. (2013) GEnomes Management Application (GEM.app): a new software tool for large-scale collaborative genome analysis. Hum Mutat 34: 842–846.
7. Bae JW, Kim DB, Choi JY, Park HJ, Lee JD, et al. (2012) Molecular and clinical characterization of the variable phenotype in Korean families with hearing loss associated with the mitochondrial A1555G mutation. PLoS One 7: e42463.
8. Guan MX, Fischel-Ghodsian N, Attardi G (1996) Biochemical evidence for nuclear gene involvement in phenotype of non-syndromic deafness associated with mitochondrial 12S rRNA mutation. Hum Mol Genet 5: 963–971.
9. Guan MX, Fischel-Ghodsian N, Attardi G (2001) Nuclear background determines biochemical phenotype in the deafness-associated mitochondrial 12S rRNA mutation. Hum Mol Genet 10: 573–580.
10. Kong A, Frigge ML, Masson G, Besenbacher S, Sulem P, et al. (2012) Rate of de novo mutations and the importance of father's age to disease risk. Nature 488: 471–475.
11. Riviere JB, van Bon BW, Hoischen A, Kholmanskikh SS, O'Roak BJ, et al. (2012) De novo mutations in the actin genes ACTB and ACTG1 cause Baraitser-Winter syndrome. Nat Genet 44: 440–444, S441–442.
12. Xu B, Ionita-Laza I, Roos JL, Boone B, Woodrick S, et al. (2012) De novo gene mutations highlight patterns of genetic and neural complexity in schizophrenia. Nat Genet 44: 1365–1369.
13. Adzhubei IA, Schmidt S, Peshkin L, Ramensky VE, Gerasimova A, et al. (2010) A method and server for predicting damaging missense mutations. Nat Methods 7: 248–249.
14. Golomb E, Ma X, Jana SS, Preston YA, Kawamoto S, et al. (2004) Identification and characterization of nonmuscle myosin II-C, a new member of the myosin II family. J Biol Chem 279: 2800–2808.
15. Chou PY, Fasman GD (1974) Conformational parameters for amino acids in helical, beta-sheet, and random coil regions calculated from proteins. Biochemistry 13: 211–222.
16. Podoly E, Hanin G, Soreq H (2010) Alanine-to-threonine substitutions and amyloid diseases: butyrylcholinesterase as a case study. Chem Biol Interact 187: 64–71.
17. Donaudy F, Snoeckx R, Pfister M, Zenner HP, Blin N, et al. (2004) Nonmuscle myosin heavy-chain gene MYH14 is expressed in cochlea and mutated in patients affected by autosomal dominant hearing impairment (DFNA4). Am J Hum Genet 74: 770–776.
18. Yang T, Pfister M, Blin N, Zenner HP, Pusch CM, et al. (2005) Genetic heterogeneity of deafness phenotypes linked to DFNA4. Am J Med Genet A 139: 9–12.
19. Yang R, Li H, Zhan CX, Mao HY, Zhan TL, et al. (2010) c.359 T>C mutation of the MYH14 gene in two autosomal dominant non-syndromic hearing impairment families with common ancestor. Zhonghua Yi Xue Yi Chuan Xue Za Zhi 27: 259–262.
20. Lesperance MM, Hall JW, 3rd, Bess FH, Fukushima K, Jain PK, et al. (1995) A gene for autosomal dominant nonsyndromic hereditary hearing impairment maps to 4p16.3. Hum Mol Genet 4: 1967–1972.
21. Inoue H, Tanizawa Y, Wasson J, Behn P, Kalidas K, et al. (1998) A gene encoding a transmembrane protein is mutated in patients with diabetes mellitus and optic atrophy (Wolfram syndrome). Nat Genet 20: 143–148.
22. Strom TM, Hortnagel K, Hofmann S, Gekeler F, Scharfe C, et al. (1998) Diabetes insipidus, diabetes mellitus, optic atrophy and deafness (DIDMOAD) caused by mutations in a novel gene (wolframin) coding for a predicted transmembrane protein. Hum Mol Genet 7: 2021–2028.
23. Hardy C, Khanim F, Torres R, Scott-Brown M, Seller A, et al. (1999) Clinical and molecular genetic analysis of 19 Wolfram syndrome kindreds demonstrating a wide spectrum of mutations in WFS1. Am J Hum Genet 65: 1279–1290.
24. Bespalova IN, Van Camp G, Bom SJ, Brown DJ, Cryns K, et al. (2001) Mutations in the Wolfram syndrome 1 gene (WFS1) are a common cause of low frequency sensorineural hearing loss. Hum Mol Genet 10: 2501–2508.

25. Young TL, Ives E, Lynch E, Person R, Snook S, et al. (2001) Non-syndromic progressive hearing loss DFNA38 is caused by heterozygous missense mutation in the Wolfram syndrome gene WFS1. Hum Mol Genet 10: 2509–2514.
26. Hogewind BF, Pennings RJ, Hol FA, Kunst HP, Hoefsloot EH, et al. (2010) Autosomal dominant optic neuropathy and sensorineual hearing loss associated with a novel mutation of WFS1. Mol Vis 16: 26–35.
27. Rendtorff ND, Lodahl M, Boulahbel H, Johansen IR, Pandya A, et al. (2011) Identification of p.A684 V missense mutation in the WFS1 gene as a frequent cause of autosomal dominant optic atrophy and hearing impairment. Am J Med Genet A 155A: 1298–1313.
28. Eiberg H, Hansen L, Kjer B, Hansen T, Pedersen O, et al. (2006) Autosomal dominant optic atrophy associated with hearing impairment and impaired glucose regulation caused by a missense mutation in the WFS1 gene. J Med Genet 43: 435–440.
29. Wasson J, Permutt MA (2008) Candidate gene studies reveal that the WFS1 gene joins the expanding list of novel type 2 diabetes genes. Diabetologia 51: 391–393.
30. Lauenborg J, Grarup N, Damm P, Borch-Johnsen K, Jorgensen T, et al. (2009) Common type 2 diabetes risk gene variants associate with gestational diabetes. J Clin Endocrinol Metab 94: 145–150.
31. Chistiakov DA, Khodyrev DS, Smetanina SA, Bel'chikova LN, Suplotova LA, et al. (2010) A WFS1 haplotype consisting of the minor alleles of rs752854, rs10010131, and rs734312 shows a protective role against type 2 diabetes in Russian patients. Rev Diabet Stud 7: 285–292.
32. Khanim F, Kirk J, Latif F, Barrett TG (2001) WFS1/wolframin mutations, Wolfram syndrome, and associated diseases. Hum Mutat 17: 357–367.
33. Middle F, Jones I, McCandless F, Barrett T, Khanim F, et al. (2000) Bipolar disorder and variation at a common polymorphism (A1832G) within exon 8 of the Wolfram gene. Am J Med Genet 96: 154–157.
34. Cryns K, Pfister M, Pennings RJ, Bom SJ, Flothmann K, et al. (2002) Mutations in the WFS1 gene that cause low-frequency sensorineural hearing loss are small non-inactivating mutations. Hum Genet 110: 389–394.
35. Lesperance MM, Hall JW, 3rd, San Agustin TB, Leal SM (2003) Mutations in the Wolfram syndrome type 1 gene (WFS1) define a clinical entity of dominant low-frequency sensorineural hearing loss. Arch Otolaryngol Head Neck Surg 129: 411–420.
36. Kunz J, Marquez-Klaka B, Uebe S, Volz-Peters A, Berger R, et al. (2003) Identification of a novel mutation in WFS1 in a family affected by low-frequency hearing impairment. Mutat Res 525: 121–124.
37. Goncalves AC, Matos TD, Simoes-Teixeira HR, Pimenta Machado M, Simao M, et al. (2014) WFS1 and non-syndromic low-frequency sensorineural hearing loss: a novel mutation in a Portuguese case. Gene 538: 288–291.
38. Fujikawa T, Noguchi Y, Ito T, Takahashi M, Kitamura K (2010) Additional heterozygous 2507A>C mutation of WFS1 in progressive hearing loss at lower frequencies. Laryngoscope 120: 166–171.
39. Lalwani AK, Jackler RK, Sweetow RW, Lynch ED, Raventos H, et al. (1998) Further characterization of the DFNA1 audiovestibular phenotype. Arch Otolaryngol Head Neck Surg 124: 699–702.
40. Gurtler N, Kim Y, Mhatre A, Schlegel C, Mathis A, et al. (2004) DFNA54, a third locus for low-frequency hearing loss. J Mol Med (Berl) 82: 775–780.
41. Bom SJ, Kunst HP, Huygen PL, Cremers FP, Cremers CW (1999) Non-syndromal autosomal dominant hearing impairment: ongoing phenotypical characterization of genotypes. Br J Audiol 33: 335–348.
42. Pennings RJ, Bom SJ, Cryns K, Flothmann K, Huygen PL, et al. (2003) Progression of low-frequency sensorineural hearing loss (DFNA6/14-WFS1). Arch Otolaryngol Head Neck Surg 129: 421–426.
43. Chaussenot A, Bannwarth S, Rouzier C, Vialettes B, Mkadem SA, et al. (2011) Neurologic features and genotype-phenotype correlation in Wolfram syndrome. Ann Neurol 69: 501–508.
44. Fuchs SA, Harakalova M, van Haaften G, van Hasselt PM, Cuppen E, et al. (2012) Application of exome sequencing in the search for genetic causes of rare disorders of copper metabolism. Metallomics 4: 606–613.
45. Tranebjærg L, Hansen L, Bille M, Eiberg H, Fagerheim T, et al. (2004) A low frequency hearing impairment due to GJB2 and WFS1 mutations shows unrecognized genetic heterogeneity. Abstract platform presentation. Bethesda, MD: Molecular Biology of Hearing and Deafness Meeting.

# Gameplay as a Source of Intrinsic Motivation in a Randomized Controlled Trial of Auditory Training for Tinnitus

**Derek J. Hoare[1,2]*, Nicolas Van Labeke[3], Abby McCormack[1,2], Magdalena Sereda[1,2], Sandra Smith[1,2], Hala Al Taher[1], Victoria L. Kowalkowski[4], Mike Sharples[3], Deborah A. Hall[1,2]**

**1** National Institute for Health Research Nottingham Hearing Biomedical Research Unit, Nottingham, United Kingdom, **2** Otology and Hearing group, Division of Clinical Neuroscience, School of Medicine, University of Nottingham, Nottingham, United Kingdom, **3** Institute of Educational Technology, The Open University, Milton Keynes, United Kingdom, **4** Medical Research Council Institute of Hearing Research, Nottingham, United Kingdom

## Abstract

***Background:*** Previous studies of frequency discrimination training (FDT) for tinnitus used repetitive task-based training programmes relying on extrinsic factors to motivate participation. Studies reported limited improvement in tinnitus symptoms.

***Purpose:*** To evaluate FDT exploiting intrinsic motivations by integrating training with computer-gameplay.

***Methods:*** Sixty participants were randomly assigned to train on either a conventional task-based training, or one of two interactive game-based training platforms over six weeks. Outcomes included assessment of motivation, tinnitus handicap, and performance on tests of attention.

***Results:*** Participants reported greater intrinsic motivation to train on the interactive game-based platforms, yet compliance of all three groups was similar (~70%) and changes in self-reported tinnitus severity were not significant. There was no difference between groups in terms of change in tinnitus severity or performance on measures of attention.

***Conclusion:*** FDT can be integrated within an intrinsically motivating game. Whilst this may improve participant experience, in this instance it did not translate to additional compliance or therapeutic benefit.

**Editor:** Berthold Langguth, University of Regensburg, Germany

**Funding:** This work was funded by the National Institute for Health Research (NIHR) Biomedical Research Unit Programme, however, the views expressed are those of the authors and not necessarily those of the NHS, the NIHR or the Department of Health. The funders had no role in study design, data collection and analysis, decision to publish, or preparation of the manuscript.

**Competing Interests:** The authors have declared that no competing interests exist.

* Email: derek.hoare@nottingham.ac.uk

## Introduction

Tinnitus refers to a person's perception of sound in the ears or head despite any corresponding sound in the external world. Affecting 10–15% of the population [1] it represents a major healthcare burden [2] yet its underlying mechanisms are not well understood, and there is no uniformly effective treatment. Hearing loss is typically comorbid with tinnitus suggesting the tinnitus percept is a direct consequence of maladaptive neuroplastic responses to hearing loss [3]. Current models of tinnitus generation therefore focus on the potential consequences of hearing loss on neuronal activity within the central auditory system [4–12], although neuronal structures or networks responsible for tinnitus that are independent of those for hearing loss are yet to be convincingly determined [13–16].

The different models of tinnitus generation provide various potential regimes for novel tinnitus intervention. One current mainstay in tinnitus management is the provision of passive sound stimulation to mask the tinnitus sound [17–18]. However, active forms of sound enrichment such as Frequency Discrimination Training (FDT) are more recently proposed as interventions to *interrupt* tinnitus generation and maintenance in a targeted way, rather than just mask it [19]. Early studies of FDT for tinnitus have all based their hypotheses on a cortical reorganization model of tinnitus typically citing the seminal work of Recanzone et al. [20], where perceptual learning through *active* listening appeared key to functional reorganisation of the auditory cortex [21–23]. A more recent animal study from Engineer et al. [10], again suggested that passive sound exposure alone was not sufficient. They reported neuroplastic and behavioural changes associated with noise-induced hearing loss were reversed through passive sound stimuli when paired with electrical stimulation of the vagus nerve. Whilst sound stimulates the auditory cortex, vagal nerve stimulation is claimed to promote neuromodulator release akin to that generated by the use of behavioural reward to reinforce behavioural or neurophysiological change due to learning [24–25].

We recently reviewed studies of auditory training for tinnitus concluding the need for good quality trials to reliably estimate its potential as a therapy [19] and have since published our own investigation of the effects of FDT in adults with tinnitus [26]. In this study we compared training at hearing loss frequencies to training at normal hearing frequencies. Whilst overall we saw a clinically significant improvement in tinnitus handicap after training, this effect was independent of whether training stimuli were in the region of hearing or hearing loss. We therefore concluded that training at *any* frequencies could equally result in some generic improvement in tinnitus self-report and hypothesised the improvement to be cognitive, by reducing deficits in attention for example, rather than physiological.

Discrepant between animal studies and human studies of FDT for tinnitus however is the use of reward. Human studies of FDT for tinnitus have thus far derived training from *n*-alternative forced-choice paradigms conventionally used to determine psychophysical threshold for discrimination [27–28]. As such, reinforcement of experience with reward was not considered. Participants were simply required to 'react' to the stimulus presentation rather than 'interact' with the training programme. Participants presumably took part because of the potential for improvement in their tinnitus (extrinsic motivation). It may be that more interactive forms of FDT that incorporate elements of gameplay such as decision making, strategy development, competition, which are intrinsically (top-down) motivating would make training more rewarding and yield significant further benefit for patients [29]. In the health domain, computer-assisted educational health interventions are shown to be more effective when they support basic patient needs such as the desire for greater autonomy [30]. Furthermore it is proposed that future intervention-focused studies evaluating the influence of video games on health should account for the need for satisfaction provided by these games [31]. In the case of FDT for tinnitus, where the 'material' used is typically short pips of pure tones, we perhaps need to meet baser needs such as measurable enjoyment and engagement with the game for maximum therapeutic benefit to be realised. For the current study therefore we developed two training platforms where the core listening task involved FDT but we systematically introduced gaming elements. These elements were expected to provide intrinsic motivation through challenge (use of point scoring, target scores), control (opportunity for developing personal game strategy), fantasy (integration of the training task and the perceived objective of the game), and curiosity, that would motivate and reward participants [32].

We hypothesised that interactive games would prove more intrinsically motivating, and lead to greater improvement in self-reported tinnitus handicap than in previous studies, and to improvement in cognitive performance. Two main questions are addressed in this study; (1) can we use gameplay to make FDT intrinsically motivating, and (2) does FDT delivered in a gaming format have significant therapeutic benefit over training delivered in a reactive task-only format?

## Methods

This work is reported according to the CONSORT statement for randomized trials of non-pharmacological treatments [33] (Checklist S1). The work was initially conceived as an experimental study but to comply with requirements for publication the study was registered as a clinical trial after enrolment of participants started (Clinicaltrials.gov ID: NCT02095262) (Protocol S1). The authors confirm that there are no ongoing or related trials for this intervention.

All testing took place at the NIHR Nottingham Hearing Biomedical Research Unit.

### Ethics statement

Ethical approval for this study was granted by the National Research Ethics Service for England (Nottingham Research Ethics Committee). Participants gave their written informed consent to take part in the study in accordance with the approval granted.

### Participants

Sixty participants were recruited through advertisement in local Ear, Nose & Throat and audiology departments, and on our departmental website. Participants were adults with chronic subjective tinnitus who had a ≥20 dB hearing loss on at least one test frequency (0.125, 0.5, 1, 1.5, 2, 3, 4, 6, 8, 9, 10, 11.25, 12.5, 14 kHz) in at least one ear, and were not currently receiving any therapy or other intervention that could impact their hearing or tinnitus. Participants with hearing loss ≥40 dB at all test frequencies were excluded as not being able to sufficiently hear the training stimuli. The screening assessment included a case history, the Beck Anxiety Index and Beck Depression Index [34] and the Hyperacusis Questionnaire [35]. Participants with clinically significant scores on any of these questionnaires were excluded as requiring clinical intervention.

### Sample size

In our previous study [26] it was estimated that 14 participants per group would be required to detect a statistical difference in mean THQ score change between two groups. Baseline tinnitus handicap was different between groups in our previous study however, suggesting that a larger sample size would be more appropriate. We therefore aimed to recruit 20 participants to each group which according to Cohen [36–37] would generally be required for significance in a one-sided test at alpha 0.05 and a power of 0.8. A one-sided test was considered appropriate as we had a directional prediction of benefit for all three groups.

### Allocation of Participants to Training Groups

Participants were randomized using a minimization protocol [38] to ensure groups were balanced with respect to (i) severity of tinnitus; THQ score; <600, 600–1200, >1200, (ii) age; 18–49, 50–69, 70+, and (iii) gender. A number of steps ensured blinding of the outcome assessment. First, the minimization was performed by an independent researcher who was not otherwise involved in the study. Second, assessment of tinnitus was carried out by a researcher who did not know which group the participant was allocated to. Third, the researcher who programmed the laptops and instructed the participants was kept unaware of any changes in the participant's tinnitus throughout the study. Participants were not blinded but received the same generic information about the purpose of the study and were required not to discuss their tinnitus or gameplay experience where it would compromise study blinding of outcome assessment. Figure 1 shows the flow of participants through the study, exclusions, and dropout.

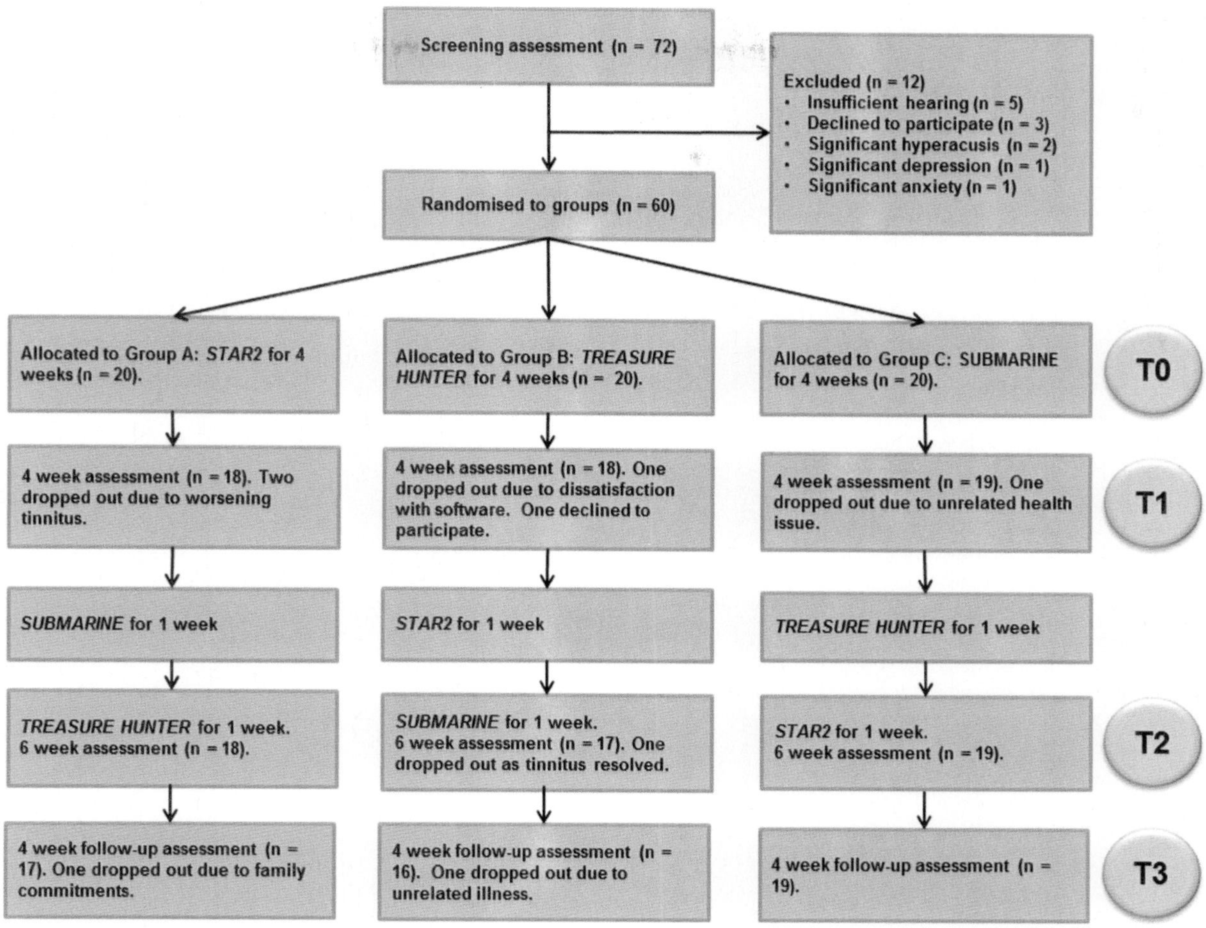


**Figure 1. Trial flow chart.**

## Audiometry

Pure-tone audiometry was conducted in a sound-proofed booth using the Siemens Unity 2 system and Sennheiser HAD 200 headphones. The frequency range tested was 0.125 kHz to 14 kHz. Pure tone average was calculated as the average threshold across 0.5, 1, 2, and 4 kHz for both ears. Audiometry was conducted at the initial assessment and again at visit three to check the stability of hearing thresholds.

## Frequency discrimination training (FDT) regimes

Participants were loaned a laptop computer with a Yoga AD-200 USB Adaptor soundcard, and Sennheiser HD 25 headphones. After 20 minutes familiarization with the program in the research unit, training was performed by participants in their own home. Participants were randomly assigned to one of three groups: Group A started training with *STAR2*, Group B started with *Treasure Hunter*, and Group C started with *Submarine* (described below, see Figure 2 for screenshots). Participants were introduced to each training platform only at the point at which they began a period of training on that game. Participants were instructed to perform the training task for 30 minutes, five times a week for four weeks. They then crossed over to train on each of the other two games for one week each in succession (Fig. 1). Training duration, date, time, and performance throughout each training session was logged by the computer. The base sound level for training was fixed at 55 dB SL according to the better ear threshold measured at the training frequency. Level was roved at random within trials by ±6 dB SPL to remove loudness cues (c.f. [39–40]). Participants were trained on a single frequency standard within the normal-hearing range one octave below the audiometric edge, derived from their audiometric profile using a 'broken-stick' fitting procedure (125 Hz to 14 kHz) (c.f. [41]).

## Game development and beta testing with experienced tinnitus participants

Five participants who had previously taken part in a trial of FDT using STAR2 software [26] took part in beta testing of two newly developed games. They were observed in real training situations, and provided feedback on the usability and playability of each game. Participants were observed playing each game and completed a semi structured interview afterwards to discuss what they liked and disliked about each game. This was an iterative process to ensure consistency in how the games responded to the actions of the participant, check the clarity and consistency of information on game status, game instructions, and other visual information, and to implement changes to overcome or remove

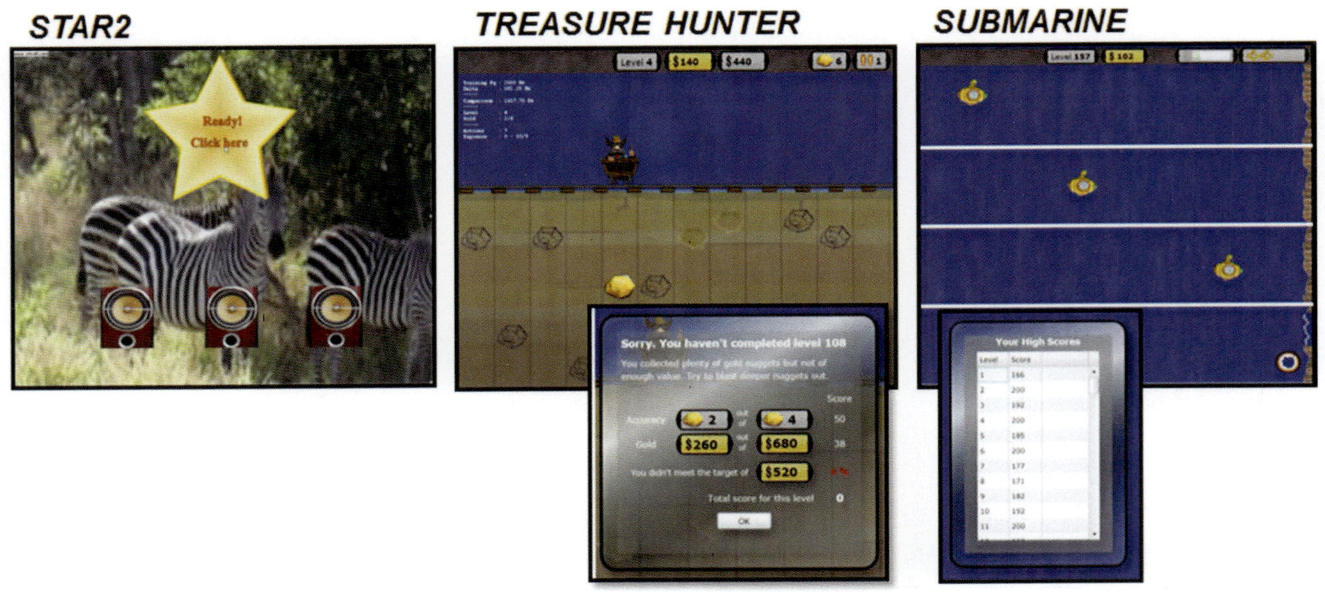


**Figure 2. Screenshots of the three training platforms.** *STAR2* background image rotates through a series of nature scenes unrelated to the task. *Treasure Hunter* is shown with an example of feedback after a level. *Submarine* is shown as successive snapshots to reflect movement across the screen, with an example of reward in the form of accrued points for each completed level.

aspects of either game that were disliked. STAR2 software was not modified for the current study.

**STAR2.** *STAR* was developed at MRC Institute of Hearing Research as a platform for assessing frequency discrimination thresholds in children [42]. Training comprised a reactive task presented in a three-interval, three-alternate forced choice (3I-3AFC) 'oddball' discrimination paradigm, delivered as a continuous block of trials. For a given individual, the 'trained' fundamental frequency (the standard) was fixed throughout, and the target (the oddball) differed by percentage (Hz) above the fundamental frequency of the standard. An adaptive staircase procedure targeted performance at 79%. *STAR2* was a modified version of this test software for use in adults. Cartoon characters and backdrops were replaced with changing nature scene backdrops and picture images of a loudspeaker. *STAR2* indicates whether a trial has been successful or not immediately following the trial using different sound cues, but no other feedback or scoring system is provided. Training comprised a single level only so each new training session started at the same fundamental frequency difference between standard and oddball.

***Treasure Hunter.*** *Treasure Hunter* was developed by co-author NVL. Training comprised of an interactive three interval task where the participant aims to progress through levels of the game by collecting sufficient reward points. Game play (selection, activation, and execution of frequency discrimination task) was participant induced. Participants had to move a mining cart left or right on the screen to 'blast out' gold nuggets buried in the ground, whilst avoiding coal nuggets. Gold nuggets had different levels of reward and nuggets buried deeper had greater reward. Coal nuggets had zero value. The 'trained' fundamental frequency was fixed throughout and the target always differed by a percentage (Hz) above the fundamental frequency of the standard; higher frequencies always corresponded to the presence of buried gold. The game had no time constraints, so participants could take a strategic approach to deciding which direction to move and when to select what they thought was a target. Rewards were earned by correctly identifying targets where the tone presented in the second interval was above the 'trained' fundamental frequency (i.e. presence of gold underneath). Participants were given a target value of reward to collect in order to progress to the next level of difficulty. Difficulty was increased in successive levels by reducing the percentage fundamental frequency difference that indicates reward. Feedback and scores were displayed after each level was attempted. Each new training session started at the level achieved in the previous session.

***Submarine.*** *Submarine* was developed by co-author MSh. Training comprised an interactive two-interval task where the participant aims to progress through levels of the game by identifying hidden exits in the sea-wall. In contrast to *Treasure Hunter*, in this instance part of the game play was system induced because the submarine continuously travelled a horizontal path across the screen from left to right. Tones were presented as repeated pairs comprising a 'sonar pulse' from the submarine (set as the 'trained' fundamental frequency) followed by a response tone from a hidden gap to the right of the screen, such that the vertical point on the screen at which the tones were of identical frequency indicated the target (gap). The participant's task was to navigate the submarine up or down, raising or lowering the fundamental frequency of the second interval tone accordingly, to the point on the screen where the two tones were identical. This allowed the submarine to pass through the gap in the wall. Participants were given four 'lives' and had to pass through five gateways to progress to the next level of difficulty. Difficulty was increased on successive levels by reducing the possible percentage fundamental frequency difference between the two tones. Feedback and scores were displayed after each level was attempted. Each new training session started at the level achieved in the previous session.

## Assessment of intrinsic motivation – interview and thematic analysis

Participant experiences of FDT using each game were evaluated qualitatively using the methods described in Benedek and Miner [43]. In the first instance, participants viewed a set of 118 product reaction cards depicting positive, negative, and neutral descriptor words (Table S1). Participants selected all words they considered applicable to their experience of the training. They were then asked to select five words from all those selected that were most relevant, and to elaborate on their word choice in an interview that centred on these five words. Interviews were recorded and transcribed, and coded using a thematic analysis approach [44–45]. A protocol for the process was developed based on Braun & Clarke [46]. Transcripts were first read and reread to familiarize the researcher with the text. Sections of text that were identified as meaningful (codes) were selected independently by two of four co-authors (DHo, MS, SS, HA). The two researchers then met to agree on which constituted codes within each transcript. In a final stage three researchers independently considered whether each code related to one of four predefined themes related to intrinsic motivation; *challenge*, *control*, *fantasy*, and *curiosity* [32], or to other themes that were not pre-defined. Those codes related to intrinsic motivation were further categorised according to whether they coded for a (positive) motivating factor, or coded for a (negative) demotivating factor.

## Usability and game preference questionnaires

Usability of each game was assessed using a three item questionnaire asking (1) what did you like the most about the game, (2) what did you dislike the most about the game? and (3) what would you like to see changed to make the game better? At the end of the 6-week training period participants completed an overall evaluation questionnaire in which they ranked the three games in order of preference (1 = liked most, 3 = liked least) and provided written comments on their selection.

## Tinnitus handicap

Two questionnaires were used to measure self-reported tinnitus handicap. The Tinnitus Handicap Questionnaire (THQ) [47] is a validated measure of change in tinnitus severity with high test-retest repeatability [48]. Twenty-seven questions provide a global measure of tinnitus handicap (maximum score = 2700). Scores > 600 indicate tinnitus severity that disrupts daily activity [49]. The THQ has two reliable subscales: Subscale 1 - physical health, emotional and social consequences of tinnitus (15 questions), Subscale 2 - hearing difficulty (8 questions). The THQ was use as our primary outcome measure.

The Tinnitus Handicap Inventory (THI) [50] is a 25 self-report item questionnaire measure of tinnitus severity. Although some argue it is insensitive to change (e.g. [51]) it is widely used and has been reported as an outcome in studies of FDT for tinnitus [23][52]. Test-retest reliability of the THI is high [53].

Questionnaires were administered at screening, T0, T1, T2, and T3.

## Psychoacoustic measures of tinnitus

Baseline tinnitus quality and changes over time were measured using the Tinnitus Tester [54], an automated computerised assessment of the qualities of the tinnitus sensation (matched loudness, dominant pitch, and bandwidth) over a 0.5–12 kHz frequency range. In addition to rating tinnitus loudness on a visual analogue scale (VAS) participants matched loudness by adjusting the level of a range of sound clips (centre frequencies 0.5–12 kHz) until each was judged to be the same as their tinnitus level. We took the loudness measure as the matched value at a single-frequency corresponding to little or no hearing loss (typically 0.5 or 1 kHz) and distant from the dominant tinnitus pitch. A profile of the individual tinnitus spectrum was generated by asking participants to rate the likeness of 11 sounds (centre frequencies 0.5–12 kHz) to the pitch of their tinnitus, using a 100-point scale. The dominant tinnitus pitch is defined as that frequency in the spectrum which had the highest likeness rating. Bandwidth was calculated as the standard deviation of all frequencies in the tinnitus spectrum, where each frequency was weighted by its percentage likeness to the tinnitus pitch of the participant (c.f. [41]). To reduce the impact of procedural learning on tinnitus outcomes the Tinnitus Tester was administered twice before training with the second measure taken as baseline (T0).

## Test of Everyday Attention (TEA)

The Test of Everyday Attention (TEA) is a standardised clinical test battery that allows for comparison across different attentional capacities in adults [55]. Two subtests were completed. Subtest 6 is a speeded visual task which measures selective attention. Participants are asked to search for and mark pairs of symbols from a list of entries in a simulated classified telephone directory (using list version A at baseline). The telephone search with counting (Subtest 7) measures divided attention by asking participants to perform the same speeded visual task (using a different version A list) whilst simultaneously counting tones presented from a loudspeaker and recalling the number of tones when prompted. Performance on the individual tasks was calculated as average time per item. Dual task detriment was then calculated as the increase in time per item required in the divided attention task compared to the sustained attention task.

The presentation level of the tone was sufficient to be clearly audible to the participant. Participants were assessed at baseline (T0) and again four weeks later (T1) when training on the first game was completed. Version B of each test was administered at T1.

## Analysis of quantitative data

For THQ and THI scores (measured at four time points) 7.9% of values were missing. For the TEA (measured at two time points) 6.7% of values were missing. These missing values were imputed using an expectation-maximisation (multiple imputation) method which assumes a normal distribution for the partially missing data and bases inferences on the likelihood under that distribution (maximum 25 iterations, SPSS v16.0).

Main analyses were conducted using analysis of variance models that included significant covariates to account for the influence of potential confounding factors (age, audiometric threshold, baseline depression and anxiety). Covariates for inclusion in the model were determined from initial analyses which included all potential covariates. Our primary analyses were (1) evidence that gameplay made FDT intrinsically motivating, (2) change in tinnitus handicap and in performance on attention tasks between T0 (baseline) and T1 (after training on the first game). Secondary analyses looked at effects across the multiple time points of this study. Clinical effect sizes were calculated as partial eta-squared ($\eta p^2$) on account of the repeated-measures design [56].

# Results

## Recruitment details

Recruitment began on 23rd July 2011 and the final follow-up assessment was completed 30th August 2012.

## Baseline characteristics

Table 1 shows mean baseline characteristics of each group. All three groups had a mean baseline tinnitus handicap sufficient to disrupt daily activity (i.e. >600; [43]).

**Table 1.** Baseline characteristics and training details.

| | Group A | Group B | Group C |
|---|---|---|---|
| **Measure** | Mean (SD) | Mean (SD) | Mean (SD) |
| **Gender** | 12 M, 8 F | 12 M, 8 F | 10 M, 10 F |
| **Age** | 60.2 (12.5) | 57.8 (14.0) | 60.6 (11.4) |
| **PTA (dB HL)** | 31.8 (17.1) | 25.2 (17.6) | 32.2 (18.0) |
| **Hearing loss slope** | 5 gradual, 15 steep | 5 gradual, 15 steep | 11 gradual, 9 steep |
| **Tinnitus duration (years)** | 12.6 (11.9) | 10 (9.7) | 11.4 (11.2) |
| **Depression** | 6.9 (8.3) | 5.2 (3.6) | 6.2 (8.1) |
| **Anxiety** | 7.7 (7.1) | 8.0 (7.1) | 5.8 (4.7) |
| **Hyperacusis** | 12.3 (7.5) | 12.1 (5.9) | 13.1 (7.3) |
| **Global THQ (/2700)** | 906 (485) | 937 (452) | 1040 (440) |
| **THQ Subscale 1 (/1500)** | 449 (323) | 467 (291) | 481 (315) |
| **THQ Subscale 2 (/800)** | 278 (176) | 289 (178) | 366 (183) |
| **VAS loudness (/100)** | 46 (20.8) | 39.8 (15.9) | 38.6 (14.9) |
| **Sensation level (dB SL)** | 29 (16) | 25 (16) | 17 (11) |
| **Dominant pitch (kHz)** | 7.6 (3.0) | 6.1 (2.7) | 6.4 (3.6) |
| **Tinnitus bandwidth (units)** | 3 (0.7) | 3.1 (0.6) | 3.3 (0.4) |
| **Training frequency (kHz)** | 0.9 (0.7) | 1.4 (1.1) | 1.3 (1.2) |

PTA: Pure Tone Average calculated as the average hearing threshold for 0.5, 1, 2 and 4 kHz, averaged across both ears. THQ: Tinnitus Handicap Questionnaire. VAS: Visual Analogue Scale.

## Compliance

Compliance with the initial block of training was calculated as a percentage of the time on task that had been prescribed (i.e. 30 min×5/week×4 weeks). For Group A *(STAR2)* compliance was 69% (SD = 21), for Group B (*Treasure Hunter*) it was 67% (SD = 22), and for Group C (*Submarine*) compliance was 75% (SD = 24). Compliance did not differ significantly between groups.

## Outcomes

**1. Motivation and preferences.** Motivations relating to participation and compliance were evaluated as part of a qualitative post-training assessment. 55 participants returned for their first post-training interview at T3. Analysis of these interviews generated 371 codes. Extrinsic motivators such as potential for improvements in tinnitus and a commitment to take part in the research were mentioned by comparable numbers of participants across all three groups but were not discussed further. We judged that 294 of the initial 371 codes related to one of the four themes under intrinsic motivation (challenge, control, fantasy, or curiosity). The pattern of reporting differed significantly across groups ($X^2 = 7.296$, $p = 0.026$, Figure 3). For *STAR2* there was a similar number of positive and negative codes related to intrinsic motivation (49 and 48 codes respectively), for *Treasure Hunter* there were more positive than negative codes (48 compared to 35), and for *Submarine* the majority of codes were positive (73 compared to 33 negative).

The most frequent positive codes were associated with the *Submarine* game and were related to the theme of 'control' (42 codes, Table 2). Participants felt *Submarine* was understandable and straightforward to use, which supported 'a desire to beat the game'. Most frequent negative codes were associated with *STAR2* and were related to the theme of 'curiosity' (33 codes, Table 2); participants felt that training on STAR2 was repetitive and boring, and that the training period (30 minutes) was too long.

Usability and game preference was determined by a brief questionnaire. Of those who had experience of all three games (n = 54), most (n = 26) expressed a preference for *Submarine*. *Treasure Hunter* was preferred by 23 participants and just five ranked *STAR2* as their preferred game. Written text provided by participants on usability and overall evaluation revealed that those who preferred *STAR2* did so because of its ease of use, finding the other games difficult or frustrating to play. For those who preferred *Treasure Hunter* or *Submarine* however, the major theme was that these games provided a sense of reward or achievement and were challenging, engaging, and stimulating.

**2. Tinnitus.** Our primary tinnitus outcome was change in THQ score (global measure of tinnitus handicap) at T1 compared to baseline (T0). Mean global THQ scores are given in Figure 4. Whereas mean THQ score increased for Group A (by 26 points) and Group B (by 20 points), for Group C THQ score was reduced by 69 points. A mixed design ANOVA was conducted with the within-subject factor of time (T0, T1) and the between-subject factor of training regime (*STAR2*, *Treasure Hunter*, or *Submarine*), with hearing loss included in the model as a significant covariate. Within-subject tests revealed a statistically significant change between T0 and T1 [$F$ (1,56) = 5.956, MSE = 117909.794, $p = 0.018$, $\eta p^2 = .096$]. Although a medium effect size, the difference in change between groups was less than is assumed to be clinically meaningful (194 points). There was no significant effect of training regime or interaction between time and training regime ($p>0.05$). Hence, we found no evidence that the type of gameplay modulates change in tinnitus handicap. Analyses of overall THQ subscale scores showed a small statistically significant effect [$F$ (1,56) = 5.931, $MSE = 208.387$, $p = 0.047$, $\eta p^2 = .047$] for THQ subscale 1 (health and psychological wellbeing) but not for THQ subscale 2 (hearing difficulties) ($p>0.05$) indicating the overall change related to change in psychological rather than functional handicap.

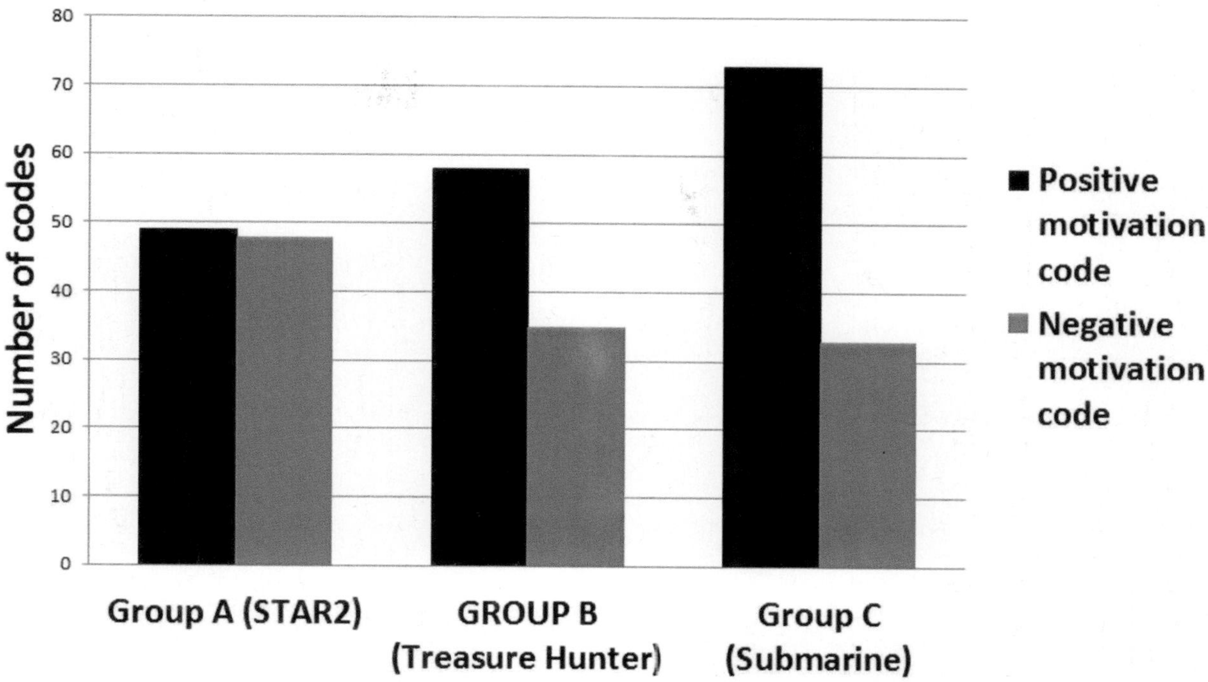


**Figure 3. Frequency of codes related to intrinsic motivation.** Data were extracted from 55 interviews in total (n = 18 for *STAR2*, 18 for *Treasure Hunter*, and 19 for *Submarine*).

In all cases the main effects above were not maintained at T3 follow-up (compared to T0 $p>0.05$ in all cases). Analysis of the THI scores revealed non-significant results, indicative of the lack of sensitivity to change of this questionnaire measure [44].

A mixed design ANOVA showed that after 4 weeks training (T1 compared to baseline T0) there was no significant effect of time or training regime on VAS loudness scores ($p>0.05$ in all cases), and no significant interaction of the main factors. Psychoacoustic measures of tinnitus quality include loudness rating, dominant tinnitus pitch, and bandwidth. For matched tinnitus loudness there was also no effect of time. There was however a significant effect of training regime [$F$ (2,57) = 3.255, MSE = 1281.258, $p = 0.046$], but no significant interaction of time and training regime. Pairwise comparisons were significant for a difference between Group A and Group C only ($p = 0.014$), where mean matched loudness level did not change, and increased by 3 dB SPL respectively. There was also no correlation between change in tinnitus loudness and change in tinnitus handicap however ($r = -0.087$, $p = 0.51$). Using the same approach to analysis, we found no significant effect of time or training regime on dominant tinnitus pitch or tinnitus bandwidth ($p>0.05$ in all cases). Neither were there significant interaction effects. As for tinnitus handicap, our results show that the type of gameplay has no impact on tinnitus quality.

**3. Attention.** A mixed-design ANOVA was used to assess the effect of training on attention. Age was included in the analysis as a significant covariate. Effects of the within-subject factor of time (T0, T1) and the between-subject factor of training regime (trained on *STAR2*, *Treasure Hunter*, or *Submarine*) were modelled.

Sustained attention (speeded visual search): There were no significant effects of time, training regime, or significant interaction (p>0.05).

Divided attention (speeded visual search while counting): There was no significant effect of time on divided attention ($p>0.05$) (Figure 5). There was a significant effect of training regime [$F(2,57) = 3.946$, MSE = 31.27, $p = 0.025$, $\eta p^2 = .122$]. Pairwise comparisons showed that the significance related to Group A

**Table 2.** Number of codes per theme.

| | Code Valence | STAR2 | TREASURE HUNTER | SUBMARINE |
|---|---|---|---|---|
| **Challenge** | Positive | 18 | 23 | 23 |
| | Negative | 13 | 9 | 6 |
| **Control** | Positive | 24 | 25 | 42 |
| | Negative | 2 | 7 | 2 |
| **Fantasy** | Positive | 0 | 2 | 1 |
| | Negative | 0 | 2 | 3 |
| **Curiosity** | Positive | 7 | 6 | 7 |
| | Negative | 33 | 17 | 22 |

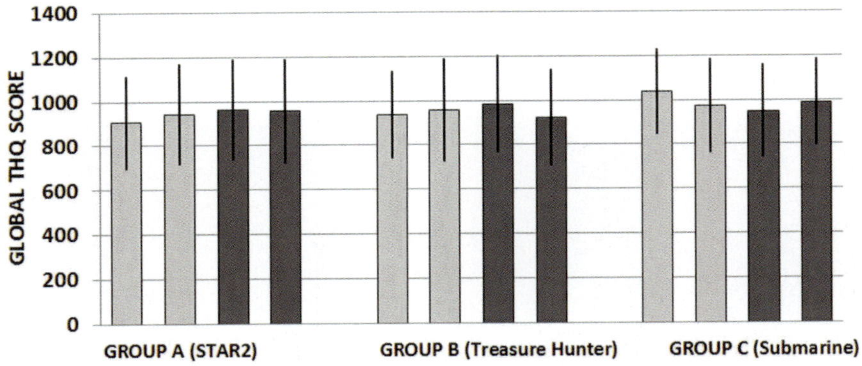


**Figure 4. Global Tinnitus Handicap Questionnaire scores.** Mean tinnitus handicap score (±95% CI) at the primary assessment points (T0 and T1 – black bars) and at follow up visits T2 and T3 (grey bars). n = 20 per group. Global score range in 0–2700.

(*STAR2*) and Group B (*Treasure Hunter*) ($p = 0.033$ after bonferroni correction), reflecting the overall differences in scores of these two groups. There was no significant interaction between time and training regime on divided attention ($p > 0.05$). Hence we found no evidence that the type of gameplay affects changes in performance on attention tasks.

Dual task detriment: As expected from the results above, there was no overall effect of time or significant interaction ($p > 0.05$) but there was a significant effect of training regime on dual task detriment [$F(2,56) = 3.841$, MSE = 23.651, $p = 0.027$, $\eta p^2 = .121$]. Pairwise comparisons again showed that the significance was between Group A (*STAR2*) and Group B (*Treasure Hunter*) ($p = 0.028$ after bonferroni correction).

This is the first study to examine the effects on FDT for tinnitus on attention. As the result was contrary to our hypothesis further analyses were conducted to investigate whether there had been any relationship between baseline tinnitus severity and performance on the attention tasks. No correlation was found between baseline tinnitus severity and either sustained or divided attention ($r = 0.04$, $p = 0.764$ and $r = 0.033$, $p = 0.8$, respectively). Partial correlation to factor in differences in audiometric threshold had no effect on the relationship ($r = -0.12$, $p = 0.93$ for sustained attention and $r = -0.13$, $p = 0.92$ for divided attention). However, audiometric threshold did correlate significantly with sustained attention ($r = 0.27$, $p = 0.037$), and approached significance for divided attention ($r = 0.244$, $p = 0.061$). So whilst there was no evidence that different levels of tinnitus severity impact on

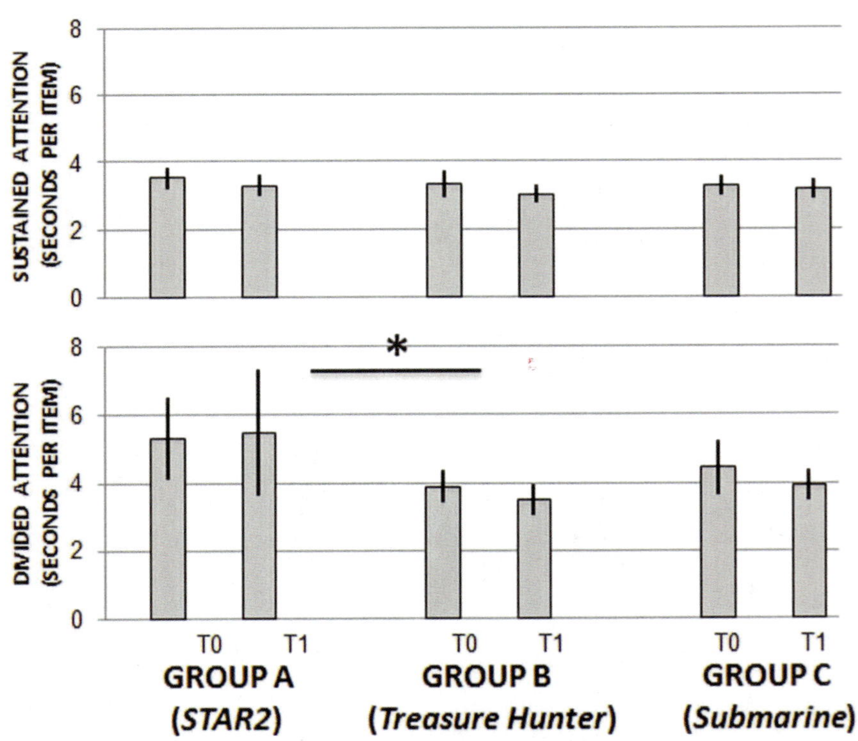


**Figure 5. Sustained and divided attention task scores before and after training.** There was no significant change in the measure of sustained attention after training. There was a significant between groups difference on the divided attention task for Group A compared to Group B but there was no effect of time or interaction (*$p < 0.05$). n = 20 per group.

attention, at baseline, better audiometric threshold was associated with better performance on these tests. Hence, we speculate that hearing loss negatively impacts cognitive performance.

## Discussion

This study addresses two questions. First, can gameplay make FDT more rewarding and intrinsically motivating? Second, would elements of intrinsic motivation that are inherent in game-play usefully increase the benefit a person with tinnitus gets from doing FDT (reduce tinnitus handicap, improve cognitive performance)?

### Intrinsic motivation in FDT

We conducted a qualitative evaluation to understand and compare intrinsic motivations to perform FDT where the FD task is delivered as a simple reactive task (as used in psychophysical testing), or where the FD task is integrated with progressing through levels of a computer game. Analysis of semi-structured interview data clearly showed that greater intrinsic motivation was associated with the gameplay on *Treasure Hunter* and particularly on *Submarine*, than with the simpler reactive task-based training of *STAR2*. Most participants reported a preference for FDT on *Treasure Hunter* and *Submarine*. Despite differences in motivation and game preference, compliance with prescribed training was similar across all groups. The intrinsic motivations identified were in any case insufficient to promote high compliance. We conclude that, whereas intrinsic motivation through gameplay may promote enjoyment and compliance with interventions in other health or educational domains (e.g. [57–58], in the case of this population (people with tinnitus) and this intervention (FDT), it promotes enjoyment but has no effect on compliance.

### Effects of training on tinnitus

Our previous work showed that the benefit derived from FDT in terms of a small reduction in tinnitus handicap was independent of the training frequency chosen and not related to a change in tinnitus quality [26]. Here again we find a small effect of FDT on our primary measure of tinnitus handicap, but within groups, mean THQ score only changes by up to 69 points (~7% of baseline) after training (T1) and there was no difference between groups.

### Effects of training on measures of attention

We also took the opportunity here to test the effect of FDT on attention in a tinnitus population. A number of studies point to deficits in cognitive processes such as attention and working memory in people with tinnitus, and for more cognitively demanding tasks in particular [59–62]. So, if FDT does improve attention then it may be useful for tinnitus. Training may reduce the amount of attention given over to the tinnitus sound and thereby increase the attentional capacity available to better perform everyday activities. Indeed, redirecting attention through movement therapy has already been applied clinically within a multi-therapy approach to tinnitus management [63].

Detrimental effects of tinnitus on measures of attention have previously been demonstrated in sub-populations of people with clinically significant tinnitus. Physiological effects were demonstrated by Delb et al. [64] who showed that tinnitus distress level impacts on the attention effects on event-related potentials (N100, phase locking), concluding that attention resources are 'captured' by tinnitus in people with higher distress levels. Rossiter et al. [61] showed there were slower reaction times on a dual task in people with moderately bothersome tinnitus compared to non-tinnitus controls. In a follow-up study Stevens et al. [62] observed slower reaction times in people with severe tinnitus in both a Stroop paradigm and a divided attention task; higher self-reported tinnitus handicap was associated with slower reaction times. Hallam et al. [59] also found that people with tinnitus show slower reaction times in a dual task condition compared to no tinnitus controls.

Here we observed no significant effect of FDT on the performance of a sustained or divided attention task. Furthermore, our results suggest that whereas the degree of hearing loss might determine performance on tasks of attention, there is no indication the degree of tinnitus handicap affects how well they perform these tasks. This is particularly contrary to the findings of Stevens et al. [62] who compared a small sample of tinnitus participants (n = 11 compared to 60 here) to a non-tinnitus control group. Stevens et al. [62] only included the degree of hearing loss at high frequencies (the average audiometric threshold for 4,6,8 kHz) in their analysis of covariance, rather than loss at the lower frequencies more relevant to speech and music perception (up to 2 kHz).

These secondary observations point to future work to fully understand the degree to which tinnitus and hearing loss contribute to performance on cognitive tasks.

### Limitations of this study

As with many studies of FDT for tinnitus, one limiting factor is the short training period prescribed and completed. The overall effect on THQ score in this study fell short of that reported in our previous study [26]. At our primary endpoint (after 4 weeks training) compliance was ~20% less than that observed in our previous study. We can speculate that this was related to factors such as (1) a longer intervention period in the current study (6 weeks compared to 4 weeks), (2) a much larger team on the current study with less continuity of the relationship between assessor and participant, or (3) ceiling effects in the previous study. Greater compliance here may have given an equal or greater effect on THQ score to that seen previously but even with identifiable extrinsic and intrinsic motivators, compliance looks likely to remain an issue for this particular intervention and participant group.

Another potential limitation, in terms of our results on the effects of attention, is that the outcome measure we chose (TEA) may not appropriately capture the changes in attentional processing that may occur as a result of FDT. A single measure of sustained attention for example may be insufficient to support or refute a main effect [65].

### Future directions

Perhaps the more challenging indications to emerge from this study are those relating the performance on attention tasks to the degree of hearing loss, and not tinnitus severity. Previous studies might suggest that cognitive training should be explored as a plausible therapeutic avenue. Indeed, psychotherapeutic approaches to tinnitus management already include elements termed attention training [66] or attention redirection [63]. Computer-based approaches to training attention, if sufficiently intrinsically motivating, may serve as an alternative self-help tool for people with tinnitus. However there is clearly first a need to explore the true impact of tinnitus on cognitive resources. The limited participant numbers and lack of control for hearing loss across previous studies on the topic mean further studies are needed to disambiguate the effect of tinnitus on cognitive performance from the effects of hearing loss or other factors. Are there subsets of tinnitus patients who show particular deficits on attention demanding tasks? If so then this may be a route for targeted management.

## Conclusion

FDT for tinnitus has now been the topic of eight published studies which taken together suggest it has a reproducible but small effect on tinnitus handicap more likely to be due to a change in cognitive representations (e.g. emotional reaction) rather than a physiological change in the auditory system (e.g. hearing) [19][26]. For most people, delivering FDT in a way that uses standard game-play approaches to intrinsically motivate the 'player' is preferred to a simple task-based training regime but this does not in itself lead to compliance or to additional improvements in self-reported tinnitus severity. The results of this study, taken in context with the limited existing literature, suggest that cognitive deficits experienced by people with tinnitus can be improved through training, if training incorporates the right intrinsically motivating elements and engages the user. It remains to be investigated whether such improvements can lead to clinically important improvements in tinnitus handicap.

## Supporting Information

**Checklist S1 CONSORT Checklist.**

**Protocol S1 Trial Protocol.**

**Table S1 Codes on product reaction cards.**

## Author Contributions

Conceived and designed the experiments: D. Hoare NVL VK M. Sharples D. Hall. Performed the experiments: D. Hoare NVL AM M. Sereda SS HA VK. Analyzed the data: D. Hoare AM M. Sereda SS HA. Wrote the paper: D. Hoare HA MS D. Hall.

## References


1. Davis A, El Rafaie A (2000) Epidemiology of tinnitus. In: Tinnitus Handbook. San Diego: Singular Publishing Group. pp. 1–24.
2. El-Shunnar SK, Hoare DJ, Smith S, Gander PE, Kang S, et al. (2011) Primary care for tinnitus: practice and opinion among GPs in England. J Eval Clin Pract 17: 684–692.
3. Moller AR. (2000) Similarities between severe tinnitus and chronic pain. J Am Acad Audiol 11: 115–124.
4. Eggermont JJ, Roberts LE (2004) The neuroscience of tinnitus. Trends Neurosci 27: 676–682.
5. Norena AJ, Eggermont JJ (2003) Neural correlates of an auditory afterimage in primary auditory cortex. J Assoc Res Otolaryngol 4: 312–328.
6. Dietrich V, Nieschalk M, Stoll W, Rajan R, Pantev C (2001) Cortical reorganization in patients with high frequency cochlear hearing loss. Hear Res 158: 95–101.
7. Weisz N, Moratti S, Meinzer M, Dohrmann K, Elbert T (2005) Tinnitus perception and distress is related to abnormal spontaneous brain activity as measured by magnetoencephalography. PLoS Med 2: e153.
8. Tass PA, Adamchic I, Freund HJ, von Stackelberg T, Hauptmann C (2012) Counteracting tinnitus by acoustic coordinated reset neuromodulation. Restor Neurol Neurosci 30: 137–159.
9. Norena AJ, Eggermont JJ (2005) Enriched acoustic environment after noise trauma reduces hearing loss and prevents cortical map reorganization. J Neurosci 25: 699–705.
10. Engineer ND, Riley RR, Seale JD, Vrana WA, Shetake JA, et al. (2011) Reversing pathological neural activity using targeted plasticity. Nature 470: 101–106.
11. Noreña AJ (2011) An integrative model of tinnitus based on a central gain controlling neural sensitivity. Neurosci Biobehav Rev 35: 1089–1109.
12. Schaette R, Kempter R (2006) Development of tinnitus-related neuronal hyperactivity through homeostatic plasticity after hearing loss: a computational model. Eur J Neurosci. 23: 3124–3138.
13. Elgoyhen AB, Langguth B, Vanneste S, De Ridder D (2012) Tinnitus: network pathophysiology-network pharmacology. Front Syst Neurosci 6: 1.
14. Rauschecker JP, Leaver AM, Mühlau M (2010) Tuning out the noise: limbic-auditory interaction in tinnitus. Neuron 66: 819–826.
15. Adjamian P, Sereda M, Hall DA (2009) The mechanisms of tinnitus: perspectives from human functional neuroimaging. Hear Res 253: 15–31.
16. Melcher JR, Knudson IM, Levine RA (2012) Subcallosal brain structure: Correlation with hearing threshold at supra-clinical frequencies (>8 kHz), but not with Tinnitus. Hear Res 295: 79–86.
17. Hoare DJ, Gander P, Collins L, Smith S, Hall DA (2012) Management of tinnitus in English NHS Audiology Departments: an evaluation of current practice. J Eval Clin Pract 18: 326–334.
18. Tyler RS (2012) Patient preferences and willingness to pay for tinnitus treatments. J Am Acad Audiol 23: 115–125.
19. Hoare DJ, Stacey PC, Hall DA (2010) The efficacy of auditory perceptual training for tinnitus: A systematic review. Ann Behav Med 40: 313–324.
20. Recanzone GH, Schreiner CE, Merzenich MM (1993) Plasticity in the frequency representation of primary auditory cortex following discrimination training in adult owl monkeys. J Neurosci 13: 87–103.
21. Flor H, Hoffmann D, Struve M, Diesch E (2004) Auditory discrimination for the treatment of tinnitus. Appl Pyschophysiol Biofeedback 29: 113–120.
22. Herraiz C, Diges I, Cobo P, Plaza G, Aparicio JM (2006) Auditory discrimination therapy (ADT) for tinnitus management: Preliminary results. Acta Otolaryngol. 126: 80–83.
23. Herraiz C, Diges I, Cobo P (2007) Auditory discrimination therapy (ADT) for tinnitus management. Prog Brain Res. 166: 467–471
24. Clark KB, Naritoku DK, Smith DC, Browning RA, Jensen RA (1999) Enhanced recognition memory following vagus nerve stimulation in human subjects. Nature Neurosci. 2: 94–98.
25. David SV, Fritz JB, Shamma SA (2012) Task reward structure shapes rapid receptive field plasticity in auditory cortex. Proc Nat Acad Sci 109: 2144–2149.
26. Hoare DJ, Kowalkowski VL, Hall DA (2012) Effects of frequency discrimination training on tinnitus: results from two randomised controlled trials. J Assoc Res Otolaryngol 13: 543–559.
27. Fu Q, Galvin JJ (2007) Computer-assisted speech training for cochlear implant patients: feasibility, outcomes and future directions. Sem Hear 28: 142–150.
28. Sweetow RW, Sabes JH (2007) Technological advance in aural rehabilitation: applications and innovative methods for service delivery. Trends Amplif 11: 101–111.
29. Amitay S, Halliday L, Taylor J, Sohoglu E, Moore DR (2010) Motivation and intelligence drive auditory perceptual learning. PLoS One 5: e9816.
30. Williams GC, Lynch MF, Glasgow RE (2007) Computer assisted intervention improves patient-centered diabetes care by increasing autonomy support. Health Psychol 26: 728–734.
31. Przybylski AK, Rigby CS, Ryan RM (2010) A Motivational Model of Video Game Engagement. Rev Gen Psychol 14: 154–166.
32. Malone TW, Lepper M (1987) Making learning fun: A taxonomy of intrinsic motivations for learning. In Aptitude, Learning and Instruction: Conative and affective process analyses. Snow& Farr (Eds.), NJ: Lawrence Erlbaum Associates. pp. 223–254.
33. Boutron I, Moher D, Altman DG, Schulz KF, Ravaud P (2008) Extending the CONSORT statement to randomized trials of nonpharmacologic treatment: explanation and elaboration. Ann Intern Med 148: 295–309.
34. Beck AT, Steer RA, Ball R, Ciervo CA, Kabat M (1997) Use of the Beck anxiety and depression inventories for primary care with medical outpatients. Assessment 4: 211–219.
35. Khalfa S, Dubal S, Veuillet E, Perez-Diaz F, Jouvent R, et al. (2002) Psychometric normalization of a hyperacusis questionnaire. Oto-Rhino-Laryngol 64: 436–442.
36. Cohen J (1998) Statistical Power Analysis for the Behavioral Sciences (second edition). Hillsdale, NJ: Lawrence Erlbaum Associates.
37. Cohen J (1992) A power primer. Psychol Bull 112: 155–159.
38. Altman DG, Bland JM (2005) Treatment allocation by minimisation. BMJ. 330: 384.
39. Thai-Van H, Micheyl C, Norena A, Collet L (2002) Local improvement in auditory frequency discrimination is associated with hearing loss slope in subjects with cochlear damage. Brain 125: 424–437.
40. Thai-Van H, Micheyl C, Moore BCJ, Collet L (2003) Enhanced frequency discrimination near the hearing loss cutoff: a consequence of central auditory plasticity induced by cochlear damage? Brain 126: 2235–2245.
41. Sereda M, Hall DA, Bosnyak DJ, Edmondson-Jones M, Roberts LE, et al. (2011) Re-examining the relationship between audiometric profile and tinnitus pitch. Int J Audiol 50: 303–312.
42. Barry JG, Ferguson MA, Moore DR (2010) Making sense of listening: the IMAP test battery. J Vis Exp 44: e2139.
43. Benedek J, Miner T (2002) Measuring Desirability: New methods for evaluating desirability in a usability lab setting. Proceedings of the Usability Professionals Association conference. Orlando, Florida.
44. Boyatzis RE (1998) Transforming Qualitative Information: Thematic Analysis and Code Development. Thousand Oaks, CA: Sage.
45. Joffe H, Yardley L (2004) Content and thematic analysis. In Research Methods for Clinical and Health Psychology (eds D. F. . Marks & L. . Yardley). London: Sage Publications Limited. pp. 56–68.

46. Braun V, Clarke V (2006) Using thematic analysis in psychology. Qual Res Psychol 3: 77–101.
47. Kuk FK, Tyler RS, Russell D, Jordan H (1990) The psychometric properties of a tinnitus handicap questionnaire. Ear Hear 11: 434–445.
48. Henry JL, Wilson PH (1998) The psychometric properties of two measures of tinnitus complaint and handicap. Int Tinnitus J 4: 114–121.
49. Sullivan M, Katon W, Russo J, Dobie R, Sakai C (1993) A randomized trial of nortriptyline for severe chronic tinnitus. Effects on depression, disability, and tinnitus symptoms. Arch Intern Med 11: 2251–2259.
50. Newman CW, Jacobson GP, Spitzer JB (1996) Development of the Tinnitus Handicap Inventory. Arch Otolaryngol Head Neck Surg 122: 143–148.
51. Meikle MB, Stewart BJ, Greist SE, Henry JA (2008) Tinnitus outcome assessment. Trends Amplif 12: 223–235.
52. Herraiz C, Diges I, Cobo P, Aparicio JM, Toledano A (2010) Auditory discrimination training for tinnitus treatment: the effect of different paradigms. Eur Arch Otorhinolaryngol 267: 1067–1074.
53. Newman CW, Sandridge SA, Jacobson G (1998) Psychometric adequacy of the Tinnitus Handicap Inventory (THI) for evaluating treatment outcome. J Am Acad Audiol. 9: 153–160.
54. Roberts LE, Moffat G, Baumann M, Ward LM, Bosnyak DJ (2008) Residual inhibition functions overlap tinnitus spectra and the region of auditory threshold shift. J Assoc Res Otolaryngol. 9: 417–435.
55. Robertson IH, Ward T, Ridgeway V, Nimmo-Smith I (1996) The structure of normal human attention: The Test of Everyday Attention. J Int Neuropsychol Soc 2: 525–534.
56. Bakeman R (2005) Recommended effect size statistics for repeated measures design. Behav Res Methods 37: 379–384.
57. Nilsson CN, Serafin S, Nordahl R (2009) Gameplay as a Source of Intrinsic Motivation for Individuals in Need of Ankle training or Rehabilitation. Presence 21: 69–84.
58. Papastergiou M (2009) Exploring the potential of computer and video games for health and physical education: A literature review. Comput Educ 53: 603–622.
59. Hallam RS, McKenna L, Shurlock L (2004) Tinnitus impairs cognitive efficiency. Int J Audiol 43: 218–226.
60. Pierce KJ, Kallogjeri D, Piccirillo JF, Garcia KS, Nicklaus JE, et al. (2012) Effects of severe bothersome tinnitus on cognitive function measured with standardized tests. J Clin Exp Neuropsychol 34: 126–134.
61. Rossiter S, Stevens C, Walker G (2006) Tinnitus and its effect on working memory and attention. J Speech Lang Hear Res 49: 150–160.
62. Stevens C, Walker G, Boyer M, Gallagher M (2007) Severe tinnitus and its effects on selective and divided attention. Int J Audiol 46: 208–216.
63. Cima RFF, maes IH, Joore MA, Scheyen DJ, El Refaie A, et al. (2012) Specialised treatment based on cognitive behaviour therapy versus usual care for tinnitus: a randomised controlled trial. Lancet 379: 1951–1928.
64. Delb W, Strauss DJ, Low YF, Seidler H, Rheinschmitt A, et al. (2008) Alterations in Event Related Potentials (ERP) associated with tinnitus distress and attention. Appl Psychophysiol Biofeedback 33: 211–221.
65. Shipstead Z, Redick TS, Engle RW (2012) Is working memory training effective? Psychol Bull 138: 638–654.
66. Delb W, D'Amelio R, Boisten CJ, Plinkert PK (2002) Evaluation of the tinnitus retraining therapy as combined with a cognitive behavioral group therapy. HNO 50: 997–1004.

# Impact of Genetic Counseling and Connexin-26 and Connexin-30 Testing on Deaf Identity and Comprehension of Genetic Test Results in a Sample of Deaf Adults: A Prospective, Longitudinal Study

**Christina G. S. Palmer[1,2,3*], Patrick Boudreault[4¤a], Erin E. Baldwin[1¤b], Janet S. Sinsheimer[2,3,5]**

**1** Department of Psychiatry & Biobehavioral Sciences, University of California Los Angeles, Los Angeles, California, United States of America, **2** Department of Human Genetics, University of California Los Angeles, Los Angeles, California, United States of America, **3** Institute for Society and Genetics, University of California Los Angeles, Los Angeles, California, United States of America, **4** Department of Deaf Studies, California State University Northridge, Northridge, California, United States of America, **5** Departments of Biomathematics and Biostatistics, University of California Los Angeles, Los Angeles, California, United States of America

## Abstract

Using a prospective, longitudinal study design, this paper addresses the impact of genetic counseling and testing for deafness on deaf adults and the Deaf community. This study specifically evaluated the effect of genetic counseling and Connexin-26 and Connexin-30 genetic test results on participants' deaf identity and understanding of their genetic test results. Connexin-26 and Connexin-30 genetic testing was offered to participants in the context of linguistically and culturally appropriate genetic counseling. Questionnaire data collected from 209 deaf adults at four time points (baseline, immediately following pre-test genetic counseling, 1-month following genetic test result disclosure, and 6-months after result disclosure) were analyzed. Four deaf identity orientations (hearing, marginal, immersion, bicultural) were evaluated using subscales of the Deaf Identity Development Scale-Revised. We found evidence that participants understood their specific genetic test results following genetic counseling, but found no evidence of change in deaf identity based on genetic counseling or their genetic test results. This study demonstrated that culturally and linguistically appropriate genetic counseling can improve deaf clients' understanding of genetic test results, and the formation of deaf identity was not directly related to genetic counseling or Connexin-26 and Connexin-30 genetic test results.

**Editor:** Francesc Palau, Centro de Investigación Príncipe Felipe – CIPF, Spain

**Funding:** CGSP received funding from the National Human Genome Research Institute (Ethical, Legal, and Social Issues Branch) (R01 HG003871, http://projectreporter.nih.gov); and from the Brocher Foundation (http://www.brocher.ch/en/brocher-fundation-in-brief/) in support of this research. The funders had no role in study design, data collection and analysis, decision to publish, or preparation of the manuscript.

**Competing Interests:** The authors have declared that no competing interests exist.

* Email: cpalmer@mednet.ucla.edu

¤a Current address: Gallaudet University, Washington, DC, United States of America
¤b Current address: ARUP Laboratories, Salt Lake City, Utah, United States of America

## Introduction

Connexin-related deafness is the most common worldwide form of hereditary deafness [1]. Furthermore, the relative frequency of Connexin-related deafness has increased several-fold over the last 100 years in the United States in the non-Hispanic white population as a result of marriages based on linguistic homogamy (signed language) [2,3]. Thus, deafness-causing variants in the genes underlying Connexin-related deafness (*GJB2* and *GJB6*, also sometimes referred to as Connexin-26 and Connexin-30, respectively) appear to play a significant role in the history and formation of the Deaf community and Deaf culture in the United States. In this article, the term Deaf (with a capital D) is used to refer to individuals who are members of the Deaf community, a distinct cultural group. The term Deaf is distinct from deaf (with a lower case d), which refers simply to an audiologic phenotype; individuals within the Deaf community may be deaf or hard-of-hearing [4]. Accordingly, Deaf identity and Deaf community (uppercase D) are used as Deaf culture descriptors only, and deaf identity and deaf community (lowercase d) are used when a collective term is needed to describe generic identity and community including Deaf and hearing affiliations.

The Deaf community has a distinct culture with its own beliefs, customs, attitudes, language (i.e., American Sign Language [ASL] in the United States), and behavioral norms. This culturally collective group views being deaf as a trait or characteristic of human diversity that is important to their culture [5]. Since the identification of deafness-causing variants in these two genes over a decade ago, a number of studies have demonstrated that some deaf individuals are interested in genetic testing to learn why they are deaf [6–9]. Although deafness-causing variants in Connexin-26 and Connexin-30 may be important for the Deaf community, the availability of deaf genetic testing raises a variety of issues for the Deaf community.

One important issue to consider is whether or not *knowing* genetic information challenges or changes an individual's deaf identity. Deaf identity is an individual's self-identification with deafness, which relates directly to and is influenced by the individual's identification with the Deaf community. Research suggests that individual differences yield four different deaf identity orientations: hearing, marginal, Deaf (also called immersion), and bicultural (sometimes referred to as equal involvement in deaf and hearing communities) [10–15]. Within this framework individuals hold a hearing identity when the mainstream hearing society is their primary frame of reference. These individuals identify with the hearing society in attitude, behavior, and communication style, and they tend to view being deaf from a medical-pathological perspective. Individuals with marginal identity are ambivalent about their deafness and their cultural frame of reference (hearing, deaf or hard-of-hearing). Individuals who are heavily engaged with the Deaf community, feel a strong sense of "Deaf" pride, view deafness as a personal characteristic, and communicate with sign language, are considered to have an immersion or culturally Deaf identity. Finally, individuals with a bicultural identity feel comfortable with both deaf and hearing people, appreciate both cultures, and may be bilingual in sign and written or spoken languages. Variation in deaf identity (and hence cultural/ community affiliations) may exist in part because most deaf individuals are not born into the Deaf community. Instead factors such as their language preference, educational experiences, and personal and social experiences play a large role in shaping their identity and affiliation with the both the Deaf and hearing communities [12,16,17].

Hence, the deaf community is composed of individuals who differ in their identity as a deaf person, that is, their cultural affiliation [18,19]. However, studies have found that identities can shift and change as a result of a variety of factors, such as demographic (e.g., age), psychological, or contextual variables [20–22]. Deaf identity is no different. Deaf identity is complex and dynamic because the development of an individual's deaf identity is a process that evolves over time, is influenced by many factors including interactions with deaf and hearing peers [23–25], and may be context-dependent or in flux [18]. Dimensional measures such as the Deaf Identity Development Scale – Revised [13] and the Deaf Acculturation Scale [11,26,27] have been developed to provide more nuanced understanding of deaf identity rather than relying on a categorical assignment.

Research has shown that the extent to which one affiliates with the Deaf culture/community affects attitudes toward genetic testing in hypothetical situations where no testing has been offered [28–32] as well as situations where actual testing is offered [6]. Not only may deaf identity affect interest, knowledge, and attitudes toward genetic information, but deaf identity may also be *affected* by genetic information provided through genetic counseling and genetic testing. Changes in deaf identity are one possible route through which the individual impact of genetic testing can affect the larger Deaf community. Sufficient concern has been raised about susceptibility to changes in deaf identity that may affect survival and growth of the Deaf community that there are studies examining effects of deaf-related technologies on deaf identity. For example, to address concern about the effects of cochlear implant use on the Deaf community/culture, several studies have examined deaf identities in cochlear implant (CI) users and non-users [33,34]. Both studies found that CI users more frequently endorsed items measuring a hearing identity compared to those without a CI. However, one study also found that CI users endorsed beliefs about deafness and Deaf culture that were similar to non-users [34], and the other study found similar number of participants with bicultural identities in both groups [33]. These results may play a role in allaying potential concerns about the impact of this particular technology on the Deaf community.

Deaf culture and the Deaf community cannot be sustained without a clear sense of identity and belonging. Changes in deaf identity are one possible route through which the individual impact of genetic testing can affect the Deaf community. Thus, an important issue to consider is whether or not genetic information challenges or changes one's deaf identity. Examining the effect of deaf genetic testing on deaf identity is important because if all prelingually deaf individuals had genetic testing, about half will be found to have a genetic explanation for why they are deaf [35]. We previously demonstrated that deaf individuals who learned that they have Connexin-related deafness experienced psychological well-being and that those who received a negative or inconclusive genetic test result experienced some psychological distress [36]. Hence, there already is empirical evidence that deaf genetic information has an impact on deaf individuals. Moreover, there is some evidence outside of the realm of deaf identity that identity may be affected by genetic information, as genetic test results have been shown to influence self-concept [37] and self-esteem [38]. Thus, if the receipt of a *genetic explanation* for deafness has a different effect on deaf identity than the receipt of *no explanation* for deafness, there could be a profound impact on the Deaf community and Deaf culture.

Individuals often learn genetic test results from a genetic counselor or geneticist through a result disclosure genetic counseling session. Genetic information can be complex to explain and understand, and the challenges of understanding the meaning of Connexin-related genetic test results have been documented among hearing parents of a deaf child [39]. As an additional layer of complexity, the unique language and culture shared by many deaf and hard-of-hearing individuals challenge the norms for both acquisition and provision of genetics information which could impact the effectiveness of result disclosure genetic counseling sessions. ASL is the primary language for culturally Deaf individuals within the U.S. Deaf community, and English is usually their second language. However, some individuals may opt to use spoken English, a combination of ASL and English, a form of signed English, or, in some rare instances, a unique signed language developed and used within the home of the deaf individual. Importantly, the use of signed language interpreting during genetic counseling to convey information between parties using two different communication modalities introduces an additional layer of complexity to the understanding of genetic concepts [40,41].

Studies specifically examining effectiveness of genetic counseling to enhance genetics knowledge outcomes in cultural and linguistic minority groups are beginning to emerge [42–44]. We recently demonstrated that deaf adults' genetics knowledge and understanding of the etiologic heterogeneity of deafness, Connexin-related deafness, inheritance, and genetic testing, are enhanced by *pre-test* genetic counseling provided in a culturally and linguistically sensitive manner [40]. Although studies have found that understanding genetic test results is challenging, particularly negative and inconclusive results, there are data on the positive effect of genetic counseling on enhancing understanding of specific genetic test results among hearing parents of a deaf child [45]. Currently there are no empirical data regarding the effects of genetic counseling on deaf individuals' understanding of their actual genetic test results. The dearth of data on deaf individuals' understanding of their genetic test results poses a barrier to the development of culturally and linguistically tailored counseling strategies and the provision of anticipatory guidance to deaf clients in general, and specifically to Deaf individuals.

This paper addresses two major aims with data collected from deaf individuals participating in a prospective, longitudinal genetic counseling and testing study. The first aim was to determine the effect of genetic counseling or Connexin-26 and Connexin-30 genetic test results on participants' deaf identity; despite having sufficient statistical power we found no evidence that the degree of change in deaf identity differs between individuals receiving a genetic explanation and individuals receiving negative genetic test results over the course of the study. The second aim was to evaluate participants' comprehension of their specific genetic test results; and we found strong evidence that participants understood their test results following result disclosure genetic counseling.

## Materials and Methods

### Research Design

The Deaf Genetics Project (DGP) is a prospective, longitudinal study to examine the impact of genetic counseling and genetic testing (Connexin-26 and Connexin-30) on deaf adults and the deaf community. A multi-institutional, multi-disciplinary team employed a collaborative research model that integrated the Deaf cultural perspective, the hearing cultural perspective, the academic cultural perspective, and the community service perspective into the research design and implementation of a genetic counseling and testing study. The research team included board-certified genetic counselors and certified project staff sign language interpreters. Details on the sample, recruitment strategies, study protocol, and research team have been previously published [6,36,40,46] and are described briefly below.

### Sample and Study Protocol

Individuals at least 18 years old, with unexplained sensorineural deafness since an early age were eligible to participate. Recruitment primarily took place in the Los Angeles, San Francisco Bay, and Riverside areas of California.

Individuals determined to be initially eligible had an audiological evaluation to confirm the presence of sensorineural deafness to ensure that Connexin-26 and Connexin-30 genetic testing was offered only to individuals for whom it was potentially relevant, i.e., those with early-onset sensorineural deafness. The first questionnaire (called the baseline questionnaire) was completed immediately following the audiology session. Individuals with confirmed sensorineural deafness then met with a genetic counselor for an in-person pre-test genetic counseling session. The genetic counselor explained the remaining study protocol, and provided general information about the genetic epidemiology of deafness, Connexin-related deafness, and genetic testing. Participants interested in pursuing genetic testing provided family and personal medical history information and a buccal sample for genetic analysis. The buccal sample was sent to a University of California, Los Angeles (UCLA) clinical laboratory for genetic analysis. The second questionnaire (called the pre-test counseling questionnaire) was completed immediately following the pre-test genetic counseling session.

Participants returned for another in-person genetic counseling session when their genetic test results were available. The genetic counselor explained the genetic test results, put them in the context of the participant's family and medical history and etiologic heterogeneity of deafness, and answered participants' questions. Participants received a copy of their genetic test report and a genetic counseling summary letter. In some cases, participants received additional information about genetics clinics in their area, either because they were interested in continuing to try to learn why they are deaf, or because something of clinical importance with a strong genetic component was noted in the family history, e.g., early onset breast cancer. About one month and six months after participants received their genetic test results, they were asked to complete the third questionnaire (1-month post-test questionnaire) and the final questionnaire (6-month post-test questionnaire), respectively. The four questionnaires assessed nearly identical information thus allowing us to examine the effect of genetic counseling and genetic information in a longitudinal framework.

The study was approved by the California State University Northridge (protocol: Deaf Genetics Study) and UCLA (protocol: 06-05-065/10-001193) institutional review boards. All research personnel obtained training on Health Insurance Portability and Accountability Act privacy rules, which provided additional protection to participants when a third party (i.e., an interpreter) was present during genetic counseling sessions. Genetic counseling and genetic testing were provided at no charge to participants in the study. All participants provided written informed consent, and as part of this process they were informed that they could pursue genetic counseling and genetic testing outside of this study on their own.

### Measures

The study questionnaires used standard as well as newly developed items to assess demographic factors, reasons for genetic testing, attitudes toward genetic testing, knowledge and understanding of genetics and genetic testing, cultural affiliation and deaf identity, and a variety of psychological and behavior measures. Questionnaires were translated into ASL using a translation-back translation procedure in which a bilingual ASL/English Deaf individual translated the original English version into ASL, another bilingual ASL/English individual back-translated the ASL version to English, and any inconsistencies in meaning were identified and resolved [47,48]. Questionnaires were available to participants in English text (paper and online versions), ASL (online video streaming), and an online dual language format of both English text and ASL video.

**Deaf Identity.** Deaf identity was assessed using the Deaf Identity Development Scale-Revised (DIDR-R) [13]. This 47-item instrument contains 4 subscales (hearing, marginal, immersion, bicultural). Each subscale is comprised of 10–13 items evaluated on a 5-point Likert scale of strongly agree to strongly disagree. Investigations of the DIDS-R demonstrate that four distinct categories can be measured [10,13]; that the subscales have good internal reliability with Cronbach's alpha ranging from 0.78–0.87; that the direction of correlations between subscales are generally consistent with the theory that deaf identity follows a developmental process [10,13]; and that there are differences in mean subscale scores between students attending Gallaudet University compared to members of the Association for Late-Deafened Adults-Boston [10], and among hard of hearing individuals, prelingually deaf individuals, and postlingually deaf individuals

[13]. An average subscale score was computed for each subject at each assessment time point by summing the individual subscale items and dividing by the total number of items in the subscale. This yielded average scores ranging from 1 (strongly agree) to 5 (strongly disagree) for each subscale and each time point.

**Understanding Specific Genetic Test Result.** Participants' understanding of their specific test result was assessed with two items: (1) *perceived chance of having Connexin-related deafness* was assessed by asking them to judge the likelihood that they have Connexin-related deafness on a 4-point Likert scale ranging from 'not at all likely' to 'definitely'; and (2) *belief about why deaf* was assessed by asking participants to select the *most likely* reason they are deaf. At baseline, respondents were presented with 6 options: "It is genetic, because other people in my family are deaf/hard-of-hearing"; "It is genetic, even though no one else in the family is deaf/hard-of-hearing"; "Something happened when my mother was pregnant with me"; "Something happened while my mother was giving birth to me"; "Something happened to me after I was born"; and "It is unknown." The first two options were then classified as "genetic," the next three options were classified as "non-genetic" and the last option was classified as "unknown" for subsequent analyses. At each of the other three timepoints, participants selected from the following options: "genetic," "not genetic," "has not been determined".

**Connexin Group Classification.** Participants were classified into one of three Connexin result groups: Connexin-positive, Connexin-negative, Connexin-inconclusive. Individuals were classified as Connexin-positive if their genetic test result clearly explained why they are deaf, i.e., they have two known Connexin-26 or Connexin-30 deafness-causing variants. Individuals were classified as Connexin-negative if their genetic test result did not identify any Connexin-26- or Connexin-30-related deafness variants. Individuals were classified as Connexin-inconclusive if their genetic test result did not provide enough information to determine if they have Connexin-related deafness (i.e., only one Connexin-related deafness variant was identified). Preliminary analyses suggested that some results were substantively changed by combining the Connexin-negative and Connexin-inconclusive groups, hence analyses do not combine these two groups.

**Demographic Characteristics.** Age, sex, ethnicity/race, high school program, income, highest level of education achieved, cultural affiliation, linguistic preference during interactions with hearing audiology and genetic counseling project staff, and family history of deaf relatives were assessed at baseline. For consistency, these variables are treated using the same categorizations described in other publications from this study [6,36,40]. Potential confounders such as enrollment site, genetic counselor, and interpreter were recorded for each participant.

## Analyses

Data from participants who completed at least one of the two post-test questionnaires are analyzed. Within that pool, responses were missing for 0.45% of the DIDS-R subscale items across the four assessment time points. To maximize the sample size, we used simple imputation to fill in missing data on individual DIDS-R subscale items, with the exception that DIDS-R subscale scores were not computed for one subject per time point because of substantial missing data.

Descriptive statistics were produced and reviewed for the presence of outliers and data errors. Bivariate analyses are performed using Fisher's exact test and ANOVA. For the primary analyses, we performed repeated measures regression analyses to determine the effect of genetic counseling or genetic test results on participants' deaf identity and their perceived chance of having Connexin-related deafness. For these analyses the interaction between Connexin group and assessment time point was the primary predictor variable in a model that included the corresponding separate main effects of Connexin group and time point. Age, education, language preference, family history of deaf relatives, and high school program were included as covariates because they are significantly associated with cultural affiliation in this sample [6]. Age was treated as a dichotomous variable as either above or below the sample median age of 45.5 years. In the case of a significant interaction term, post-hoc two-way comparisons were conducted to identify specific group differences using Tukey's HSD test [49], which controls for Type I experiment-wise error rate. Secondary or subset analyses were also performed as additional checks on participants' understanding of the genetic test results. Analyses were conducted using SAS version 9.3 [50]. Statistical significance was set at $\alpha = 0.05$.

Analyses that include language preference exclude individuals who were categorized in the "other" language group as there were too few ($n = 2$) in this group for meaningful comparison. The number of individuals self-reported as non-white was relatively small ($n = 40$) and consisted of a number of ethnic groups, prohibiting using ethnicity/race as a covariate. Instead, to address the robustness of the results, we re-ran the repeated measures regression analyses with the subset of participants who marked white as their ethnic/racial category. These analyses yielded similar parameter estimates, providing evidence that the results from the larger sample are robust with respect to race/ethnic heritage.

For the repeated measures analysis of deaf identity, we conducted power analyses using PASS 11's mixed model procedure to determine the minimally detectable interaction between Connexin group and assessment time point for each DIDS-R subscale with 80% power and a two-sided significance level of 0.05. Because the Connexin inconclusive group was small and it is difficult to hypothesize the direction of change in values for this group, we limited our power assessments to compare two levels of the factor Connexin, positive and negative, in order to determine the minimum detectable group by time interaction. The mixed model power repeated measures procedure relies on simulations; with each power analysis conducted we used 500 simulation iterates providing us with precision of +/−2%. We used the same covariance structures that were used in actual data analyses and all parameter estimates, except the interaction effect sizes, were fixed to those observed values from the actual data analyses.

## Results

### Sample Demographics

A total of 271 participants completed the audiology evaluation portion of the study, of which 263 were determined to be eligible to participate in the genetic counseling and testing part of the study. Figure 1 depicts the sample size and questionnaire completion rates at each step in the research protocol.

Among the 263 eligible individuals, 241 (91.6%) continued through the protocol to receive their genetic test results; 22 (8.4%) did not. Of those 22 subjects, 15 stopped participation after audiology evaluation (3 subjects withdrew after the audiology evaluation and all collected data on these individuals was destroyed; 3 declined to continue; 9 were not able to be scheduled for a pre-test genetic counseling session after at least one attempt), while the other 7 stopped participation after the pre-test genetic counseling session in which they provided a DNA sample for

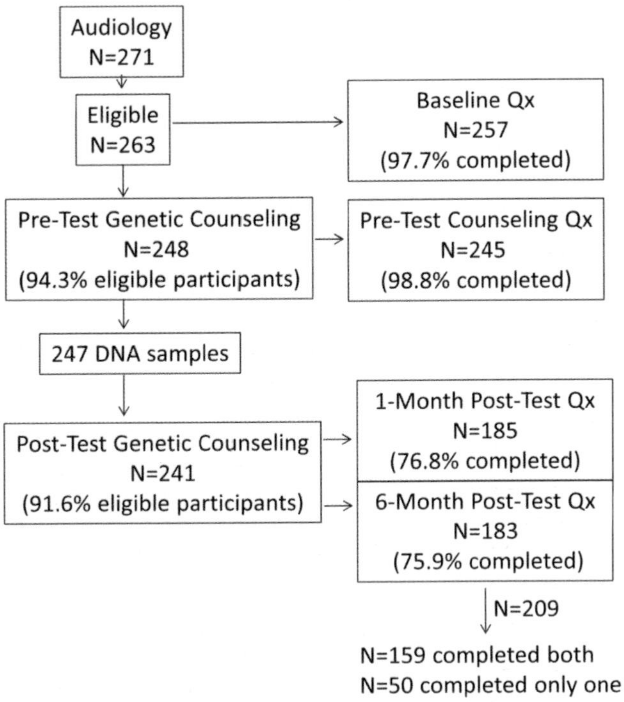


**Figure 1. Study sample and questionnaire completion rates.** Qx = questionnaire.

testing (3 declined to continue, 3 were not able to be scheduled for a test result disclosure session after at least one attempt, and 1 did not attend a scheduled test result disclosure session).

We compared subjects who received their genetic test results ($n = 241$) to those who ceased participation prior to that point (data available on $n = 19$) on the demographic variables evaluated in this study, DIDS-R subscale scores, enrollment site, genetic counselor, and interpreter. The results demonstrated that those who ceased participation were more likely to be male ($p = 0.001$) and to use ASL ($p = 0.03$), were less likely to self-identify as non-Hispanic white ($p = 0.01$), and more strongly endorsed the DIDS-R immersion subscale items ($p = 0.004$) than those who continued through the protocol to receive their genetic test results. About a quarter (26.2%) of participants were enrolled in the last six months of the study, and individuals who ceased participation were disproportionately represented in this group (63.1%) ($p = 0.0005$).

Among the 241 subjects who received their genetic test results, 100% completed the baseline and pre-test counseling questionnaires. Among these 241 subjects, 209 completed at least one post-test questionnaire, with the following breakdown: 159 completed both post-test questionnaires (complete responders), 50 completed only one post-test questionnaire (partial responders), and 32 (13.3%) did not complete any post-test questionnaires (non-responders). One individual provided unusable questionnaire data and was excluded from all analyses. Comparisons of complete, partial, and non-responders did not reveal statistically significant differences on any of the demographic variables evaluated in this study, on DIDS-R subscale scores, in the distribution of Connexin test results, or as a function of enrollment site, genetic counselor, interpreter, or length of time between providing a DNA sample and Connexin result disclosure ($p$'s$>0.05$), thus allowing us to treat the data as missing at random. Cronbach's $\alpha$ was computed from our sample for the DIDS-R subscales and found to be acceptable at each of the four time points (hearing subscale: $\alpha$'s ranged from 0.85–0.87, marginal subscale: $\alpha$'s ranged from 0.88–0.91, immersion subscale: $\alpha$'s ranged from 0.80–0.84, bicultural subscale: $\alpha$'s ranged from 0.77–0.84).

Responses from the 209 subjects who completed at least one post-test questionnaire are the focus of our analyses, and demographic characteristics of this sample are provided in Table 1 by Connexin result category. In this study sample, 39.2% were classified as Connexin-positive ($n = 82$), 13.4% as Connexin-inconclusive ($n = 28$), and 47.4% as Connexin-negative ($n = 99$). The Connexin groups were compared on the demographic variables in Table 1 and found to be comparable on all but preferred language ($p = 0.03$) and family history ($p<0.0001$). Not surprisingly, the three Connexin groups differed in terms of the presence of deaf relatives where 75.6% of those in the Connexin-positive group had at least one closely related deaf relative compared to 57.1% and 37.4% of those in the Connexin-inconclusive and Connexin-negative groups, respectively. Furthermore, 73.2% of those in the Connexin-positive group preferred to use ASL with an interpreter with the genetic counselor, compared to 67.9% and 53.5% in the Connexin-inconclusive and Connexin-negative groups, respectively.

## Deaf Identity

Prior to investigating the effect of genetic counseling or Connexin test results on participants' deaf identity we performed ANOVA to determine if change in DIDS-R subscale scores from pre-test (prior to learning the Connexin results) to 1-month post-test (after learning the Connexin results) was associated with a specific genetic counselor or sign language interpreter. No association was found between genetic counselor and any of the four DIDS-R subscale difference scores ($p$'s$>0.05$). There was a significant association between sign language interpreter and change on immersion subscale scores ($p = 0.03$); however, results were not substantively altered when interpreter was included as a covariate in the regression analysis described below, therefore genetic counselor and interpreter are not considered further in this subsection.

Repeated measures regression analysis with covariates was then performed to determine if participants' responses to these deaf identity subscales changed over the course of the study, particularly after they learned their genetic test results. Figures 2A–2D plot participants' least square estimates of the DIDS-R subscale scores by Connexin result group before and after receiving their genetic test results; and Table S1 provides the least square estimates and standard errors for the main effects, covariates, and interaction term. Regardless of Connexin result, endorsement of the bicultural subscale was strongest, and endorsement of the hearing and marginal subscales was weakest, at each time point.

**Hearing Subscale (Figure 2A).** While controlling for the main effects of Connexin result ($F_{(2,189)} = 0.17$, $p = 0.84$) and time ($F_{(2,538)} = 2.29$, $p = 0.08$), we found that the interaction between Connexin and time was significantly associated with hearing subscale scores ($F_{(6,538)} = 2.44$, $p = 0.02$). The covariates preferred language ($F_{(2,189)} = 9.78$, $p<0.0001$), age ($F_{(1,189)} = 7.59$, $p = 0.006$), education ($F_{(1,189)} = 31.78$, $p<0.0001$), and family history ($F_{(1,189)} = 6.18$, $p = 0.01$) also were significantly associated with these scores. Individuals expressing stronger endorsement of this subscale tended to be English-users, older than 45.5 years, not have college degrees, and have no first or second degree deaf relatives. Although the Connexin and time interaction term was statistically significant, post-hoc pairwise analyses did not demonstrate significant group differences at $\alpha = 0.05$ at any of the four timepoints.

**Table 1.** Sample demographics by Connexin result.

| | | Connexin result | | | $p$ |
|---|---|---|---|---|---|
| | | Positive | Inconclusive | Negative | |
| Sample size | | 82 | 28 | 99 | |
| Average age (SD), years | | 44.6 (15.9) | 48.0 (17.4) | 46.3 (15.3) | 0.58 |
| Female, % (n) | | 54.9 (45) | 67.9 (19) | 66.7 (66) | 0.23 |
| Ethnicity/race, % (n) | non-Hispanic white | 85.4 (70) | 82.1 (23) | 76.8 (76) | 0.34[a] |
| | Hispanic | 7.3 (6) | 3.6 (1) | 12.1 (12) | |
| | Asian | 4.9 (4) | 14.3 (4) | 9.1 (9) | |
| | Other | 2.4 (2) | 0 | 2.0 (2) | |
| High school program[b], % (n) | Deaf | 42.5 (34) | 28.6 (8) | 28.4 (27) | 0.31 |
| | Hearing | 23.8 (19) | 32.1 (9) | 38.9 (37) | |
| | Mainstream | 25.0 (20) | 25.0 (7) | 21.1 (20) | |
| | Mixed | 8.8 (7) | 14.3 (4) | 11.6 (11) | |
| Median income, thousands of $ | | 35–50 | 50–65 | 35–50 | 0.27 |
| ≥Bachelor degree, % (n) | | 57.3 (47) | 53.6 (15) | 56.1 (55) | 0.93 |
| Cultural affiliation, % (n) | Deaf community | 63.4 (52) | 53.6 (15) | 48.5 (47) | 0.20[c] |
| | Hearing community | 6.1 (5) | 14.3 (4) | 7.2 (7) | |
| | Both communities | 29.3 (24) | 32.1 (9) | 42.3 (41) | |
| | Neither community | 1.2 (1) | 0 | 2.1 (2) | |
| Language, % (n) | ASL, interpreter present | 73.2 (60) | 67.9 (19) | 53.5 (53) | 0.03[d] |
| | ASL and English, interpreter present | 19.5 (16) | 14.3 (4) | 29.3 (29) | |
| | English, no interpreter present | 6.1 (5) | 17.9 (5) | 16.2 (16) | |
| | Other | 1.2 (1) | 0 | 1.0 (1) | |
| Deaf 1st - or 2nd -degree relatives, % (n) | | 75.6 (62) | 57.1 (16) | 37.4 (37) | <0.0001 |

*Note.* [a]Compares non-Hispanic white group to all other ethnic groups;
[b]As in Boudreault et al. 2010, deaf-based high school indicates predominantly ASL or coded communication in the classroom; hearing-based high school indicates predominantly oral instruction in the classroom without interpreter/support services; mainstream high school indicates public school that predominantly provides sign instruction with interpreter/support services; and mixed indicates attending two or more of the previously described high school programs;
[c]Individuals in "Neither Community" excluded from all analyses involving this variable due to small sample size;
[d]Individuals in "Other" indicated signed English or Pidgin Signed English and are excluded from analyses involving this variable due to small sample size.

**Marginal Subscale (Figure 2B).** While controlling for the main effects of Connexin result ($F_{(2,189)} = 0.81$, $p = 0.45$) and time ($F_{(3,538)} = 0.61$, $p = 0.61$), we found no evidence that responses to marginal subscale items changed by genetic test result category before or after learning results [non-significant interaction between Connexin and time ($F_{(6,538)} = 1.31$, $p = 0.25$)]. However, the main effects of education ($F_{(1,189)} = 38.59$, $p<0.0001$) and family history ($F_{(1,189)} = 10.50$, $p = 0.001$) were significantly associated with marginal subscale scores averaged over the four assessment time points. On average an individual without a college degree and without deaf relatives more strongly endorsed items on the marginal subscale than an individual with a college degree and deaf family members. Age ($F_{(1,189)} = 1.25$, $p = 0.26$), language ($F_{(2,189)} = 0.15$, $p = 0.85$), and high school program ($F_{(3,189)} = 2.48$, $p = 0.06$) were not significant predictors of marginal subscale scores.

**Immersion Subscale (Figure 2C).** While controlling for the main effects of Connexin result ($F_{(2,189)} = 1.14$, $p = 0.32$) and time ($F_{(3,538)} = 1.16$, $p = 0.32$), we found no evidence that responses to immersion subscale items changed by genetic test result category before or after learning results [non-significant interaction between Connexin and time ($F_{(6,538)} = 1.43$, $p = 0.20$)]. However, the main effects of preferred language ($F_{(2,189)} = 32.90$, $p<0.0001$) and high school program ($F_{(3,189)} = 4.23$, $p = 0.006$) were significantly associated with immersion subscale scores averaged over the four assessment time points. ASL-users and individuals who attended a deaf-based high school more strongly endorsed items on the immersion subscale than English-users or those who attended a hearing-based high school. Age ($F_{(1,189)} = 0.61$, $p = 0.44$), education ($F_{(1,189)} = 0.46$, $p = 0.50$), and family history ($F_{(1,189)} = 0.24$, $p = 0.63$) were not significant predictors of immersion subscale scores.

**Bicultural Subscale (Figure 2D).** While controlling for the main effects of Connexin result ($F_{(2,189)} = 0.13$, $p = 0.88$) and time ($F_{(3,538)} = 1.43$, $p = 0.23$), we found no evidence that responses to immersion subscale items changed by genetic test result category before or after learning results [non-significant interaction between Connexin and time ($F_{(6,538)} = 1.27$, $p = 0.27$)]. However, the covariate preferred language ($F_{(2,189)} = 20.36$, $p<0.0001$) was significantly associated with bicultural subscale scores averaged over the four assessment time points. Individuals who use both ASL and English or predominantly ASL more strongly endorsed items on the bicultural subscale than English-users. Age ($F_{(1,189)} = 0.09$, $p = 0.76$), education ($F_{(1,189)} = 0.54$, $p = 0.46$), family history ($F_{(1,189)} = 1.35$, $p = 0.25$), and high school program ($F_{(3,189)} = 1.41$, $p = 0.24$) were not significant predictors of bicultural subscale scores.

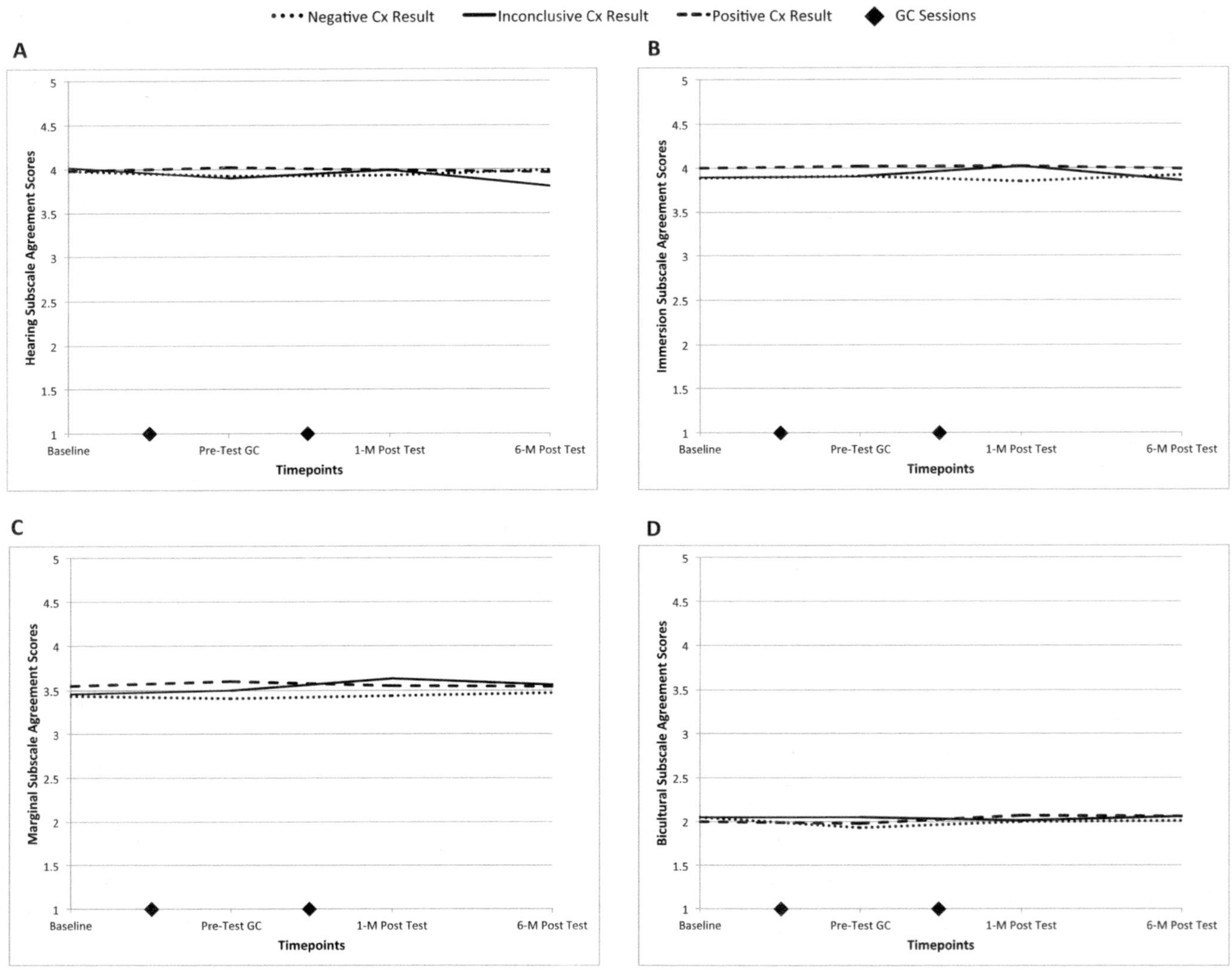


**Figures 2. 2A–2D: DIDS-R subscale agreement score least squares estimates by Connexin result group before and after genetic testing.** A. hearing subscale, main effects: Connexin $p = 0.84$, time $p = 0.08$; interaction: Connexin x time $p = 0.02$. Non-significant pairwise comparisons at $\alpha = 0.05$ at each timepoint. B. marginal subscale, main effects: Connexin $p = 0.45$, time $p = 0.61$; interaction: Connexin x time $p = 0.25$. C. immersion subscale, main effects: Connexin $p = 0.32$, time $p = 0.32$; interaction: Connexin x time $p = 0.20$. D. bicultural subscale, main effects: Connexin $p = 0.88$, time $p = 0.23$; interaction: Connexin x time $p = 0.27$. 1 = strongly agree, 5 = strongly disagree. Cx = connexin; GC = genetic counseling; M = month.

**Power Analysis.** Power analyses demonstrate that our sample size is sufficient to detect moderate group by time interactions within the four subscales. Specifically, there is at least 80% power to detect an interaction between Connexin group and time that would result in an individual with a Connexin negative result experiencing on average a 0.14 unit greater shift towards *endorsement* of a hearing identity during their participation in the study than an individual receiving a Connexin-positive result would experience in the same amount of time. That is, as an example, after adjustment for the covariates, we could expect the change for a Connexin-negative individual to be −0.10 units (increased endorsement of the hearing identity) and the change for a Connexin-positive individual to be 0.04 units (increased rejection of the hearing identity). Similarly, there is at least 80% power to detect an interaction between Connexin group and time that would result in an individual with a Connexin-negative result experiencing on average a 0.14 unit greater shift towards *endorsement* of a marginal identity during their participation in the study than an individual receiving a Connexin-positive would experience in the same amount of time. Reflecting the anticipated direction of change, there is at least 80% power to detect an interaction between Connexin group and time that would result in an individual with a Connexin-negative result experiencing on average a 0.16 unit greater shift towards *rejection* of an immersion identity than an individual receiving a Connexin-positive would experience in the same amount of time. As an example, after adjustment for the covariates, we would expect the change for a Connexin-negative individual to be 0.11 units (a decrease in endorsement of an immersion identity) and the change for a Connexin-positive individual to be -0.05 units (a slight increase in endorsement of an immersion identity). Finally there is at least 80% power to detect an interaction between Connexin group and time that would result in an individual with a Connexin-negative result experiencing on average a 0.12 unit greater shift towards *rejection* of a bicultural identity during their participation in the study than an individual receiving a Connexin-positive would experience in the same amount of time.

Visual inspection of Figures 2A–2D supports the conclusions of the statistical analyses that the subscale scores are essentially unchanged over the four assessment time points. Unsolicited comments provided by participants at the end of the post-test questionnaires further bolster the conclusion that participants' deaf identity was not changed as a result of genetic testing.

"Thank you for doing this project. It *helped me re-affirm my view of myself as a proud Deaf person*." – Participant with Connexin-positive result (italics added for emphasis)

"I decided to participate in the genetics test to see why I am Deaf. My family and I had a hunch that it was genetic, but this helped proved that and *really had no immediate effect on my life*. Thanks for doing this!" Participant with Connexin-positive result (italics added for emphasis)

"I didnt [sic] know what to think when I got the test results. Whether to be exhilarated, excited, upset or confused. *I just felt sort quiet*." Participant with Connexin-negative result (italics added for emphasis)

**Cultural Affiliation and Number of Connexin Deafness-Causing Variants.** Although these analyses provide support that Connexin result does not appear to *change* deaf identity in this sample of deaf adults, we hypothesized that culturally Deaf individuals would be more likely to be Connexin-positive, i.e., that cultural affiliation is associated with Connexin result. This hypothesis is based on evidence that the frequency of Connexin-related deafness has increased several-fold over the last 100 years in the US in the non-Hispanic white population as a result of marriages based on linguistic homogamy (signed language) [2] which is important for Deaf culture. Given the observed stability of the DIDS-R subscale scores over time in this sample, we categorized participants by their self-reported cultural affiliation at baseline to test this hypothesis. This categorical measure of cultural affiliation has been shown to correlate well with relevant variables such as preferred language, high school program, and involvement in the Deaf community, as well as responses to the DIDS-R subscales at baseline in this sample [6].

We found a significant correlation between participants' cultural affiliation and number of Connexin deafness-causing variants (FE $p = 0.04$), focusing on the non-Hispanic white subsample ($n = 165$) to avoid confounding with ethnic ancestry or potential cross-cultural differences. Specifically, 50.53% (48/95) of those who reported affiliation with the Deaf community had two Connexin deafness-causing variants (i.e., Connexin-related deafness) compared to 30.51% (18/59) of those who reported affiliation with both Deaf and hearing communities and 27.3% (3/11) of those who reported affiliation with the hearing community. When re-analyzed in the presence of language, age, education, family history, and high school program, the association between cultural affiliation and number of deafness-causing variants remained significant ($p = 0.05$). Overall these results suggest that the Connexin-26 and Connexin-30 genes are intimately connected to Deaf culture in the US, but individuals who have genetic counseling, Connexin testing, and learn their results do not experience a change in their deaf identity.

## Understanding Specific Connexin Result

**Perceived Chance.** We next assessed participants' understanding of their specific Connexin result by examining whether their responses to the *perceived chance* item "How likely is it that you have Connexin-related deafness?" was consistent with their actual Connexin test result, with the expectation that those who received a Connexin-positive result would be more likely to indicate that they have Connexin-related deafness than those who received a Connexin-inconclusive or Connexin-negative result. The majority of participants felt it was at least somewhat likely that they had Connexin–related deafness at baseline and immediately following the *pre-test* genetic counseling session (83.7%, 82.4%, respectively), but prior to learning their Connexin results. At 1- and 6- months after receiving the genetic test results, 74% of those who received a Connexin-positive result indicated that they *definitely* have Connexin-related deafness. In contrast, among those who received a Connexin-negative test result, 71.3% at 1-month and 68.6% at 6-months post-test result indicated that they felt it was *not at all likely* that they have Connexin-related deafness. The responses of the Connexin-inconclusive group are spread across all four response categories at 1-month and 6-months post-test result (not at all likely: 26.1%, 36.4%; somewhat likely: 43.5%, 27.3%; very likely: 17.4%, 22.7%; definitely: 13.0%, 13.6%), revealing the challenge of personalizing the meaning of an inconclusive test result.

Repeated measures regression analysis with covariates was then performed to determine if participants' responses to *perceived chance* changed over the course of the study, particularly after they learned their genetic test results. Figure 3 plots participants' least square estimates of *perceived chance* responses before and after receiving their genetic test results by Connexin result group; and Table S1 provides the least square estimates and standard errors for the main effects, covariates, and interaction term. The analysis demonstrated a statistically significant interaction between Connexin result and time ($F_{(6,530)} = 50.26$, $p<0.0001$) indicating that participants' perceived chance of having Connexin-related deafness changed by Connexin result category over the course of the study, while controlling for the main effects of Connexin result ($F_{(2,189)} = 110.15$, $p<0.0001$) and time ($F_{(3,530)} = 3.65$, $p = 0.01$), language preference ($F_{(2,189)} = 0.79$, $p = 0.46$), age ($F_{(1,189)} = 0.25$, $p = 0.62$), education ($F_{(1,189)} = 0.38$, $p = 0.54$), family history ($F_{(1,189)} = 29.25$, $p<0.0001$), and high school program ($F_{(3,189)} = 5.14$, $p = 0.002$). Posthoc pair-wise Tukey tests demonstrated that the perceived chance ratings of the three Connexin result groups did not differ at baseline, but significantly differed at the other three timepoints (Figure 3). Unexpectedly, the Connexin-positive group rated their chance of having Connexin-related deafness higher than the other two groups following pre-test genetic counseling. This finding could reflect that pre-test genetic counseling facilitated a good understanding of the meaning of participants' medical history and family history and set appropriate expectations for a participant's test result. The perceived chance ratings differed among all three groups at 1-month post-test and 6-month post-test. At both of these time-points, the Connexin-positive group indicated a high level of certainty that they have Connexin-related deafness, the Connexin-negative group indicated a high level of certainty that they do not have Connexin-related deafness, and the Connexin-inconclusive group yielded an average score indicative that there remains some chance that they have Connexin-related deafness. These results provide evidence that participants' subjective assessments of Connexin-related deafness are consistent with the actual test results.

**Connexin Result and Belief Why Deaf.** As a check on participants' understanding of their genetic test results, we performed two additional analyses. First, we evaluated the relationship between Connexin result and belief about why deaf, with the expectation that those with a Connexin-positive result

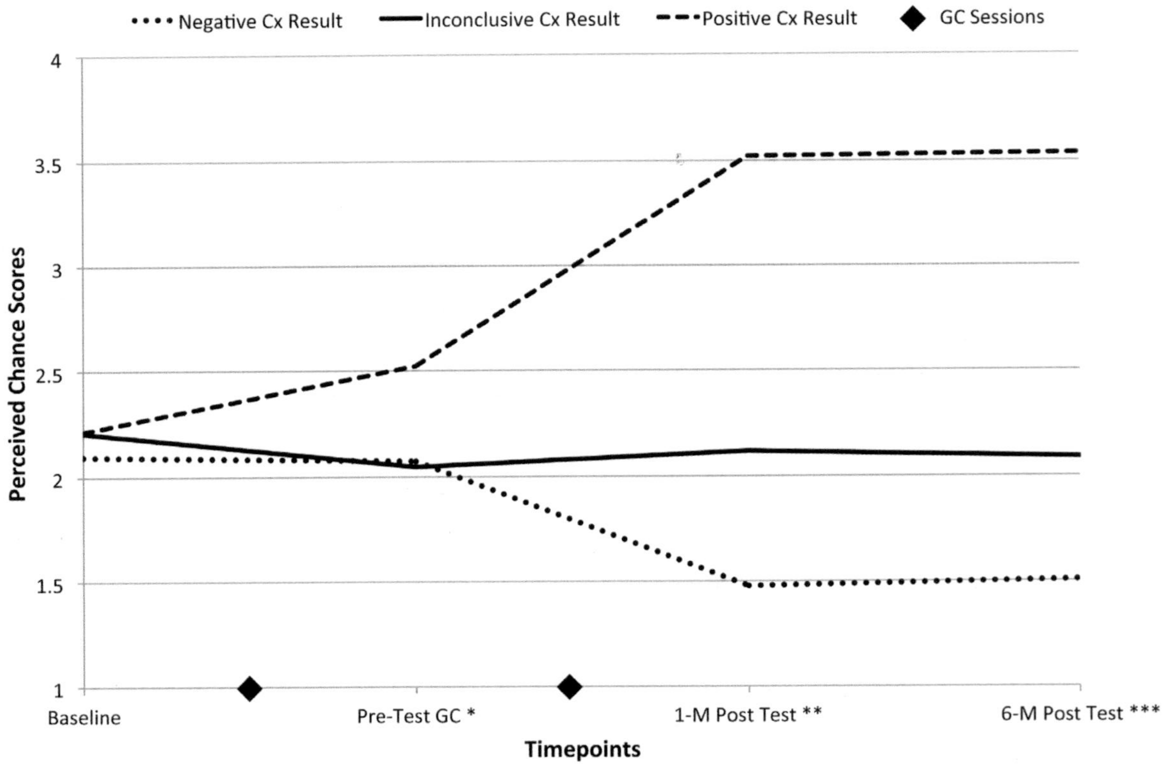


**Figure 3.** ***Perceived chance*** **least squares estimates by Connexin result group before and after genetic testing.** How likely is it that you have Connexin-26 related deafness? 1 = not at all likely, 2 = somewhat likely, 3 = highly likely, 4 = definitely. Main effects: Connexin $p<0.0001$, time $p=0.01$; interaction Connexin x time $p<0.0001$; *Significant difference between Connexin-positive and Connexin-negative groups $p=0.02$, and Connexin-positive and Connexin-inconclusive groups $p=0.02$; **Significant difference between Connexin-positive and Connexin-negative groups $p<0.0001$, Connexin-positive and Connexin-inconclusive groups $p<0.0001$, and Connexin-negative and Connexin-inconclusive groups $p=0.0003$; ***Significant difference between Connexin-positive and Connexin-negative groups $p<0.0001$, Connexin-positive and Connexin-inconclusive groups $p<0.0001$, and Connexin-negative and Connexin-inconclusive groups $p=0.0006$. Cx = connexin; GC = genetic counseling; M = month.

would be more likely to report that they have a genetic form of deafness, and those with a Connexin-negative and Connexin-inconclusive result would be more likely to report that they are deaf for reasons 'not determined' after they learned their genetic test results. As shown in Figure 4, at baseline the distribution of participant responses for the reason they are deaf did not differ as a function of their underlying Connexin result (FE $p=0.16$), and nearly a third reported that the reason they are deaf was undetermined. While the percentage of participants reporting an undetermined reason for their deafness increased to ~60% at the pre-test genetic counseling assessment time point, prior to knowing their Connexin test result, those in the Connexin-negative group were less likely to indicate a genetic explanation compared to the Connexin-positive and inconclusive groups (FE $p=0.02$). This result provides additional evidence that pre-test genetic counseling appropriately set expectations about genetic test results. One-month following receipt of Connexin results, >95% of participants with a Connexin-positive result reported a genetic explanation for their deafness; the Connexin-inconclusive group was fairly evenly split between attributing a genetic explanation and reporting that the etiology of their deafness was undetermined; and the Connexin-negative group was least likely to report that they have a genetic type of deafness (FE $p<0.0001$). Of note both the Connexin-negative and Connexin-inconclusive groups were more likely to report that the reason they are deaf is 'undetermined' than 'not genetic'. This result suggests that communication between the genetic counselor and participant was effective in conveying the important concepts of genetic heterogeneity and that ruling out one genetic explanation does not imply 'not genetic'. Results were similar at 6-months following receipt of Connexin results (FE $p<0.0001$).

Second, we examined the how participants' understood their Connexin result in light of their family history of deaf relatives. Although we demonstrated that those who received Connexin-negative results were less likely to report that they have Connexin-related deafness, it is clear that those with deaf relatives have more reason to believe they have a *genetic* form of deafness than those without deaf relatives. On the other hand, although those with Connexin-positive results were more likely to indicate that they have Connexin-related deafness, they also should believe that they have a genetic form of deafness *regardless* of their family history.

Irrespective of Connexin result category, it is clear at baseline that family history was associated with participants' beliefs about why they are deaf. Specifically, those with deaf relatives were more likely to attribute a genetic explanation to the reason they are deaf compared to those with no deaf relatives (Connexin-negative group, $p<0.0001$; Connexin-inconclusive group, $p<0.0001$; Connexin-positive group, $p=0.01$). Following pre-test genetic counseling, this association continued to be statistically significant for the Connexin-negative and Connexin-inconclusive groups ($p<0.0001$, $p=0.02$, respectively). Although the Connexin-positive group followed the same trend (40% of those with deaf relatives attributed a genetic explanation to their deafness compared to 20% of those without deaf relatives), the association was not

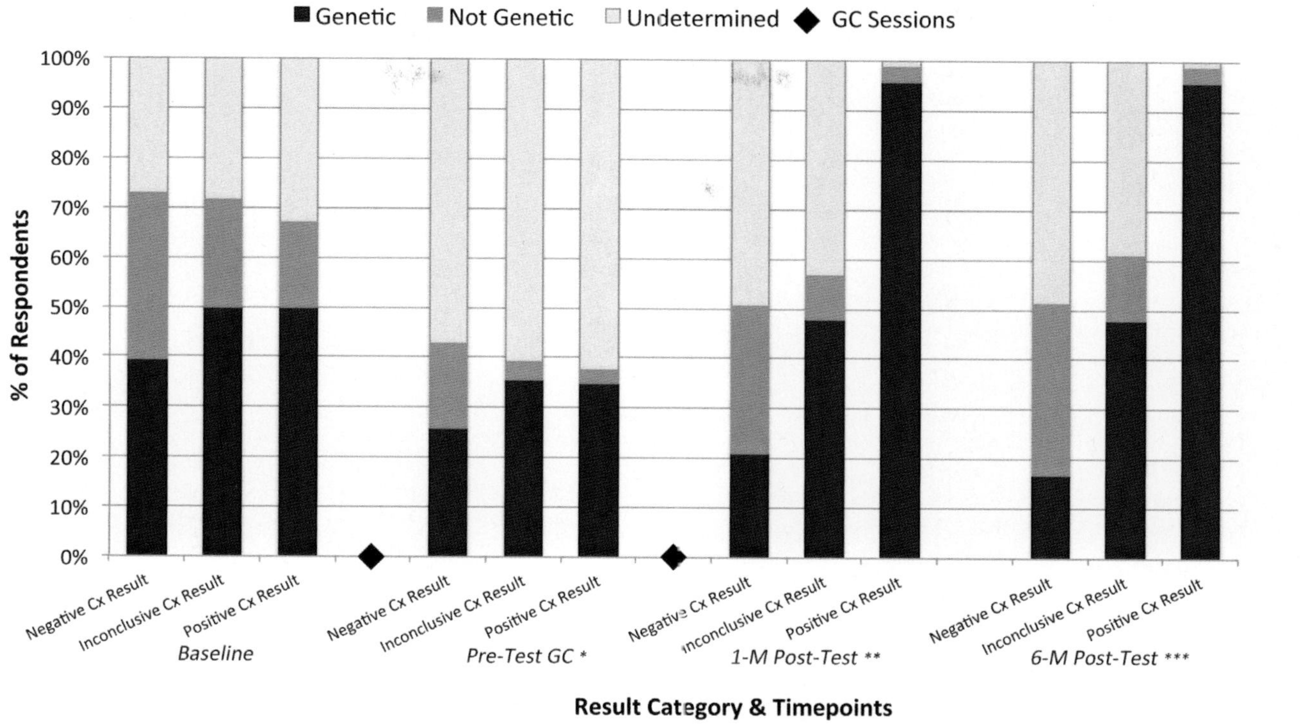


**Figure 4. Responses to "belief about why deaf" by assessment timepoint.** $*p = 0.02$; $**p<0.0001$; $***p<0.0001$; Cx = connexin; GC = genetic counseling; M = month.

statistically significant ($p = 0.17$). One-month following disclosure of Connexin test results, the role of family history continued to be a significant factor for attributing a genetic explanation to deafness for participants who received Connexin-negative or Connexin-inconclusive results (FE $p<0.0002$, FE $p = 0.03$, respectively). Specifically, in the Connexin-negative group, 42.4% with deaf family members marked that their deafness is genetic in origin compared to 7.69% without deaf relatives; and in the Connexin-inconclusive group, 66.7% with deaf family members marked that their deafness is genetic compared to 12.5% without deaf relatives. In contrast, there was no association between family history and reason why deaf for the Connexin-positive group at 1-month post-test (FE $p = 1.0$) and>95.0% of these individuals marked that their deafness is genetic in origin. Results are nearly identical at 6-months post test result (Connexin-negative group FE $p = 0.005$; Connexin-inconclusive group FE $p = 0.003$; Connexin-positive group FE $p = 0.14$). Overall, these results provide evidence that participants have good understanding of their Connexin results, i.e., they understood their Connexin results in the context of the terms 'Connexin-related deafness' and 'genetic,' and in the context of their family history.

## Discussion

Deaf genetic testing raises a variety of ethical, social, and genetic counseling issues, yet there is a lack of empirical data on the actual impact of genetic counseling and genetic testing on deaf adults and the culturally Deaf community from which to address these issues. This article reports results from the only prospective, longitudinal study to address outcomes of deaf genetic testing and genetic counseling, in a sample of 209 deaf adults who underwent actual genetic counseling and Connexin-26 and Connexin-30 genetic testing and received their genetic test results. Our results provide insight into the effects of genetic counseling and testing on deaf individuals' identity and understanding of their genetic test results, for the period including pre- and post-test genetic counseling through six months after receipt of genetic test results. We found evidence that pre-test genetic counseling set appropriate expectations about test results and that participants understood their specific Connexin results following genetic counseling. However, we found no evidence that genetic information, provided in the context of linguistically and culturally appropriate genetic counseling, altered participants' deaf identity, despite having adequate power to detect moderate differences in identity change over time.

Deaf genetic testing raises questions about the psychological and social impact of genetic information on deaf individuals. In a recent article, we demonstrated that Connexin-26 and Connexin-30 test results can alter deaf adults' feelings of perceived personal control and anxiety, but that these results have no effect on feelings of depression [36]. Importantly, we found that deaf genetic testing can promote psychological well-being in deaf individuals who receive a positive Connexin result. In the current study we examined the effect of genetic counseling or Connexin-26 and Connexin-30 genetic testing on deaf identify using the DIDS-R subscales to measure four orientations of deaf identity: hearing, marginal, immersion, and bicultural. Consistent with other studies [12,51], we found that language, age, family history, education level, and high school program were significantly associated with deaf identity, and hence are important for the formation of deaf identity. However, despite adequate power, we found no evidence that genetic counseling and Connexin genetic testing, or the nature of that result (e.g., Connexin-positive, Connexin-negative) meaningfully *changed* participants' deaf identity, at least out to 6-months post-test result. Furthermore, unsolicited comments from participants were consistent with the statistical results and provided some context for understanding these results. Because we found clear evidence that participants understood their genetic test results, the lack of impact of the Connexin result on deaf identity cannot be explained by "not understanding their results." Our findings suggests that *knowing* the underlying reason why an individual is deaf is less relevant to the formation of deaf identity/cultural affiliation than socio-cultural and educational factors and that those individuals receiving positive genetic results are no more likely to change their identity/cultural affiliation than those individuals receiving negative genetic results.

In light of evidence that the relative frequency of Connexin-related deafness has increased in the non-Hispanic population in the United States in the last 100 years due to marriages between sign language users (linguistic homogamy), a language valued by the Deaf community, we hypothesized that Connexin-positive results would be enriched in our sample of non-Hispanic white culturally Deaf adults. Our results demonstrated that individuals self-reporting as affiliated with the Deaf community were significantly more likely to have Connexin-positive results than individuals reporting affiliation with the hearing community or with both Deaf and hearing communities. These results reveal the importance of deafness-causing variants in the Connexin-26 and Connexin-30 genes, albeit indirectly, to Deaf culture and the Deaf community in the United States, because these genetic variants are reflective of ethnic ancestry, family history, degree of deafness, age of onset, and language preference. It is interesting to note that participants indicated an interest in deaf genetic testing to strengthen the Deaf community [6]. [The survey item used lowercase d (…strengthen the deaf community…) but we use uppercase D here because analyses demonstrated that subjects who self-identified as affiliating with the Deaf community or with both Deaf and hearing communities more strongly endorsed this item than those self-identifying with the hearing community [6].] Our data suggest that the effects of Connexin-26 and Connexin-30 on strengthening the Deaf community will not come from changing deaf identity, but may come from the presence of deafness-causing variants in the population expanding the pool of hearing (children of Deaf adults) and deaf sign language users through the generations.

Deaf genetic testing is also complex for scientific reasons, and thus introduces complexity into genetic counseling for deafness. The scientific complexity arises because deafness is etiologically heterogeneous and because there are limits to our current ability to interpret some genetic test results. The current study underscores this complexity because 39.2% of participants received Connexin-positive results, 47.4% received Connexin-negative results, and 13.4% received Connexin-inconclusive results.

A Connexin-positive result reveals that the individual's deafness is genetic in origin, whereas, negative or inconclusive results do not provide definitive information about why an individual is deaf. Importantly, negative or inconclusive results do not rule out a genetic form of deafness because there are many untested genes that can explain why a person is deaf. Several studies of parents of a deaf child have documented that, in the absence of genetic counseling, this scientific complexity adversely affects parents' ability to understand inheritance of deafness, genetic information, and empiric recurrence chances when genetic testing or other clinical evaluation does not provide an explanation for why their child is deaf [39,52,53]. A common finding is that individuals tend to equate a negative genetic test result with 'not genetic' and a zero percent recurrence chance, reflecting the recognized phenomenon of misinterpretation of "residual chance" [54]. However, when genetic counseling is provided, parental understanding of their child's genetic test results is improved [45].

Deaf individuals' understanding of genetic test results may be additionally influenced by uneven access to information related to genetics concepts and genetics topics in ASL, and the use of sign language interpreters during encounters between deaf clients and non-ASL proficient genetics professionals. In a previous analysis of this study sample, we demonstrated that deaf adults' general knowledge and understanding of genetics concepts, heterogeneity of deafness, and genetic testing are enhanced by pre-test genetic counseling provided in a culturally and linguistically sensitive manner [40].

Here we demonstrate other outcomes of the effectiveness of genetic counseling because we found in this sample of deaf adults that individuals who received positive test results felt this was a more likely outcome of genetic testing immediately following the pre-test genetic counseling session than those who did not receive positive results. Furthermore, we found at 1- and 6-months after result disclosure that those who received positive test results understood that they have Connexin-related deafness and that this is genetic in origin even if they do not have any deaf relatives, which suggests that through genetic counseling one aspect of the meaning of positive test results was successfully conveyed. Moreover, individuals who received an inconclusive test result accurately reported that the reason they are deaf is undetermined, that it is still somewhat likely that they have Connexin-related deafness, and that the presence of deaf relatives is a meaningful predictor of having a genetic type of deafness. Finally, participants who received negative test results accurately reported that it was unlikely that they have Connexin-related deafness, that the reason they are deaf is undetermined, and that the presence of deaf relatives is a meaningful predictor of having a genetic type of deafness. Similar results were observed in a sample of hearing parents of a deaf child following genetic counseling [45], suggesting that the knowledge outcomes of genetic counseling for deaf genetic testing are generalizable across deaf and hearing clients.

This study has several strengths, including the high response rate at each assessment time point, and the lack of evidence for response bias between questionnaire responders and non-responders. However, there are several limitations that warrant discussion. First, the individuals who chose to participate in this study may differ in important ways from those who did not participate. As one example, our study participants were more highly educated and had a higher median income than a national sample of prelingually deaf adults [55]. Second, ~8% of individuals determined eligible to participate in the study ceased participation either prior to submitting a DNA sample or prior to receiving results. These individuals were more likely to be male, more likely to be ASL-users, less likely to self-identify as white, and more strongly endorsed the DIDS-R immersion subscale items than those who continued through the protocol to receive their genetic test results. These factors raise questions about whether these participants were uncomfortable with lack of direct communication with the researchers, a non-ethnically diverse research team, or potential medicalization of deafness. Hence, generalizing our findings to the general deaf population should be done with caution. However, because the majority of this group was enrolled in the final six months of the study compared to those who continued to receive their genetic test results, it is possible that the most relevant factor for discontinued participation was simply related to timing of participation.

Another important limitation is that the average age of the sample was 45.9 years at enrollment, and baseline assessment of the deaf identity subscales indicated that most of the participants endorsed the bicultural identity and rejected the other three identities. Deaf identity is conceptualized as a construct that develops over time culminating in the bicultural identity, and since our sample was composed of adults we may have been less likely to observe changes to deaf identity due to genetic test results. It would be important to assess the effect of deaf genetic testing on the development of deaf identity in younger deaf individuals. In addition, this study evaluated whether participants' view of their own deaf identity changed, but it would also be interesting to study if others within the Deaf community view a persons' identity differently if they are found to have Connexin-positive result. Finally, this study did not specifically measure participants' views about a connection between Deaf culture and the Connexin-related genes. Thus, one potential explanation for our results is that our participants were not aware of this potential connection. If this connection was widely known in the Deaf community then there is a chance that learning Connexin results would change deaf identity, and this is a topic for future research.

## Conclusions

In summary, this is a prospective, longitudinal study to determine the impact of genetic counseling or genetic testing on deaf identity and understanding of genetic test results. To date, we have demonstrated that some deaf individuals are interested in deaf genetic testing [6], that pre-test genetic counseling enhances participants' general knowledge outcomes regarding genetics concepts, heterogeneity of deafness, and genetic testing [40]; and that individuals who receive a Connexin-positive result experience psychological well-being [36]. This study demonstrates that pre-test genetic counseling appropriately sets expectations about Connexin results; that post-test genetic counseling enhances participants' understanding of their specific Connexin results; that deaf identity is not changed as a function of genetic counseling or learning a Connexin result; and that the formation of or change in deaf identity is not directly related to Connexin results, but it is based on other variables such as age, language, family history, education level, and high school program. We hypothesize that deafness-causing variants in Connexin-26 and Connexin-30 play an important indirect role on the Deaf community.

## Supporting Information

**Table S1 Repeated measures regression analyses: Least square estimates and standard errors for main effects, interaction term, and covariates.**

## Acknowledgments

Thanks to the Deaf, deaf and hard-of-hearing individuals of California for their participation in this research.

## Author Contributions

Conceived and designed the experiments: CGSP PB JSS. Performed the experiments: CGSP JSS. Analyzed the data: CGSP PB EEB JSS. Contributed reagents/materials/analysis tools: CGSP PB EEB JSS. Wrote the paper: CGSP PB EEB JSS.

## References

1. Prasad S, Cucci RA, Green GE, Smith RJ (2000) Genetic testing for hereditary hearing loss: connexin 26 (GJB2) allele variants and two novel deafness-causing mutations (R32C and 645-648delTAGA). Hum Mutat 16: 502–508.
2. Arnos KS, Welch KO, Tekin M, Norris VW, Blanton SH, et al. (2008) A comparative analysis of the genetic epidemiology of deafness in the United States in two sets of pedigrees collected more than a century apart. Am J Hum Genet 83: 200–207.
3. Blanton SH, Nance WE, Norris VW, Welch KO, Burt A, et al. (2010) Fitness among individuals with early childhood deafness: studies in alumni families from Gallaudet University. Ann Hum Genet 74: 27–33.
4. Senghas RJ, Monaghan L (2002) Signs of their times: Deaf communities and the culture of language. Annu Rev Anthropol 31: 69–97.
5. Padden C, Humphries T (1988) Deaf in America: Voices from a culture. Cambridge, MA: Harvard University Press.
6. Boudreault P, Baldwin EE, Fox M, Dutton L, Tullis L, et al. (2010) Deaf adults' reasons for genetic testing depend on cultural affiliation: results from a prospective, longitudinal genetic counseling and testing study. J Deaf Stud Deaf Educ 15: 209–227.
7. Burton SK, Withrow K, Arnos KS, Kalfoglou AL, Pandya A (2006) A focus group study of consumer attitudes toward genetic testing and newborn screening for deafness. Genet Med 8: 779–783.
8. Withrow KA, Tracy KA, Burton SK, Norris VW, Maes HH, et al. (2009) Impact of genetic advances and testing for hearing loss: results from a national consumer survey. Am J Med Genet A 149A: 1159–1168.
9. Withrow KA, Tracy KA, Burton SK, Norris VW, Maes HH, et al. (2009) Provision of genetic services for hearing loss: results from a national survey and comparison to insights obtained from previous focus group discussions. J Genet Couns 18: 618–621.
10. Glickman NS, Carey JC (1993) Measuring deaf cultural identities: a preliminary investigation. Rehabil Psychol 38: 275–282.
11. Leigh IW, Marcus A, Dobosh P, Allen T (1998) Deaf/hearing cultural identity paradigms: modification of the deaf identity development scale. J Deaf Stud Deaf Educ 3: 329–338.
12. Bat-Chava Y (2000) Diversity of deaf identities. Am Ann Deaf 145: 420–428.
13. Fischer LC, McWhirter JJ (2001) The deaf identity development scale: a revision and validation. J Clin Psychol 48: 355–358.
14. Holcomb TK (1997) Development of Deaf bicultural identity. Am Ann Deaf 142: 89–93.
15. Kannapell B (1993) Language choice - identity choice. Burtonsville, MD: Linstok Press, Inc.
16. Nikolaraizi M, Hadjikakou K (2006) The role of educational experiences in the development of deaf identity. J Deaf Stud Deaf Educ 11: 477–492.
17. Bat-Chava Y (1994) Group identification and self-esteem of deaf adults. Pers Soc Psychol Bull 20: 494–502.
18. Sheridan M (2000) Inner lives of deaf children. Washington, DC: Gallaudet University Press.
19. Hole R (2007) Narratives of identity: A poststructural analysis of three Deaf women's life stories. Narrat Inq 17: 259–278.
20. Hormuth SE (1990) The ecology of the self: relocation and self-concept change. Cambridge, England: Cambridge University Press.
21. Deaux K (1993) Reconstructing social identity. Pers Soc Psychol Bull 19: 4–12.
22. Ethier K, Deaux K (1994) Negotiating social identity when contexts change. J Pers Soc Psychol 67: 243–251.
23. Ohna SE (2004) Deaf in my own way: identity, learning, and narratives. Deafness Educ Int 6: 20–38.
24. Padden C, Humphries T (2005) Inside deaf culture. Cambridge, MA: Harvard University Press.
25. Leigh IW (1999) Inclusive education and personal development. J Deaf Stud Deaf Educ 3: 330–338.
26. Maxwell-McCaw D, Zea MC (2011) The Deaf Acculturation Scale (DAS): development and validation of a 58-item measure. J Deaf Stud Deaf Educ 16: 325–342.
27. Maxwell-McCaw D (2001) Acculturation and psychological well-being in Deaf and hard of hearing people. Washington DC: The George Washington University.
28. Middleton A, Hewison J, Mueller RF (1998) Attitudes of deaf adults toward genetic testing for hereditary deafness. Am J Hum Genet 63: 1175–1180.
29. Middleton A, Hewison J, Mueller RF (2001) Prenatal diagnosis for inherited deafness - what is the potential demand? J Genet Couns 10: 121–131.
30. Stern SJ, Arnos KS, Murrelle L, Welch KO, Nance WE, et al. (2002) Attitudes of deaf and hard of hearing subjects towards genetic testing and prenatal diagnosis of hearing loss. J Med Genet 39: 449–453.
31. Martinez A, Linden J, Schimmenti LA, Palmer CGS (2003) Attitudes of the broader hearing, deaf, and hard-of-hearing community toward genetic testing for deafness. Genet Med 5: 106–112.
32. Taneja PR, Pandya A, Foley DL, Nicely LV, Arnos KS (2004) Attitudes of deaf individuals towards genetic testing. Am J Med Genet A 130A: 17–21.
33. Leigh IW, Maxwell-McCaw D, Bat-Chava Y, Christiansen JB (2000) Correlates of psychosocial adjustment in deaf adolescents with and without cochlear implants: a preliminary investigation. J Deaf Stud Deaf Educ 14: 244–259.
34. Wald RL, Knutson JF (2000) Deaf cultural identity of adolescents with and without cochlear implants. Ann Otol Rhinol Laryngol Suppl 185: 87–89.
35. Gorlin RJ, Toriello HV, Cohen Jr MM (1995) Hereditary hearing loss and its syndromes. New York: Oxford University Press.

36. Palmer CG, Boudreault P, Baldwin EE, Fox M, Deignan JL, et al. (2013) Deaf genetic testing and psychological well-being in deaf adults. J Genet Couns 22: 492–507.
37. Klitzman R (2009) "Am I my genes?": Questions of identity among individuals confronting genetic disease. Genet Med 11: 880–889.
38. Michie S, Bobrow M, Marteau TM, FAP Collaborative Research Group (2001) Predictive genetic testing in children and adults: a study of emotional impact. J Med Genet 38: 519–526.
39. Brunger JW, Murray GS, O'Riordan M, Matthews AL, Smith RJH, et al. (2000) Parental attitudes toward genetic testing for pediatric deafness. Am J Hum Genet 67: 1621–1625.
40. Baldwin EE, Boudreault P, Fox M, Sinsheimer JS, Palmer CGS (2012) Effect of pre-test genetic counseling for deaf adults on knowledge of genetic testing. J Genet Couns 21: 256–272.
41. Malcolm K (2005) Contact sign, transliteration and interpretation in Canada. In: Janzen T, editor. Topics in signed language interpreting: theory and practice. Amsterdam: J. Benjamins Pub. Co. pp.107–133.
42. Halbert CH, Kessler LJ, Troxel AB, Stopfer JE, Domcheck S (2010) Effect of genetic counseling and testing for BRCA1 and BRCA2 mutations in African American women: a randomized trial. Public Health Genomics 13: 440–448.
43. Pal T, Stowe C, Cole A, Lee J, Zhao X, et al. (2010) Evaluation of phone-based genetic counselling in African American women using culturally tailored visual aids. Clin Genet 78: 124–131.
44. Sussner K, Jandorf L, Thompson H, Valdimarsdottir H (2010) Interest and beliefs about BRCA genetic counseling among at-risk Latinas in New York City. J Genet Couns 19: 255–268.
45. Palmer CGS, Martinez A, Fox M, Zhou J, Shapiro N, et al. (2009) A prospective, longitudinal study of the impact of GJB2/GJB6 genetic testing on the beliefs and attitudes of parents of deaf and hard-of-hearing infants. Am J Med Genet A 149A: 1169–1182.
46. Kobayashi Y, Boudreault P, Hill K, Sinsheimer JS, Palmer CGS (2013) Using a social marketing framework to evaluate recruitment of a prospective study of genetic counseling and testing for the deaf community. BMC Med Res Methodol 13: 145.
47. Samady W, Sadler GR, Nakaji M, Malcarne VL, Trybus R, et al. (2008) Translation of the multidimensional health locus of control scales for users of American sign language. Public Health Nurs 25: 480–489.
48. Brislin RW (1970) Back-translation for cross-cultural research. J Cross Cult Psychol 1: 185–216.
49. Box GEP, Hunter WG, Hunter JS (1978) Statistics for experimenters. New York: John Wiley & Sons.
50. SAS (2002) SAS. 9.1 ed. Cary, North Carolina: SAS Institute Inc.
51. Hadjikakou K, Nikolaraizi M (2007) The impact of personal educational experiences and communication practices on the construction of deaf identity in Cyprus. Am Ann Deaf 152: 398–414.
52. Parker MJ, Fortnum HM, Young ID, Davis AC (2000) Genetics and deafness: what do families want? J Med Genet 37: 37–40.
53. Steinberg A, Kaimal G, Ewing R, Soslow LP, Lewis KM, et al. (2007) Parental narratives of genetic testing for hearing loss: audiologic implications for clinical work with children and families. Am J Audiol 16: 57–67.
54. Lewis S, Curnow L, Ross M, Massie J (2006) Parental attitudes to the identification of their infants as carriers of cystic fibrosis by newborn screening. J Paediatr Child Health 42: 533–537.
55. Barnett S, Franks P (1999) Smoking and deaf adults: Associations with age at onset of deafness. Am Ann Deaf 144: 44–50.

# 21

# Hair Cell Regeneration after ATOH1 Gene Therapy in the Cochlea of Profoundly Deaf Adult Guinea Pigs

**Patrick J. Atkinson[1,2], Andrew K. Wise[1,2,3], Brianna O. Flynn[1], Bryony A. Nayagam[1,2,4], Rachael T. Richardson[1,2,3]***

**1** Bionics Institute, East Melbourne, Victoria, Australia, **2** Department of Otolaryngology, University of Melbourne, East Melbourne, Victoria, Australia, **3** Department of Medical Bionics, University of Melbourne, East Melbourne, Victoria, Australia, **4** Department of Audiology and Speech Pathology, University of Melbourne, Parkville, Victoria, Australia

## Abstract

The degeneration of hair cells in the mammalian cochlea results in permanent sensorineural hearing loss. This study aimed to promote the regeneration of sensory hair cells in the mature cochlea and their reconnection with auditory neurons through the introduction of ATOH1, a transcription factor known to be necessary for hair cell development, and the introduction of neurotrophic factors. Adenoviral vectors containing ATOH1 alone, or with neurotrophin-3 and brain derived neurotrophic factor were injected into the lower basal scala media of guinea pig cochleae four days post ototoxic deafening. Guinea pigs treated with ATOH1 gene therapy, alone, had a significantly greater number of cells expressing hair cell markers compared to the contralateral non-treated cochlea when examined 3 weeks post-treatment. This increase, however, did not result in a commensurate improvement in hearing thresholds, nor was there an increase in synaptic ribbons, as measured by CtBP2 puncta after ATOH1 treatment alone, or when combined with neurotrophins. However, hair cell formation and synaptogenesis after co-treatment with ATOH1 and neurotrophic factors remain inconclusive as viral transduction was reduced due to the halving of viral titres when the samples were combined. Collectively, these data suggest that, whilst ATOH1 alone can drive non-sensory cells towards an immature sensory hair cell phenotype in the mature cochlea, this does not result in functional improvements after aminoglycoside-induced deafness.

**Editor:** Bruce Riley, Texas A&M University, United States of America

**Funding:** The authors wish to acknowledge the generous support of the Garnett Passe and Rodney Williams Memorial Foundation (PJA), the National Health and Medical Research Council (GNT1024350) (RTR), Action on Hearing Loss (RTR), the Royal Victorian Eye and Ear Hospital (PJA) and the University of Melbourne (PJA). The Bionics Institute acknowledges the support it receives from the Victorian Government through its Operational Infrastructure Support Program. The funders had no role in study design, data collection and analysis, decision to publish, or preparation of the manuscript.

**Competing Interests:** The authors have declared that no competing interests exist.

* Email: rrichardson@bionicsinstitute.org

## Introduction

Hearing loss is a major health concern which affects over 5% of the world's population. This equates to approximately 360 million people suffering from a disabling hearing impairment (World Health Organisation, 2013), a number that is expected to grow with an ageing population. Sensorineural hearing loss (SNHL), the most common cause of hearing loss, can occur as a result of a congenital defect or be acquired through exposure to excessive noise, exposure to certain classes of antibiotics, infections or ageing. The loss of hearing in many of these cases is permanent due to the irreversible degeneration of the sensory hair cells (HCs) in the cochlea [1]. Currently, the only clinical treatment for a severe-to-profound SNHL (characterised by a hearing threshold of 70 dB or above) is a cochlear implant, which bypasses the damaged or lost HCs and electrically stimulates the remaining auditory neurons. Despite their success, however, there is variable patient performance with a cochlear implant, especially in relation to speech perception in noisy environments and for music appreciation, where performance can be markedly decreased [2,3]. As such, in the last decade there has been a strong research focus on alternative treatments for SNHL, in particular, the use of novel techniques to restore the degenerated elements of the cochlea.

Hair cell regeneration is thought to be the panacea for restoring function to the cochlea after SNHL, however, this is not without challenges. For example, it is known from developmental studies that the initial formation, patterning and correct connection of HCs to auditory neurons requires a complex cascade of molecular signaling with precise timing [4]. One of these molecular signals is the expression of the basic helix-loop-helix transcription factor ATOH1, a factor which has been found to be necessary for HC development and is thought to be the earliest determinant of HC fate [5,6]. Indeed, ATOH1 null mice lack both cochlear HCs and the supporting cells that comprise the sensory epithelium known as the organ of Corti (OC) [7]. Moreover, the overexpression of ATOH1 has been shown to result in ectopic and supernumerary HCs, which is thought to occur through the direct transdifferentiation of non-sensory supporting cells in the OC towards a HC fate [7–9]. Experimental manipulations reintroducing ATOH1 into the deaf cochlea has also highlighted the role of this transcription factor in HC development. An initial study in the short-term (four day) ototoxically deafened guinea pig (GP), demonstrated both a greater number of HCs in the viral-mediated ATOH1-treated cochlea (as noted by the expression of a known HC marker, myosinVIIa) and also a significant improvement in hearing thresholds (as measured by auditory brainstem responses; ABRs) [10]. These results in the mature GP provided evidence that it is possible to manipulate non-sensory cells to generate sensory HCs, which subsequently leads to improved auditory function. These findings were further bolstered by a gain-of-function study, which demonstrated that *in utero* gene transfer of ATOH1 not only forced the production of supernumerary and ectopic HCs, but also that these additional HCs were functional [8]. Whilst, these results were very promising, recent studies have underscored the complex nature of HC regeneration. Indeed, the ability to regenerate HCs, particularly within the mature cochlea, has been variable [10–13]. Further to this, a recent study demonstrated that ATOH1-induced HC regeneration after HC loss is possible in neonatal and juvenile mice but not in adult mice [13]. Moreover, little is known about the ability of these newly generated HCs to form synaptic connections with remaining auditory neurons, especially within the mature cochlea, which is critical for the effectiveness of this strategy. A recent study, however, has demonstrated that the presence of NTs significantly enhanced synaptogenesis between HCs and the regrowing peripheral fibres after deafferentation [14].

Experiments carried out in this study examined the ability of ATOH1 gene therapy alone or in combination with NT-gene therapy, to induce transdifferentiation of non-sensory cells towards a HC phenotype in the mature deaf cochlea and promote the regrowth of peripheral fibres towards the new HCs. Transduced cells were further characterised, with a particular focus on the ability of these cells to generate complex ribbon synaptic proteins, attract auditory neuron peripheral fibres and improve hearing.

## Materials and Methods

### Ethics Statement

National Health and Medical Research Council (NHMRC) and Nation Institutes of Health (NIH) Guidelines for the Care and Use of Laboratory Animals were observed. The Animal Research Ethics Committee of the Royal Victorian Eye and Ear Hospital approved the care and use of the animals in this study (ethics #09/180AB).

### Adenoviral vectors

Adenoviral vectors were generated as previously described [15]. Briefly, replication deficient adenovirus type 5 was genetically modified to expression green fluorescent protein (GFP) in concert with mouse brain derived neurotrophic factor (BDNF), mouse neurotrophin-3 (NT-3) or mouse ATOH1. Adenoviral vectors were diluted 1:5 in artificial endolymph (120 mmol/l KCL, 2.5 mmol/l NaCl, 0.5 mmol/l $MgCl_2$, 028 mmol/l $CaCl_2$, 7.6 mmol/l $K_2HPO_4$, 2.7 mmol/l $KH_2PO_4$, pH 7.4) to final concentrations of $3.0\times10^{10}$ OPU/ml (Ad-NT-3), $4.3\times10^{10}$ OPU/ml (Ad-BDNF) and $2.1\times10^{11}$ OPU/ml (Ad-ATOH1). Ad-NT-3 and Ad-BDNF were mixed in a 1:1 ratio just prior to injection and will hereafter be referred to as Ad-NTs. When required Ad-NTs was mixed in a 1:1 ratio with Ad-ATOH1 (Ad-ATOH1+Ad-NTs).

### Experimental animals

Male and female adult pigmented Dunkin-Hartley GPs (n = 26, average weight 365±12 g) were used in this study. Each gene therapy group had five animals while the normal and four day deaf groups had three animals (in the normal and four day deaf groups data was used from left and right cochleae as there was no difference in HC number observed). Viral administration was performed with the approval of the Office of the Gene Technology Regulator Australia (Licence #444), and under approval of the Royal Victorian Eye and Ear Hospital Animal Ethics Committee.

### Deafening

The hearing status of each GP was assessed prior to deafening by measuring ABRs to computer-generated click and tone-pip stimuli (1, 2, 8, 16, 24 and 32 kHz) [16]. For inclusion in the study, GPs were required to have normal hearing, which was defined as an auditory brainstem response (ABR) threshold <43 dB peak-equivalent sound pressure level. Animals meeting this criterion were deafened under gaseous anaesthesia via intravenous infusion of 100 mg/kg furosemide (Troy Laboratories, Smithfield, Australia) and subcutaneous injection of 400 mg/kg kanamycin sulphate (Applichem, Taren Point, Australia; [17]). Deafness was confirmed four days post-procedure using ABRs, where animals with threshold shifts of >50 dB were considered profoundly deaf.

### Cochlear injection of viral sample

In order to target the supporting cells of the OC two microliters of Ad-GFP, Ad-NTs, Ad-ATOH1 or Ad-NTs+Ad-ATOH1 were unilaterally injected into the lower basal scala media of the cochlea four days post-deafening as previously described [15]. Briefly, a retroauricular approached was used to expose the bulla. An opening was made in the bulla with a drill and a small cochleostomy was made into the otic capsule of the cochlear basal turn. Perilymph was removed using gentle suction to visualise basilar membrane. A glass recording micropipette was advanced via a stepper motor (Kopf, model 2662) through the basilar membrane until an endocochlear potential was measured, after which the viral preparation was injected using a rate controlled micropump system (WPI), over 5 minutes. This approach was selected to specifically target the OC for gene transfection. The pipette was then retracted and the cochleostomy sealed with connective tissue, the bulla sealed with dental cement and the wound closed in layers with dissolvable sutures.

### Functional assessment and histology

Four days post-deafening and three weeks post-injection GP hearing was assessed with click and tone-pip ABRs as described above. Animals were then euthanised with 1.5 ml pentobarbitone and intracardially perfused with 0.9% (wt/vol) saline containing 0.1% (vol/vol) heparin sodium and 0.025% (wt/vol) sodium nitrite, followed by 10% (vol/vol) neutral buffered formalin. The bullae were removed and the cochleae visualised. Cochleae were decalcified, embedded in optimal cutting temperature compound and sectioned in the pre-modiolar and mid-modiolar planes as previously described [18]. Half of the cochlea was retained for surface preparations as described [15,19]. The following primary antibodies were used: anti-neurofilament (1:200, NF; Merck Millipore, Australia), rabbit anti-myosinVIIa (1:100, Proteus Bioscience), mouse anti-myosinVIIa (1:100, Developmental Studies Hybridoma Bank, University of Iowa) anti-calbindin (1:500, Merck Millipore), anti-parvalbumin (1:200, Sigma), anti-prestin (1:50, Santa Cruz Biotechnology), anti-oncomodulin (1:200, Swant), anti-CtBP2 (1:50, BD Biosciences). AlexaFluor secondary antibodies (1:200–1:500, Life Technologies) were used to visualise several antibodies in the same sample and mounted in media with or without DAPI. Sections were examined on a Zeiss Axioplan fluorescence microscope and imaged using Axiovision v4.8 (Carl Zeiss, Germany). Cochlear half-turn surface preparations and pre mid-modiolar sections were viewed on a Zeiss LSM Meta 510

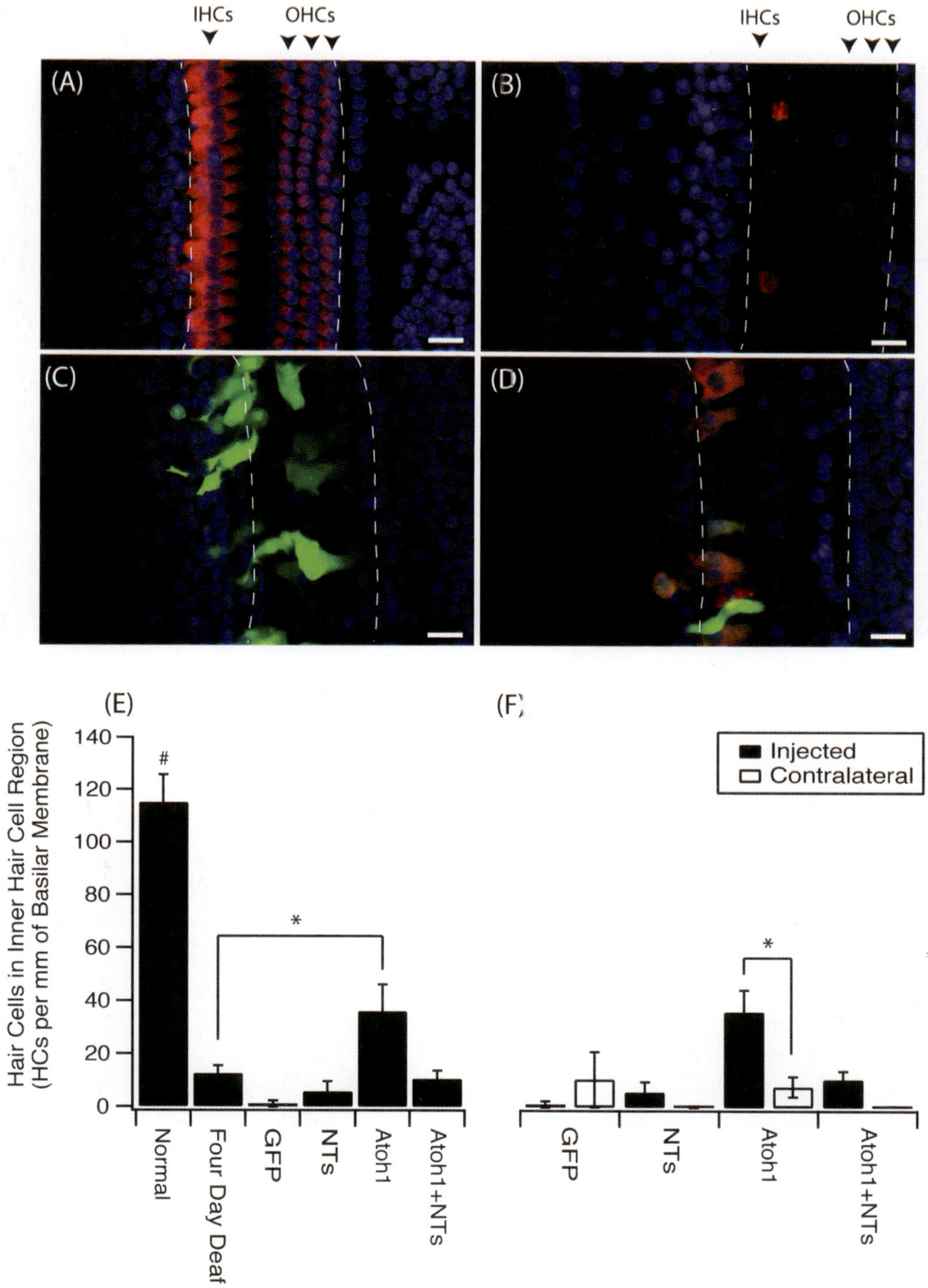


**Figure 1. An increase in hair cells in the inner hair cell region after ATOH1 gene therapy.** Example photomicrographs of surface preparations of the basal turn of the cochlea from (A) normal, (B) four day deaf, (C) Ad-GFP treated, (D) Ad-ATOH1 treated animals (red = myosinVIIa, green = GFP, blue = DAPI, dashed lines mark the sensory region, scale bar = 20 μm). (E) When quantified there was a significant loss of IHCs after four days of deafness compared to normal hearing animals. Three weeks post ATOH1-gene therapy there were significantly more myosinVIIa positive cells in the IHC region compared with the four day deaf group (*$p<0.05$, ANOVA). This number however remained below that observed in normal cochleae which had a greater number of IHCs compared to any other treatment group (#$p<0.05$, ANOVA). (F) A comparison of treated (injected) versus non-treated (contralateral) cochleae showed ATOH1-injected cochleae to have a significantly greater number of IHCs relative to the contralateral control cochleae (§$p<0.05$ paired t-test).

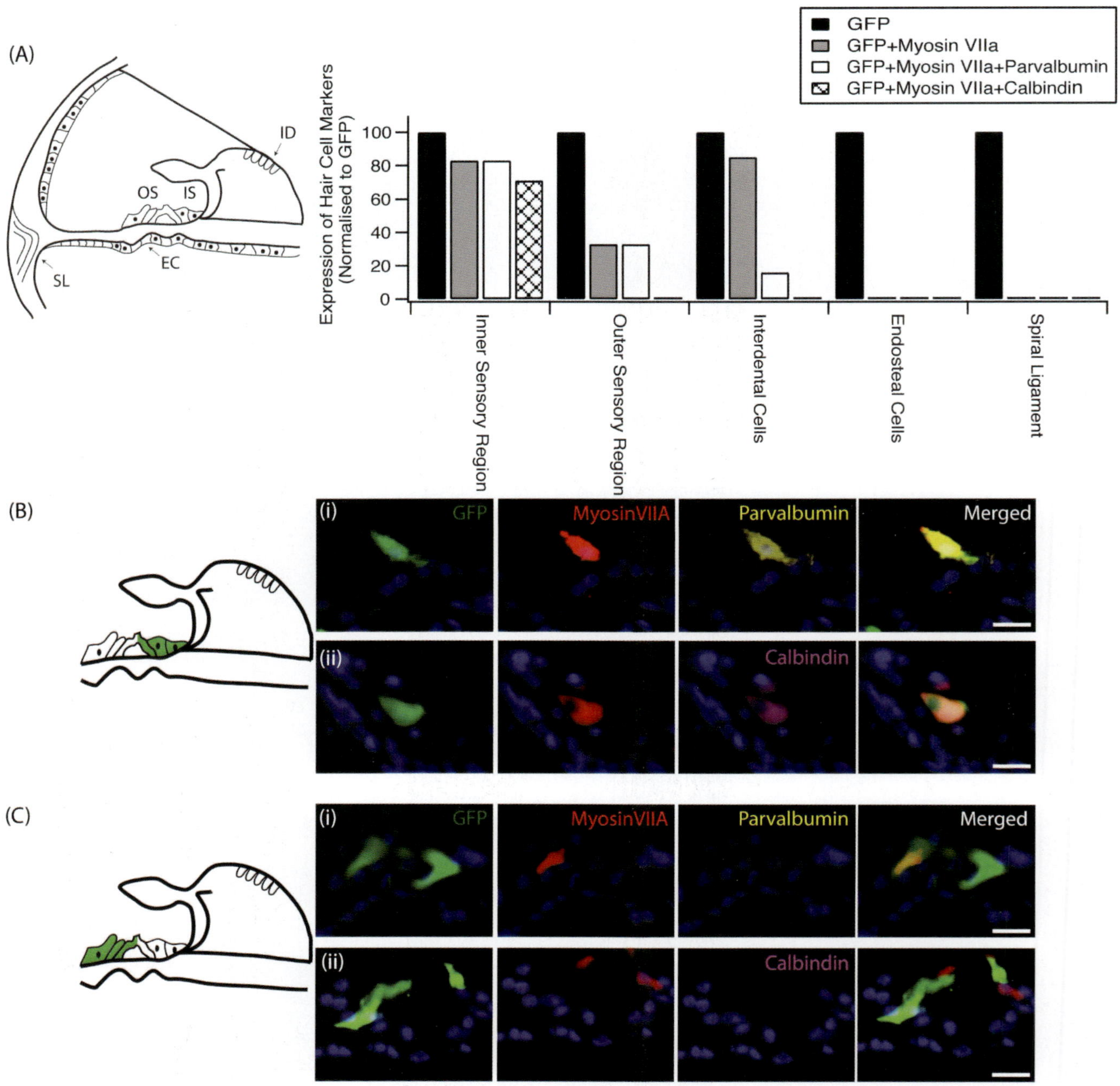


**Figure 2. HC marker expression following ATOH1 treatment.** (A) The transduction of cells with ATOH1 resulted in cells expressing HC markers to varying degrees depending on their location (EC: endosteal cells, ID: interdental cells, IS: inner sensory region, OS: outer sensory region, SL: spiral ligament). Transduced cells (green) in the inner sensory region (B) had the highest percentage of cells that expressed the HC markers myosinVIIa (red), parvalbumin (yellow) and calbindin (magenta). A high proportion of myosinVIIa-positive transduced cells in this region co-labelled with (i) parvalbumin or (ii) calbindin. Fewer cells in the outer sensory region (C) expressed HC markers. ATOH1-transduced cells within the spiral ligament or endosteal cell region did not express any HC markers. Scale bar = 20 μm.

confocal microscope and images captured using Zen software (2009 edition).

## Data Analysis

### Hair cell quantification

Hair cells were analysed in basal turn surface preparations. Cells which expressed MyosinVIIa, had a nucleus, and resided within the organ of Corti were categorised as HCs. These cells were quantified along the entire length of the basilar membrane. The length of the basilar membrane was measured and the total number of HCs was expressed per mm of basilar membrane.

### Quantification of presynaptic ribbons

Inner hair cell synaptic ribbon quantification was conducted using basal turn surface preparations. Optical sections in the z-axis were imaged and recorded at 0.6 μm intervals for high resolution. Pre-synaptic ribbon synapses were visualised as CtBP2 immuno-reactive puncta. The number of synaptic ribbons observed in each

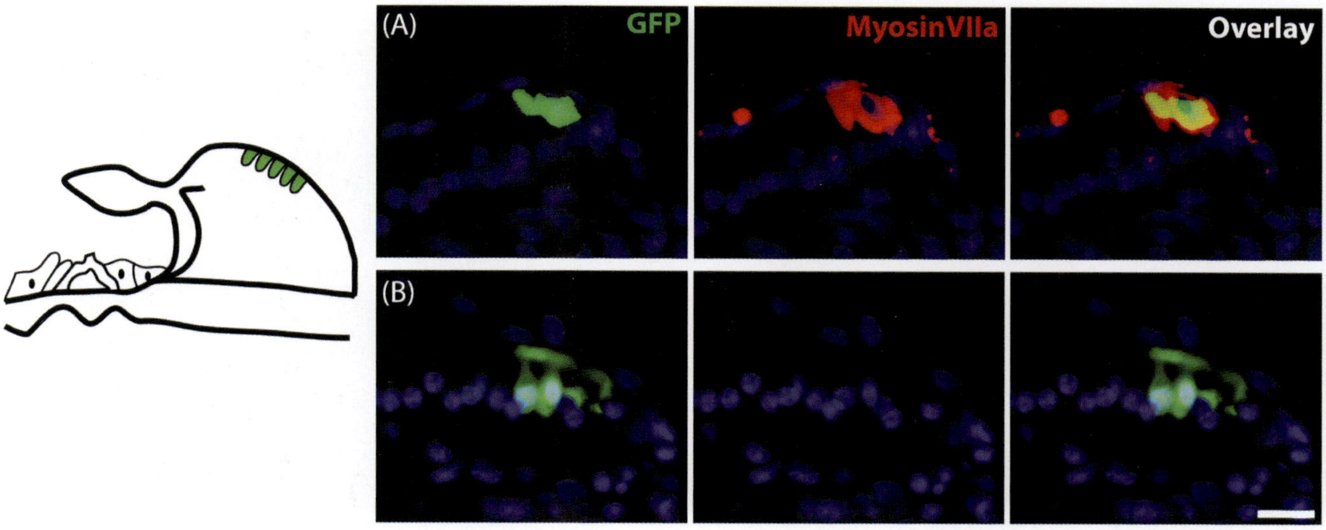


**Figure 3. Transduction of interdental cells following ATOH1 or GFP treatment.** Schematic at left illustrates the region of the interdental cells within the spiral limbus. The transduction of interdental cells (green) with ATOH1 (A) resulted in the expression of the HC marker myosinVIIa (red) in 85% of the cells. (B) MyosinVIIa expression was not detected following transduction of interdental cells with the GFP control vector. Scale bar = 20 μm.

inner hair cell (IHC) was quantified by counting CtBP2 puncta within an IHC. The percentage of IHCs with CtBP2 puncta was also quantified. For all Ad treatment groups, every HC was imaged for quantification.

## Quantification of peripheral fibre regrowth towards transduced cells

The growth of auditory neuron peripheral fibres towards transduced cells in the scala media was analysed from confocal images that contained GFP-positive cells, as previously described [18]. Briefly, confocal images were initially split into their individual channels using ZEN software. These images were converted to 32-bit and thresholded using the "moments" algorithm in ImageJ. This was done for each image within the stack. The GFP-positive channel image was opened in Gimp software (GNU image manipulation software) and a 10 pixel border was drawn around the GFP-positive cell. This border was then copied and pasted on the NF-positive image, such that only those NF-positive fibres that fell within this area were visible. The pixel density of these fibres was then measured using ImageJ software. Four consecutive Z-planes with the highest pixel density were averaged to give a final result. Only GFP-expressing cells within the OC region and distal to the IHCs were used for analysis to avoid including fibres that are normally observed in the inner spiral bundle, as such, not all animals could be included in this analysis (n = 5 GPs for Ad-GFP, n = 4 GPs for Ad-NTs). Measurements from Ad-GFP injected GPs and Ad-NTs injected GPs were compared using a student's t-test.

## Auditory neuron density

Spiral ganglion neuron density was analysed blindly from three non-consecutive (greater than 72 μm apart) mid-modiolar sections from each cochlea as outlined previously [18]. Briefly, density was calculated by counting co-labelled NF and DAPI-positive auditory neuron cell bodies within Rosenthal's canal, and then dividing the number of auditory neurons by the area of Rosenthal's canal using ImageJ software. Lower and upper basal, middle and apical turn densities were averaged to calculate the overall density for each cochlear region. Statistical analyses of auditory neuron density data were performed using a paired student's t-test and presented as mean ± SEM.

# Results

## Hair cell regeneration with ATOH1 gene therapy

In normal hearing cochleae there was a well-defined single row of myosinVIIa-positive IHCs displaying stereotypical pear-shaped morphology and three rows of myosinVIIa-positive outer hair cells (OHCs), along the entire length of the surface preparation (Figure 1A). Animals that were sacrificed four days post-deafening showed a complete bilateral loss of OHCs and a near-complete loss of IHCs in the basal turn. The few remaining IHCs in these animals had atypical spherical morphology (Figure 1B). Deafened cochleae examined three weeks after Ad-GFP (Figure 1C) or Ad-NTs treatment also had very few HCs compared normal hearing animals, despite significant regions of GFP expression. In contrast, cochleae treated with Ad-ATOH1 displayed myosinVIIa and GFP co-positive HCs in the lower basal turn. These HCs had a varied morphology with some displaying a typical pear-shaped morphology and others with a more spherical morphology (Figure 1D). The HCs observed in ATOH1 treated cochleae were generally located proximal to the IHC region with some ectopic expression observed near the inner spiral bundle and in the outer sensory region, proximal to the location of the OHCs.

There were no significant differences detected between the number of HCs observed after four days of deafness alone compared to Ad-GFP or Ad-NTs treated animals (Figure 1E). The Ad-mediated introduction of ATOH1, in contrast, resulted in significantly more myosinVIIa-positive cells compared to the four day deaf cohort (Mann-Whitney test, $p<0.05$; Figure 1E) and their contralateral non-treated cochleae (Student t-test, $p<0.05$; Figure 1F). The overall numbers of HCs in ATOH1 treated cochleae was still significantly lower than those observed in normal cochleae. The combined treatment of ATOH1 and NTs did not result in an increase in HCs compared to the four day deaf group. However, the ATOH1 and NT viral titres in this group were halved, limiting the inferences that can be made for this group.

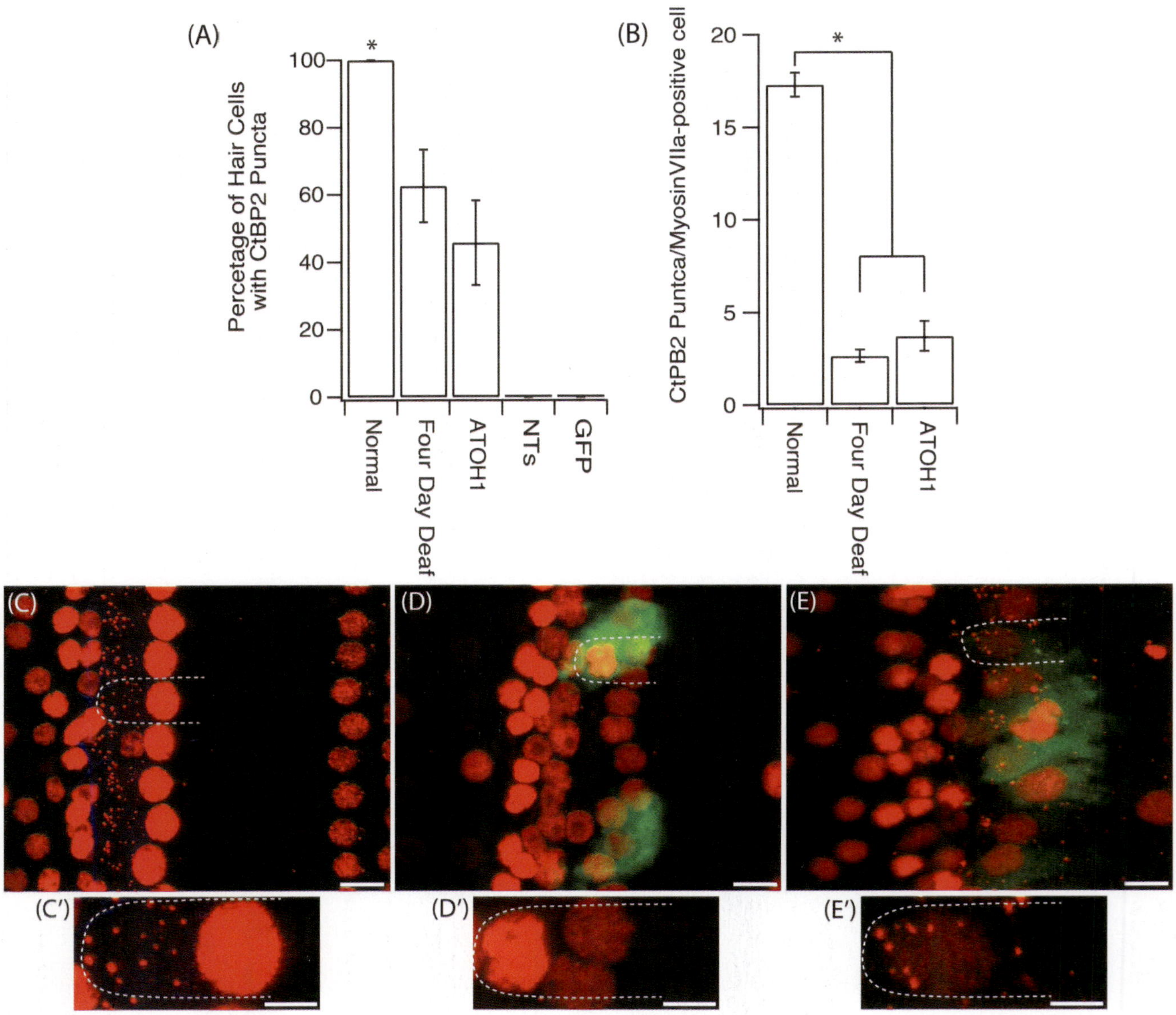


**Fure 4. CtBP2 expression in IHCs.** (A) There was a significant decrease in the percentage of HCs that were positive for CtBP2 puncta after four days of deafness and after treatment with ATOH1 when compared to the normal hearing cochlea (*p<0.05, one way ANOVA). (B) There were also significantly less CtBP2 puncta per IHC after four days of deafness or ATOH1 treatment. Examples of CtBP2 staining (red) in the (C) normal, (D) GFP treated and (E) ATOH1 treated cochlea with their respective magnified image (C′-E′), green = GFP. Scale bar =10 μm (main image) and 5 μm (magnified image)

## Characterisation of ATOH1 transduced cells

**Immunohistochemical characterisation.** To more thoroughly characterise cells that had been transduced by ATOH1, mid-modiolar sections were double-labelled with myosinVIIa and either parvalbumin, calbindin, oncomodulin or prestin (Figure 2). The location of transduced cells was further divided into five regions consisting of the inner sensory region (proximal to the location of the IHCs), the outer sensory region (proximal to the location of the OHCs), the interdental cell region of the spiral limbus, the spiral ligament region and finally the endosteal cell region. In ATOH1-transduced cells in the inner sensory region, which had the most transduced cells, parvalbumin was found to co-label with myosinVIIa 83% of the time and calbindin co-labelled with myosinVIIa 71% of the time. In the outer sensory region this percentage dropped to 33% of transduced cells for myosinVIIa and parvalbumin co-labelling, and cells were no longer positive for calbindin. The myosinVIIa, parvalbumin and calbindin HC markers were not expressed in any ATOH1-transduced cell in the endosteal and spiral ligament regions. Moreover, regardless of location, ATOH1-transduced cells failed to express the mature HC markers oncomodulin or prestin (data not shown). When transduced with Ad-GFP only, no co-localisation with any HC marker was observed.

The interdental cells of the spiral limbus were often transduced and interestingly, when transduced by ATOH1, 85% of those GFP positive cells were also myosinVIIa-positive (Figure 3A). In only one instance was an interdental cell co-labelled with parvalbumin. When transduced with Ad-GFP only, no co-localisation with myosinVIIa or any other HC marker was observed in the interdental cells (Figure 3B).

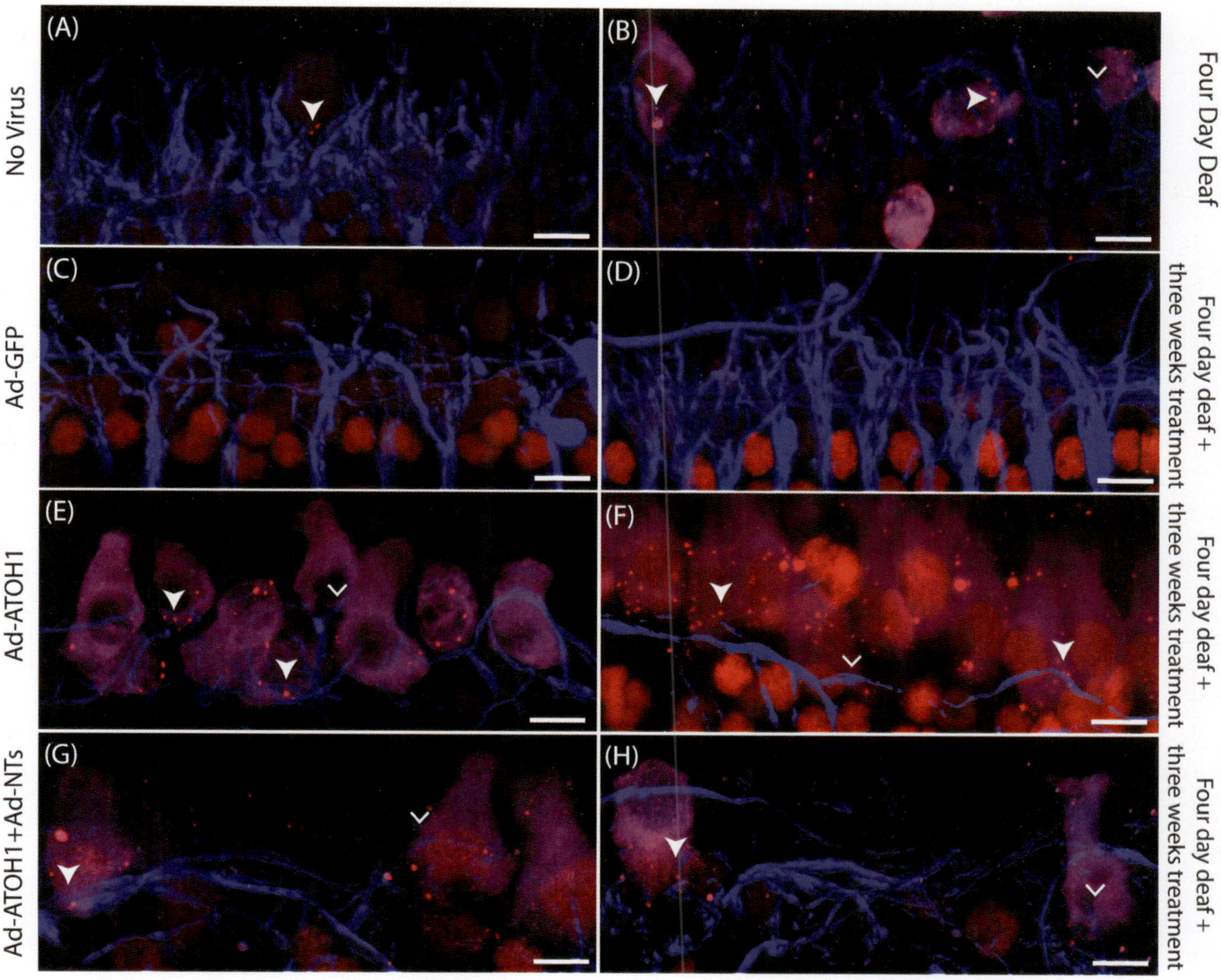


**Figure 5. Surface preparations illustrating peripheral fibres in close proximity to HCs with ribbon synapses.** Examples of peripheral fibres (blue) close to myosinVIIa-positive cells (magenta) with CtBP2 puncta (red; filled arrowhead) or without CtBP2 puncta (arrowhead) in the four day deafened (A&B), GFP treated (C&D), ATOH1 treated (E&F) or ATOH1+NTs (G&H) treated cochleae. Scale bar = 10 µm.

**Synaptic ribbon detection and quantification.** A unique feature of IHCs in the cochlea is their ribbon synapse, which is critical for HC function. With the evidence that ATOH1 transduction induces cells to differentiate towards a HC phenotype, as noted by the expression of multiple HC markers, we next sought to determine if the transduced cells could also generate these highly specialised synaptic proteins. In normal cochleae all IHCs contained ribbon synapses, as indicated by the presence of CtBP2 puncta located on the basolateral surface of the HC (Figure 4A). When assessed four days post-deafening, of the IHCs that remained, only 62.5±10.7% (11 cells across 3 animals) had CtPB2 puncta. When examined three weeks post-ATOH1 gene therapy, 45.8±1.2% of myosinVIIa-positive cells were observed to have CtBP2 puncta. In total there were 21 myosinVIIa-positive cells with CtBP2-positive puncta in ATOH1 transduced cochleae across five animals (Figure 4A). In contrast, CtBP2 puncta were absent in the few remaining HCs observed after GFP or NTs treatment (Figure 4A). To further quantify the presence of synaptic ribbons in the normal hearing, four day deaf and ATOH1 treatment groups, the number of CtBP2 puncta per IHC was examined. In the cochleae of normal hearing animals there was a mean of 17.3±0.7 puncta/IHC, a value similar to that found in other species [14]. This number decreased 2.6±0.3 puncta/IHC in the four day deaf cohort and after ATOH1 treatment there were 3.7±0.8 puncta/IHC (Figure 4B). In the four day deaf animals and ATOH1 treated animals, the location of CtBP2 puncta also differed when compared to normal hearing animals. In the normal hearing cochlea, puncta were localised to the basolateral pole of the HC (Figure 4C). CtBP2 puncta were absent after treatment with GFP only (Figure 4D), whilst in the ATOH1-treated group puncta were observed in the middle and the apex as well as in the basolateral pole of the HC (Figure 4E).

## Peripheral fibre innervation of hair cells

Synapses were examined further to determine if peripheral auditory neuron fibres innervated myosinVIIa and CtBP2 puncta-positive cells. When examined four days post deafening there were very few remaining IHCs, and even fewer with CtBP2-positive puncta (Figure 5A, B). Of the HCs that were CtBP2-positive, there was a marked reduction in the density of peripheral fibres

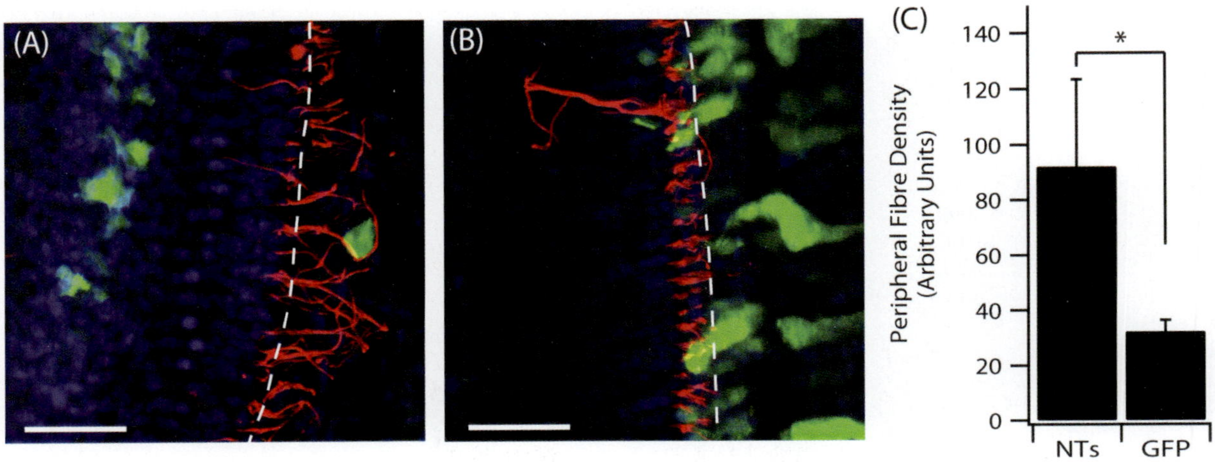


**Figure 6. Resprouting peripheral fibres.** Cochlear surface preparations were stained with anti-NF (red) and DAPI (blue). (A) Peripheral fibre responses to NT-expressing cells in the OC post Ad-NTs treatment. (B) Peripheral fibre response to GFP only expressing cells in the OC post Ad-GFP treatment. The perforated lines indicate the approximate medial edge of the inner pillar cells of the OC. Scale bar = 50 μm. (C) Significantly greater fibre density was observed in close proximity (≤10 μm) to NT-secreting cells compared to GFP-only transduced cells ($p<0.05$, t-test).

proximal to the remaining HCs, compared to the dense innervation pattern in the normal cochlea. Cochleae treated with Ad-GFP (Figure 5C, D) or Ad-NTs (not shown) did not have any CtBP2-positive puncta within transduced cells. In ATOH1 (Figure 5E, F) and the ATOH1+NTs (Figure 5G, H) cochleae, a number of peripheral fibres were observed to co-localise with HCs expressing CtBP2 puncta. There were also fibres observed within close proximity to myosinVIIa-positive cells without CtBP2 co-localisation. Interestingly, the peripheral fibres in the ATOH1 treated groups appeared to be travelling laterally along the myosinVIIa-positive cells, which is characteristic of OHC innervation rather than IHC innervation.

Whilst treatment with Ad-NTs did not lead to an increase in the number of myosin-positive cells or CtBP2 puncta-positive cells, the density of peripheral fibres in close proximity to transduced cells was significantly greater in GPs treated with Ad-NTs (92.27±31.18 NF-pixels/GFP-positive cell) compared to GPs treated with Ad-GFP (32.34±4.04 NF pixels/GFP-positive cell; $p<0.05$, t-test). These peripheral fibres were observed to loop around the NT-expressing cells (Figure 6).

## Functional assessment of ATOH1 gene therapy

To test the functional effect resulting from the increase in HCs observed after ATOH1 gene therapy in the deaf cochlea, ABR thresholds were measured prior to aminoglycoside deafening, four days post deafening, and also three weeks post-gene therapy treatment (Figure 7). ABRs measured four days after deafening showed that all animals were profoundly deaf across all frequencies measured, indicating a loss of functional HCs (one way repeated measures ANOVA, $p<0.001$). When thresholds were remeasured three weeks post gene therapy treatment, there was no improvement in hearing thresholds in any of the treatment

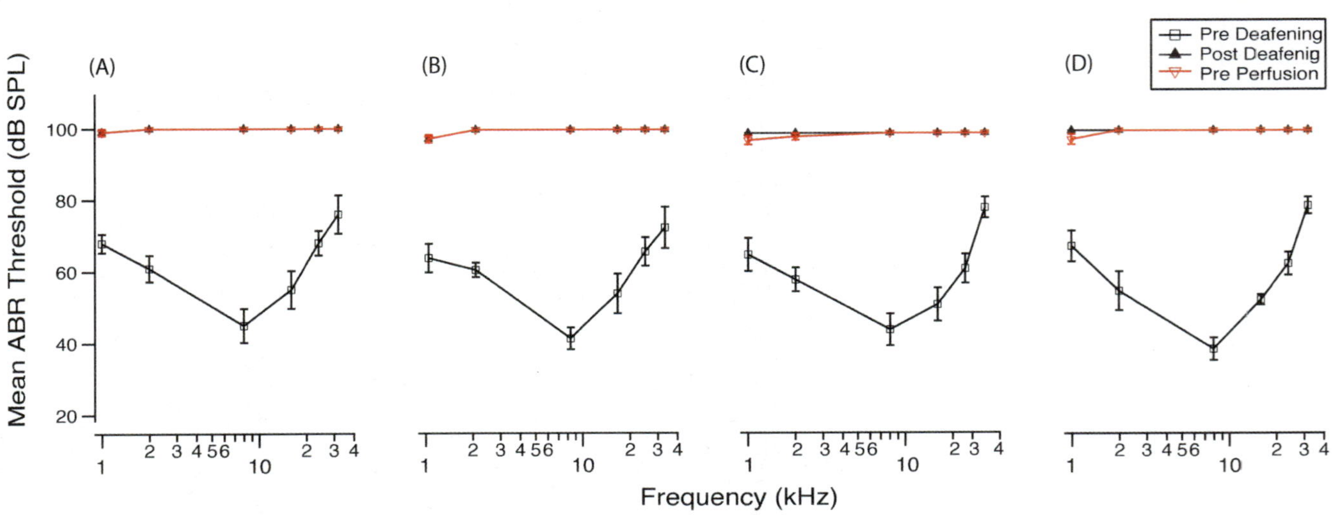


**Figure 7. Mean ABR thresholds pre-deafening, post-deafening and post-treatment.** There was a profound hearing loss across all frequencies measured (1, 2, 8, 16, 24, 32 kHz) four days post aminoglycoside deafening for all animals. Three weeks after treatment with either (A) Ad-GFP, (B) Ad-NTs, (C) Ad-ATOH1 or (D) Ad-ATOH1+Ad-NTs there was no change in hearing thresholds compared to those measured post-deafening ($p>0.05$, repeated measured ANOVA).

groups (one way repeated measures ANOVA, $p>0.05$). No differences were detected between hearing thresholds in the treated compared to the contralateral non-treated ear (data not shown), indicating no functional recovery due to ATOH1 or NT-gene therapy.

### Auditory neuron densities

To determine if the introduction of ATOH1 and the subsequent increase in HCs was able to promote the survival of auditory neurons after deafness, auditory neuron density was measured in the basal, middle and apical turns after Ad-injections. Statistical comparisons were made between injected and the non-injected contralateral cochlea for each cochlear region. There was no significant difference in auditory neuron density between the Ad-GFP treated cochleae and the contralateral cochleae ($1101\pm29$ versus $1125\pm53$ auditory neurons/$mm^2$), nor was there any difference in auditory neuron density between the treated and contralateral sides in the Ad-ATOH1 group ($947\pm60$ versus $933\pm57$ auditory neurons/$mm^2$). There was, however, a significant increase in auditory neuron density in the basal turn on the treated side compared to the contralateral side in the Ad-NTs group ($1254\pm42$ versus $1079\pm51$ auditory neurons/$mm^2$) and the Ad-ATOH1+NTs group ($1168\pm84$ versus $994\pm108$ auditory neuron s/$mm^2$; paired t-test, $p<0.05$).

## Discussion

The key finding of this study is that ATOH1-gene therapy results in an increase in the number of HCs, defined as myosinVIIa-positive cells with non-pyknotic nuclei residing within the OC, after profound aminoglycoside-induced SNHL in the mature GP. This study also demonstrated that cells transduced with ATOH1 expressed a multitude of HC proteins, however, these cells did not regenerate a full complement of synaptic ribbons nor was hearing function restored after severe SNHL.

### ATOH1 gene therapy was unable to restore hearing after deafness in the mature GP cochlea

Deafening resulted in a profound and rapid hearing loss across all frequencies, when measured four days post-deafening. In contrast to a previous study [10], the current study did not show any hearing recovery after the introduction of ATOH1. One possible explanation for this contrasting result is the differences in the severity of deafness and therefore the extent OC degeneration prior to ATOH1 introduction. The differing degree of severity of OC damage is illustrated by the contrasting ABR results. In a previous study there was a hearing response recorded in the contralateral ear when remeasured 8 weeks post-deafening [10], suggesting that there was a degree of recovery without treatment, unlike in the current study where complete hearing loss persisted in the non-treated contralateral ear when re-examined at all time points post-deafening. The level of recovery observed in this previous study, however, was greater in the ATOH1 treated ear suggesting, when viewed in the context of the current findings, that ATOH1 may have played a protective or repair role as well as a role in generating new HCs.

### ATOH1 gene therapy results in an increase in the number of HCs in the profoundly deaf cochlea

Whilst ATOH1 gene therapy was unable to restore hearing after aminoglycoside-induced SNHL, it did result in an increase in the number of HCs compared to cochleae examined four days post-deafening and compared to the contralateral non-treated cochleae. The number of HCs in the ATOH1 treated animal was, as expected, significantly less than that of the normal hearing animal. The numbers of HCs observed after ATOH1 therapy in this study, however, was less than that reported previously [10], where the number of IHCs observed in the inoculated ear was much closer to the number of IHCs observed in the normal hearing GP cochlea, again most likely reflecting the higher severity of damage to the OC in this study, limiting the number of protected or repaired HCs and the number of viable supporting cells that were able to undergo transdifferentiation after the deafening procedure used in this current study.

The HCs observed in the ATOH1 treated cochleae in the present study had a varied morphology; some displayed the more stereotypical mature pear-shaped IHC morphology, whilst others had a more spherical morphology (Figure 1). These observations are supported by an earlier study where ATOH1 treatment-induced HCs also lacked a mature morphology [13]. Given that there were occasional HCs present at the time of inoculation, it is possible that ATOH1 expression could be promoting the survival of existing HCs. As such, HCs with the more typical morphology might be existing HCs that were protected rather than regenerated HCs. Indeed, expression of ATOH1 within the supporting cells of the damaged OC was recently shown to repair stereocilia and improve hearing thresholds, suggesting that ATOH1 may be able to maintain and repair injured HCs [20]. However, the findings that the overall density of HCs in the ATOH1 inoculated cochleae were significantly greater than that observed in the four day deaf cohort (e.g. at the time point of ATOH1 inoculation), suggests that these new additional HCs were transdifferentiated from other cell types in the OC.

### ATOH1-transduced cells of the OC express multiple immature HC proteins

Upon further characterisation of the HCs observed after ATOH1 treatment, it was noted that the expression of HC markers was related to the location of the transduced cells, even within the OC region itself. Transduced cells in the inner sensory region, for example, expressed a multitude of HC markers (myosinVIIa, parvalbumin, calbindin), whilst expression of these HC markers by transduced cells was lower in the outer sensory region. It has been previously demonstrated that ectopic ATOH1 expression in the outer sensory region of the immature cochlea can lead to the generation of new HCs, which expressed myosinVIIa, parvalbumin and calbindin [13]. Interestingly, in both the current study and that conducted by Liu and colleagues (2012), cells that underwent transdifferentiation towards HC in the outer sensory region failed to express mature OHC proteins such as oncomodulin and prestin.

The varied expression observed within the OC region is thought to reflect both a location specific effect of ectopic ATOH1 expression within the OC region and the level of degeneration at the time of treatment, factors which have been previously shown to be a critical determinate in the ability of ATOH1 to manipulate non-sensory cells towards a HC fate [11,21]. Specifically, the range of cells within the OC that are able to undergo ATOH1-mediated HC differentiation has been shown to decrease with age. By post-natal day eight in mice the subpopulation of supporting cells able to be driven towards a HC phenotype was restricted to the medial side of the IHC row. This location correlates to the location of the inner sensory region described in the present study. The lack of expression of HC markers by transduced endosteal cells and cells of the spiral ligament, most likely reflect an inherent inability of these cells to be transdifferentiated by ATOH1. Interestingly, the transduction of the interdental cells with Ad-ATOH1 resulted in expression of myosinVIIa, a marker not observed within these cells when transduced with the control (Ad-GFP) vector or in non-treated cochleae. The results presented demonstrate that ATOH1 is capable of forcing the transdifferentiation of some mature cochlear cells towards a HC phenotype. Not all HCs observed were the result of a protective effect afforded by ATOH1 treatment, as indicated by the greater number of HCs (as quantified by myosinVIIa positive cells in the sensory epithelium) after ATOH1 treatment, compared to the number of HCs present at the time of intervention. The direct transdifferentiation of non-sensory cells towards a HC phenotype through the introduction of ATOH1 has been further confirmed in another study, where approximately 97% of non-sensory cells that newly expressed myosinVIIa after the forced expression of ATOH1 were BrdU-negative, demonstrating that these myosinVIIa-positive cells did not undergo mitotic division prior to conversion towards a HC phenotype [9].

### ATOH1 gene therapy does not restore a full complement of synaptic ribbons in the deaf cochlea

The expression of the cohort of HC markers described herein demonstrates that the introduction of ATOH1 results in at least a partial change in phenotype towards a HC. The conversion of non-sensory cells to HCs has been observed in multiple studies [7,10,22,23]. However, one requirement for mature functional connections is for HCs to have synaptic ribbons, which were assessed in this study by quantifying CtBP2-positive puncta staining. Of the remaining HCs observed after four days of hearing loss there was a significant decrease in the number of HCs that expressed CtBP2-positive puncta. Furthermore, the absolute number of puncta per HC was also significantly decreased at four days post deafening. A decrease in CtBP2-puncta positive HCs and in the number of synaptic ribbons per HC has been previously described after a reversible noise-induced hearing loss, suggesting that ribbon synapses are extremely sensitive to damage [24]. Treatment with ATOH1 was unable restore synaptic ribbons to normal levels, nor generate new HCs with synaptic ribbons at normal levels. Furthermore, the percentage of HCs that had CtBP2 puncta after ATOH1 treatment was not different to those examined after four days of deafness. Interestingly, no CtBP2 puncta were observed in HCs in the NTs or GFP treated cochleae. Collectively, these findings suggest that the ATOH1 may confer a level of protection on residual HCs and the delicate ribbon synapse as well forcing supporting cells to undergo transdifferentiation towards a HC phenotype.

While synaptic ribbons, albeit at a much lower number, were observed after ATOH1 treatment (alone and when combined with NTs) the regrowth of peripheral fibres towards the HCs and evidence of synaptogenesis between these HCs and auditory neurons still warranted investigation. We aimed to assess the connection between peripheral fibres and HCs, however, it was not possible to quantify synaptogenesis in this study due to the low number of remaining HCs that were positive for ribbon synapses combined with the low number of fibres observed. Unlike previous studies, which have qualitatively shown ectopic HC innervation [22,23] and synaptic connections [8], there was no clear trend for the growth of peripheral fibres towards ectopic HCs nor towards HCs that where positive for CtBP2-positive puncta. Moreover, most fibres that were observed within close proximity of HCs appeared to travel laterally along the HCs, rather than form the synaptic boutons normally observed between auditory neuron afferent fibres and IHCs. In contrast, peripheral fibres in the Ad-NTs group did appear to respond to the gene therapy treatment. There were significantly more fibres within close proximity of the NT producing cell compared to GFP-only producing cells, indicating that NTs are able to influence the growth of peripheral fibres, similar to previous findings [15]. Interestingly, the combined treatment of ATOH1 and NTs did not result in an increase in HCs when compared to the four day deaf cohort, nor did this combined treatment appear to result in an increase in fibre resprouting. This effect is somewhat unexpected as the two vectors are unlikely to inhibit the effects on HC formation and fibre outgrowth observed when the vectors were injected alone. Therefore, the lack of HC regeneration and the lack of any apparent increase in fibre resprouting is likely to be due to the lower concentration of the individual viral titres, as when combined, the effective volume of each virus (Ad-ATOH1 and Ad-NTs) was halved.

## Conclusions

Collectively, the results presented in this study suggest that ATOH1-gene therapy may lead to an increase in HCs in the deaf cochlea in two ways; by promoting the survival and/or repair of the remaining HCs and by the direct transdifferentiation of supporting cells towards an immature HC phenotype. ATOH1 gene therapy alone, however, is unable to fully rescue the phenotype of surviving HCs. Nor is it able to cause the full conversion of non-sensory cells into mature HCs after severe aminoglycoside-induced deafness in the mature GP. The further examination of ATOH1 gene therapy should not be dismissed, as it still provides a powerful tool for the manipulation of non-sensory cells in the cochlea. When combined with other treatments such as manipulation of the Notch signalling pathway to decrease inhibitory signalling [25] or after forms of deafness that result in less severe damage to the OC, ATOH1 gene therapy may lead to functional improvement.

## Supporting Information

**Data S1 Data for supporting figures.** Hair cell counts: Number of hair cells in the inner sensory region of individual animals. This data was used to generate Figure 1. Hair cell expression: Number of GFP-positive cells co-expressing hair cell markers. This data was used to generate Figure 2. CtBP2 expression: Number of CtBP2 puncta per myosinVIIa-positive cell. This data was used to generate Figure 4. Peripheral fibres: Area of neurofilament-positive pixels within 10 mm of GFP-positive cells. This data was used to generate Figure 6. ABRs: Hearing thresholds of each animal pre-deafening, post-deafening and pre-perfusion. This data was used to generate Figure 7. SGN density: Density of spiral ganglion neurons in the basal, middle and apical turns of the cochleae of all animals. This data was used in the "Auditory Neuron Densities" section of the results.
(XLSX)

## Acknowledgments

The authors would like to acknowledge and thank Associate Professor Clifford Hume from the University of Washington, for the adenoviral vectors used in this paper.

## Author Contributions

Conceived and designed the experiments: PJA AKW BAN RTR. Performed the experiments: PJA AKW BOF RTR. Analyzed the data: PJA AKW RTR. Contributed to the writing of the manuscript: PJA AKW BAN RTR.

## References


1. Feghali JG, Lefebvre PP, Staecker H, Kopke R, Frenz DA, et al. (1998) Mammalian auditory hair cell regeneration/repair and protection: a review and future directions. Ear Nose Throat J. 77: 276, 280, 282–275.
2. Fu QJ, Nogaki G (2005) Noise susceptibility of cochlear implant users: the role of spectral resolution and smearing. J Assoc Res Otolaryngol 6: 19–27.
3. Kong YY, Cruz R, Jones JA, Zeng FG (2004) Music perception with temporal cues in acoustic and electric hearing. Ear Hear 25: 173–185.
4. Kelly MC, Chen P (2009) Development of form and function in the mammalian cochlea. Curr Opin Neurobiol 19: 395–401.
5. Bermingham NA, Hassan BA, Price SD, Vollrath MA, Ben-Arie N, et al. (1999) Math1: an essential gene for the generation of inner ear hair cells. Science 284: 1837–1841.
6. Chen P, Johnson JE, Zoghbi HY, Segil N (2002) The role of Math1 in inner ear development: Uncoupling the establishment of the sensory primordium from hair cell fate determination. Development 129: 2495–2505.
7. Woods C, Montcouquiol M, Kelley MW (2004) Math1 regulates development of the sensory epithelium in the mammalian cochlea. Nat Neurosci 7: 1310–1318.
8. Gubbels SP, Woessner DW, Mitchell JC, Ricci AJ, Brigande JV (2008) Functional auditory hair cells produced in the mammalian cochlea by in utero gene transfer. Nature 455: 537–541.
9. Yang J, Cong H, Han Z, Huang Y, Chi F (2013) Ectopic hair cell-like cell induction by Math1 mainly involves direct transdifferentiation in neonatal mammalian cochlea. Neurosci Lett. 549: 7–11
10. Izumikawa M, Minoda R, Kawamoto K, Abrashkin KA, Swiderski DL, et al. (2005) Auditory hair cell replacement and hearing improvement by Atoh1 gene therapy in deaf mammals. Nat Med 11: 271–276.
11. Izumikawa M, Batts SA, Miyazawa T, Swiderski DL, Raphael Y (2008) Response of the flat cochlear epithelium to forced expression of Atoh1. Hear Res 240: 52–56.
12. Kraft S, Hsu C, Brough DE, Staecker H (2013) Atoh1 induces auditory hair cell recovery in mice after ototoxic injury. Laryngoscope 123: 992–999.
13. Liu Z, Dearman JA, Cox BC, Walters BJ, Zhang L, et al. (2012) Age-dependent in vivo conversion of mouse cochlear pillar and Deiters' cells to immature hair cells by Atoh1 ectopic expression. J Neurosci 32: 6600–6610.
14. Wang Q, Green SH (2011) Functional role of neurotrophin-3 in synapse regeneration by spiral ganglion neurons on inner hair cells after excitotoxic trauma in vitro. J Neurosci 31: 7938–7949.
15. Wise AK, Hume CR, Flynn BO, Jeelall YS, Suhr CL, et al. (2010) Effects of localized neurotrophin gene expression on spiral ganglion neuron resprouting in the deafened cochlea. Mol Ther 18: 1111–1122.
16. James DP, Eastwood H, Richardson RT, O'Leary SJ (2008) Effects of Round Window Dexamethasone on Residual Hearing in a Guinea Pig Model of Cochlear Implantation. Audiol Neurootol 13: 86–96.
17. Richardson RT, Wise AK, Thompson BC, Flynn BO, Atkinson PJ, et al. (2009) Polypyrrole-coated electrodes for the delivery of charge and neurotrophins to cochlear neurons. Biomaterials 30: 2614–2624.
18. Atkinson PJ, Wise AK, Flynn BO, Nayagam BA, Hume CR, et al. (2012) Neurotrophin Gene Therapy for Sustained Neural Preservation after Deafness. PLoS One 7: e52338.
19. Wise AK, Richardson R, Hardman J, Clark G, O'Leary S (2005) Resprouting and survival of guinea pig cochlear neurons in response to the administration of the neurotrophins brain-derived neurotrophic factor and neurotrophin-3. J Comp Neurol 487: 147–165.
20. Yang SM, Chen W, Guo WW, Jia S, Sun JH, et al. (2012) Regeneration of stereocilia of hair cells by forced Atoh1 expression in the adult mammalian cochlea. PLoS One 7: e46355.
21. Kelly MC, Chang Q, Pan A, Lin X, Chen P (2012) Atoh1 directs the formation of sensory mosaics and induces cell proliferation in the postnatal mammalian cochlea in vivo. The Journal of neuroscience: the official journal of the Society for Neuroscience 32: 6699–6710.
22. Kawamoto K, Ishimoto S-I, Minoda R, Brough DE, Raphael Y (2003) Math1 Gene Transfer Generates New Cochlear Hair Cells in Mature Guinea Pigs In Vivo. J Neurosci 23: 4395–4400.
23. Yang J, Bouvron S, Lv P, Chi F, Yamoah EN (2012) Functional features of trans-differentiated hair cells mediated by Atoh1 reveals a primordial mechanism. J Neurosci 32: 3712–3725.
24. Lin HW, Furman AC, Kujawa SG, Liberman MC (2011) Primary neural degeneration in the Guinea pig cochlea after reversible noise-induced threshold shift. J Assoc Res Otolaryngol 12: 605–616.
25. Mizutari K, Fujioka M, Hosoya M, Bramhall N, Okano HJ, et al. (2013) Notch inhibition induces cochlear hair cell regeneration and recovery of hearing after acoustic trauma. Neuron 77: 58–69.

# 22

# Identifying MicroRNAs Involved in Aging of the Lateral Wall of the Cochlear Duct

**Qian Zhang, Huizhan Liu, Garrett A. Soukup*, David Z. Z. He***

Department of Biomedical Sciences, Creighton University School of Medicine, Omaha, Nebraska, United States of America

**Abstract**

Age-related hearing loss is a progressive sensorineural hearing loss that occurs during aging. Degeneration of the organ of Corti and atrophy of the lateral wall of the cochlear duct (or scala media) in the inner ear are the two primary causes. MicroRNAs (miRNAs), a class of short non-coding RNAs that regulate the expression of mRNA/protein targets, are important regulators of cellular senescence and aging. We examined miRNA gene expression profiles in the lateral wall of two mouse strains, along with exploration of the potential targets of those miRNAs that showed dynamic expression during aging. We show that 95 and 60 miRNAs exhibited differential expression in C57 and CBA mice during aging, respectively. A majority of downregulated miRNAs are known to regulate pathways of cell proliferation and differentiation, while all upregulated miRNAs are known regulators in the pro-apoptotic pathways. By using apoptosis-related gene array and bioinformatic approaches to predict miRNA targets, we identify candidate miRNA-regulated genes that regulate apoptosis pathways in the lateral wall of C57 and CBA mice during aging.

**Editor:** Manuel S. Malmierca, University of Salamanca- Institute for Neuroscience of Castille and Leon and Medical School, Spain

**Funding:** This work has been supported by NIH grant R01 DC004696 to DH. QZ has been supported by a graduate student scholarship from Creighton University School of Medicine. GS is supported by NIH grant R01 DC 009025 from the NIDCD. We acknowledge the use of the Integrated Biological Imaging Facility (supported by the Creighton University School of Medicine and C06 Grant RR17417-01 from the NCRR, NIH) and the University of Nebraska Microarray Facility (supported by P20 Grant RR 018788 from the NCRR, NIH). The funders had no role in study design, data collection and analysis, decision to publish, or preparation of the manuscript.

**Competing Interests:** The authors have declared that no competing interests exist.

* Email: GarrettSoukup@creighton.edu (GS); hed@creighton.edu (DH)

## Introduction

Age-related hearing loss (ARHL), also known as presbycusis, is a progressive sensorineural hearing loss. It has been reported that as many as 30 to 35% of the population aged between 65 and 75 have ARHL [1,2]. The prevalence and severity of hearing loss are much higher in populations older than 80 [3]. A recent study shows that more than 95% of centenarians suffer from severe to profound hearing loss [4]. Schuknecht classified the etiology of presbycusis into six distinct causes [5]. The two major causes are due to degeneration of the organ of Corti (OC) and the lateral wall (LW) of the scala media, which includes the stria vascularis (SV) and the spiral ligament [6,7]. The OC contains mechanosensitive hair cells that transduce mechanical vibration into electrical signal, while SV pumps potassium ions to the scala media and generates endocochlear potential (EP), which is essential for hair cell mechanotransduction. Stria-originated ARHL is usually characterized by reduction of EP and atrophy/degeneration of the LW.

MicroRNAs (miRNAs) are a class of post-transcriptional regulators. They are short ~22 nucleotide RNA sequences that bind to complementary sequences in the 3′ UTR of multiple target mRNAs, usually resulting in their silencing. miRNAs, collectively targeting ~60% of all genes, are abundantly present in all human cells and able to repress hundreds of target genes each [8,9,10,11]. miRNAs are required for the fine-tuning and tight regulation of a wide range of cellular processes and biological functions, including cell differentiation, proliferation, apoptosis, mobility, migration, metabolism, and self-renewal [12]. Recent studies have established a direct correlation between miRNA regulation and aging in worms (*Caenorhabditis elegans*), mice, and humans [13,14]. Several miRNAs have been implicated in the occurrence and progression of age-related diseases, such as Alzheimer's disease, type II diabetes, pulmonary heart disease, and cardiovascular diseases [15,16].

Since miRNA expression is cell/tissue-specific and time-dependent, which is consistent with the specific functions of different signaling pathways in different cells/tissues at different stages during development and aging [17], the analysis of miRNAs that are differentially expressed with aging has led to the discovery of numerous miRNAs that are important for controlling aging processes [13,18,19]. By comparing the expression profiles of miRNAs in the OC from younger and old mice, we identified approximately 100 miRNAs that exhibited differential expression, with downregulated miRNAs significantly outnumbering upregulated miRNAs [20]. The goal of the current study was to identify miRNAs that are differentially expressed in the LW during aging and to explore their potential apoptosis-related target genes. We first examined strial morphology and measured EP at different stages during aging from two mouse strains, C57BL/6J and CBA/J. We then used GeneChip microarray technology to identify differentially expressed miRNAs in the LW. Quantitative real-time

PCR (q-PCR) and *in situ* hybridization techniques were used to determine the temporal and spatial expression of several subsets of miRNAs identified by the microarray analysis. We subsequently used a quantitative PCR array to examine apoptosis-related gene expression in the LW. Finally, we used target prediction algorithms and bioinformatics tools to explore potential regulatory networks of apoptosis signaling pathways composed of miRNAs and mRNAs in the LW.

## Materials and Methods

### SV tissue collection and RNA extraction

C57BL/6J and CBA/J mice were bred in-house, with breeding pairs purchased from the Jackson Laboratory (Bar Harbor, ME, USA). Care and use of the animals in this study were approved by the Creighton University Institutional Animal Care and Use Committee.

Cochleae were rapidly dissected in cold phosphate-buffered saline (PBS) with 10 mM $Na_2HPO_4$, 1.7 mM $KH_2PO_4$, 137 mM NaCl, 2.7 mM KCl, and pH 7.4. The LW of scala media from all cochlear turns was isolated. Ten cochleae from five mice were pooled to generate each sample, and three independent samples were prepared for triplicate GeneChip miRNA array analyses. The animal ages for microarray analysis were postnatal 21 days (P21), 9 months (9 m) and 16 months (16 m) for both strains of mice. The isolated LW tissue was stored at −20°C in RNAlater stabilization reagent (Ambion, Austin, TX, USA). Total RNA including miRNAs was isolated using mirVana miRNA Isolation Kit (Ambion) and dissolved in 20–30 µl of RNase free water. RNA concentration was determined by UV spectrophotometry (Nanodrop ND-1000), and the quality of each RNA sample was verified by measuring the ratio of 28*S* to 18*S* rRNA using an Agilent 2100 BioAnalyzer. Additional samples of total RNA from the LW were prepared for quantitative PCR assays using the same procedure.

### Microarray analysis of miRNAs

The miRNA expression profile for each total RNA sample of the LW was determined using GeneChip miRNA 1.0 arrays (Affymetrix, Santa Clara, CA, USA). Synthesis of cDNA, hybridization to chips, and washes were performed according to the manufacturer's protocol. GeneChip arrays were scanned at 3-µm density using a GeneArray Scanner (Affymetrix). Images were inspected to ensure that all 18 chips had low background and bright hybridization signals. Mean signal fluorescence signal intensity for each probe was quantile normalized. Each miRNA probe was assessed for detection based on a Wilcoxon Rank-Sum test of the miRNA probe set signals compared to the distribution of signals from the background. One-way ANOVA test was used to determine significant differences in miRNA expression between P21 and older age groups, where $p<0.05$ was interpreted as significant. The raw data of the miRNA array has been submitted to the National Center for Biotechnology Information-Gene Expression Omnibus (GEO) (GEO submission number: GSE57782).

### Quantitative real-time PCR

For q-PCR analysis of miRNAs, the LW from five additional animals was obtained. Q-PCR detection of miRNAs was performed using mirVana q-PCR miRNA Primer sets (Ambion). 100 ng total RNA from each group was reverse transcribed using SuperScript Reverse Transcriptase (Invitrogen) in a 20 µl reaction to produce cDNA. q-PCR was performed using a 7500 Fast Real-Time PCR System (Applied Biosystems) to analyze triplicate reactions (20 µl) containing 2× SYBR Green PCR Master Mix (Applied Biosystems), a 10-fold dilution of mirVana q-PCR Primer Set, and cDNA. After incubation at 95°C for 20 s, PCR products were analyzed throughout 40 cycles consisting of incubation at 95°C for 3 s and 60°C for 30 s. U6 RNA was detected as an internal relative control for each group. The threshold cycle ($C_T$) was defined as the PCR cycle number at which the fluorescence intensity was appreciably above the background level but was still in the early exponential phase of amplification. The change in $C_T$ between a given miRNA and U6 RNA for each reaction was defined as $\Delta C_T$ and averaged for each group. The change in $\Delta C_T$ between two groups was defined as $\Delta\Delta C_T$, which represents the relative difference in expression of miRNA. Fold difference in miRNA expression between groups was calculated as $2^{-\Delta\Delta CT}$. We compared the $\Delta C_T$ values for each miRNA from older groups with those for the P21 group using the one-way ANOVA test, where $p<0.05$ was interpreted as significant.

### In Situ Hybridization

Control digoxigenis (DIG)-labeled beta-actin mRNA riboprobe (633 nt) was prepared by *in vitro* transcription from DNA templates using T7 RNA polymerase and DIG-UTP (Roche) and purified using RNAeasy spin columns (Qiagen). DNA templates for *in vitro* transcription of the beta-actin riboprobe were generated by PCR using primers 5′-TAATACGACTCAC-TATAGGG ACCGCTCGTTGCCAATAGTG and 5′-TGGTGGGAATGGGTCAGAAG and random-hexamer-primed mouse cDNAs.

Cross-section preparations were used for *in situ* hybridization as previously described [21,22,23]. Anesthetized mice were transcardially perfused with PBS followed by PBS containing 4% PFA. Inner ears were dissected, fixed in PBS containing freshly dissolved 4% paraformaldehyde (PFA), and decalcified with 0.5M EDTA for 24–48 h. The cochleae were cryoprotected and embedded in cutting temperature compound (O.C.T. Tissue-Tek, Sakura Finetek, Torrance, CA) for frozen sectioning. After incubated in PBS with diluted Proteinase K (Sigma catalog # P4850) and defatted through a graded ethanol series and rehydrated in PBS containing 0.1% TWEEN 20, the serial cross-sections (6 µm) were pre-hybridized in 2 mL hybridization solution (50% formamide, 2× SSC, 0.1% Tween 20, and 150 µg/ml denatured herring sperm DNA) for 1–3 h at 53°C. Hybridizations were incubated overnight at 53°C following the addition of 12 pmol DIG-labeled LNA probe or 1 pmol DIG-labeled beta-actin mRNA riboprobe denatured for 10 min at 68°C in hybridization buffer. Tissues were washed at 50°C in 0.5× SSC, and RNA was digested by incubation for 1 h at 37°C with RNase A (100 mM Tris–HCl pH 7.5, 500 mM NaCl, 0.1% TWEEN 20, and 10 µg/ml RNase A). After the digestions were terminated, tissues were incubated in wash and block for 1 h at 4°C and incubated overnight in a 1000-fold dilution of sheep anti-DIG-AP Fab fragment (Roche Diagnostics Corporation, Indianapolis, IN) in block buffer. Samples were washed at 4°C with wash buffer, and alkaline phosphatase activity was detected using BM Purple AP Substrate (Roche) by incubation for 2–16 h at 25°C. Reactions were terminated for at least 1 h in PBS (pH 5.5) containing 10 mM EDTA. Tissues were fixed by incubation overnight at 4°C in PBS containing 4% PFA. Fixed tissues were mounted in glycerol under glass cover slips for image acquisition as described previously [24]. Localization of BM purple was visualized by differential interference contrast optics.

### q-PCR Array of Apoptosis-Related Genes

Total RNA isolated from LW of each type of mouse at two ages was used to examine apoptosis-related gene expression by reverse transcription and RT-PCR using an RT2 Profiler q-RT-PCR Array (SABiosciences, Frederick, MD, USA). The 84 apoptosis-related genes contained in the array are listed in Table S1. Details of the procedures were provided in a previous study [25]. Upon completion of total RNA extraction from the LW and quality assessment, first strand cDNA was synthesized using oligodT-primed reverse transcription supplied with the RT2 first strand kit (SABiosciences). This kit contains genomic DNA elimination buffer and a built-in external RNA control. Total RNA used for cDNA synthesis was 500 ng for each sample. Expression of 84 apoptosis-related genes was evaluated in the LW tissue at the ages of P21 and 16 month in a 96-well plate (including five housekeeping and seven control genes; Mouse Apoptosis RT2 Profiler PCR Array, SABiosciences, PAMM-012C). $RT^2$Real-TimeTM SYBR Green/fluorescein PCR Master Mix was used to monitor the fluorescence signal during each cycle of PCR using a 7500 Fast Real-Time PCR Detection System (Applied Biosystems). Each reaction started with an initial denaturation cycle at 95°C for 10 min, followed by 40 cycles consisting of 15 s at 95°C, and 1 min at 60°C for annealing. Each sample was repeated three times. Upon completion of the PCR, threshold cycle ($C_T$) values were calculated automatically. The $C_T$ value of each apoptosis-related gene was normalized by the average $C_T$ value of five housekeeping genes to determine $\Delta C_T$. The change in $\Delta C_T$ for each gene between groups ($\Delta\Delta C_T$) represents the relative difference in expression, and fold difference was calculated as $2^{-\Delta\Delta Ct}$. One-way ANOVA test was used to compare $\Delta C_T$ values for each gene from older groups with those for the P21 group, where $p<0.05$ was interpreted as significant.

### miRNA Target Prediction of Apoptosis Related Genes

The potential mRNA targets of differentially expressed miRNAs were predicted by the TargetScan mouse version 6.2 (http://www.targetscan.org/mmu_61/). Analyses were based on expression profiles from GeneChip microarray and apoptosis q-PCR array. Both conserved and non-conserved targets for conserved miRNA families were considered. TargetScan predictions were used to construct a bipartite network graph in which miRNAs were connected to their predicted targets.

### Recording of EP

Animal were anesthetized with a combined regimen of ketamine (16.6 mg/ml) and xylazine (2.3 mg/ml) and supplemented as needed to maintain a surgical level of anesthesia. An incision was then made in the inferior portion of the right postauricular sulcus. The bulla was perforated allowing for exposure of the stapedial artery, basal turn, and upper turn of the cochlea. A basal turn location was chosen to record EP. This location was approximately 2 mm from the basal end, corresponding to the region with best frequency of 20–30 kHz, based on the cochlear frequency map for the mouse [26]. A hole was made using a fine drill. A glass capillary pipette electrode (10–20 MΩ) filled with 150 mM KCl was mounted on a hydraulic micromanipulator and advanced until a stable positive potential was observed. The ground electrode was implanted in the dorsal neck muscles. The biological signals (filtered at 1 kHz) were amplified under current-clamp mode using an Axopatch 200B amplifier (Molecular Devices, Sunnyvale, CA, USA) and acquired by software pClamp 9.2 (Molecular Devices) running on an IBM-compatible computer with a 16-bit A/D converter (Digidata 1322B, Molecular Devices). The voltage changes during a penetration were continuously recorded under the Gap-free model using the Clampex in the pClamp software package. The sampling frequency was 10 kHz. Data were analyzed using Clampfit and Igor Pro (WaveMetrics, Portland, OR, USA).

### Morphology of LW

Cochleae were isolated at the age of P21, 9 m, and 16 m and fixed in 4% paraformaldehyde in PBS at 4°C overnight and decalcified with 0.5 M EDTA for 2 days. The cochleae were embedded in celloidin. Serial cross sections (8–10 μm) were prepared with a microtome (CM3050, Leica, Nussloch, Germany) and collected on microslides. The sections were stained with Hematoxylin and Eosin and then washed. The slides were mounted with regular mounting solution (glycerol) and examined under a microscope. Images at 10× and 25× magnification were taken from middle turns. The area of the spiral ligament and the SV was determined using ImageJ (version 1.47) from captured images.

## Results

### 1. Changes of EP magnitude during aging

The CBA and C57 mice are commonly used for the study of ARHL [27,28]. Hearing threshold and EP are often measured to assess the functional status of the OC and the LW of the scala media. Both hearing threshold and EP of the two strains have been examined before [29,30,31]. We and others have shown that C57 mice display an onset and rapid progression of hearing loss starting from high frequencies as early as 3 m, and by 16 m profound hearing loss greater than 100 dB is observed across the frequency range tested [20]. In contrast, CBA mice exhibit minimal hearing loss (less than 20 dB) between P21 and 16 m. To determine the functional status of the LW during aging and to provide guidance for tissue collection for molecular biology studies, we measured basal turn EP at P21 and 3 m, 6 m, 9 m, 12 m, and 16 m. Seven animals (seven ears) from each age/strain were used. Fig. 1A shows some representative responses from such recordings. The EP response was a constant polarization with a magnitude of 80–100 mV when the electrode penetrated the endolymphatic spaces. The mean value of EP at different ages was determined and is presented in Fig. 1B. The EP magnitude of CBA mice did not display any significant change between P21 and 16 m ($p>0.05$ in all cases). In contrast, the EP magnitude of C57 mice exhibited a significant elevation at 3 m ($p<0.05$ between P21 and 3 m) and remained elevated between 3 m and 16 m. Thus, while the hearing thresholds of C57 mice began to deteriorate at high frequency from 3 m, the EP magnitude showed a paradoxical increase from 3 m. The elevation at 3 m and beyond is the result of progressive hair cell loss beginning at 3 m [20].

### 2. Morphological changes of the LW during aging

We examined morphological changes of the LW during aging. Decrease in thickness of the SV and spiral ligament is often regarded as a sign of atrophy. As shown in Fig. 2, there are no apparent decrease in the thickness of the SV and the spiral ligament in C57 and CBA mice between P21 to 16 m. However, hyperpigmentation (Fig. 2B) and reduction in the number of capillaries (Fig. 2A) were observed in the SV at 16 m.

### 3. Differential expression of miRNAs in the LW during aging

Total RNA isolated from LW of C57 and CBA mice was analyzed by miRNA microarray analysis that included 7,788 miRNA gene probe sets covering a variety of species. Our analyses were performed on all included mouse miRNAs (mmu-miRNAs). There were 609 probe sets for mmu-miRNAs. For comparison,

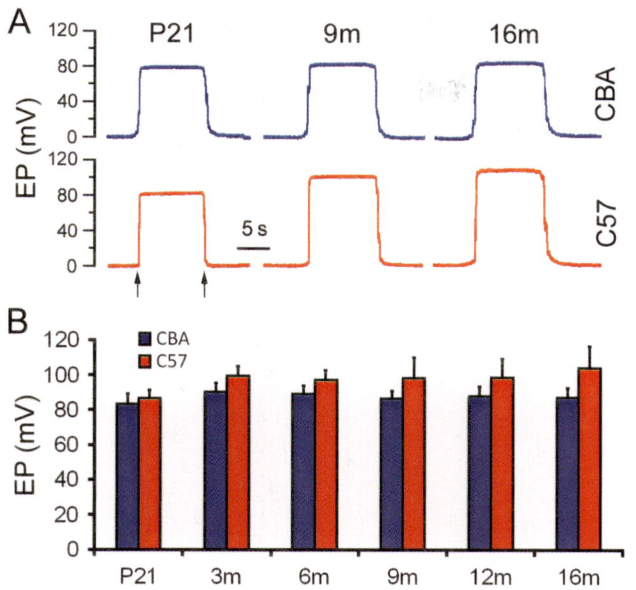


**Figure 1. EP waveforms and magnitude change during aging.** A. Representative waveforms of EP at three different ages. B. Mean and SD of EP magnitude at different time points during aging. Arrows indicate electrode penetrated into and withdrawn from the scala media.

the present study used the same criteria as those in our prior study of differentially expressed miRNAs in the OC [20]. The two criteria were: 1) the miRNA had to be "expressed" in each of the three repeats for each age group, and 2) the expression level of the miRNAs had to be significantly different from that of the youngest group ($p<0.05$, Student's t-test). miRNAs that met the two criteria are presented in Figs. 3 and 4.

We examined miRNA differential expression between P21 and 9 m as well as between P21 and 16 m in both strains. The rationale for selecting these time points is provided in our previous publication [20]. Selection of the same time points for collecting the OC and LW tissues made it possible to compare miRNA profiles between the two important structures in the inner ear. Fig. 3 depicts differential expression profiling of miRNAs from CBA mice between P21 and 9 m (in blue) as well as between P21 and 16 m (in red). A total of 60 miRNAs were identified as significantly differentially expressed during aging. Fifty miRNAs (83%) exhibited changes in the same direction (upregulation or downregulation) at the two different ages. Among the 50 miRNAs, downregulated miRNAs outnumbered upregulated miRNAs by a ratio of 3.5:1 (39/11). Eleven miRNAs had their expression level downregulated by more than 50%, whereas 9 miRNAs were upregulated by more than twofold.

Fig. 4 presents differential expression profiles of miRNAs from C57 mice between P21 and 9 m (in blue) as well as between P21 and 16 m (in red). A total of 95 miRNAs were identified as significantly differentially expressed. Sixty-nine miRNAs (73%) showed changes in the same direction (upregulation or downregulation) at the two different ages. Among the 69 miRNAs, 33 were downregulated while 36 were upregulated, with a downregulation versus upregulation ratio of 0.9:1. Thirty-four miRNAs had their expression level upregulated by more than twofold, whereas 7 miRNAs were downregulated by more than 50%. Comparison of miRNA expression profiles between C57 and CBA mice showed that the number of miRNAs indicated in aging of the LW of C57 mice is substantially greater than that of CBA mice during aging.

The early onset and rapid progression of hearing loss seen in C57 mice are due to *Ahl* gene mutation. As a result, the miRNA profiles for LW of C57 mice were expectedly different from those of CBA mice. However, C57 and CBA strains should share some common miRNAs associated with apoptosis and degeneration of LW. Fig. 5 depicts 21 common miRNAs that were differentially expressed during aging in both strains. Among the list, members of the miR-29 family, miR-203, miR-762, and miR-1224, showed upregulation, whereas members of the miR-107 family, miR-127 and miR-130a/b, miR-342-3p, miR-351, miR-379, miR-455, and miR-467a, were downregulated in both strains.

## 4. Temporal and spatial expression of four subsets of miRNAs in the LW

Q-PCR was used to validate some of the differentially expressed miRNAs indicated by the high-throughput microarray techniques. Two upregulated (miR-29a and miR-203) and two downregulated (miR-342 and miR-455) miRNAs shown in the microarray analyses were selected for q-PCR analysis. These miRNAs were selected since these four miRNAs are known to be involved in the

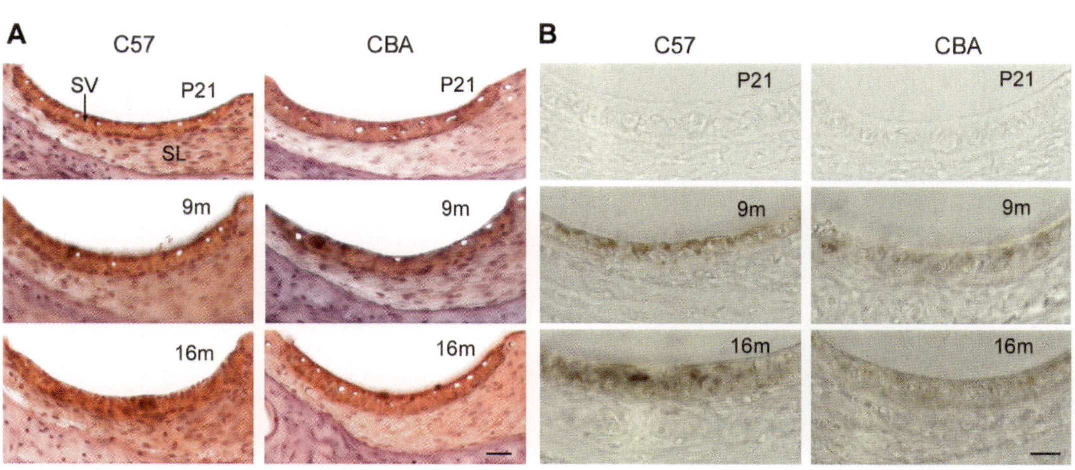


**Figure 2. Cross sections of the LW at three different times points during age.** Sections were obtained from cochlear middle turns at P21, 9 m, and 16 m. A. Cross sections stained with Hematoxylin and Eosin. Scale bars: 20 μm. B. Cross sections without any staining. Hyperpigmentation and reduction in the number of capillaries are apparent in the SV at 16 m.

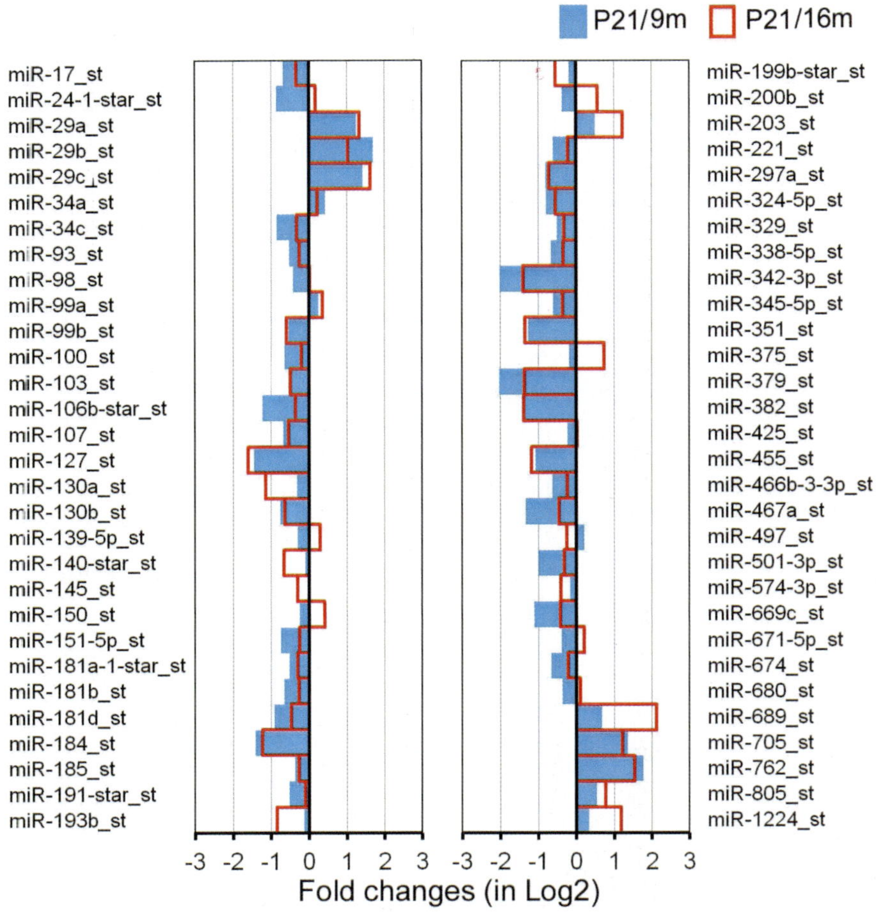


**Figure 3. Differentially expressed miRNAs in the LW of CBA mice during aging.** The X-axis relates Log2 transformed fold change in miRNA expression at 9 m (in blue) and 16 m (in red) compared to P21. Only those miRNAs whose levels were statistically different ($p<0.05$) from P21 were included.

pro-apoptotic and anti-apoptotic processes in other cells and diseases. miR-29a is also differentially expressed in the OC during aging in both strains of mice [20]. The fold change was determined from $\Delta\Delta C_T$ using the U6 as the internal control. Fig. 6A exhibits the dynamic changes of these miRNAs during aging by q-PCR assay. For comparison, changes in these four miRNAs from microarray analyses are also included. As shown, the expression levels of miR-342 and miR-455 in SV were significantly downregulated, while miR-29a and miR-203 were upregulated when compared to those of the P21 mice. The changes in miRNA expression determined by q-PCR were consistent with trends observed by microarray analyses.

We also examined the spatial expression of approximately 20 miRNAs in the LW of 3 m C75 mice using *in situ* hybridization. Four miRNAs showed strong expression in the SV (Fig. 6B). miR-107 and miR-200a were found in all three cell types in the SV. miR-203 was expressed in all cell types with weak expression in the marginal cells, while miR-145 was expressed in all cell types in the SV with strongest expression in the marginal cells.

## 5. Apoptosis-related gene expression in the LW

To elucidate the possible functional relevance of age-affected miRNAs, we next examined expression of genes that are associated with apoptosis and that were differentially expressed during aging. To determine which apoptosis-related genes are dynamically expressed in the LW during aging, a PCR-based apoptosis-related gene array (Table S1) was utilized. The array included 84 apoptosis-related genes in known extrinsic and intrinsic apoptotic pathways. Five stable housekeeping genes (Gusb, Hprt, Hsp90ab1, Gapdh, and Actb) were used as controls. We compared the expression levels of apoptosis-related genes in P21- and 9m-old C57 mice and in P21- and 16m-old CBA mice. Table 1 presents differentially expressed apoptosis-related genes in the LW with the fold change and p-value included in parenthesis. Atf5, Bid, Naip1, Birc2, Casp14, Dapk1, Mcl1, Nol3, Tnf, Cd40, Tnfsf10, and Zc3hc1 were significantly upregulated, while Xiap, Birc5, Bok, and Casp3 were significantly downregulated in C57 mice. Most anti-apoptotic genes, such as Xiap and Birc5, were downregulated, while pro-apoptotic genes, such as Bid, Tnf and Tnfsf10, were upregulated in C57 mice. It is also apparent that more apoptosis-related genes were expressed in C57 mice than in CBA mice, despite the fact gene expression in C57 mice was assessed at 9 m (as opposed to 16 m for CBA mice).

## 6. miRNAs and their target apoptosis-related mRNAs in the LW

In order to assess whether differential miRNA expression with age has an impact on putative target gene expression, we next examined the relationship between differentially expressed miRNAs and mRNAs. It is generally accepted that perfect miRNA

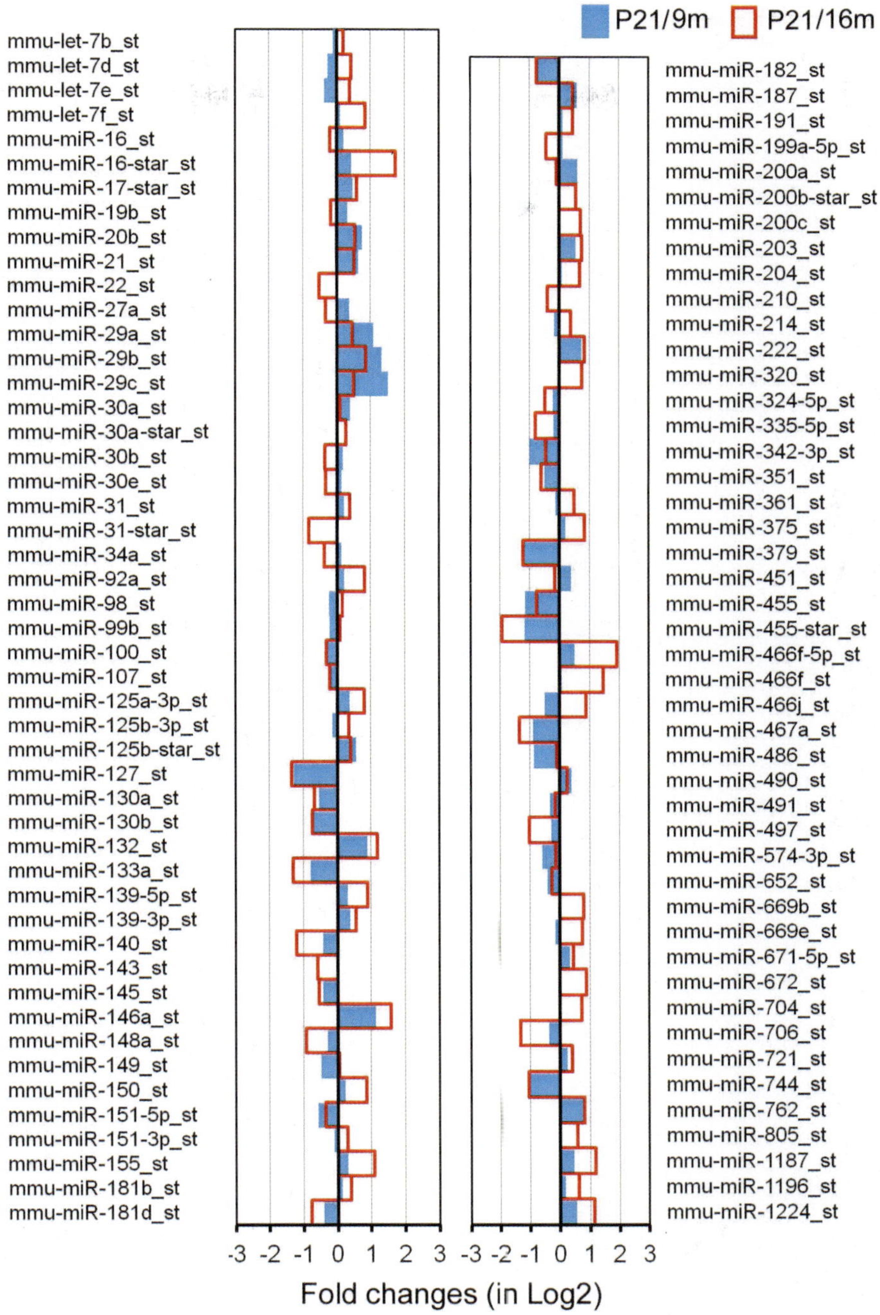


**Figure 4. Differentially expressed miRNAs in the SV of C57 mice during aging.** The X-axis relates Log2 transformed fold change in miRNA expression at 9 m (in blue) and 16 m (in red) compared to P21. Only those miRNAs which showed a statistically significant different in expression ($p < 0.05$) compared to P21 are shown.

seed region/target complementarity is predominantly associated with the destabilization of target mRNAs [32]. Accordingly, the level of a miRNA should be inversely correlated to the levels of its target gene transcripts. Differentially expressed miRNAs and their predicted target mRNAs were analyzed using TargetScan 6.2.

Our analyses identified 8 upregulated mRNAs (Atf5, Bid, Birc2, Casp14, Tnfsf10, Zc3hcl, Cd40, and Niap1) and 4 downregulated mRNAs (Birc5, Bok, Casp3, and Xiap) that contained binding sites for differentially expressed miRNAs identified in the LW of C57 mice. Fig. 7 presents the networks of potential interaction between the miRNAs and mRNAs. The coincident relationships that pro-apoptotic miRNAs regulate anti-apoptotic genes, and anti-apoptotic miRNAs regulate pro-apoptotic genes, are exhibited in the networks. For example, Tnfsf10, a critical pro-apoptotic gene whose expression was upregulated by 1.9-fold in the LW of C57 mice, is predicted to be regulated by two anti-apoptotic miRNAs, miR-145 and miR-107, which were downregulated at 9 m. Also, Birc5, an anti-apoptotic gene downregulated in both

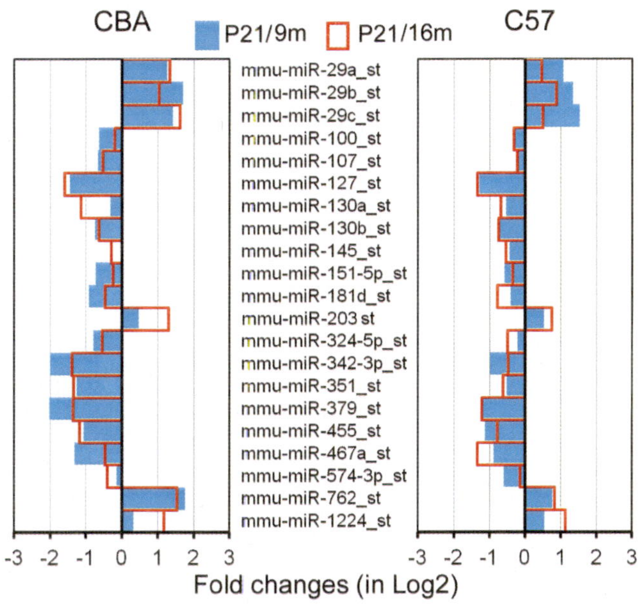


**Figure 5. miRNAs that are commonly expressed in the LW of C57 and CBA mice during aging.** Only those miRNAs that showed dynamic changes in the same direction (upregulated or downregulated) in both strains are included.

strains during aging, is predicted to be regulated by miR-200a, a known pro-apoptotic miRNA that was upregulated at 9 m in the LW of C57 mice.

## Discussion

This is the first study that examines the extent and specificity of miRNA expression in the LW of scala media during aging in two strains of mice. We detected 95 and 60 miRNAs that exhibited significant differential expression in the LW of C57 and CBA mice, respectively, with aging. Many of those differentially expressed miRNAs are predicted to target pathways and processes relevant to aging. Most miRNAs that were significantly upregulated are pro-apoptotic, while most of those downregulated are anti-apoptotic or pro-proliferative. Although the precise function of these individual miRNAs in regulating cellular senescence and aging in the LW is yet to be determined, it is conceivable that the underlying process and regulatory mechanism might involve a gradual and collective action of repression of miRNAs important for proliferation and differentiation, and concomitant enhancement of miRNAs that promote apoptosis during aging. Such changes of miRNA expression precede morphological and functional changes that can be detected.

In our previous study, we identified 111 and 71 miRNAs that exhibit differential expression in the OC of C57 and CBA mice, respectively [20]. Comparison of miRNA expression profiles in the OC and LW shows that several miRNAs are expressed in both tissues. These miRNAs include miR-29a/b, miR-100, miR-107, miR-130b, miR-193b, miR-343-3p, miR-351, and miR-455. miRNAs that were differentially expressed only in the LW during aging include miR-29c, miR-705, miR-99a, miR-127, miR-130a, miR-145, miR-151-5p, miR-379, miR-467a, and miR-574-3p. While miR-29c and miR-705 were upregulated, the rest were downregulated. Members of the miR-29 family (miR-29a/b/c) were significantly upregulated in the LW of both strains (Fig. 5). More than a two-fold increase of miR-29a/b was reported in the OC during onset and progression of ARHL [20]. This family is involved in cellular senescence and apoptosis in several cell lines, tissues, and organisms during aging [33–36]. miR-203, a transcriptional target of p53/TA-p73/p63 [37], is an anti-proliferative/pro-apoptotic miRNA involved in regulation of proliferation, differentiation, and apoptosis in several cell types (including epithelia and melanocyte) through p16/Rb and p53 pathways [38,39]. It also targets E2F3 and ZBP-89, inducing cell cycle arrest by inhibiting p16 expression [40]. In melanocytes, miR-203 acts as a tumor suppressor by inducing senescence, and ABL1 is the target of miR-203, suggesting an anti-proliferative function of this miRNA [41]. miR-203 exhibited significant upregulation in the LW of both strains, and its expression was confirmed by both q-PCR and *in situ* hybridization (Figs. 6A, B). Since miR-203 is an anti-proliferative/pro-apoptotic miRNA and was upregulated, it is likely this miRNA is involved in degeneration of the SV.

It is interesting to observe the enhanced expression of miR-762 and miR-1224 in the LW. Although little is known about the role of these two miRNAs, two recent studies show that these two miRNAs are upregulated during infection and inflammatory responses. miR-762 has been found ubiquitously distributed in murine ocular tissues [42] and negatively regulates the expression of genes encoding the antimicrobial RNase7, the immunomodulator ST2, and the RhoGTP-binding protein Rab5a [43]. miR-1224 is highly expressed in mouse spleen, kidney, and lung [44]. Transfection of miR-1224 results in a decrease in basal tumour necrosis factor-$\alpha$ (TNF-$\alpha$) promoter reporter gene activity and a downregulation of LPS-induced TNF-$\alpha$ mRNA in RAW264.7 cells [44]. If these two miRNAs are involved in inflammatory responses, it suggests that inflammation of the SV might be a component of degeneration in the SV during aging.

A number of miRNAs were downregulated in the LW during aging. These miRNAs include miR-107, miR-127, miR-130a/b, miR-145, miR-342, miR-351, miR-379, miR-455, and miR-467. These miRNAs have been detected in other tissues. Although a miRNA can have different roles and even opposite functions in different tissues, these miRNAs are, in general, pro-proliferative or anti-apoptotic. miR-127 is part of the miRNA signature that is upregulated in acute myeloid leukaemia [45] and in nodal diffuse large B-cell lymphomas [46]. miRNA-130a is oncogenic, contributing to colon tumorigenesis by regulating TGF-$\beta$/Smad signaling [47]. miR-351 is detected during myogenic progenitor cell differentiation and inhibits E2f3 expression, a key regulator of cell cycle progression and proliferation [48]. miR-379 is expressed in breast cancer, regulating interleukin-11 and Cyclin B1 [49]. The expression of miRNA-455 is detected in adrenal, ovarian granulosa, and model Leydig cell lines, and its expression is downregulated by trophic hormones or their second messenger, cyclic AMP [50]. miRNA-455 is also important for chondrogenesis [51]. miR-467a, an abundant member of the Sfmbt2 cluster, can promote cell proliferation. Finally, miR-467a can promote growth and survival of mouse ES cells [52].

Four miRNAs among the downregulated miRNAs in the LW deserve some discussion, since they may be related to function and maintenance of intermediate cells (melanocytes) in the SV. Intermediate cells play an important role for maintenance of endolymph and generation of EP. Mutations in melanocytes result in loss of EP and hair cells [53–55]. The four downregulated miRNAs are miR-107, miR-145, miR-342, and miR-455. miR-107, together with miR-15a/b, miR-16, miR-103, miR-195, miR-424, miR-497, miR-503, and miR-646, belongs to the miR-15-107 group. This cluster of miRNAs regulates gene expression involved in cell division, metabolism, and stress response [56,57]. This

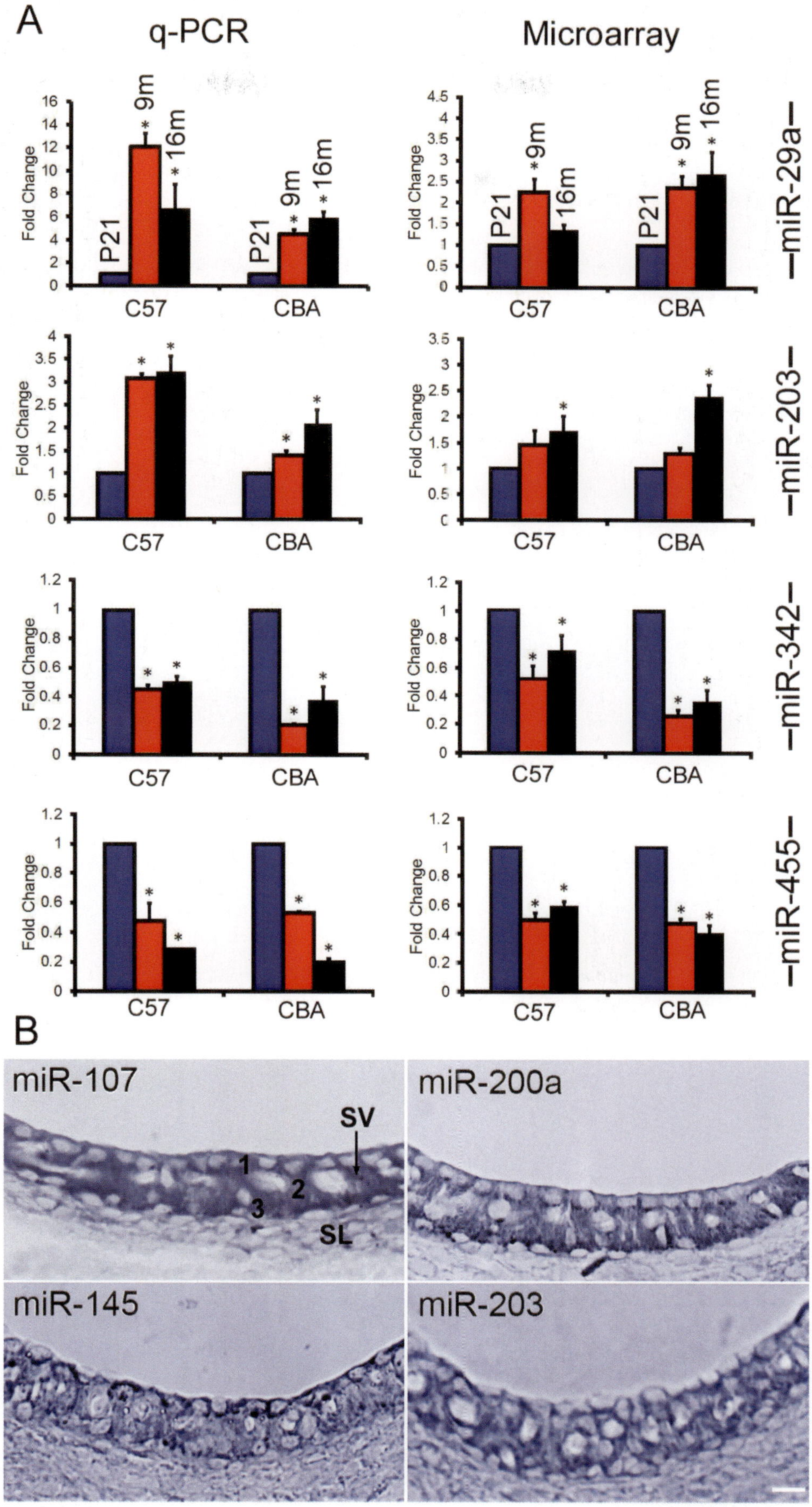
A
q-PCR
Microarray
miR-29a
miR-203
miR-342
miR-455
Fold Change
P21
9m
16m
C57
CBA
B
miR-107
miR-200a
miR-145
miR-203
SV
SL
1
2
3

**Figure 6. miRNA expression detected by q-PCR and *in situ* hybridization.** A: Comparison of changes in miRNA expression detected by q-PCR versus microarray analyses for four miRNAs in the SV of C57 and CBA mice. Asterisks indicate statistically significant differences ($p<0.05$) compared to P21. Each q-PCR plot represents means from three repeats. B: Expression of four miRNAs in the LW of C57 mice using *in situ* hybridization technique. SV: Stria vascularis. SL: Spiral ligament. 1, 2, and 3 mark the three cell types in the SV (marginal, intermediate, and basal cells), respectively. Bar: 20 μm.

group has been implicated in some age-related diseases, such as cardiovascular disease and neurodegenerative disease including Alzheimer's [58,59]. miR-107 is expressed abundantly in brain tissue [60]. Our *in situ* hybridization showed miR-107 was expressed in the SV (Fig. 6B). Intermediate cells in the SV are derived from neural crest cells. Downregulation of miR-107 during aging in the SV is coincident with its anti-apoptotic function, suggesting that decline of its regulatory pathways might contribute to stria degeneration.

miR-145 was also detected in the SV by *in situ* hybridization (Fig. 6B). Previous studies demonstrated miR-145 is abundantly expressed in the smooth muscle tissues and critical for vascular smooth muscle cell differentiation [61,62]. miR-145 expression is also found in the vascular wall of the capillaries in the SV [63,64] and in the intermediate cells. Dynoodt et al. [65,66] demonstrated that miR-145 is a key regulator in melanogenesis. The expression of miR-145 in melanocytes exhibits a negative relationship with the expression of Sox9, Mitf, Tyr, Trp1, Myo5a, Rab27a, and Fscn1. Downregulation of this miRNA during aging is consistent with its role in regulating vascular smooth muscle and melanocytes in the SV.

One of the putative targets of miR-455 is PAX6, which has been shown to play a critical role in the self-renewal and differentiation of neural stem cells. miR-455 is also detected in primary melanoma cell lines and metastatic melanomas [51,67–69]. It is speculated that the loss of miR-455 and its subsequent effect on PAX6 expression may disrupt the normal progression of melanogenesis. Reduced expression of miR-455 was evident in our microarray analysis and q-PCR validation, and it might reflect a reduction of intermediate cells in the SV during aging. Similarly, miR-342 was also downregulated and has been shown to regulate melanogenesis [70].

Apoptosis-related q-PCR arrays are often used to analyze gene expression related to known apoptosis pathways. In the auditory system, such analyses have been used to examine gene expression after ototoxic drug treatment or after noise exposure [25,71]. We combined apoptosis-related q-PCR array results with miRNA microarray analyses and bioinformatics approaches to explore potential miRNA-mRNA networks in the LW during aging. While the relationship between some of these miRNAs and mRNAs have been shown before in other tissues and cell lines, this is the first time that their relationship (Fig. 7) has been examined in the LW during aging.

Notably, our data revealed that expression of Tnfsf10 (upregulated by ~2-fold) is likely influenced by several miRNAs including miR-107, miR-145, miR-342-3p, miR-491, miR-494, miR-182, and miR-467a. miR-107 and miR-145 were found to be expressed in the SV and downregulated during aging in both strains. Tnfsf10 is a pro-apoptotic cytokine that belongs to the tumor necrosis factor ligand family. It predominantly induces apoptosis in transformed and tumor cells [72,73]. Tnfsf10 binds to several members of the TNF receptor superfamily and triggers the activation of MAPK8/JNK, caspase-8, and caspase-3. Tnfsf10 is upregulated in cochlear spiral ganglion cells in the early stage of salicylate-induced degeneration [25]. This suggests that TNF receptor families play an important role in cochlear degeneration by eliciting caspase-mediated cell death. Tnfsf10 is predicted to be directly targeted by miR-107 and miR-145, which were found to be expressed in the SV and downregulated during aging in both strains. miR-145 additionally targets the insulin receptor substrate-1 (IRS1), a factor in the insulin/insulin-like growth factor-1 (IGF-1) signaling pathway, the first established aging pathway [74].

Some other apoptosis-related genes identified in our study have been linked to degeneration and cell death in the inner ear. For example, BH3 interacting domain death agonist, or Bid, a

**Table 1.** Differential expression of apoptosis-related genes in the LW of C57 and CBA mice.

| Strain | Upregulated (Fold change, P value) | Downregulated (Fold change, P value) |
|---|---|---|
| C57BL/6 J: 9 m/P21 | *Atf5 (3.053, 0.013)* | *Xiap (0.675, 0.034)* |
| | **Bid (3.239, 0.012)** | *Birc5 (0.305, 0.042)* |
| | *Naip1 (4.968, 0.015)* | **Bok (0.302, 0.033)** |
| | *BirC2 (2.281, 0.027)* | **Casp3 (0.593, 0.015)** |
| | **Casp14 (8.589, 0.004)** | |
| | *Dapk1 (3.697, 0.001)* | |
| | *Mcl1 (1.634, 0.0238)* | |
| | *Nol3 (5.795, 0.019)* | |
| | **Tnf (3.047, 0.025)** | |
| | **Cd40 (2.121, 0.008)** | |
| | **Tnfsf10 (1.886, 0.002)** | |
| | *Zc3hcl (2.440, 0.045)* | |
| CBA/J: 16 m/P21 | *Dapk1 (4.385, 0.001)* | *Birc5 (0.103, 0.049)* |
| | | **Casp3 (0.449, 0.034)** |

Bold and Italics fonts represent pro-apoptotic and anti-apoptotic genes, respectively.

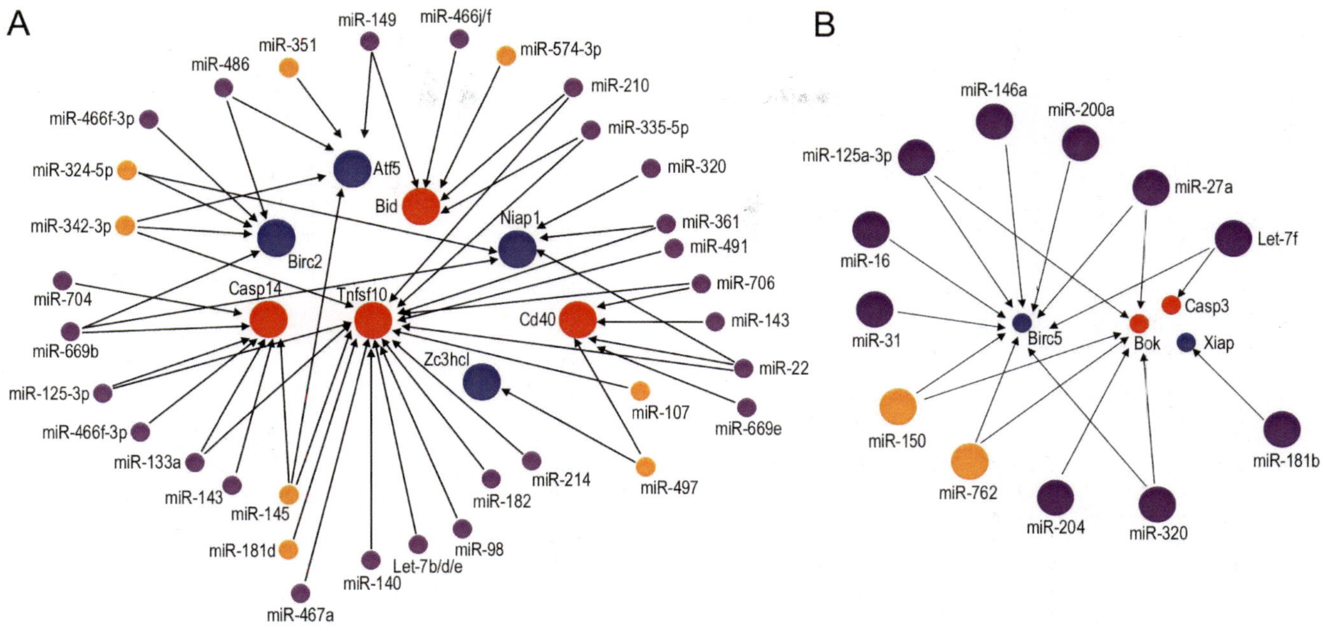


**Figure 7. Network analysis of the relationship between differentially expressed miRNAs and mRNAs in the LW.** A: Upregulated apoptosis-related genes predicted to be targeted by downregulated miRNAs. B: Downregulated apoptosis-related genes predicted to be targeted by upregulated miRNAs. Small circles represent downregulated miRNAs or mRNAs while large circles represent upregulated miRNAs or mRNAs. Purple and orange circles denote differentially expressed miRNAs in C57 and CBA mice, respectively. Red and blue circles represent pro-apoptotic and anti-apoptotic genes, respectively.

member of the Bcl-2 family of cell death regulators and a mediator of mitochondrial pathway induced caspase-8, is a predicted target of miR-574-3p and miR-494. Bid is activated following enhanced caspase-8 activity in cisplatin-induced apoptosis of auditory cells *in vitro* through both the death receptor mechanisms and mitochondrial pathways of apoptosis [75]. Co-expression of Bid and its predicted miRNA regulators in both OC (our unpublished observation) and LW during aging indicates that regulation of Bid and its related signaling pathways are crucial during cochlear ARHL. Another example is Birc5, a member of the inhibitor of apoptosis gene family that encodes negative regulatory proteins that prevent apoptotic cell death. Birc5 was significantly downregulated during aging. Previous studies demonstrated an otoprotective role of Birc5 against ototoxic and noise insults [76,77]. Birc5 is predicted to be regulated by miR-27b, miR-125b-3p, miR-150, miR-200a, miR-146a, miR-709, miR-705, and miR-762.

A number of issues deserve some discussion. First, the selection of the two mouse strains for the current study. We are fully aware that neither mouse strain shows a stria-originated ARHL. We used CBA mice as a model to identify miRNAs involved in physiological aging. C57 mice have an early onset and rapid progression of hearing loss due to *Ahl* gene mutation. This strain is not an ideal model to study molecular mechanism of aging in the LW. However, since C57 has a progressive hair cell loss during aging, it would be interesting to determine how degeneration of the OC would affect strial function and miRNA expression profile in this strain. Furthermore, we examined miRNA expression profiles of the OC during aging in CBA and C57 mice. Comparison of miRNA expression profiles between the OC and the LW during aging in the same strain and between the two strains would allow us to identify common pathways involved in the degeneration of the OC and LW during aging. Second, we observed an increase in EP magnitude in C57 mice during aging, which has never been reported before. Most studies that have examined EP magnitude change during aging often started at later stage (i.e., after 3 m) and therefore did not observe the change. Progressive hair cell loss is most likely responsible for the elevation in EP magnitude, although a delay in stria development could not be ruled out either. Hair cells have a standing (leak) current through mechanotransduction channels at rest [78] which reduces the voltage difference between scala media and scala tympani. Early hair cell loss diminishes the leak current and increases the resistance between the scala media and scala tympani, resulting the increase in EP. Third, we observed no significant reduction in EP magnitude during aging although some minor morphological changes were observed in the LW of C57 mice. However, significant change in miRNA expression was already detected. The fact that differential expression of miRNAs occurred well before morphological and functional changes in both strains of mice supports our previous conclusion that changes in miRNA expression precede morphological and functional changes [20]. Fourth, we showed that downregulated miRNAs outnumber upregulated miRNAs by a wide margin in the OC of both strains during aging in our previous study. This global decline of miRNA during aging was also observed in the LW of CBA mice and was consistent with the trend observed in other studies [79]. For example, in the aging brain, 85 miRNAs are downregulated, while only 8 are upregulated [79]. The vast majority of *C. elegans* miRNAs that are differentially expressed during aging are also downregulated [80]. Interestingly, the number of upregulated and downregulated miRNAs was essentially equal in the LW of C57 mice (Fig. 4). Therefore, it appears that there was a significant increase in upregulated miRNAs in C57 during aging. Two previous studies examining miRNAs in the aging brain and liver also reported predominant miRNA upregulation [81,82]. It is important to note that different degrees of cochlear deterioration in two different strains may provide a possible explanation for the different results. Comparison of miRNA expression profiles between C57 and CBA mice showed that the number of miRNAs involved in the LW of C57 mice is significantly greater than in CBA mice during aging. This is consistent with the fact that the onset of hearing loss occurs much earlier and progresses more rapidly in C57 mice than in the CBA strain. Fifth, we are fully aware that miRNAs function as post-transcriptional regulators of gene expression that might only effect protein expression. We only examined target mRNA levels for proteins that are part of apoptosis-related pathways, and other effects have undoubtedly been missed. Although Western blotting can be used to examine protein expression, it was technically impractical to examine many proteins involved in apoptosis in these small tissue samples. Finally, aging is a multidimensional process that involves multiple molecular mechanisms and pathways. While apoptosis-related cell loss and atrophy maybe part of the mechanisms involved in aging, other mechanisms and pathways are also involved. The present study only examined genes associated with apoptosis. Future experiments will examine other pathways associated with aging.

The differential expression of many miRNAs during aging in the LW supports their involvement in a complex process of age-related degeneration of stria function that is not molecularly well understood. The pattern of altered miRNA expression we observe here suggests that multiple gene regulatory relationships are affected during aging. These findings point to novel functions for miRNAs in the molecular mechanisms of aging. The present work is the first step in an effort to elucidate the roles of miRNAs and their regulatory networks in age-related degeneration of the LW. It also lays the groundwork for future experiments that can explore whether suppression or overexpression of some miRNAs can slow the onset and progression of stria degeneration.

## Supporting Information

**Table S1 84 apoptosis related genes contained in the apoptosis RT$^2$ Profiler PCR Array.**

## Author Contributions

Conceived and designed the experiments: DH QZ GS. Performed the experiments: QZ HL. Analyzed the data: QZ DH HL GS. Contributed reagents/materials/analysis tools: GS. Wrote the paper: QZ DH.

## References


1. Gilad O, Glorig A (1979) Presbycusis: the aging inner ear. Part I. J Am Audit Soc 4: 195–206.
2. Gilad O, Glorig A (1979) Presbycusis: the aging ear. Part II. J Am Audit Soc 4: 207–217.
3. Schacht J, Hawkins JE (2005) Sketches of otohistory. Part 9: presbycusis. Audiol Neurootol 10: 243–247.
4. Mao Z, Zhao L, Pu L, Wang M, Zhang Q, et al. (2013) How well can centenarians hear? PLoS One 8: e65565.
5. Ohlemiller KK (2004) Age-related hearing loss: the status of Schuknecht's typology. Curr. Opin. Otolaryngol. Head Neck Surg 12: 439–443.
6. Nelson EG, Hinojosa R (2006) Presbycusis: a human temporal bone study of individuals with downward sloping audiometric patterns of hearing loss and review of the literature. Laryngoscope 116: 1–12.
7. Lee RC, Feinbaum RL, Ambros V (1993) The C. elegans heterochronic gene lin-4 encodes small RNAs with antisense complementarity to lin-14. Cell 75: 843–854.
8. Reinhart BJ, Slack FJ, Basson M, Pasquinelli AE, Bettinger JC, et al. (2000) The 21-nucleotide let-7 RNA regulates developmental timing in Caenorhabditis elegans. Nature 403: 901–906.
9. Pasquinelli AE, Reinhart BJ, Slack F, Martindale MQ, Kuroda MI, et al. (2000) Conservation of the sequence and temporal expression of let-7 heterochronic regulatory RNA. Nature 408: 86–89.
10. Gregory RI, Yan KP, Amuthan G, Chendrimada T, Doratotaj B, et al. (2004) The microprocessor complex mediates the genesis of microRNAs. Nature 432: 235–240.
11. Bartel DP (2004) MicroRNAs: genomics, biogenesis, mechanism and function. Cell 116: 281–297.
12. Kato M, Slack FJ (2008) microRNAs: small molecules with big roles - C. elegans to human cancer. Biol Cell 100: 71–81.
13. Bates DJ, Liang R, Li N, Wang E (2009) The impact of noncoding RNA on the biochemical and molecular mechanisms of aging. Biochim Biophys Acta 1790: 970–979.
14. Provost P (2010) Interpretation and applicability of microRNA data to the context of Alzheimer's and age-related diseases. Aging 2: 166–169.
15. van Rooij E, Sutherland LB, Liu N, Williams AH, McAnally J, et al. (2006) A signature pattern of stress-responsive microRNAs that can evoke cardiac hypertrophy and heart failure. Proc Natl Acad Sci USA 103: 18255–18260.
16. Holzenberger M, Dupont J, Ducos B, Leneuve P, Géloën A, et al. (2003) IGF-1 receptor regulates lifespan and resistance to oxidative stress in mice. Nature 421: 182–187
17. de Lencastre A, Pincus Z, Zhou K, Kato M, Lee SS, et al. (2010) MicroRNAs both promote and antagonize longevity in C. elegans. Curr Biol 20: 2159–2168.
18. Ibáñez-Ventoso C, Yang M, Guo S, Robins H, Padgett RW, et al. (2006) Modulated microRNA expression during adult lifespan in Caenorhabditis elegans. Aging Cell 5: 235–246.
19. Kato MI, Slack FJ (2008) microRNAs: small molecules with big roles - C. elegans to human cancer. Biol Cell 100: 71–81.
20. Zhang Q, Liu H, McGee J, Walsh EJ, Soukup GA, et al. (2013) Identifying microRNAs involved in degeneration of the organ of Corti during age-related hearing loss. PLoS One 8: e62786.
21. Judice TN, Nelson NC, Beisel CL, Delimont DC, Fritzsch B, et al. (2002) Cochlear whole mount in situ hybridization: identification of longitudinal and radial gradients. Brain Res Protoc 9: 65–76.
22. Wienholds E, Kloosterman WP, Miska E, Alvarez-Saavedra E, Berezikov E, et al. (2005) MicroRNA expression in zebrafish embryonic development. Science 309: 310–311.
23. Kloosterman WP, Wienholds E, de Bruijn E, Kauppinen S, Plasterk RH (2006) In situ detection of miRNAs in animal embryos using LNA-modified oligonucleotide probes. Nat Methods 3: 27–29.
24. Pauley S, Wright TJ, Pirvola U, Ornitz D, Beisel K, et al. (2003) Expression and function of FGF10 in mammalian inner ear development. Dev Dyn 227: 203–215.
25. Wei L, Ding D, Salvi R (2010) Salicylate-induced degeneration of cochlea spiral ganglion neurons-apoptosis signaling. Neuroscience 68: 288–299.
26. Müller M, von Hünerbein K, Hoidis S, Smolders JW (2005) A physiological place-frequency map of the cochlea in the CBA/J mouse. Hear Res 202: 63–73.
27. Spongr VP, Flood DG, Frisina RD, Salvi RJ (1997) Quantitative measures of hair cell loss in CBA and C57BL/6 mice throughout their life spans. J Acoust Soc Am 101: 3546–3553.
28. Willott JF (1986) Effects of aging, hearing loss, and anatomical location on thresholds of inferior colliculus neurons in C57BL/6 and CBA mice. J Neurophysiol 56: 391–408.
29. Sha SH, Kanicki A, Dootz G, Talaska AE, Halsey K, et al. (2008) Age-related auditory pathology in the CBA/J mouse. Hear Res 243: 87–94.
30. Ohlemiller KK, Lett JM, Gagnon PM (2006) Cellular correlates of age-related endocochlear potential reduction in a mouse model. Hear Res 220: 10–26.
31. Ohlemiller KK, Rosen AD, Rellinger EA, Montgomery SC, Gagnon PM (2011) Different cellular and genetic basis of noise-related endocochlear potential reduction in CBA/J and BALB/cJ mice. J Assoc Res Otolaryngol 12: 45–58.
32. Filipowicz W, Bhattacharyya SN, Sonenberg N (2008) Mechanisms of post-transcriptional regulation by microRNAs: are the answers in sight? Nat Rev Genet 9: 102–114.
33. Pekarsky Y, Santanam U, Cimmino A, Palamarchuk A, Efanov A, et al. (2006) Tcl1 expression in chronic lymphocytic leukemia is regulated by miR-29 and miR-181. Cancer Res 66: 11590–11593.
34. Fabbri M, Garzon R, Cimmino A, Liu Z, Zanesi N, et al. (2007) MicroRNA-29 family reverts aberrant methylation in lung cancer by targeting DNA methyltransferases 3A and 3B. Proc Natl Acad Sci USA 104: 15805–15810.
35. Mott JL, Kobayashi S, Bronk SF, Gores GJ (2007) miR-29 regulates Mcl-1 protein expression and apoptosis. Oncogene 26: 6133–6140.
36. Park SY, Lee JH, Ha M, Nam JW, Kim VN (2009) miR-29 miRNAs activate p53 by targeting p85a and CDC42. Nat Struct Mol Biol 16: 23–29.
37. McKenna DJ, McDade SS, Patel D, McCance DJ (2010) MicroRNA 203 expression in keratinocytes is dependent on regulation of p53 levels by E6. J Virol 84: 10644–10652.
38. Lena AM, Shalom-Feuerstein R, Rivetti di Val Cervo P, Aberdam D, Knight RA, et al. (2008) miR-203 represses 'stemness' by repressing DeltaNp63. Cell Death Differ 15: 1187–1195.
39. Boominathan L (2010) The tumor suppressors p53, p63, and p73 are regulators of microRNA processing complex. PLoS One 5: e10615.
40. Noguchi S, Mori T, Otsuka Y, Yamada N, Yasui Y, et al. (2012) Anti-oncogenic microRNA-203 induces senescence by targeting E2F3 protein in human melanoma cells. J Biol Chem 287: 11769–11777.
41. Bueno MJ, Pérez de Castro I, Gómez de Cedrón M, Santos J, Calin GA, et al. (2008) Genetic and epigenetic silencing of microRNA-203 enhances ABL1 and BCR-ABL1 oncogene expression. Cancer Cell 13: 496–506.

42. Karali M, Peluso I, Gennarino VA, Bilio M, Verde R, et al. (2010) miRNeye: a microRNA expression atlas of the mouse eye. BMC Genomics 11: 715–741.
43. Mun J, Tam C, Chan G, Kim JH, Evans D, et al. (2013) MicroRNA-762 is upregulated in human corneal epithelial cells in response to tear fluid and Pseudomonas aeruginosa antigens and negatively regulates the expression of host defense genes encoding RNase7 and ST2. PLoS One 8: e57850.
44. Niu Y, Mo D, Qin L, Wang C, Li A, et al. (2011) Lipopolysaccharide-induced miR-1224 negatively regulates tumour necrosis factor-α gene expression by modulating Sp1. Immunology 133: 8–20.
45. Dixon-McIver A, East P, Mein CA, Cazier JB, Molloy G, et al. (2008) Distinctive patterns of microRNA expression associated with karyotype in acute myeloid leukaemia. PLoS One 3: e2141.
46. Yang Z, Zhang Y, Wang L (2013) A feedback inhibition between miRNA-127 and TGFβ/c-Jun cascade in HCC cell migration via MMP13. PLoS One 8: e65256.
47. Liu L, Nie J, Chen L, Dong G, Du X, et al. (2013) The oncogenic role of microRNA-130a/301a/454 in human colorectal cancer via targeting Smad4 expression. PLoS One 8: e55532.
48. Chen Y, Melton DW, Gelfond JA, McManus LM, Shireman PK (2012) MiR-351 transiently increases during muscle regeneration and promotes progenitor cell proliferation and survival upon differentiation. Physiol Genomics 44: 1042–1051.
49. Khan S, Brougham CL, Ryan J, Sahrudin A, O'Neill G, et al. (2013) miR-379 regulates cyclin B1 expression and is decreased in breast cancer. PLoS One 8: e68753.
50. Hu ZG, Shen WJ, Kraemer FB, Azhar S (2012) MicroRNAs 125a and 455 repress lipoprotein-supported steroidogenesis by targeting scavenger receptor class B type I in steroidogenic cells. Mol Cell Biol 32: 5035–5045.
51. Swingler TE, Wheeler G, Carmont V, Elliott HR, Barter MJ, et al. (2012) The expression and function of microRNAs in chondrogenesis and osteoarthritis. Arthritis Rheum 64: 1909–1919.
52. Sun Z, Wei Q, Zhang Y, He X, Ji W, et al. (2011) MicroRNA profiling of rhesus macaque embryonic stem cells. BMC Genomics 12: 276.
53. Steel KP, Barkway C (1989) Another role for melanocytes: their importance for normal stria vascularis development in the mammalian inner ear. Development 107: 453–463.
54. Cable J, Jackson IJ, Steel KP (1993) Light (Blt), a mutation that causes melanocyte death, affects stria vascularis function in the mouse inner ear. Pigment Cell Res 6: 215–225.
55. Ni C, Zhang D, Beyer LA, Halsey KE, Fukui H, et al. (2013) Hearing dysfunction in heterozygous Mitf(Mi-wh)/+ mice, a model for Waardenburg syndrome type 2 and Tietz syndrome. Pigment Cell Melanoma Res 26: 78–87.
56. Chen L, Chen XR, Chen FF, Liu Y, Li P, et al. (2013) MicroRNA-107 inhibits U87 glioma stem cells growth and invasion. Cell Mol Neurobiol 33: 651–657.
57. Nelson PT, Wang WX, Mao G, Wilfred BR, Xie K, et al. (2011) Specific sequence determinants of miR-15/107 microRNA gene group targets. Nucleic Acids Res 39: 8163–8172.
58. Yao J, Hennessey T, Flynt A, Lai E, Beal MF, et al. (2010) MicroRNA-related cofilin abnormality in Alzheimer's disease. PLoS One 5: e15546.
59. Augustin R, Endres K, Reinhardt S, Kuhn PH, Lichtenthaler SF, et al. (2012) Computational identification and experimental validation of microRNAs binding to the Alzheimer-related gene ADAM10. BMC Med Genet 13: 35–35.
60. Trivellin G, Butz H, Delhove J, Igreja S, Chahal HS, et al. (2012) MicroRNA miR-107 is overexpressed in pituitary adenomas and inhibits the expression of aryl hydrocarbon receptor-interacting protein in vitro. Am. J. Physiol. Endocrinol Metab 303: E708–719.
61. Albinsson S, Swärd K (2013) Targeting smooth muscle microRNAs for therapeutic benefit in vascular disease. Pharmacol Res 75: 28–36.
62. Hutcheson R, Terry R, Chaplin J, Smith E, Musiyenko A, et al. (2013) MicroRNA-145 restores contractile vascular smooth muscle phenotype and coronary collateral growth in the metabolic syndrome. Arterioscler Thromb Vasc Biol 33: 727–736.
63. Santovito D, Mandolini C, Marcantonio P, De Nardis V, Bucci M, et al. (2013) Overexpression of microRNA-145 in atherosclerotic plaques from hypertensive patients. Expert Opin Ther Targets 17: 217–223.
64. Jakob P, Landmesser U (2012) Role of microRNAs in stem/progenitor cells and cardiovascular repair. Cardiovasc Res 93: 614–622.
65. Dynoodt P, Mestdagh P, Van Peer G, Vandesompele J, Goossens K, et al. (2013) Identification of miR-145 as a key regulator of the pigmentary process. J Invest Dermatol 133: 201–209.
66. Dynoodt P, Speeckaert R, De Wever O, Chevolet I, Brochez L, et al. (2013) miR-145 overexpression suppresses the migration and invasion of metastatic melanoma cells. Int J Oncol 42: 1443–1451.
67. Kaur P, Armugam A, Jeyaseelan K (2012) MicroRNAs in neurotoxicity. J Toxicol 2012: 870150.
68. Cammarata G, Augugliaro L, Salemi D, Agueli C, La Rosa M, et al. (2010) Differential expression of specific microRNA and their targets in acute myeloid leukemia. Am J Hematol 85: 331–339.
69. Segura MF, Belitskaya-Lévy I, Rose AE, Zakrzewski J, Gaziel A, et al. (2010) Melanoma MicroRNA signature predicts post-recurrence survival. Clin Cancer Res 16: 1577–1586.
70. Pichiorri F, De Luca L, Aqeilan RI (2011) MicroRNAs: new players in multiple myeloma. Front Genet 2: 22–41.
71. Hu BH, Cai Q, Manohar S, Jiang H, Ding D, et al. (2009) Differential expression of apoptosis-related genes in the cochlea of noise-exposed rats. Neuroscience 161: 915–925.
72. Zhou DH, Yang LN, Roder C, Kalthoff H, Trauzold A (2013) TRAIL-induced expression of uPA and IL-8 strongly enhanced by overexpression of TRAF2 and Bcl-xL in pancreatic ductal adenocarcinoma cells. Hepatobiliary Pancreat Dis Int 12: 94–98.
73. Jin CY, Park C, Hong SH, Han MH, Jeong JW, et al. (2012) Synergistic induction of TRAIL-mediated apoptosis by anisomycin in human hepatoma cells via the BH3-only protein Bid and c-Jun/AP-1 signaling pathway. Biomed Pharmacotherapy 67: 321–328.
74. Law PT, Ching AK, Chan AW, Wong QW, Wong CK, et al. (2012) MiR-145 modulates multiple components of the insulin-like growth factor pathway in hepatocellular carcinoma. Carcinogenesis 33: 1134–1141.
75. Devarajan P, Savoca M, Castaneda MP, Park MS, Esteban-Cruciani N, et al. (2002) Cisplatin-induced apoptosis in auditory cells: role of death receptor and mitochondrial pathways. Hear Res 174: 45–54.
76. Habtemichael N, Heinrich UR, Knauer SK, Schmidtmann I, Bier C, et al. (2010) Expression analysis suggests a potential cytoprotective role of Birc5 in the inner ear. Mol Cell Neurosci 45: 297–305.
77. Knauer SK, Heinrich UR, Bier C, Habtemichael N, Docter D, et al. (2010) An otoprotective role for the apoptosis inhibitor protein survivin. Cell Death Dis 1: e51.
78. Farris HE, Wells GB, Ricci AJ (2006) Steady-state adaptation of mechanotransduction modulates the resting potential of auditory hair cells, providing an assay for endolymph [Ca2+]. J Neurosci 26: 12526–12536.
79. Inukai S, de Lencastre A, Turner M, Slack F (2012) Novel microRNAs differentially expressed during aging in the mouse brain. PloS One 7: e40028.
80. Boehm M, Slack F (2005) A developmental timing microRNA and its target regulate life span in C. elegans. Science 310: 1954–1957.
81. Li N, Bates DJ, An J, Terry DA, Wang E (2011) Up-regulation of key microRNAs, and inverse down-regulation of their predicted oxidative phosphorylation target genes, during aging in mouse brain. Neurobiol Aging 32: 944–955.
82. Maes OC, An J, Sarojini H, Wang E (2008) Murine microRNAs implicated in liver functions and aging process. Mech Ageing Dev 129: 534–541.

# 23

# Lexical Variation and Change in British Sign Language

**Rose Stamp[1]*, Adam Schembri[2], Jordan Fenlon[1], Ramas Rentelis[1], Bencie Woll[1], Kearsy Cormier[1]**

**1** Deafness, Cognition and Language Research Centre (DCAL), University College London, London, United Kingdom, **2** Linguistics program and The Centre for Research on Language Diversity, La Trobe University, Melbourne, Australia

## Abstract

This paper presents results from a corpus-based study investigating lexical variation in BSL. An earlier study investigating variation in BSL numeral signs found that younger signers were using a decreasing variety of regionally distinct variants, suggesting that levelling may be taking place. Here, we report findings from a larger investigation looking at regional lexical variants for colours, countries, numbers and UK placenames elicited as part of the BSL Corpus Project. Age, school location and language background were significant predictors of lexical variation, with younger signers using a more levelled variety. This change appears to be happening faster in particular sub-groups of the deaf community (e.g., signers from hearing families). Also, we find that for the names of some UK cities, signers from outside the region use a different sign than those who live in the region.

**Editor:** Howard Nusbaum, The University of Chicago, United States of America

**Funding:** The data for this study were collected as part of the British Sign Language Corpus Project, supported by the Economic and Social Research Council (ESRC) (Grant RES- 062-23-0825 and postgraduate award, Stamp, 2013). Additional work was supported by the Economic and Social Research Council of Great Britain grants RES-620- 28-6001 and RES-620-28-0002: Deafness Cognition and Language Research Centre. The funders had no role in study design, data collection and analysis, decision to publish, or preparation of the manuscript.

**Competing Interests:** The authors have declared that no competing interests exist.

* E-mail: rose_stamp@hotmail.com

## Introduction

Variation is an intrinsic part of all languages whether spoken or signed. It is apparent at all levels of language organisation: for example, there are several lexical variants in British Sign Language (BSL) which all mean 'America' (see Figure 1) (following the glossing convention used in sign language literature, examples of sign variants are represented by a corresponding English word written in small capitals, e.g., MONDAY; lexical variants, which have the same meaning, are represented with numbers following the gloss, e.g., MONDAY, MONDAY2 - as outlined by Cormier, Fenlon, Johnston, Rentelis, Schembri, et al. in 2012, [1], the gloss used in this paper reflects the glossing system used in the BSL Corpus Project and the BSL lexical database arising from it). Similar lexical variation has been observed in various sign languages studied to date, including American Sign Language (ASL) [2] and newly emerged sign languages, such as Nicaraguan Sign Language [3]. Variation in lexis may be systematically used by speakers to index their affiliation with particular social groups [4]. Recently, work has shown that this is also true for sign languages [2]. This variation may function as an index of social variables such as region, gender, ethnicity, and social class, or social factors that are distinctive to sign language communities [2], such as the language policy of the school attended during childhood or the language background of the signer's family. It may also be indicative of a language change in progress [5].

In an earlier study, sociolinguistic variation and change in BSL numeral signs was investigated. Stamp, Schembri, Fenlon and Rentelis [6] found that lexical variation in signs for the numerals 1 to 20 was systematically constrained by several social factors. Age, school location and language background (whether a signer is from a deaf or hearing family) were found to be significant predictors of a signer's lexical choice. Younger signers used a decreasing proportion of regionally distinct number signs, suggesting that levelling may be taking place. It had previously been suggested that this change may be a result of increased dialect contact [7] and increased exposure to regional variants through the media [8]. Stamp et al.'s study [6] formed part of the larger investigation of lexical variation undertaken as part of the BSL Corpus Project [9]. In this paper, we look at sign variants for colour terms, foreign and UK place names as well as numerals in data from a lexical elicitation task. Variants for these four semantic categories were elicited from 249 deaf native, near-native and early learner BSL users recruited from eight UK cities (we use the term 'native signers' here to refer to those individuals who acquired BSL from birth, 'near-native signers' as those who acquired the language before beginning school, and 'early learners' to refer to deaf adults who report acquiring BSL during primary school). Forty-one lexical items are analysed and correlated with the semantic category of the sign and the following social factors: region, age, gender, social class, language background and school location. The sign variants produced for colours, countries and numbers were coded as either 'traditional' or 'non-traditional' for the signer's region of residence in order to determine whether there is empirical evidence for *levelling* – i.e. the reduction in use of regionally marked variants which is thought to be the outcome of regular face-to-face interactions between speakers of differing linguistic repertoires [10–11]. Anecdotal reports from the deaf community indicate that BSL may be undergoing levelling, given previous suggestions of change in the past thirty years because of increased exposure to lexical variants through the media [8],[12–13]. For UK place names, we were interested in finding evidence related to anecdotal reports that signers use different variants depending on their in-group and out-group status (i.e., residents of

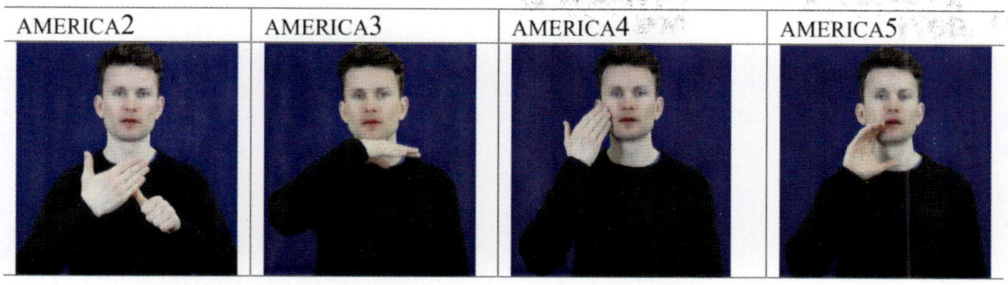


**Figure 1. Four regional lexical variants for the concept 'America' in BSL.**

a specific urban centre use a different sign to refer to their city from the one used by non-residents). The most comparable research on lexical variation to date was conducted on New Zealand Sign Language (NZSL), a sign language closely related to BSL [14]. McKee and McKee [14] found that variation in the NZSL lexicon had become increasingly levelled following the introduction of the Australasian Signed English system (from Australia) into New Zealand deaf education, with younger signers making greater use of the lexical variants associated with this system. The research aims of the current study are to investigate: (1) the extent of lexical variation in the target lexical items in BSL; (2) the degree to which this variation reflects social factors such as age, region, gender and language background; and (3) whether there is evidence for a language change in progress, including possible levelling in BSL.

This paper is organised into five parts: first, we discuss the history of BSL regional variation. Next, we present a brief review of the literature on spoken and signed language lexical variation. We then explain the methodology for the BSL Corpus Project and present the results of this study. Finally, we discuss the findings in relation to other relevant sign language studies and consider their implications for an understanding of variation in BSL.

## The British deaf community

The 2011 Census for England and Wales reports that between 15,000–20,000 people in the UK use BSL as their main language [15]. BSL, the sign language of the British deaf community, is also closely related to the sign languages used in Australia (Auslan) and New Zealand (NZSL), with some researchers even suggesting that they are dialects of the same sign language: BANZSL (British-Australian-New Zealand Sign Language) [16].

**Schools and the development of BSL regional variation.** Typically language is transmitted from caregiver to child. However, the vast majority of deaf children are born to hearing parents (Mitchell & Karchmer [17] found 92% of deaf children in the USA have two hearing parents; Uus & Bamford [18] found 10.6% of congenitally deaf children in the UK have a family history of deafness). Hearing parents are unlikely to know a sign language, and a deaf child may have limited access to the spoken language. Acquisition of a first language may thus be delayed for many deaf children [19–20]. Schools for deaf children, especially residential schools, have therefore long been associated with sign language transmission [21]. Since the first deaf schools were opened in 1760, sign language has been used as a form of communication among deaf children and passed on from older to younger peers [22]. Because there was minimal interaction between schools and no standard or written form of BSL, these 'school-lects' continued to develop separately in each community [13]. It is believed that deaf school-leavers maintained the use of these school variants in the local community and they became the basis for current regional varieties of BSL [13],[23]. These regional varieties have been found to vary most obviously at a lexical level (although see Fenlon, Schembri, Rentelis, & Cormier [24] for a study on phonological variation from the same regions reported here).

**Changes in the British deaf community.** In recent years, anecdotal claims within the British deaf community suggest that traditional regional variation is in decline, and there is some evidence for these claims, e.g., in numeral signs [6]. Several recent changes in the British deaf community have been offered as possible causes. Perhaps the most important of these changes has been the closure of centralised schools for deaf children. In the late 1970s, the Warnock Report recommended that deaf children be sent to integrated schools alongside their hearing counterparts [25]. As a result, many residential schools for deaf children closed [26], and deaf children have been increasingly sent to mainstream schools [21]. Centralised schools for deaf children, which would have once served as an opportunity for deaf children from hearing families to acquire signing from their native signing peers [23], are being replaced by the mainstreaming of deaf children where hearing educational and communication support workers enable deaf children to participate in classroom activities alongside hearing children. In the absence of deaf peers, these communication support workers sometimes serve as language models for the children, despite the fact that they may have limited sign language skills themselves [27–30].

In addition, increased mobility and transnational contact have exposed deaf and hearing British people alike to a multitude of languages, dialects and social practices. Research on British English accents has shown how increased mobility within the UK has resulted in dialect levelling [31–32]. Whilst levelling has not been widely researched in sign languages, there is evidence that increased international interaction has influenced the lexicon of a number of sign languages [33–34]. Advances in technology such as the use of webcams and online video have substantially increased exposure to BSL signers outside an individual's local community. Broadcast media have had an impact on the lexicon, with younger signers reported to incorporate new signs seen on television into their BSL [8], and the suggestion that some Scottish regional signs have gained more widespread currency through the influence of Scottish presenters on the BBC deaf community programme *See Hear* [12].

Changes in BSL resulting from the emergence of TV programmes for the deaf community and sign language interpreting on television may have led to an increased preoccupation with political correctness since the 1990s. Signs for foreign countries which portray physical features have sometimes been perceived as 'racist' by the hearing non-signing community [35–36]. As a result, it has been claimed that traditional BSL signs meaning 'China', 'Africa', 'gay' and 'India', for example, may have become less commonly used by younger signers because of concern that their form was strongly associated with stereotypical images or actions associated with these groups [12–13]. However, some of the country name signs in the lexicon appear to be changing for reasons that cannot be attributed to political correctness (e.g., the traditional variants meaning 'America' cannot be considered offensive). Thus, political correctness alone cannot explain all the patterns of lexical change, even within this specific semantic domain.

**Lexical variation in signed and spoken languages.** Sociolinguistic research has identified the following social factors as providing important insights into the nature of language variation and change in spoken and signed languages: age [14],[37], gender [38–40] and social class [2],[41]. Age-related variation in lexis has been reported for BSL [42]. As a broad generalisation, for example, older deaf people of the late 1980s used more fingerspelling (the use of a manual alphabet to spell out English words) than younger deaf people of the late 1980s, reflecting previous educational practices (a more recent study indicated this is also true of Auslan, see [43]). Iconicity as a factor in sign creation may also result in age differences. As new technology has replaced old, lexical items used by younger signers may reflect the changed appearance or means of operating new appliances, while older signers may maintain the sign in its earlier form [44]. For example, an earlier sign meaning 'telephone' represented how a person would hold a candlestick phone whilst a newer variant resembles how a person holds a mobile phone.

Although sociolinguistic investigations have tended to concentrate on variation and change in the phonology and grammar, lexical variables are also an important point of sociolinguistic investigation [45–50]. Nevertheless, it has been argued that the lexicon cannot tell us anything about language change, since speakers continually adopt new concepts into their vocabularies [51–53].

In contrast to the focus in contemporary studies in the sociolinguistics of spoken languages on sociophonetic variation, the obvious presence of considerable variation in sign language lexicons has meant that studies of variation in sign language have emphasised lexical variation and change. In contrast to spoken languages, regional and social sign language 'accents' have not been described, although some subtle variation in the application of phonological processes to specific sublexical elements does appear to be correlated with region [2],[24],[54].

Theories of regional dialects often implicitly presuppose that there was once a single, uniform language, which diverged until identifiable regional varieties arose, either through spontaneous evolution or language mixing, or both processes [55]. There is no evidence, however, that there was once a single variety of BSL, which split up as deaf people spread throughout the country. We can also probably dismiss the idea that regional variants in BSL differ primarily because of mixing with other languages (although there is evidence that some Scottish and Northern Irish varieties have been influenced by Irish Sign Language and American Sign Language, see [56–57].

Woll et al. [58] identified considerable lexical variation between the varieties of BSL used in Glasgow, Newcastle, Manchester, London and Bristol. Regional differences were seen in culturally significant signs (e.g., 'deaf', 'hearing', 'interpreter'), everyday lexical items (e.g., 'British', 'business', 'theatre') and forms new to the deaf community (e.g., 'discrimination', 'community'). In some core semantic areas (such as colour terms, days of the week, and numerals), signs exhibited substantial regional variation. It was the case, however, that while there were regional differences, there was usually one variant recognised across all regions, suggesting gradual emergence of a national standard [2].

In contrast to the evidence of considerable traditional lexical variation in BSL, it has been claimed that ASL may have a relatively more standardised lexicon than other documented sign languages [59]. In their lexical variation study, Lucas and colleagues [2] found that of the 34 target concepts they studied, 27 included a variant that appeared in the data from all seven sites across the USA. Lucas et al. [2] suggested that historical patterns of ASL transmission account for the existence of widely shared variants. The residential schools in each of regions they studied all had direct or indirect links with the American School for the Deaf in Hartford, Connecticut, which had trained deaf graduates as teachers who then were sent out across the USA to establish new schools during the 19$^{th}$ century, leading to the spreading of a single variety of ASL across the continent.

## Methodology

The lexical data in this paper was elicited as part of the BSL Corpus Project. Here we briefly introduce the BSL Corpus Project by outlining the sites of collection, participant characteristics and the methods used in data collection, coding and analysis (for more detail, see [60]).

### Ethics Statement

Participants in this research were all deaf with British Sign Language as their main/preferred language. Participants were all aged 16 or over. The University College London (UCL) Research Ethics Committee guidelines state that "young people aged 16–18 with sufficient understanding are able to give their full consent to participate in research independently of their parents and guardians" so no additional consent was obtained from those under 18. It cannot be assumed that members of this language community (deaf BSL users) have fluent or full comprehension of written English. Therefore the comprehensive information statement and consent form in written English which are required by the UCL Research Ethics Committee were translated into British Sign Language by local deaf fieldworkers and deaf researchers working on the project. Questions were clarified in person in BSL and consent obtained in writing. This project including the consent procedure was approved by the UCL Research Ethics Committee (project ID 0864/001). All individuals pictured in this manuscript have given written informed consent to publish their images.

### British Sign Language Corpus Project

The BSL Corpus Project, which began in 2008, was the first large-scale corpus project to be undertaken for BSL. The aim of the project was to create a corpus of elicited and spontaneous BSL digital video data from deaf native, near-native and early learners of BSL. The project has established an online, open-access video dataset available for researchers and the sign language community [60], and has provided data for a number of studies which have thus far investigated sociolinguistic variation and change, language contact and lexical frequency [61–62].

**Sites.** In order to obtain samples of regional variation, data were collected from eight sites across the UK: Belfast, Birmingham, Bristol, Cardiff, Glasgow, London, Manchester and Newcastle. These sites were selected because they are, or were previously, locations of a centralised school for deaf children, and because, as relatively large urban centres, it was assumed that they would provide a sufficiently large deaf community from which to recruit.

**Participants.** Thirty participants were filmed at most sites, although slightly larger samples were collected in Bristol and

London, with 32 and 37 participants respectively. In total, 249 deaf individuals were filmed. Figure 2 shows the regional distribution of the BSL Corpus Project participants, based on their home address at the time of filming. We attempted to recruit 'lifelong' users of BSL (cf., [2]) who were representative of the regional signs used in their particular region. Target participants were British-born, exposed to BSL before the age of seven, and had lived in the region where they were filmed for the previous 10 years, but a small number of people who did not fit these criteria were included. Five individuals were not British-born and 12 reported learning BSL after age seven (all but one, however, learned BSL before age 12). Participants were recruited by deaf community fieldworkers who were native or fluent BSL signers and familiar with the local deaf community. Fieldworkers recruited local deaf people they knew personally (e.g., friends, family, work colleagues) and who matched the project criteria. In recruitment we attempted to balance the sample for age groups, gender and social class and to represent deaf individuals from both deaf and hearing family backgrounds. Table 1 shows the participant characteristics in each site.

**Data collection.** The methodology for the BSL Corpus Project was based on two similar large-scale investigations of ASL [2] and Auslan [54] with some key differences. Unlike the other projects where participants were filmed in groups, all British participants were filmed in pairs with a person from the same region and of a similar age (in London, one participant was filmed a second time with a different partner). Four types of data were collected: a personal experience narrative, a free conversation of 30 minutes, responses to interview questions and responses to a lexical elicitation task.

In the lexical elicitation task, fieldworkers showed participants PowerPoint slides or flashcards for 102 concepts. Each slide displayed an image of the referent or something associated with it, and the equivalent English word underneath (see Figure 3 for examples). The concepts chosen were based on previous BSL lexical variation studies, existing dictionaries, and also following suggestions from the BSL Corpus Project Deaf Advisory Group [58],[63]. Responses for 41 of the 102 items are analysed here: five colour terms ('brown', 'green', 'grey', 'purple', 'yellow'); eight countries ('America', 'Britain', 'China', 'France', 'Germany', 'India', 'Ireland', 'Italy'); the numerals one to twenty; and eight UK place names ('Belfast', 'Birmingham', 'Bristol', 'Cardiff', 'Glasgow', 'London', 'Manchester', 'Newcastle'). These 41 items were chosen as they represent the complete set of signs elicited for the four domains; colours, countries, numbers and UK place names. The specific signs were selected on the basis of existing lexicographical work on BSL, as well as a result of suggestions from the BSL Corpus Project Deaf Advisory Group (http://www.bslcorpusproject.org/team/). Numbers and colours are known to be highly variable according to region. Countries are believed to be a semantic field affected by lexical change and UK place names are believed to represent examples of exonymy/endonymy.

Stimulus items were also selected in order to investigate anecdotal reports about variation and change in their usage. Observation suggests that signs for country names, for example, have been undergoing considerable change in recent years. For UK placenames, anecdotal reports from BSL teachers indicated that lexical variants differ according to in-group and out-group membership.

For each target concept, participants were asked to produce the sign variant they use most on a daily basis. One limitation of this

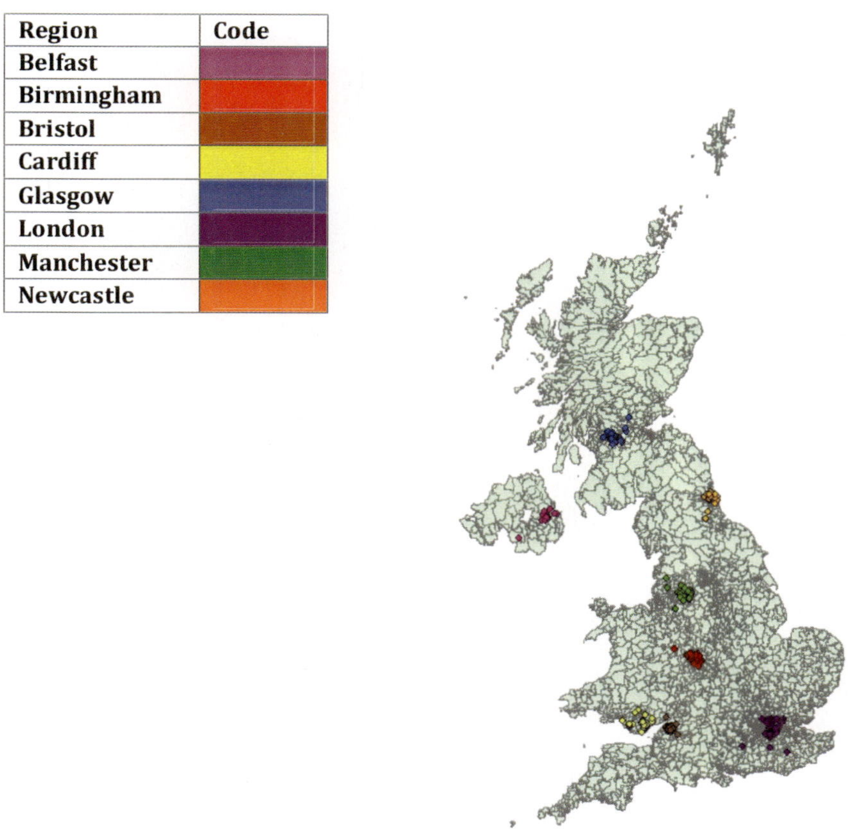


**Figure 2. Regional distribution of the BSL Corpus Project participants.**

**Table 1.** Participant characteristics.

| Sites | Total | Age | | | Gender | | Ethnicity | | Language background | | Social class | | School location (*some metadata missing) | |
|---|---|---|---|---|---|---|---|---|---|---|---|---|---|---|
| | | Younger 16–39 | Middle 40–59 | Older 60+ | Female | Male | White | Other | Deaf | Hearing | Working class | Middle class | Local | Non-local |
| Belfast | 30 | 10 | 12 | 8 | 17 | 13 | 30 | 0 | 7 | 23 | 26 | 4 | 21 | 9 |
| Birmingham | 30 | 12 | 9 | 9 | 13 | 17 | 27 | 3 | 12 | 18 | 16 | 14 | 21 | 9 |
| Bristol | 32 | 9 | 14 | 9 | 17 | 15 | 30 | 2 | 17 | 15 | 16 | 16 | 16 | 16 |
| Cardiff | 30 | 10 | 12 | 8 | 17 | 13 | 28 | 2 | 6 | 24 | 22 | 8 | 10* | 19* |
| Glasgow | 30 | 10 | 13 | 7 | 15 | 15 | 27 | 3 | 6 | 24 | 17 | 13 | 20 | 10 |
| London | 37 | 8 | 19 | 10 | 17 | 20 | 31 | 6 | 13 | 24 | 15 | 22 | 20* | 16* |
| Manchester | 30 | 12 | 6 | 12 | 16 | 14 | 27 | 3 | 8 | 22 | 23 | 7 | 13* | 16* |
| Newcastle | 30 | 6 | 11 | 13 | 17 | 13 | 29 | 1 | 7 | 23 | 19 | 11 | 18* | 11* |
| TOTAL | 249 | 77 | 96 | 76 | 129 | 120 | 229 | 20 | 76 | 173 | 154 | 95 | 139* | 106* |

task is that sign variants are elicited in isolation and signers may respond to normative pressures or perceptions about what is appropriate for their region rather than offer the sign they actually use most. Therefore, a subset of the conversational data was also analysed to investigate whether the sign variants from the lexical elicitation task correspond to those used in the free conversation data (collected prior to the lexical elicitation task).

**Data Coding (Signs for colours, countries & numbers).** Lexical variants for colours, countries and numbers (33 concepts) were elicited from 249 participants, producing a total of 8, 217 tokens. All tokens were annotated in ELAN [64]. Many participants produced multiple examples of signs and, as a result, either the variant stated to be the sign, or if not stated, the first variant produced, was coded. A small number of participants omitted or incorrectly identified some target concepts (e.g., one participant produced a sign meaning 'eighteen' in response to '16' on the slide). For this reason, 18 tokens were excluded from the coding process. Our dataset included only one lexical variant for the numerals 'one', 'two' and 'five'. As a result, these number signs were also excluded from the coding process, representing 747 tokens in the dataset. A further 120 tokens were excluded as some essential demographic information was missing from individual participants' background questionnaires, and thus social factors for those participants could not be coded. In total, 7332 tokens were analysed.

Phonological variants were grouped together as one lexeme [65–66]. Following previous work [1],[65], variants which were formationally related and differed only in one parameter (handshape, location, movement, orientation, or non-manual features) were considered to be phonological variants.

The lexical elicitation task produced an extremely complex dataset in which each of the individual stimuli represent a variable that could be investigated in detail. As a means to capturing overall patterns in the data, we coded each response as either a 'traditional' or 'non-traditional sign' for the signer's region. This would make it possible to investigate whether there is any evidence that levelling is taking place in BSL, and whether or not this language change is more strongly associated with any specific subgroup(s) (e.g., young males) in the British deaf community. The traditional signs for colours, countries and numbers for each region were determined by two methods. First, there are existing teaching resources about BSL lexical variation that make claims about the association of certain BSL signs with particular regions in the UK. For example, the lexical variant AMERICA4 (shown in Figure 1) has been claimed to be traditionally associated with the London/south-eastern region of England [67]. In addition, earlier studies in BSL describe a number of regional signs [68]. Secondly, the signs produced by elderly signers in each region were examined and each local deaf community fieldworker was consulted to confirm which of these represented traditional signs in their region (usually this was the most frequent variant in the data from the older signers). In cases where the actual productions of the oldest group of signers contradicted what signs were claimed to be traditional for the region by the fieldworker, these examples (a total of 610 tokens) were then excluded from the analysis.

Each token was coded for the following social factors: age, gender and social class of the signer. For this study, participants were categorised into three age groups: 16–39 years (younger), 40–59 years (middle) and 60 years and above (older) to reflect the different educational policies experienced by deaf children throughout the twentieth century (and thus our age groups reflect emic criteria [69]). Most of the participants in the older category would have attended residential schools and been educated predominantly using lip-reading and fingerspelling [13]. Those

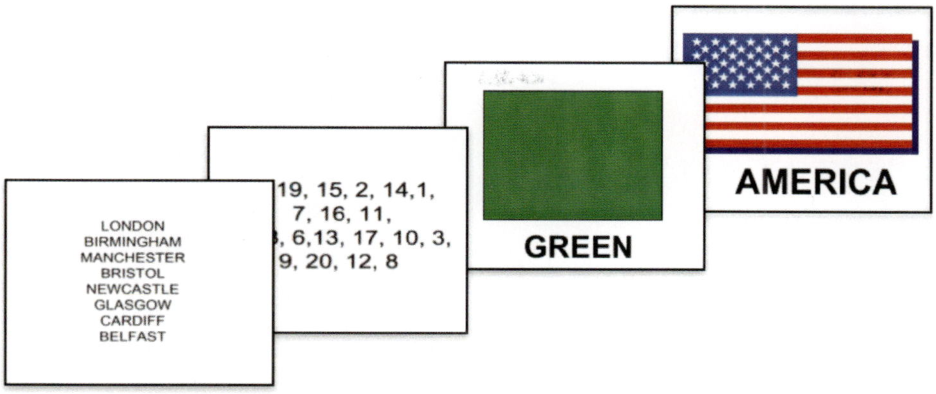


**Figure 3. Example of the stimuli shown to participants.**

in the middle age group would have experienced an increasing emphasis on speech and lip-reading and the beginning of mainstreaming of deaf students into schools with hearing children. Younger signers are more likely to have attended mainstream schools with communication support workers, or experienced the shift to bilingual education following the increasing acceptance of BSL as a language. For social class, participants were classified as either working or middle class based on occupation and/or education (i.e., 'working class' referred to individuals working in unskilled, semi-skilled or skilled manual jobs, while 'middle class' were those who had a university education and/or worked in skilled non-manual jobs or professional/managerial positions). Whether an adult signer grew up signing from birth or acquired sign language later in life has been found to be an important predictor of lexical variation in sign languages [2]. Responses were thus coded as being from participants with hearing or deaf language backgrounds according to their parents' audiological status (whilst the assumption here is that only participants with deaf parents will have learnt sign language natively, this is not always the case as some deaf parents may be non-signers and some hearing parents may be fluent sign language users). Finally, the regional background of each signer was also included in the analysis. In Quinn's [23] study on BSL regional variation (unlike previous studies of sociolinguistic variation and change in sign languages), a signer's regional background was determined by the location of the school they attended rather than the region of the UK in which they lived at the time of data collection. For the purposes of the current study, participants' responses were coded both for their region of residence and their school location. A participant's school location was classified as 'local' if he or she had attended a school at any point in their education (primary and/or secondary school) located in the region in which they were currently living.

In addition to these social factors, the semantic category of the elicited sign (signs for countries, numbers or colours) was coded to see whether subcategories of signs were changing at a different rate than others.

In summary, sign variants produced for colours, countries and numbers were coded as traditional or non-traditional for the signer's region. The following social factors were investigated: region (Belfast, Birmingham, Bristol, Cardiff, Glasgow, London, Manchester, Newcastle), age (16–39, 40–59, 60+), gender (female, male), social class (middle, working), language background (deaf, hearing), school location (local, non-local). The semantic category of the sign was also coded (colour, country, number).

**Data coding: sub-sample (UK placenames).** The UK placename data were analysed separately to investigate anecdotal claims about their usage. Such claims suggest that place name signs may work to index local, in-group versus non-local, out-group identity. For example, it is claimed that Bristol signers use a different lexical variant for 'Bristol' than those living elsewhere. To investigate this claim, fieldworkers from each of the eight regions were asked to identify which lexical variants were considered to be the local variants. The elicited forms for these UK placenames were analysed and the variants produced were coded as either local or non-local for the particular placename. In most cases, the local sign is a lexicalised form of fingerspelling consisting of the first letter and possibly some subsequent letters (e.g., the Manchester variant meaning 'Manchester' is formed by producing the manual letter 'M' followed by 'C') (for more discussion of lexicalised fingerspelling, see [70–71]). This is also the case for the following placenames: 'Birmingham' (B-H-M), 'Bristol' (B-L), 'Cardiff' (C-F-F), 'Glasgow' (G-W), and 'Newcastle' (N-C). For the placenames 'London' and 'Belfast', a different sign unrelated to fingerspelling is used locally. The data were analysed to investigate if there was a correlation between the use of a variant local to the region and participants' place of residence.

**Data coding: sub-sample (Conversational data).** The effects of the observer's paradox were likely to be greater during the lexical elicitation task than the conversational task, due to the relatively greater attention to sign language production in the former compared to the latter activity [5]. Annotation work on the conversational data is ongoing, and only a subset of 500 tokens from 50 signers in Birmingham and Bristol have been annotated, making a total of 25,000 searchable tokens [72]. In this dataset, we searched for tokens of those colour, numeral, and country lexical items elicited in the lexical elicitation task to investigate whether participants produced identical or different lexical variants in the two datasets. In total, 570 different tokens were identified and analysed.

**Data Analysis.** For the current study, we carried out multivariate statistical analyses of the data using Rbrul [73]. Like the program GoldVarb, developed by [74], Rbrul can quantitatively evaluate the influence of multiple factors on variation. In addition, Rbrul uses mixed-effects modeling to group individual responses accounting for the effects of individual differences [75–76].

## Results

The results for the colour, country and number signs study are discussed first. This study investigates the relationship between the use of traditional regional signs and social factors (e.g., signers' age, gender, etc.). Following this, the results for the UK placenames study will be presented. Finally, the comparison between the conversational and lexical elicitation data will be discussed.

### Variables of analysis: Social factors

Of the 6722 tokens analysed, 5279 (79%) were classified as traditional for the signer's region. Participant and lexical item were included in the analysis as random effects. Table 2 presents the results, including the log odds, number of tokens analysed, percentage of traditional variants and the centred weight for each factor (with the use of traditional sign variants as the application value). Results with a positive log-odd and a factor weight over 0.5 (shown in bold) indicate that this factor results in an increased likelihood that the traditional variants will be used while a negative log-odd and a factor weight below 0.5 indicate an increased likelihood that non-traditional variants will be found in the data.

We tested for interactions between the seven variables under investigation and found that region and school location were not independent of each other (region/school, $p>0.05$); as a result, we excluded region of residence from the analysis. Of the six factor groups remaining, the following three, in order from greater to lesser importance, predict the use of traditional signs: age, school location and language background. Participants in the older age group strongly favour the use of traditional signs (0.693), while those in the younger age group strongly disfavour the use of traditional signs (0.275). Those who were educated locally slightly favour the use of traditional signs (0.57) compared to those who were educated outside of the region where they reside (0.43). The third most significant predictor was language background, with participants with hearing parents slightly disfavouring the use of traditional signs (0.444). Participants with deaf parents slightly favour the use of traditional signs (0.556). The semantic category of the sign, social class and gender were not found to be significant. The results for each category (in increasing order of their proportion of traditional signs: signs for countries, numbers and colours) were analysed separately to look at the patterns of traditional sign use.

**Signs for countries.** In the country names dataset, a total of 1623 tokens were analysed. Table 3 presents the results. Language background, school location, social class and gender were not significant factors. Age was found to be an important factor, however. Older signers favoured the use of traditional signs (0.635) and younger signers disfavoured the use of traditional country signs (0.303).

**Signs for numbers.** Age, school location and language background were significant predictors of the use of traditional number signs (see Table 4). Older signers strongly favoured the use of traditional number variants (.778) and younger signers strongly disfavoured the use of traditional number variants (.211). A chi-square analysis revealed a significant difference ($\chi^2=49.53$, $p<0.001$) in the use of traditional variants between the younger and middle age groups but no significant difference between the middle and older age groups ($\chi^2=0.857$, $p=0.835$). School location was the second most significant factor. Signers who attended a school in the same region in which they currently reside favour the use of traditional number signs (.601) to a greater extent than signers who attended a school outside of their region (.399). Signers from a hearing family slightly disfavour the use of traditional number signs (.418) while signers with deaf parents slightly favour the use of traditional number signs (.582). Social class and gender were not found to be significant.

**Signs for colours.** Of the 1222 colour tokens analysed, only 16% (201 tokens) were non-traditional sign variants. The signer's age and school location were important in predicting the use of traditional colour signs (see Table 5). Gender, language background and social class were not significant predictors for the lexical variant chosen. Similar to results for the other semantic categories, older signers showed a preference for the use of traditional forms (0.594) compared to younger signers (0.334).

**Table 2.** Multiple logistic regression results for signs for colours, countries and numbers.

| Factor Group | Factor | Log odds | Tokens | % of traditional signs | Centred weight |
|---|---|---|---|---|---|
| *Age (in years) | **60+** | **0.815** | **2042** | **87.6** | **0.693** |
| | **40–59** | **0.154** | **2606** | **81.4** | **0.538** |
| | 16–39 | −0.969 | 2074 | 66.1 | 0.275 |
| *School location | **Local** | **0.281** | **3798** | **81.3** | **0.570** |
| | Non-local | −0.281 | 2924 | 75.0 | 0.430 |
| *Language Background | **Deaf** | **0.223** | **2099** | **78.1** | **0.556** |
| | Hearing | −0.223 | 4623 | 78.7 | 0.444 |
| Semantic category | **Colours** | **0.420** | **1222** | **83.6** | **0.603** |
| | **Numbers** | **0.006** | **3877** | **79.4** | **0.501** |
| | Countries | −0.426 | 1623 | 72.6 | 0.395 |
| Social class | **Middle** | **0.09** | **2599** | **77.6** | **0.522** |
| | Working | −0.09 | 4123 | 79.1 | 0.478 |
| Gender | **Male** | **0.018** | **3221** | **78.0** | **0.505** |
| | Female | −0.018 | 3501 | 79.0 | 0.495 |

Application value: Traditional signs.
*Factor groups significant at $p<.05$. 6722 tokens.
Input probability = 0.866, Mean = 0.785, Intercept = 1.868, Deviance = 5752.805. Random (participant) standard deviation = 1.064. Random (lexical item) standard deviation = 0.809.

**Table 3.** Multiple logistic regression results for signs for countries.

| Factor Group | Factor | Log odds | Tokens | % of traditional signs | Centred weight |
|---|---|---|---|---|---|
| *Age (in years) | **60+** | **0.555** | **492** | **80.9** | **0.635** |
| | **40–59** | **0.278** | **630** | **77.0** | **0.569** |
| | 16–39 | −0.832 | 501 | 58.9 | 0.303 |
| Language Background | **Deaf** | **0.212** | **515** | **73.4** | **0.535** |
| | Hearing | −0.212 | 1108 | 72.2 | 0.499 |
| School location | **Local** | **0.165** | **916** | **74.2** | **0.541** |
| | Non-local | −0.165 | 707 | 70.4 | 0.459 |
| Social class | **Working** | **0.005** | **1003** | **73.5** | **0.501** |
| | Middle | −0.005 | 620 | 71.1 | 0.499 |
| Gender | **Female** | **0.04** | **841** | **74.0** | **0.51** |
| | Male | −0.04 | 780 | 71.1 | 0.49 |

Application value: Traditional signs.
*Factor groups significant at p<.05. 1623 tokens.
Input probability = 0.793, Mean = 0.726, Intercept = −1.342, Deviance = 1646.468. Random effects (participant) standard deviation = 0.809. Random effects (lexical item) standard deviation = 1.131.

Also, those signers who were educated locally favoured the use of traditional signs (0.556) while those who were educated outside of the region slightly disfavoured the use of traditional signs (0.444).

**Signs for UK placenames.** To investigate anecdotal reports that individuals who reside within a given urban centre use a different sign variant to refer to that city than non-residents do, a total of 1992 tokens were classified as either local or non-local for the particular placename analysed. The results revealed that, with the exception of 'Glasgow', 'London' and 'Manchester', the use of the local placename variant significantly correlated with residency in that location, with residents found to strongly favour the use of the local variant: Belfast (>0.999), Birmingham (0.673), Bristol (0.736), Cardiff (0.724) and Newcastle (0.794). Table 6 presents the results of each significant Rbrul run for the UK placenames data including the log odds, the number of tokens and the centred weight.

## Extent of lexical variation in BSL

This study has investigated the lexical variants produced by 249 signers for 41 concepts within the semantic fields of colours, numerals, countries, and UK placenames. In total, 10, 209 tokens were elicited. Of these, 295 separate lexical variants were identified for the 41 stimuli. Thus, the variation for these concepts in BSL is considerable, mirroring the findings of previous studies [58]. This was most true of the signs for colours: we found 22 variants for 'purple'. It is likely that this range is not exhaustive, given that it is based on data collected in only eight sites across the UK. Importantly, 79% of responses (5279 tokens) maintained the use of traditional signs for each region, suggesting that any loss of regional variation in this part of the BSL lexicon is limited. Some semantic fields are, however, undergoing greater loss of variation than others. Only 72% of signs for countries (1178 tokens) were traditional variants, compared to 79% of signs elicited for numbers

**Table 4.** Multiple logistic regression results for signs for numbers.

| Factor Group | Factor | Log odds | Tokens | % of traditional signs | Centred weight |
|---|---|---|---|---|---|
| *Age | **60+ years** | **1.256** | **1181** | **90.3** | **0.778** |
| | **40–59 years** | **0.060** | **1501** | **81.3** | **0.515** |
| | 16–39 years | −1.316 | 1195 | 66.3 | 0.211 |
| *School location | **Local** | **0.408** | **2195** | **82.7** | **0.601** |
| | Non-local | −0.408 | 1682 | 75.2 | 0.399 |
| *Language Background | **Deaf** | **0.33** | **1194** | **79.0** | **0.582** |
| | Hearing | −0.33 | 2683 | 79.6 | 0.418 |
| Social class | **Middle** | **0.169** | **1506** | **78.6** | **0.542** |
| | Working | −0.169 | 2371 | 80.0 | 0.458 |
| Gender | **Male** | **0.1** | **1849** | **79.2** | **0.525** |
| | Female | −0.1 | 2028 | 79.6 | 0.475 |

Application value: Traditional signs.
*Factor groups significant at p<.05. 3877 tokens.
Input probability = 0.909, Mean = 0.794, Intercept = 2.301, Deviance = 3018.346. Random (participant) standard deviation = 1.654. Random (lexical item) standard deviation = 0.697.

**Table 5.** Multiple logistic regression results for signs for colours.

| Factor Group | Factor | Log odds | Tokens | % of traditional signs | Centred weight |
|---|---|---|---|---|---|
| *Age (in years) | **60+** | **0.380** | **369** | **87.5** | **0.594** |
| | **40–59** | **0.312** | **475** | **87.2** | **0.577** |
| | 16–39 | −0.692 | 378 | 75.1 | 0.334 |
| *School location | **Local** | **0.224** | **687** | **86.0** | **0.556** |
| | Non-local | −0.224 | 535 | 80.4 | 0.444 |
| Gender | **Male** | **0.045** | **590** | **83.4** | **0.511** |
| | Female | −0.045 | 632 | 83.7 | 0.489 |
| Language background | **Deaf** | **0.035** | **390** | **81.8** | **0.509** |
| | Hearing | −0.035 | 832 | 84.4 | 0.491 |
| Social class | **Middle** | **0.032** | **473** | **82.9** | **0.508** |
| | Working | −0.032 | 749 | 84.0 | 0.492 |

Application value: Traditional signs.
*Factor groups significant at p<.05. 1222 tokens.
Input probability = 0.885, Mean = 0.836, Intercept = 2.037, Deviance = 990.857. Random effects (participant) standard deviation = 0.898. Random effects (lexical item) standard deviation = 0.682.

(3080 tokens) and 84% of signs for colours (1021 tokens). Table 7 shows the number of lexical variants per item: over half of the items investigated (21 lexical items) exhibited eight or more lexical variants. Six of the stimuli have ten lexical variants and three have more than thirteen lexical variants ('grey', 'purple', 'thirteen').

**Conversational data.** To consider the use of traditional signs across settings all examples of the signs for colours, countries and numbers from the LFS conversational data were compared to those elicited as part of the lexical elicitation task. A total of 570 tokens were coded for analysis. Of these, 124 tokens (22%) were not the same sign variant as those elicited during the lexical elicitation task, suggesting that 78% of elicitations as part of the lexical elicitation task were an accurate representation of the signer's actual lexical use when there is less attention paid to their language production. There were 26 instances in which a response involved a signer using a traditional variant in one setting and another traditional variant in a different setting, or a non-traditional variant in one setting and a different non-traditional variant in another setting. Twelve percent of responses (15 of 124) involved the use of a non-traditional variant in the lexical elicitation task and a traditional variant in the conversational task. In sixty-seven percent of responses (83 of 124) a signer used a traditional variant in the lexical elicitation task and a non-traditional variant in the conversational task. Overall, the results indicate that the majority of signers used the same variant across different settings (conversation and the lexical elicitation tasks). In conversation, the more naturalistic setting, a minority of participants produced more non-traditional variants.

## Discussion

### Variation according to social factors and semantic category

Participants' use of traditional signs was conditioned by a number of social factors, in order of significance: age, school location, and language background. In this section, we discuss these findings in relation to previous sign language research, explore whether the results reveal language change in progress, and finally suggest what this study can tell us about the BSL variation in the future.

**Table 6.** Multiple logistic regression results for UK placenames.

| Lexical item | Factor | Log odds | Tokens | Centred Weight |
|---|---|---|---|---|
| Belfast | **Residents** | **8.395** | **30** | **>0.999** |
| | Non-residents | −8.395 | 219 | <0.001 |
| Birmingham | **Residents** | **0.72** | **30** | **0.673** |
| | Non-residents | −0.72 | 219 | 0.327 |
| Bristol | **Residents** | **1.024** | **32** | **0.736** |
| | Non-residents | −1.024 | 217 | 0.264 |
| Cardiff | **Residents** | **1.017** | **30** | **0.724** |
| | Non-residents | −1.017 | 217 | 0.266 |
| Newcastle | **Residents** | **1.347** | **30** | **0.794** |
| | Non-residents | −1.347 | 219 | 0.206 |

Application value: Local variant for region. All factor groups significant at p<.05.

**Table 7.** Number of lexical variants per concept.

| | **Number of stimuli** | | | | | | | |
|---|---|---|---|---|---|---|---|---|
| **Number of variants** | **0** | **1** | **2** | **3** | **4** | **5** | **6** | **7** |
| 1 | | | | x | | | | |
| 2 | | x | | | | | | |
| 3 | | | x | | | | | |
| 4 | | | | x | | | | |
| 5 | | | | x | | | | |
| 6 | | | | x | | | | |
| 7 | | | | | | x | | |
| 8 | | | | | | | | x |
| 9 | | | | x | | | | |
| 10 | | | | | | | x | |
| 11 | | | x | | | | | |
| 12 | x | | | | | | | |
| 13+ | | | | x | | | | |
| TOTAL | | | | | | | | |

The results suggest that age is the most significant factor predicting the use of traditional signs with a decline in use from older to younger signers. This was true, to differing degrees, across all regions. Some variants were found to be unique to certain age groups. For example, some number sign variants which originate from Irish Sign Language were not present at all in the data elicited from younger participants. These variants are associated with St. Vincent's School for deaf children in Glasgow, a Catholic school in which teachers used Irish Sign Language as the language of instruction until the 1950s [56]. This finding suggests that these variants may, with time, disappear from the BSL lexicon.

School location is the second most important factor predicting the use of traditional signs in BSL. Those individuals who were educated locally in our study used a higher proportion of regional signs than those individuals who had attended a school outside the region. The findings do suggest that, although individuals may have lived in a given region for the last 10 years, they do not entirely adapt their lexicon to the local variety. This finding appears to confirm the importance of schooling in the maintenance of regional variation in BSL, supporting Quinn's [23] findings that the BSL variants acquired at school strongly influence the variants used in adulthood. It also suggests that the geographical location of a participant's school might be a better predictor of lexicon in adulthood than current region of residence.

Language background is also a significant factor in predicting the use of non-traditional signs. Signers with deaf parents favour the use of traditional signs, supporting previous work on ASL which found that signers with deaf parents favour the use of 'conservative' variants [2]. The significance of language background is not surprising given that our age-related findings indicated that older signers use more traditional forms. It is likely that deaf children learning BSL from deaf parents will be exposed to a higher proportion of traditional variants compared to their counterparts from hearing families (since most hearing parents have not learned BSL before the birth of their deaf child). These findings highlight the importance of deaf native signers in maintaining and transmitting BSL regional variation.

Although semantic category was not a significant factor in predicting the use of traditional signs, the results indicate that some semantic categories are undergoing greater change than others. In this study, signs for countries are changing at a faster rate than signs for numbers and colours.

**Signs for countries.** Signs for countries appear to have undergone the most dramatic change. Around half of the responses by younger participants in the lexical elicitation task (302 tokens) were not traditional signs for their region. Younger and older signers may have adopted a different lexical variant later in life from the variant acquired in their early years. This is quite evident from the discussions between participants during the lexical elicitation task in which many older and younger signers explicitly mention the sign they formerly used and the sign they use now.

By comparing the traditional variant for each region to the most frequent non-traditional variant used amongst younger signers, we can observe the direction of change in some country name signs. For example, the traditional BSL sign meaning 'China' is produced at the eyes with a twist of the wrist of both hands (see CHINA, Figure 4). The use of this sign has been perceived by some both within the deaf community and outside it as 'politically incorrect', presumably because the sign depicts the characteristic eye shape of east Asian people [35–36]. The traditional variant glossed as CHINA, shared across all eight regions in the BSL Corpus dataset, is produced by 67% (164 participants) overall, although younger signers produce only 12% of this variant. Instead, a variant glossed as CHINA2 (Figure 4), which portrays an aspect of the country's national costume, is the most frequent non-traditional variant amongst younger signers. The sign variant CHINA2 was reported by Sutton-Spence and Woll [13] to have been introduced into BSL as a 'politically correct' alternative and is used by 61% of the younger corpus participants (47 participants) compared with only 24% of the older signers (18 participants).

The change in progress for signs meaning 'China' appears to be the same across all eight regions in the BSL Corpus Project. This shift in signs representing China co-occurred with the introduction of signs for other east Asian countries. The pattern of change (from

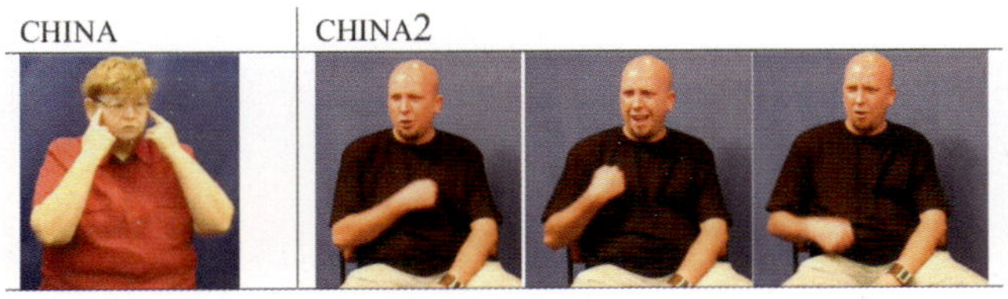


**Figure 4. Examples of variants for 'China' in BSL.**

a sign representing physical characteristics to one representing clothing) is not observed for other country name signs. For example, the BSL variant INDIA (Figure 5) is the traditional variant for 'India' in five of the eight collection sites of the BSL Corpus Project. This variant is produced at the forehead to represent the bindi or tilak worn by followers of the Hindu religion in India. This sign is perceived as inappropriate by some signers (see [13]), as it is seen to exclude Indian Muslims. In these five regions, 40% of participants (n = 75) do not report using this traditional sign, instead using INDIA2 (Figure 5), which is thought to depict the shape of the country. Of this 40%, 21% (n = 39) are younger signers, 10% (n = 19) are middle-aged signers, and 9% (n = 17) are older signers. In the remaining three regions, where the sign variant INDIA is not traditional, a similar proportion of participants are not using their traditional regional sign (38%, n = 23). Despite this, however, the most frequent non-traditional variant (used by 85%, n = 23 of participants) is INDIA. This suggests that political correctness does not explain all examples of language change in this component of the BSL lexicon.

Additionally, a small number of signers in the younger and middle groups are using a sign variant borrowed from Indian Sign Language [77]. It is interesting that this variant (INDIA5, Figure 5), referring to the same iconic feature as INDIA, is spreading while the traditional BSL sign appears to be falling out of favour. Thus the process of lexical change for this particular example is complex, and we could speculate that because of concerns about excluding Muslims (as noted above), some signers adopt the newer sign INDIA2, while others prefer to use lexical borrowing. This is consistent with work by Lucas and colleagues, [2] who suggested that similar changes in ASL were a means of showing respect for other cultures. Some signers may be making such choices consciously, following media coverage that has raised deaf community awareness of these changes (e.g., *See Hear* - [62]).

Lexical borrowing may be the source of several of the country signs in this study as we have seen with 'India'. Like 'India', the traditional variants for 'America' in all regions have been replaced amongst younger signers with the borrowed ASL form AMERICA (as in Figure 6). This can be seen in all regions except Belfast where AMERICA is already the traditional sign used amongst older signers (possibly reflecting known earlier language contact with ASL). Similarly in the case of 'Germany', lexical borrowing may have occurred much earlier than signs for the other countries, given that the sign used in DGS (Deutche Gebärdensprache, German Sign Language) to represent 'Germany' is also used by the oldest generation of BSL signers from four regions in the BSL Corpus dataset.

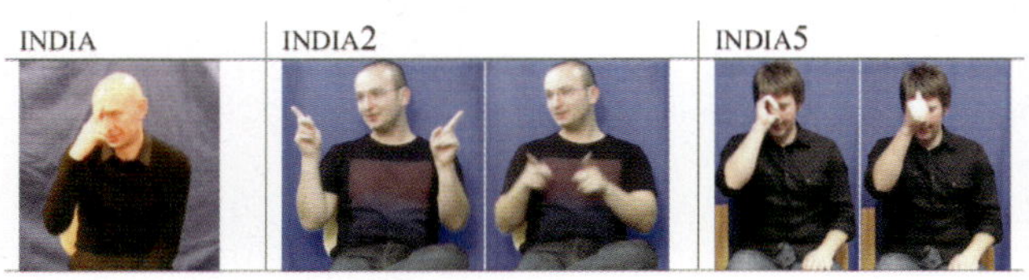


**Figure 5. Examples of sign variants for 'India' in BSL.**

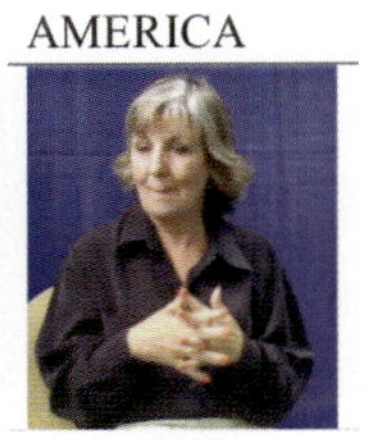


**Figure 6. Example of borrowed variant for 'America'.**

Finally, not all borrowed forms may come from the corresponding country's sign language. For example, we find that seven regions (again, except for Belfast which already uses IRELAND2, see Figure 7) share the traditional variant IRELAND produced with a flicking movement at the chest area (a popular anecdotal explanation for this sign is that it represents a shamrock). However, of these seven regions we find that 81% of signers (n = 44) who do not use the traditional variant, instead using a variant associated with ASL (see IRELAND2, Figure 7). Younger signers do not show any preference for IRELAND3, a form borrowed from Irish Sign Language (ISL).

To summarise, signs for countries in BSL have experienced rapid lexical innovation. This may, in some cases, be linked to pressures from political correctness but it may also reflect increased contact between deaf communities around the world leading to the borrowing of signs. The language change processes for signs for numbers and colours will be discussed in the next section.

## Language change & levelling

**Signs for numbers and colours.** Previous research has suggested that signs acquired first are generally maintained over a signer's lifetime [23]. The use of a high proportion of traditional signs for colours and numbers was also correlated with having been educated locally (unlike signs for countries, for which school location was not significantly associated with use of traditional signs), reinforcing the observation that signers maintain their school variants over the course of their lifetime. We adopt here the apparent time hypothesis to interpret the age-related results. A decrease in traditional number signs in younger age groups is an indicator that levelling may be taking place [11]. With number signs, younger signers appear to be adopting the two systems used in southern England (London or Bristol), both of which are widely known. Our levelling results resemble the findings of McKee and McKee [14] for NZSL. They concluded that there was evidence of increasing standardisation towards Australasian Signed English

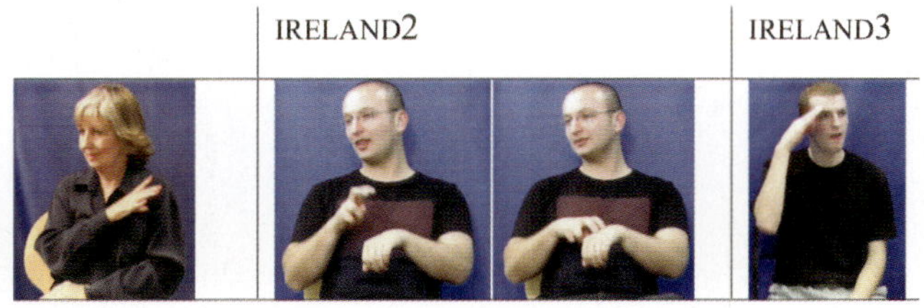


**Figure 7. Examples of the sign variants for the concept 'Ireland' in BSL.**

variants following the introduction of this signed English system in New Zealand deaf education from 1979. While the reasons for levelling in the current study remain unexplored, one possible cause for the rapid change is the loss of transmission following the closure of deaf schools.

In the dataset presented here, we have analysed the changes in colour signs as well as number signs. Results must be viewed with caution as the colour dataset is significantly smaller than the number dataset (17 target numeral stimuli compared to 5 target colour stimuli), but the results indicate that there have been fewer changes in colour signs than number signs. Age was found to be a contributing factor in the use of colour signs with younger signers using a decreasing proportion of traditional signs compared to older signers. Instead, those younger signers who used non-traditional signs used variants associated with the London region (e.g., BROWN3); variants associated with more than one region (e.g., GREEN1 in Manchester and London, GREY1 in Birmingham and London); or single manual letter forms, where the first letter of the corresponding lexical item in English is fingerspelled (e.g., GREY1, PURPLE1 and YELLOW1 are produced by using the fingerspelled letters 'g', 'p' and 'y' respectively, and in some cases modifying the movement). Overall, the patterns suggest that younger signers are using a variant that is widely used and/or reflects English influence.

**Signs for UK placenames.** With UK placenames, we were interested in the folk belief that residents of a city use a different sign variant for their city's name than non-residents. The only exceptions were the signs for 'Glasgow', 'London' and 'Manchester': almost all signers in all regions used the same lexical variant for 'Glasgow' (221 tokens), 'London' (244 tokens) and 'Manchester' (209 tokens). In most cases, the endonym, or local name for the city, was a reduced fingerspelled form, as described above, with the exception of the sign for 'Belfast'. The exonym, or name used for the city by individuals from outside that city, in some cases was a calque – i.e. a literal translation of the equivalent English words. For example, one exonym variant for 'Manchester' consists of a compound of individual signs MAN and CHEST. Other exonyms include the use of signs PISTOL or PETROL to refer to 'Bristol', perhaps because of similarities in the mouthing of these English words.

## Conclusion

In this investigation of lexical variation and change in signs for 41 key concepts in BSL, we have identified a number of processes taking place in the language that reflect different conditioning factors operating on different subsets of the data. Age is an important predictor of lexical variation and change across all groups of signs in this study. Signs for countries are subject to a number of external influences, including political correctness, changing attitudes towards lexical borrowing, and greater international mobility and transnational contact. The change we see here is age-graded, with anecdotal evidence of some older signers also adopting newly introduced variants. Changes in the use of traditional regional signs for colours and numbers, however, do not appear to be subject to changes in attitudes to language, but appear to reflect changes in the transmission of BSL as well as increased mobility within the UK and exposure to lexical variation in BSL via the media.

This descriptive and quantitative analysis of a large dataset of BSL provides a 'snapshot' of BSL lexical variation and change synchronically and suggests how societal changes have directly influenced BSL. This study lays the groundwork for more detailed ethnographic studies and investigations into the relationship between variation, change and language attitudes in the British deaf community.

## Acknowledgments

We gratefully acknowledge the following people: the project co-investigators (Margaret Deuchar, Frances Elton, Donall O'Baoill, Rachel Sutton-Spence, Graham Turner); Daniel Ezra Johnson for his continued support with the data analysis using RBrul; the Deaf Community Advisory Group members for their advice and assistance (Lorna Allsop, Linda Day, Clark Denmark, Helen Foulkes, Melinda Napier, Tessa Padden, Gary Quinn and Kate Rowley); the project's research associate (Sally Reynolds) and to our deaf community fieldworkers who made the data collection possible (Jeff Brattan-Wilson, Mischa Cooke, Avril Hepner, Sarah Lawrence, Dawn Marshall, Evelyn McFarland, Carolyn Nabarro, Melinda Napier, Mark Nelson, Jacqueline Parker, and Jenny Wilkins). We are grateful to Jackie Carcillo for cross-checking the data coding for this study and to John Holliday for his continued support in using ArcGIS mapping. Finally, we extend special thanks to all of the deaf individuals who participated in the BSL Corpus Project: without their participation, none of this research would have been possible.

## Author Contributions

Conceived and designed the experiments: AS. Performed the experiments: AS JF RR. Analyzed the data: RS AS. Contributed reagents/materials/analysis tools: RS AS JF RR KC. Wrote the paper: RS AS JF RR KC BW.

## References

1. Cormier K, Fenlon J, Johnston T, Rentelis R, Schembri A, et al. (2012) From Corpus to Lexical Database to Online Dictionary: Issues in Annotation of the BSL Corpus and the Development of BSL SignBank. In Crasborn O, Efthimiou E, Fotinea E, Hanke T, Kristoffersen J, et al., editors. 5th Workshop on the Representation of Sign Languages: Interactions between Corpus and Lexicon [workshop part of 8th International Conference on Language Resources and Evaluation, Turkey, Istanbul LREC 2012. Paris: ELRA. pp. 7–12.
2. Lucas C, Bayley R, Valli C (2001) Sociolinguistic Variation in American Sign Language. Washington, D.C.: Gallaudet University Press.
3. Katseff S (2004) From Symbol to System: The Development of Number Signs in Nicaraguan Sign Language. Presentation at the Theoretical Issues in Sign Language Research (TISLR 8). Barcelona.
4. Weinreich U, Labov W, Herzog MI (1968) Empirical foundations for a theory of language change. University of Texas Press.
5. Labov W (1972) Sociolinguistic Patterns. Philadelphia: University of Pennsylvania Press.
6. Stamp R, Schembri A, Fenlon J, Rentelis R (under review) Sociolinguistic Variation and Change in British Sign Language Number Signs. Journal of Sociolinguistics.
7. Woll B (1987) Historical and Comparative Aspects of British Sign Language. In Kyle J, editor. Sign and School: Using Signs in Deaf Children's Development. Clevedon: Multilingual Matters Ltd. pp. 12–34.
8. Woll B (1994) The Influence of Television on the Deaf Community in Britain. In Ahlgren I, Bergman B, Brennan M, editors. Perspectives on Sign Language Use: Papers from the Fifth International Symposium on Sign Language Research: Volume 2. Durham: The International Sign Linguistics Association. pp. 293–301.
9. Schembri A, Fenlon J, Rentelis R, Reynolds S, Cormier K (2013) Building the British Sign Language Corpus. Language Documentation and Conservation 7: 136–154.
10. Giles H, Powesland P (1997) Accommodation theory. In Coupland N, Jaworski A, editors. Sociolinguistics: A reader. Basingstoke: Macmillan. pp. 232–239.
11. Trudgill P (1986) Dialects in Contact. Oxford: Basil Blackwell.
12. Elton F (2010) Changing the Way we Sign: An Analysis of the Signing Style used by Translators in the Queen's Christmas Speech since the 1980s. Birkbeck College, University of London.
13. Sutton-Spence R, Woll B (1999) The Linguistics of British Sign Language: An Introduction. Cambridge: Cambridge University Press.
14. McKee R, McKee D (2011) Old Signs, New Signs, Whose Signs? Sociolinguistic Variation in the NZSL Lexicon. Sign Language Studies 11(4): 485–527.

15. Office for National Statistics UK (2011) 2011 Census: Quick Statistics for England and Wales, March 2011. Available: http://www.ons.gov.uk/ons/rel/census/2011-census/key-statistics-and-quick-statistics-for-wards-and-output-areas-in-england-and-wales/STB-2011-census-quick-statistics-for-england-and-wales-march-2011.html. Accessed 2014 Feb 1.
16. Johnston T (2003) BSL, Auslan and NZSL: Three Signed Languages or One? In Baker A, Van den Bogaerde B, Crasborn O, editors. Cross-linguistic Perspectives in Sign Language Research, Selected Papers from TISLR 2000. Hamburg: Signum Verlag. pp. 47–69.
17. Mitchell RE, Karchmer MA (2004) Chasing the Mythical Ten Percent: Parental Hearing Status of Deaf and Hard of Hearing Students in the United States. Sign Language Studies 4(2): 138–163.
18. Uus K, Bamford JM (2006) Effectiveness of Population-Based Newborn Hearing Screening in England: Ages of Interventions and Profile of Cases Pediatrics 117(5): e887–e893.
19. Bonvillian RJ, Folven JD (1993) Sign Language Acquisition: Developmental Aspects. In Marschark M, Clark DM, editors. Psychological Perspective on Deafness. Hillsdale, NJ: Lawrence Erlbaum Associates. pp. 229–265.
20. Woll B, Sutton-Spence R, Elton F (2001) Multilingualism: The Global Approach to Sign Languages. In Lucas C, editor. The Sociolinguistics of Sign Languages. Cambridge: Cambridge University Press. pp. 8–32.
21. Ladd P (2003) Understanding Deaf Culture: In Search of Deafhood. Clevedon: Multilingual Matters Ltd.
22. Jackson P (1990) Britain's Deaf Heritage. Michigan: The Pentland Press.
23. Quinn G (2010) Schoolization: An Account of the Origins of Regional Variation in British Sign Language. Sign Language Studies 10(4): 476–501.
24. Fenlon J, Schembri A, Rentelis R, Cormier K (2013) Variation in Handshape and Orientation in British Sign Language: The Case of the "1" Hand Configuration. Language and Communication 33: 69–91.
25. The Warnock Report (1978) Report of the Committee of Enquiry into the Education of Handicapped Children and Young People. Retrieved from http://www.educationengland.org.uk/documents/warnock/ Accessed January 22 2014.
26. Kyle J, Woll B (1993) Language in Sign: The Development of Deaf Children's Communication in Sign Language. Bristol: University of Bristol.
27. Lane H (1992) The Mask of Benevolence: Disabling the Deaf Community. New York: Alfred A. Knopf.
28. Marschark M (2007) Raising and Educating a Deaf Child: A Comprehensive Guide to the Choices, Controversies, and Decisions faced by Parents and Educators (2nd ed.). Oxford: Oxford University Press.
29. Schembri A (2010) Documenting Sign Languages. In Austin PK, editor. Language Documentation and Description, Volume 7. London: SOAS. pp. 105–143.
30. Schembri A, Cormier K, Johnston T, McKee D, McKee R, et al. (2010) Sociolinguistic Variation in British, Australian and New Zealand Sign Language. In Brentari D, editor. Sign Languages. Cambridge: Cambridge University Press. pp. 476–498.
31. Watt D (2002) "I don't speak with a Geordie accent, I speak, like, the Northern accent": Contact-induced Levelling in the Tyneside Vowel System. Journal of Sociolinguistics 6 (1): 44–63.
32. Williams A, Kerswill P (1999) Dialect Levelling: Change and Continuity in Milton Keynes, Reading and Hull. In Foulkes P, Docherty G, editors. Urban Voices: Accent Studies in the British Isles. London: Arnold. pp. 141–162.
33. Hiddinga A, Crasborn O (2011) Signed Languages and Globalization. Language in Society 40: 483–505.
34. Hoyer K (2007) Albanian Sign Language: Language Contact, International Sign, and Gesture. In Quinto-Pozos D, editor. Sign Languages in Contact. Washington, D.C.: Gallaudet University Press. pp. 195–234.
35. Mickelburgh R, Syal R (2004, March 21) Limp wrists and slant eyes must go as political correctness demands new signs for the deaf. The Telegraph. Retrieved from http://www.telegraph.co.uk/news/uknews/1457400/Limp-wrists-and-slant-eyes-must-go-as-political-correctness-demands-new-signs-for-the-deaf.html Accessed on January 21 2014 .
36. The Sun Newspaper (2004, March 22) Sign of times. The Sun, p. 8.
37. Bayley R (2002) The Quantitative Paradigm. In Chambers JK, Trudgill P, Schilling-Estes N, editors. The Handbook of Language Variation and Change. Oxford: Blackwell. pp. 312–322.
38. Cheshire J (2002) Sex and Gender in Variationist Research. In Chambers JK, Trudgill P, Schilling-Estes N, editors. The Handbook of Language Variation and Change. Oxford: Blackwell. pp. 423–443.
39. Coates J, Sutton-Spence R (2001) Turn-taking Patterns in Deaf Conversation. Journal of Sociolinguistics 5(4): 507–529.
40. Le Master B, Dwyer JP (1991). Knowing and Using Female and Male Signs in Dublin. Sign Language Studies 73: 361–369.
41. Ash S (2002) Social Class. In Chambers JK, Trudgill P, Schiling-Estes N, editors. The Handbook of Language Variation and Change. Oxford: Blackwell. pp. 402–422.
42. Sutton-Spence R, Woll B, Allsop L (1990) Variation and Recent Change in Fingerspelling in British Sign Language. Language Variation and Change 2: 313–330.
43. Johnston T, Schembri A (2007) Australian Sign Language (Auslan): An Introduction to Sign Language Linguistics. Cambridge: Cambridge University Press.
44. Kyle J, Woll B (1985) Sign Language: The Study of Deaf People and their Language. Cambridge: Cambridge University Press.
45. Armstrong N (2001) Social and Stylistic Variation in Spoken French: A Comparative Approach. Amsterdam: Benjamins.
46. Chambers JK (1999) Converging features in the Englishes of North America. Cuadernos de Filologia Inglesa 8: 117–127.
47. Chambers JK (2000) Region and Language Variation. English World-wide 21: 1–31.
48. Chambers JK (2004) "Canadian Dainty": the rise and decline of Briticisms in Canada. In Hickey R, editor. The Legacy of Colonial English: A Study of Transported Dialects. Cambridge: Cambridge University Press. pp. 224–241.
49. Lodge RA (2004) A Sociolinguistic History of Parisian French. Cambridge: Cambridge University Press.
50. Sankoff D (1988) Sociolinguistics and Syntactic Variation. In Newmeyer F, editor. Language: The Socio-cultural Context. Cambridge: Cambridge University Press. pp. 140–161.
51. Bayard D (1989) "Me say that? No way!": The Social Correlates of American Lexical Diffusion in New Zealand English. Te Reo 32: 17–60.
52. Nagy N (2011) Lexical Change and Language Contact: Faetar in Italy and Canada. Journal of Sociolinguistics 15(3): 366–382.
53. Tagliamonte S, D'Arcy A (2007) Frequency and Variation in the Community Grammar: Tracking a New Change through the Generations. Language Variation and Change 19(2): 199–217.
54. Schembri A, McKee D, McKee R, Pivac S, Johnston T, et al. (2009) Phonological Variation and Change in Australian and New Zealand Sign Languages: The Location Variable. Language Variation and Change 21: 193–231.
55. Francis WN (1983) Dialectology: An Introduction. London: Longman.
56. Foran C (1995) Vincentian Ministry to Deaf People in Scotland. Contact: Voice of the Irish Deaf Community. 23.
57. Matthews PA (1996) The Irish Deaf Community Volume 1: Survey Report, History of Education, Language and Culture. Dublin: Linguistics Institute of Ireland.
58. Woll B, Allsop L, Sutton-Spence R (1991) Variation and Recent Change in British Sign Language: Final Report to the ESRC. Bristol.
59. Valli C, Lucas C, Mulrooney K (2005) Linguistics of American Sign Language: An Introduction. Washington, D.C.: Gallaudet University Press.
60. Schembri A, Fenlon J, Rentelis R, Cormier K (2011) British Sign Language Corpus Project: A Corpus of Digital Video Data of British Sign Language 2008–2010 (First Edition). Retrieved from http://www.bslcorpusproject.org Accessed on December 2 2013.
61. Schembri A (2008) The British Sign Language Corpus Project: Open Access Archives and the Observer's Paradox. Presented at the Conference on Construction and Exploitation of Sign Language Corpora. Marrakesh.
62. Schembri A, Fenlon J, Rentelis R (2009) The British Sign Language (BSL) Corpus Project: Sociolinguistic variation, language change, language contact and lexical frequency in BSL. See Hear, BBC.
63. Brien D (1992) Dictionary of British Sign Language/English. London: Faber and Faber.
64. Crasborn O, Sloetjes H (2008) Enhanced ELAN functionality for sign language corpora. Proceedings of 3rd Workshop on the Representation and Processing of Sign Languages: Construction and Exploitation of Sign Language Corpora. pp. 39–43.
65. Johnston T, Schembri A (1999) On defining lexeme in a signed language. Sign Language & Linguistics 2(2): 115–185.
66. Johnston T (2010) From Archive to Corpus: Transcription and Annotation in the Creation of Signed Language Corpora. International Journal of Corpus Linguistics 15: 106–131.
67. Elton F, Squelch L (2008) British Sign Language: London and South-East Regional Signs. London: Lexisigns.
68. Woll B, Allsop L, Sutton-Spence R, Walker S (1990) Sign Language Varieties in British Television: An Historical Perspective. In Prillwitz S, Vollhaber T, editors. Current Trends in European Sign Language Research. Hamburg: Signum. pp. 60–72.
69. Eckert P (1997) Age as a Sociolinguistic Variable. In Coulmas F, editor. The Handbook of Sociolinguistics. Oxford: Blackwell. pp. 151–167
70. Sutton-Spence R (1994) The Role of the Manual Alphabet and Fingerspelling in British Sign Language. University of Bristol: Bristol, Unpublished Ph.D. thesis.
71. Cormier K, Schembri A, Tyrone M (2008) One hand or two? Nativisation of fingerspelling in ASL and BANZSL. Sign Language and Linguistics11(1): 3–44.
72. Cormier K, Fenlon J, Rentelis R, Schembri A (2011) Lexical Frequency in British Sign Language Conversation: A Corpus-Based Approach. Proceedings of the Conference on Language Documentation and Linguistic Theory 3 (LDLT3). London: School of Oriental and African Studies.
73. Johnson DE (2009) Getting off the GoldVarb Standard: Introducing Rbrul for Mixed-Effects Variable Rule Analysis. Language and Linguistics Compass 3(1): 359–383.

74. Rand D, Sankoff D (1991) GoldVarb 2.1: A Variable Rule Application for Macintosh. Montreal: Centre de recherches mathematiques.
75. Baayen RH, Davidson DJ, Bates DM (2008) Mixed Effects Modeling with Crossed Random Effects for Subjects and Items. Journal of Memory and Language 59: 390–412.
76. Jaeger TF (2008) Categorical Data Analysis: Away from ANOVAs (Transformation or Not) and Towards Logit Mixed Models. Journal of Memory and Language 59: 434–446.
77. The World Federation of the Deaf (2003) Country Name Sign Book. Helsinki: World Federation of the Deaf.

# 24

# Sign Language Ability in Young Deaf Signers Predicts Comprehension of Written Sentences in English

**Kathy N. Andrew, Jennifer Hoshooley, Marc F. Joanisse***

Department of Psychology and Brain and Mind Institute, The University of Western Ontario, London, Ontario, Canada

## Abstract

We investigated the robust correlation between American Sign Language (ASL) and English reading ability in 51 young deaf signers ages 7;3 to 19;0. Signers were divided into 'skilled' and 'less-skilled' signer groups based on their performance on three measures of ASL. We next assessed reading comprehension of four English sentence structures (actives, passives, pronouns, reflexive pronouns) using a sentence-to-picture-matching task. Of interest was the extent to which ASL proficiency provided a foundation for lexical and syntactic processes of English. Skilled signers outperformed less-skilled signers overall. Error analyses further indicated greater single-word recognition difficulties in less-skilled signers marked by a higher rate of errors reflecting an inability to identify the actors and actions described in the sentence. Our findings provide evidence that increased ASL ability supports English sentence comprehension both at the levels of individual words and syntax. This is consistent with the theory that first language learning promotes second language through transference of linguistic elements irrespective of the transparency of mapping of grammatical structures between the two languages.

**Editor:** Frederic Dick, Birkbeck College, United Kingdom

**Funding:** This research was supported by an NSERC Canada Graduate Scholarship to KNM and an NSERC operating grant to MFJ. The funders had no role in study design, data collection and analysis, decision to publish, or preparation of the manuscript.

**Competing Interests:** The authors have declared that no competing interests exist.

* E-mail: marcj@uwo.ca

## Introduction

Learning to read is a difficult task for most deaf individuals. Sign languages like American Sign Language (ASL) do not have a written form, and a written language like English is not an orthographic code for a signed language. Thus, a deaf individual who is learning to read is literally learning a foreign language through a modality that is only partially accessible (i.e., through orthography but not phonology).

One of the principal explanations for reading difficulties in deaf signers is their lack of access to the phonological code of a written language [1–2]. Hearing individuals learn a spoken language through the auditory modality prior to learning to read, and subsequently learn to map the written word onto their knowledge of this spoken code. Thus, when a hearing reader sees a word on the page they have access to the word's orthographic form and, at least in alphabetic orthographies like English, can compute its phonological form. This access to phonology allows hearing readers to parse written words into their individual phonemes making the semantics of even unfamiliar words accessible through decomposition. Deaf readers on the other hand must rely more heavily on orthography to access meaning in written language (notwithstanding evidence suggesting that some higher-achieving deaf readers have some limited access to phonology [3–5]).

Although learning to read is difficult for all deaf individuals, there can be significant variation in this respect, and for reasons that are not always transparent. That said, degree of ASL proficiency has been repeatedly shown to be the single best predictor of English reading outcomes in the deaf population (for a review and meta-analysis, see [6]). For instance, Strong and Prinz [7] compared ASL signers with low, medium and high signing ability on English proficiency, where proficiency in either language was operationalized as a composite score of a variety of comprehension and production tasks. They found that ASL skill was significantly correlated with English ability, such that the high ability group outperformed both the medium and low ability groups, and the medium ability group outperformed the lowest ability group. The authors present this finding as evidence that increased levels of ASL ability lead to increased English proficiency. Padden and Ramsey [8] drew similar conclusions defining English ability via a collection of subtasks from the Stanford Achievement Test (adapted for deaf participants).

Several others have reported similar findings, where ASL proficiency is correlated with English reading outcomes, both in children [9–11] and adults [12]. However these studies all examined the relationship between ASL and English in a relatively broad sense, using general comprehension and production tasks spanning a range of language abilities.

In contrast, studies have not tended to investigate this issue with regard to finer-grained aspects of language processing. An exception here is Mayberry and Lock [13], who assessed performance on specific English sentence constructions including a passive sentence construction, and found that deaf adults who had early language exposure performed similarly to native English speakers, whereas deaf adults without early language exposure performed more poorly on this construction.

The present study takes a closer look at English syntactic comprehension in deaf signers of ASL, with regard both to individuals' comprehension accuracy as well as the types of errors produced by both deaf individuals and hearing native English speakers. Our goal was to investigate in a more detailed manner whether ASL proficiency predicts learning specific elements of English grammar, or whether it is limited to a more basic transfer like vocabulary learning.

This investigation builds on two models of second language learning that focus on the role of first language (L1) proficiency in determining second language (L2) outcomes. Cummins' Linguistic Interdependence Hypothesis [14] proposes that L2 learning is dependent on the degree to which the individual has learned L1 before extensive exposure to L2 begins. Accordingly, for primarily unilingual children to effectively learn L2, it is essential that a concretely link first be established between real world concepts and L1 lexical items. MacWhinney's Unified Competition Model [15] represents a more comprehensive view of this relationship where not only lexical items transfer between languages. Elaborating on the earlier Competition Model of learning [16], it proposes that initially, learners infer that L2 properties map directly onto L1, regardless of actual fit, and that this occurs across multiple levels of linguistic analysis including lexical knowledge but also sensory processing, and sentence comprehension (described by MacWhinney as: 'grammatical role decoding' plus 'comprehension'). For the purposes of our study, we focus on the lexical and sentence comprehension levels since there is no clear mechanism by which one can gauge the sensory processing similarities of an ASL sign and a printed English word.

Transference in lexical knowledge takes place when there is high conceptual overlap between lexical items in L1 and L2. ASL learners should find it easier to comprehend English words when they can be directly mapped onto known signs. In both Cummins' and MacWhinney's models, L1 acts as an intermediary between the lexical item in L2 and the concept itself. This raises the first question of the present study: is the relationship between L1 and L2 learning in ASL strictly due to better signers having larger vocabularies, and thus being better able to map known concepts onto written English words?

The alternative is that L2 facilitation occurs at both the lexical and sentence comprehension (syntactic) levels. The task of understanding a full sentence goes well beyond assigning meaning to the individual words in a sentence. In order to extract the full meaning of the sentence, readers must also understand the language's syntactic constructions. According to the Unified Competition Model successful transference of L2 syntactic structures to L1 depends on the degree of syntactic match between those structures. Transference in sentence comprehension can thus be described as the extent to which syntactic principles of L1 reflect syntactic principles in L2.

As it turns out, English syntactic constructions vary with respect to how transparently they map onto ASL constructions. This permits us to examine whether the relative similarity of an ASL and English construction affects signers' ability to learn the construction in English. In this study we addressed this via four sentence types, active, passive, pronoun, reflexive pronoun, which map between languages to differing degrees. We group these sentence types into two separate syntactic investigations: pronoun binding trials (pronouns, reflexives) and word order trials (actives, passives).

Non-reflexive and reflexive pronouns exist in both ASL and English: while ASL uses spatial cues, inflections on agreeing verbs and even eye gaze to bind a pronoun or reflexive to its antecedent, in English this is achieved through a syntactic relationship. In English, non-reflexive pronouns refer back to an earlier antecedent that is indicated by a different word at an earlier point in a sentence (e.g., *him* refers back to *John* in "John said that Alice likes him"). Sometimes understanding who is being referred to by the pronoun is non-ambiguous, as in the example above. Other times, the relationship is more ambiguous (e.g., *him* refers back to *John* in "John said that Jack likes him"). In contrast, ASL pronoun use is accomplished by indexing the exact location in which the entity was previously set up in physical space. Since all possible referents occupy their own unique position in the signing space, identifying the antecedent of a pronoun is non-ambiguous in ASL [17]. As such, we propose that non-reflexive English pronoun sentences may be difficult for signers due to the potential for ambiguity in these constructions, which does not map clearly onto ASL pronouns.

Reflexive pronouns also exist in both English and ASL. In English they take the form, *herself*, *itself* etc., always ending in the marker, *self*. ASL employs a specific handshape (the 'A' handshape) that indicates the idea of SELFNESS when articulated in the direction of the referent's spatial location as established by the signer, (e.g., HIMSELF, MYSELF). Thus reflexives are produced similarly in the two languages, both using a specific marker (*self* in the case of English, and the *A* handshape in the case of ASL) to clearly identify the reflexive pronoun. We expect that these sentences will be less difficult for signers than the non-reflexive pronouns because the mapping between languages is more straightforward.

The most prominent description of the structure of pronouns comes from Chomsky's Binding Theory [18]. The theory explains why *mother*, but not *girl*, is an acceptable antecedent to *herself* in the reflexive pronoun sentence, "The girl says the mother washes herself", and why *father*, but not *boy*, is an acceptable antecedent to *him* in the non-reflexive pronoun sentence, "The father says the boy pushed him." Previous research suggests that children typically acquire comprehension of reflexives earlier and more consistently than non-reflexives [19–21].

The second syntactic manipulation of interest in this study involved the active/passive alternation in word order. This is of interest since ASL permits some freedom in choice of word order. However, the principle of economization demands clarity and efficiency in ASL [17] such that signers tend to focus production on content, exclude function words, and minimize the use of word orders that add unnecessary lexical items and ambiguity to utterances. Indeed in both English and ASL the most typical way to express a transitive relationship is S-V-O [22]. Note that there are reports of passive-like constructions in ASL, where a signer takes on the role of the object of the sentence, thereby shifting focus toward the object. For instance, Janzen et al. [23] suggest the example of "a girl punching a boy." In order to explain what is happening in the picture, the signer might use the location of signs relative to their own body position in order to set up the girl on the right (with body facing slightly left) and the boy on the left (with body facing slightly right). The signer then reassumes the position of the girl and produces a punching motion in the direction of the boy, then quickly switches *to become the body of the boy while the signer's oncoming fist is understood to be that of the girl's*. The italicized portion of the above sentence where the boy is looking towards the oncoming fist from the direction of the girl might be taken as an equivalent to the English passive: "the boy was punched by the girl". While this shift in focus is what we consider to be a passive in English, when it is used in ASL there is much set up before the production of the passive-like formation. That is, the passive-like construction does not stand alone as a full sentence but rather is part of the sentence that serves to emphasize focus on the object at a particular point within the sentence. A true ASL equivalent of the English passive construction is thus difficult to positively identify and has gone largely unmentioned in studies of ASL acquisition. Since it does not compare well to English passives it seems reasonable to assume that the mapping between the constructions (if ASL does in fact have such a construction) in the two languages is non-obvious at best.

There is good evidence that hearing children acquire passives later than active sentences [24] especially 'reversible' passives (e.g., "The mother was hugged by the daughter") where the subject and object can only be inferred through syntactic means. There is also some evidence that deaf signers perform poorly on passives relative to same age hearing children, though less is known as to whether this is due to a general difficulty in word recognition, or a more specific difficulty with processing English syntactic structures [25].

### Rationale of present study

We examined how general ASL proficiency relates to increased English sentence comprehension in school-age deaf signers. The Linguistic Interdependence Hypothesis and the Unified Competition Model both predict that skilled signers should show better reading outcomes than less-skilled signers because increased ASL ability should facilitate English reading ability in a concrete manner: transference of lexical items should allow for comprehension of individual English words. Further, the Unified Competition Model predicts that facilitation should also occur at the level of sentence comprehension, such that more advanced ASL signers should have improved ability to decode English syntax. We examined the key assumption in both theories, that L2 proficiency reflects L1 proficiency, as well as the ways in which L1 proficiency constrains L2 learning with the Unified Competition Model in mind. Of interest was distinguishing advantages due to improved single word reading skill from more advanced syntactic comprehension strategies.

In order to investigate these questions, participants performed an assessment of ASL abilities (which included vocabulary, sign decision, and story comprehension measures) and an English sentence comprehension task that spanned four sentence structures (active, passive, pronoun and reflexive). Participants were divided into two groups based on signing achievement, and English sentence comprehension (accuracy and error tendencies) was compared across groups. We expected to see increased syntactic processing ability by skilled signers relative to less-skilled signers marked by increased accuracy on across the syntactic structures. This finding would be consistent with the Linguistic Interdependence Hypothesis where second language acquisition reflects first language proficiency. Additionally, we expected less-skilled signers to make both word recognition and syntactic parsing errors, but skilled signers to tend towards syntactic parsing errors only. This finding would be consistent with the Unified Competition Model such that even when syntax becomes an obstacle less-skilled signers continue to use their lexical knowledge to approach the correct answer. Further in line with the Unified Competition Model, we expected passive sentences to be particularly difficult for all deaf readers, since there is no obvious analogue in ASL, and exposure to English passives is limited in the deaf population [26]. While both the Linguistic Interdependence Hypothesis and the Unified Competition Model were conceived of to explain L2 learning in relation to L1 proficiency in spoken languages, here the models are used in a novel fashion—to explain L2 learning of a written language in relation to L1 proficiency of a signed language.

In addition to the deaf participants, ten hearing children were assessed on the English sentence comprehension task. These children were included in the study not as a control group *per se*, but only to provide a baseline of how hearing children perform on this task. Our goal was not to draw direct comparisons between the hearing and deaf groups, only to have the hearing group serve as a qualitative indicator of what should be expected in terms of native English sentence reading ability.

## Methods

### Participants

All procedures were approved by The University of Western Ontario Office of Research Ethics. A total of 51 deaf children and adolescents, ages 7;3 to 19;0, were recruited from two Schools for the deaf in southern Ontario. Six were children of deaf parents, and all reported first exposure to ASL before the onset of puberty. Written informed consent was obtained from individuals older than 18 years, or from a parent for all individuals younger than 18 years of age. ASL was the exclusive language of instruction and communication inside and outside the classroom, the one exception being English literacy training, which occurred through reading and writing activities. All students used ASL to communicate and were severe to profoundly deaf (70+ dB hearing thresholds).

A group of ten hearing children, ages 8;02 to 8;11 were also included in the study. These children were recruited through The University of Western Ontario Participant Pool and were assessed in our laboratory.

### Procedures

The deaf children were tested individually in a private room in their school, over two sessions. Session one consisted of the ASL and English reading tasks, and took approximately 40 minutes to complete. Session two consisted of a hearing assessment and a nonverbal intelligence test. Note that this study was part of a larger research project that investigated the factors influencing English and ASL proficiency in deaf children, and included some additional tasks intended to test phonological and single-word knowledge in ASL and English. Those tasks did not involve sentence recognition skills and so data from them are not reported in the present study.

Stimuli for the language tasks in session one were presented via a 12-inch Macintosh PowerBook or a 13-inch MacBook computer placed directly in front of the seated participant. The researcher sat next to the participant and recorded responses on prepared score sheets. As described below, all language tasks were receptive in nature, and therefore the experimenter was not required to interpret children's signs. However the experimenter was a fluent (hearing) signer and was able to answer any questions that arose during the sessions. Sequence of task presentation was held constant across participants, in the order indicated below.

**ASL assessment.** Three receptive sign language proficiency tasks were administered. We used receptive ASL tasks to maximize comparability to written English comprehension, which is itself a receptive task. Standardized language measures exist for both ASL [27] and English [28]. However, the following tasks were used here since the present experiment was part of a larger study that selectively assessed specific aspects of ASL and English proficiency in a way that was matched across both languages. This is somewhat harder to do using standardized tests, which tend to be quite lengthy and/or conflate different aspects of processing into a single score.

In the *ASL Vocabulary Task*, participants saw four pictures (one target picture and three distractors) arranged into each corner of the computer screen. A video clip appeared at the center of the screen, depicting a native signer producing an ASL sign. The participant was asked to point to the picture that correctly matched the sign. The researcher provided feedback on four practice items, 16 test items followed without feedback (Appendix S1 in File S1).

In the *ASL Sign Decision Task*, participants saw pairs of video clips, each depicting a single ASL sign. In each pair, one clip contained a true ASL sign; the other contained a permutation of that true sign making it invalid. Incorrect foils were created by changing either the handshape, point of articulation or movement feature of the valid sign [29]. In this task the participant was asked to point to the correct sign in the pair. The researcher provided feedback on four practice items, 18 test items followed without feedback (Appendix S2 in File S1). One of these items contained a potentially ambiguous sign pair, and was removed from analyses.

In the *ASL Story Comprehension Task*, participants viewed videos of short stories told in ASL, each of which was followed by five multiple-choice comprehension questions also presented in ASL. The stories and questions were adapted by a native deaf signer from items in Form A of the Gray Oral Reading Test version 4 (GORT-4 [30]; items 1, 2, 4, 6 & 8), ordered with respect to story length and difficulty. We chose to adapt an existing English test to ASL only because it provided a set of stories and questions that are known to be age-appropriate and minimize effects of real-world knowledge that can potentially contaminate story comprehension measures. Moreover, the new task did not assess English reading or the comprehension of syntactic structures in ASL, only ASL story comprehension ability. To begin each trial, the signer presented a short story. Signed instructions indicated that the story could not be repeated—participants had only one opportunity to become familiar with each story. At the end of each story, five new ASL clips appeared on screen; at the center was a video of a question pertaining to the story, and at each corner was a video presenting one of four possible answers. The question and possible answers were played in succession thereby allowing participants to see all of the options. Participants responded by pointing to the video depicting the correct answer. Participants were allowed to view the question and the possible answers as many times as they wished. Prior to the test items, participants viewed a practice story complete with questions and potential answers, to ensure that they understood the task. Feedback was provided during the practice story and questions only. The task was terminated early if a participant answered incorrectly to four or more questions on any one story.

Of primary interest in this study was the degree to which overall receptive ASL proficiency is related to English sentence comprehension. To this end, we obtained a composite score of ASL ability by calculating the average proportion of items correct across all three tasks, with all tasks weighted equally. This composite score was then used to group participants into two groups, henceforth skilled and less-skilled signers. Note that a median split was used to divide signers into these separate groups, and therefore the labels are used in a strictly relative sense rather than to suggest an objective judgment of unusually poor signing ability in the less-skilled group. However, since the goal of the study was to examine differences in English syntactic comprehension between the lower and higher ends of the ASL ability, the distinction serves as a useful way to examine these differences.

**English sentence comprehension.** Participants were presented with four pictures (one target picture and three distractors; Figure 1) arranged into each corner of the computer screen. At the same time, a written English sentence appeared across the center of the screen in 44 point sans serif font, without obstructing the pictures. Picture stimuli were cartoon illustrations depicting transitive actions (e.g., washing, pinching, pointing) being performed by humans or other animate creatures (e.g., dogs, cats, turtles). The participant's task was to read the sentence and point to the picture that correctly depicted it. The researcher provided feedback on four practice items, followed by 16 test items presented without feedback. (Appendix S3 in File S1). Both deaf and hearing children participated in this task whereas only the deaf children participated in the previously described ASL measures.

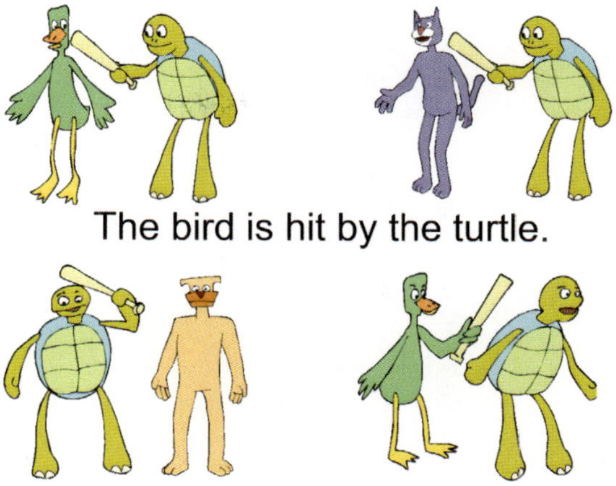


**Figure 1. English Sentence Comprehension task.** Individuals viewed a written English sentence and chose among four cartoon depictions. Foils included near-miss items (bottom right – agent and patient are reversed) and other-miss items (e.g., top-right and bottom-left picture, which involve actors that are not mentioned in the sentence).

The task was designed to assess comprehension of four types of syntactic constructions: active, passive, pronoun and reflexive pronoun sentences. Examples of each construction were presented four times each throughout the task, for a total of 16 sentences. Each sentence involved a variety of actors and actions including male and female humans, and also common animals. Note that plausibility was maintained for all items, for instance by having all actors variably depicted as subject or object of the verbs, and by depicting animals in a cartoon-like way such that it was possible for them to be pictured either as agent or patient. Sentences were designed so that both proportion correct and proportion of error types could be analyzed. There were two possible types of errors represented on each trial: 'near-misses' (at a rate of .25 per trial) and 'other-misses' (at a rate of .50 per trial). As explained more fully below and in Figure 1, a 'near-miss' involved pointing to a picture that included the mentioned actor(s) and action but did not involve the correct configuration of agent and patient. These errors were considered closer to the correct response than the 'other miss' since selection of this picture foil demonstrated recognition of the lexical items in the sentence in spite of incorrectly parsing its syntactic form. In contrast, 'other-miss' errors depicted characters, or relationships between the characters, that were unrelated to the target sentence, and thus illustrated a relatively weaker comprehension of the written English sentence.

A near-miss took on two possible forms in this experiment depending on which type of sentence was presented. In the case of active and passive sentences, a near-miss was one in which the patient and the agent were switched (i.e., a word order error). For example, in a sentence that read, "The mother washes the girl" (or in the passive sentences, "The girl is washed by the mother") the near-miss would be the picture that instead showed the girl washing the mother. Near-misses on the pronoun sentences depicted a misinterpretation of the Binding Principles (i.e., a binding error [18]). For example in a sentence that read, "The mother washes her" the near-miss was a picture that showed the mother washing herself as opposed to the mother washing the girl (vice versa for the reflexive pronoun sentences).

It might be useful to think of the error analysis in terms of educated guesses, which would result in mostly near-misses, versus guessing at random which would result in a proportional mixture of near- and other-misses. Other-misses always depicted more gross departures from the given sentence, and depending on the sentence, included depictions of characters that were not mentioned, characters that represented gender-pronoun mismatches or by pictures that depicted a self-orienting action when non-reflection action is indicated (or vice versa).

**Hearing and nonverbal intelligence measures.** Measures of hearing ability and nonverbal intelligence (NVIQ) were obtained in session two, which took approximately 15 minutes to complete. Both deaf and hearing children also completed the NVIQ portion of session two. Pure-tone hearing thresholds were obtained at 500, 1000, 2000 and 4000 Hz using a standard audiometric procedure [31]. For the purpose of statistical analyses we computed an overall hearing threshold for each child by averaging across all four frequencies. We also averaged across the 500 and 1000 Hz levels, and the 2000 and 4000 Hz levels to obtain low and high frequency thresholds respectively. In our analyses, we operationalized hearing threshold as the lowest dB threshold in the better ear within each frequency range (overall, low, high). NVIQ was assessed using Form A of the Test of Nonverbal Intelligence, version 3 (TONI-3; [32]). This test was specifically designed to eliminate the confound of verbal ability in assessing intelligence, thus it was the ideal intelligence measure for our study. For some of the children, audiometric and TONI-3 scores were available on file at their school. In these cases, the existing scores were used instead, and the children were only assessed on session one (the language measures).

## Results

Our first analysis examined the overall relationship between ASL and English using a Pearson correlation between ASL ability (defined as the composite score on the three ASL tasks) and English reading ability (defined as accuracy on the sentence comprehension task). ASL composite scores positively correlated with average accuracy across the four sentence types, $r = .74$, $p < .001$. This initial finding provided justification for the remaining analyses, which examine the ASL/English relationship in finer detail with special attention paid to the relationship between ASL proficiency and English sentence comprehension.

Deaf children were divided into skilled and less-skilled signer groups (Table 1) using a median split on the ASL composite score. Use of a median split represented a data-driven approach to dividing group into two ability groups. While a median value conceptually divides a sample into two groups, here we obtained somewhat different samples sizes for the two groups due to several individuals' scores falling exactly at the median. We thus included individuals scoring on or above median in the skilled group, and individuals scoring below the median were placed in the less-skilled group. Groups did not differ on age, $t(49) = 0.99$, $p = .33$, or hearing threshold (low frequency threshold: $t(45) = 0.89$, $p = .38$; high frequency threshold: $t(43) = 0.51$, $p = .62$; overall threshold: $t(43) = 0.90$, $p = .38$). The group difference in NVIQ approached significance, $t(49) = 1.95$, $p = .06$; to guard against the possibility that this factor was confounding results, subsequent analyses used ANCOVAs with NVIQ included as the covariate.

Group accuracy on the sentence comprehension task (Figure 2) was compared using a two-way mixed ANCOVA for the effects of group (skilled, less-skilled) and sentence-type (active, passive, pronoun, reflexive pronoun). This revealed main effects of group, $F(1, 48) = 25.88$, $p < .001$, and sentence type, $F(3, 144) = 11.88$, $p < .001$, and a significant interaction, $F(3, 144) = 2.99$, $p < .05$. Post hoc tests revealed that skilled signers outperformed less-skilled signers on active, $F(1, 166) = 18.39$, $p < .001$, pronoun, $F(1, 166) = 13.58$, $p < .001$, and reflexive sentences, $F(1, 166) = 25.18$, $p < .001$, but not on passives, $F(1, 166) = 1.75$, $p = .19$.

Within groups, we examined performance on each sentence type using one-sample t-tests that compared accuracy rates to a chance level of .25. The skilled signers performed significantly above chance on active, $t(27) = 20.77$, $p < .001$, pronoun, $t(27) = 6.47$, $p < .001$, and reflexive pronoun sentences, $t(27) = 11.94$, $p < .001$, but not on the passive sentences, $t(27) = .28$, $p = .78$. The less-skilled group showed a different pattern, performing significantly above chance on actives, $t(22) = 5.25$, $p < .001$, and reflexive pronouns, $t(22) = 2.65$, $p < .05$, but not on pronouns, $t(22) = .625$, $p = .54$, or passive sentences, $t(22) = -2.01$, $p = .06$.

Further, we noted that the skilled group performed more accurately on actives than passives $t(27) = 9.83$, $p < .001$, and more accurately on the reflexives than pronouns $t(27) = 4.50$, $p < .001$. Likewise, the less-skilled signer group performed more accurately on actives than passives $t(22) = 4.36$, $p < .001$, however no accuracy difference existed between the reflexive pronouns and pronouns sentences in this group, $t(22) = 1.59$, $p = .13$.

We also compared the types of errors made on the two trial types (word order, pronoun binding) using two mixed ANCOVAs for the effects of group and error type (near-miss vs. other-miss; Figure 3, 4). On word order trials there was a main effect of group, $F(1, 48) = 17.58$, $p < .001$, and a group by error type interaction, $F(1, 48) = 10.89$, $p < .05$. There was no main effect of error type, $F(1,48) = .27$, *ns*. Post hoc tests revealed that signers in the less-skilled group made significantly more other-miss errors than skilled signers, $F(1, 97) = 24.15$, $p < .001$, on word order trials. No group difference was found with respect to near-miss errors, $F(1, 97) = .119$, *ns*. On pronoun binding trials there was a main effect of group, $F(1, 48) = 19.93$, $p < .001$, and a group by error type interaction, $F(1, 48) = 12.09$, $p < .01$. There was no main effect of error type, $F(1,48) = 1.40$, *ns*. Post hoc tests again revealed fewer other-miss errors in skilled signers, $F(1, 97) = 36.98$, $p < .001$. As above, no group difference was found with respect to the near-miss errors on the pronoun binding sentences, $F(1, 97) = .246$, *ns*.

### Hearing Children

As noted above, deaf children showed better performance on actives vs. passives, and reflexive pronouns vs. pronouns. To summarize, the signers in the high-skilled group performed above chance on all English sentences types except for passives, whereas the signers in the low-skilled group performed above chance on the actives and reflexive pronouns only. Of interest was how these patterns compared to the typical progression of syntactic development shown by first language hearing learners of English. Importantly, this group did not differ with respect to NVIQ from either of the signer groups, $F(2, 60) = 1.98$, $p = .15$. Hearing children showed higher accuracy rates for actives vs. passives, $t(9) = 4.30$, $p < .01$, and reflexive pronouns vs. pronouns, $t(9) = 11.00$, $p < .001$, and performed above chance on all four sentence types, all $p < .05$. They also made significantly more near-miss than other-miss errors on both word order and pronoun binding trials, $t(9) = 3.09$, $p < .05$; $t(9) = 2.586$, $p < .05$, similar to the pattern that what was found in the skilled signers group.

**Table 1.** Characteristics of the deaf signer groups.

| | Skilled signers (n = 28) | Less-skilled signers (n = 23) |
|---|---|---|
| Age (yy;mm) | 13;02 (2.70) | 12;04 (3.34) |
| TONI-3 percentile | 44.71 (26.60) | 30.30 (25.93) |
| ASL Composite (/58) | 43.07 (4.37) | 30.95 (4.96) |
| Vocabulary (/16) | 14.68 (1.19)* | 10.70 (1.69) |
| Sign Decision (/17) | 16.82 (0.39)* | 15.26 (1.81) |
| Story Comprehension (/25) | 11.57 (3.99)* | 5.00 (2.32) |
| Hearing threshold (dB) | 92.10 (7.57) | 89.91 (8.82) |
| low frequencies (dB) | 88.69 (10.41) | 86.14 (8.92) |
| high frequencies (dB) | 95.52 (7.87) | 93.97 (11.45) |
| Number of children born to deaf parents | 4 | 2 |

*Note.* All values represent group mean, with standard deviation in parentheses.
*Skilled group significantly greater than less-skilled group, $p<.05$.

## Discussion

It is well established that deaf individuals are generally delayed in learning to read English, performing on average at a fourth-grade level [10]. Interestingly, across a large number of studies ASL ability has been shown to be the single best predictor of their English reading ability [6]. In light of this, the contribution of the present study was to consider whether how this relationship specifically holds for processing of the syntactic structure of written English, and also whether such effects are best explained as the direct transfer of ASL knowledge to congruent structures in English.

As predicted, there was a strong association between ASL proficiency and English sentence comprehension, marked by differences in sentence reading performance in the skilled vs. lower-skilled group overall. The differences in performance were manifest as both higher accuracy scores across three of the four sentence types (excluding only passives), and as function of the types of errors being committed across trial types. One explanation for these results is that higher-achieving signers have improved single word knowledge of English, and that this alone leads to improved English sentence comprehension. The error analysis seems consistent with this to some extent: the lower-skilled signer group made significantly more other-miss errors, which reflected difficulty in recognizing individual words in a written sentence both on word order and pronoun binding trials. We interpret this as evidence of a general lexical identification difficulty in those

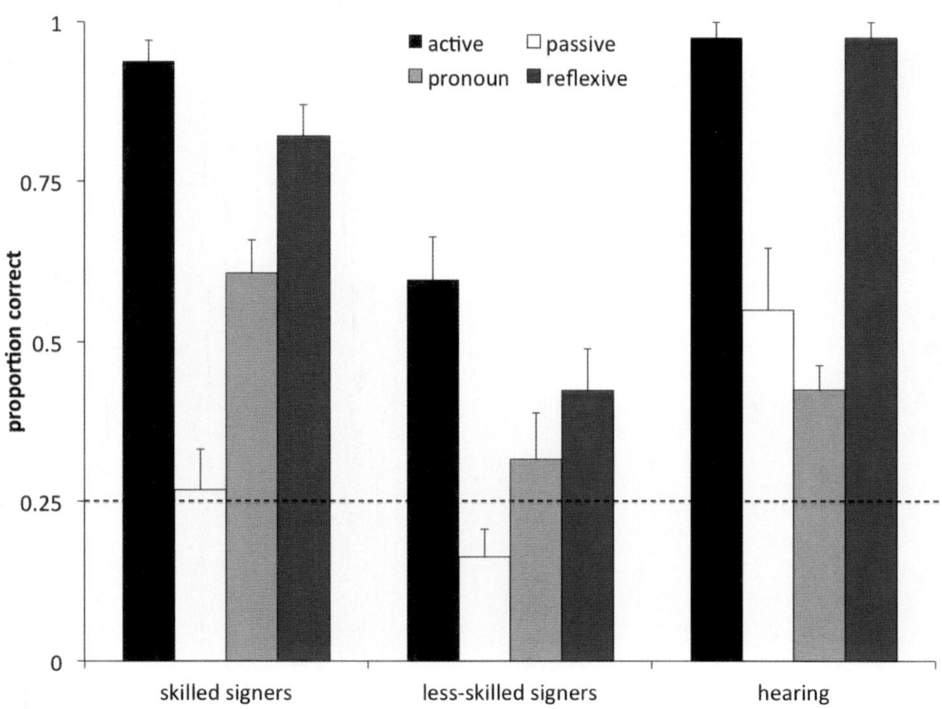


**Figure 2. Sentence comprehension scores by group.** Proportion of sentences correctly comprehended per group by sentence type. Chance performance equals .25. Error bars indicate standard errors; dotted line indicates chance performance of 25% correct.

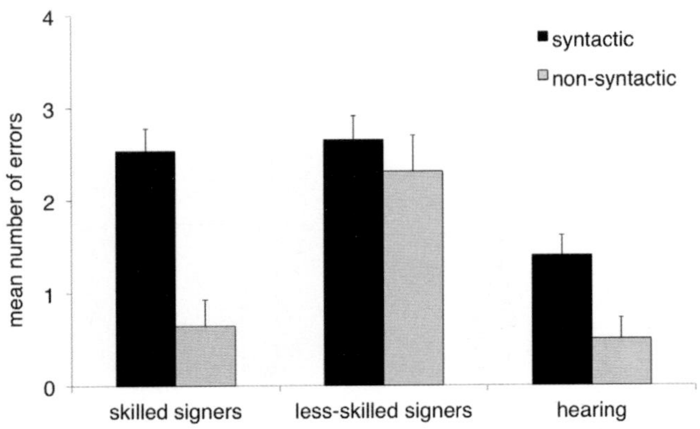


**Figure 3. Error analysis for sentence comprehension task – word order trials.** Mean number of near-miss and other-miss errors on the word order trials. Error bars indicate standard errors.

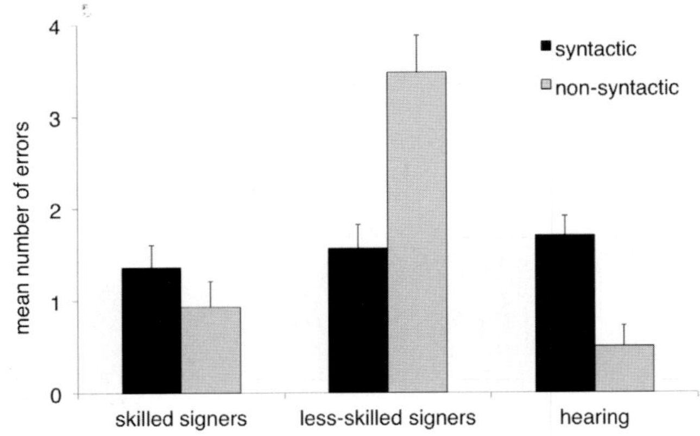


**Figure 4. Error analysis for sentence comprehension task – pronoun trials.** Mean number of near-miss and other-miss errors on pronoun binding trials. Error bars indicate standard errors.

individuals. This in itself might explain apparent difficulties in sentence comprehension in that group. Skilled signers on the other hand made proportionally more near-miss errors, indicating that they were able to revert to a strategy of matching written words to the pictures when a syntactic analysis failed. As such, it appears that even when syntax became an obstacle, these better signers were able to fall back on their lexical knowledge in order to select a response that more closely reflected the correct answer. That is, the near-miss errors reflect generally good single-word reading ability, even in the absence of difficulties processing the syntactic form of the sentence. From this we conclude that increased ASL ability supports single word reading.

Indeed, it may be that better ASL proficiency yields better English sentence comprehension reading because of direct cross-language transfer effects in which deaf readers use written English words to access their ASL translation equivalents [33]. On this view, improved ASL ability would predict better English reading ability through the formation of direct links between the two codes. Such a finding would be consistent with the predictions of Cummins' Linguistic Interdependence Hypothesis [14], which proposes that specific L1 knowledge potentiates L2 learning through a process of directly translating lexical features from one language to the next.

That said, the present dataset suggests single word reading ability cannot be the whole story, and thus the effects extend beyond a strict lexical mapping account. If increased ASL ability affects only the lexical level of English reading, then when difficulty of English syntax increases (as in non-reflexive pronouns and passives) the skilled signers should look like the lower-skilled signers in terms of accuracy, because in these sentence structures both lexical identification and syntactic comprehension are required in order to select the correct answer. On a pure mapping account, we should only expect to see increased comprehension in the skilled signer group on sentences where the mapping is transparent (as in actives and reflexives). In fact, we observed skilled signers had stronger performance on the pronoun sentences as well. This suggests that proficiency in ASL promotes the development of word-order knowledge that allows skilled signers to move beyond the one-to-one mapping of lexical items and syntactic structures of L1 to L2. Consistent with the Unified Competition Model our results indicate that L1 proficiency promotes both lexical and syntactic abilities in L2, even across sensory modalities (i.e., signed vs. written language).

That said, we did not find support for increased syntactic abilities on the passive sentences. We are not the first to report passive construction difficulties in young deaf signers [25]. One explanation for this is that deaf children receive very limited exposure to passive structures in English. Thus, while we argue that increased ASL ability relates to increased syntactic proficiency in second language learning, we concede that passives appear to be sufficiently difficult that they defy this explanation. On the other hand we also note that newer work examining sentence processing in deaf adults failed to identify significant differences in reading times for passive versus active sentences [34], suggesting that this represents a delay in development rather than a wholesale failure to master learn these English constructions.

We also examined how hearing children performed on the sentence comprehension task. These children showed the same pattern of performance as deaf individuals: actives were easier than passives, and reflexives were easier than pronouns, suggesting that similar constraints operate on how deaf and hearing children learn syntactic principles in English. Similarly, acquisition of English syntax in deaf readers does not appear to be qualitatively different from how it is learned in hearing readers, and is instead delayed to different extents, largely as a function of their sign ability. Note also that the error pattern of the hearing children resembled that of the skilled signers, but not the lower-skilled signers. This finding further highlights the idea that the skilled signers' English sentence comprehension ability more resembles that of normally hearing children.

Some limitations from the present study are worth mentioning. First, deaf participants were drawn from a relatively wide age band spanning early school years through adolescence. The age range is admittedly not optimal for studying questions of language and reading development given that that both abilities can improve significantly with age. However the population of individuals fitting the criteria for inclusion in this study in the southern/southwestern Ontario areas is already quite small, and additional participants are simply not available in this geographic region. Examining a smaller group of children within a narrower age band would thus have severely limited statistical power in this study. Instead, we chose to obtain the largest sample size possible, rather than limiting the pool of potential participants. This more inclusive strategy also maximized the range of ASL abilities, which was important given our interest in identifying individuals with relatively high vs. low proficiency in this regard. One possibility could have been to divide participants into separate age bands, although preliminary analyses suggested that the patterns of responses across age groups did not yield additional information beyond the typical increase in overall performance with age while limiting statistical power by increasing the number of factors being included in our analyses. Finally, we noted that our two ASL proficiency groups did not differ with respect to age, such that the age ranges were relatively stable across the two proficiency levels. This suggests our strategy of including a wide age range did not confound the findings observed in our study.

We also did not preclude children from the study on the basis of nonverbal difficulties. This raises the possibility that children performed more poorly than expected on certain tasks due to cognitive delays. We did observe a non-significant difference between the skilled and less-skilled signer groups in terms of nonverbal IQ scores. However, we noted that the observed sentence processing differences between groups persisted even when these scores were taken into account statistically using ANCOVAs. Thus, this factor alone seems unlikely to explain the differences we observed.

## Conclusions

We examined the relationship between ASL proficiency and English reading ability specifically with respect to how young deaf readers process written English sentences. We found significant differences between higher- and lower-proficiency signers on sentence comprehension accuracy for active, pronoun and reflexive pronoun sentences in favor of the skilled signers. We also found significant differences in the types of errors committed by each group. Together these findings indicate that the ability to extract lexical and syntactic information from written sentences increases as a function of sign ability. Note that this effect was maintained while holding NVIQ constant. We interpret these results as support for theories suggesting that L2 learning is influenced at both lexical and grammatical levels by L1, even across linguistic modalities. Specifically, ASL proficiency in young signers predicted both English word recognition and English syntactic comprehension abilities.

## Supporting Information

**File S1 Supporting appendices.**

## Acknowledgments

We thank Daphne Bavelier and Elizabeth Hirshorn for useful comments on an earlier version of this article. We also acknowledge Dr. Cathy Chovaz for her assistance developing the ASL materials and recruiting participants.

## Author Contributions

Conceived and designed the experiments: MFJ KA. Performed the experiments: KA. Analyzed the data: MFJ KA JH. Wrote the paper: KA MFJ JH.

## References

1. Beech JR, Harris M (1997) The prelingually deaf young reader: A case of reliance on direct lexical access? J Res Read 20: 105–121.
2. Transler C, Leybaert J, Gombert J (1999) Do deaf children use phonological syllables as reading units? J Deaf Stud Deaf Educ 4: 124–143.
3. Friesen DC, Joanisse MF (2012) Homophone effects in deaf readers: Evidence from lexical decision. Read Writ 25: 375–388.
4. Hanson VL, Fowler CA (1987) Phonological coding in word reading: Evidence from hearing and deaf readers. Mem Cognit 15: 199–207.
5. Nielsen DC, Luetke-Stahlman B (2002) Phonological awareness: One key to the reading proficiency of deaf children. Am Ann Deaf 147: 11–19.
6. Mayberry RI, del Giudice AA, Lieberman AM (2011) Reading achievement in relation to phonological coding and awareness in deaf readers: A meta-analysis. J Deaf Stud Deaf Educ 16: 164–188.
7. Strong M, Prinz P (1997) A study of the relationship between American Sign Language and English literacy. J Deaf Stud Deaf Educ 2: 37–46.
8. Padden C, Ramsey C (1998) Reading ability in signing deaf children. Top Lang Disord 18: 30–46.
9. Hoffmeister RJ (2000) A piece of the puzzle: ASL and reading comprehension in deaf children. In: Chamberlain C, Morford JP & Mayberry RI, editors. Language acquisition by eye.Mahwah, New Jersey: Lawrence Erlbaum Associates Inc.pp.143–163.
10. Goldin-Meadow S, Mayberry RI (2001) How do profoundly deaf children learn to read? Learn Disabil Res Pract 16: 222–229.
11. Mayberry RI, Lock E, Kazmi H (2002) Linguistic ability and early language exposure. Nature 417: 38.
12. Chamberlain C, Mayberry RI (2008) American Sign Language syntactic and narrative comprehension in skilled and less skilled readers: Bilingual and bimodal evidence for the linguistic basis of reading. Appl Psycholinguist: 29: 367–388.
13. Mayberry RI, Lock E (2003) Age constraints on first versus second language acquisition: Evidence for linguistic plasticity and epigenesis. Brain and Lang 87:369–383.
14. Cummins J (1979) Linguistic interdependence and the educational development of bilingual children. Rev Educ Res 49: 222–251.
15. MacWhinney B (2005) New directions in the competition model. In Tomasello M, Slobin DI, editors. Beyond Nature-Nurture Mahwah, New Jersey: Lawrence Erlbaum Associates, Publishers. pp. 79–110.
16. MacWhinney B, Bates E (1989) The crosslinguistic study of sentence processing. New York: Cambridge University Press.
17. Isenhath JO (1990) The linguistics of American Sign Language. Jefferson, NC: McFarland.
18. Chomsky N (1981) Lectures on government and binding: the Pisa lectures. Berlin: Mouton de Gruyter.
19. Deutsch W, Koster C, Koster J (1986) What can we learn from children's errors in understanding anaphora? Linguistics 24: 203–225.
20. Chien YC, Wexler K (1990) Children's knowledge of locality conditions in binding as evidence for the modularity of syntax and pragmatics. Lang Acq 1: 225–295.
21. van der Lely HKJ, Stollwerck L (1997) Binding theory and grammatical specific language impairment in children. Cognition 62: 245–290.
22. Chen Pichler D (2001) Word order variation and acquisition in American Sign Language. Doctoral Dissertation, University of Connecticut.
23. Janzen T, O'Dea B, Shaffer B (2001) The construal of events: Passives in American Sign Language. Sign Language Studies 1: 281–310.
24. Baldie BJ (1976) The acquisition of the passive voice. J Child Lang 3: 331–348.
25. Power DJ, Quigley SP (1973) Deaf children's acquisition of the passive voice. J Speech Lang Hear Res 16: 5–11.
26. Vasilyeva M, Huttenlocher J, Waterfall H (2006) Effects of language intervention on syntactic skill levels in preschoolers. Dev Psychol 42: 164–174.
27. Hoffmeister RJ (1999) American Sign Language Assessment Instrument (ASLAI) Boston University: Center for the Study of Communication & The Deaf.
28. Semel E, Wiig EH, Secord WA (1995) Clinical evaluation of language fundamentals 3 (CELF-3) San Antonio, TX: The Psychological Corporation.
29. Klima E, Bellugi U (1979) The signs of language. Cambridge, MA: Harvard University Press.
30. Wiederholt JL, Bryant BR (2001) Gray oral reading test, version 4. Pearson Education, Inc.
31. American National Standards Institute (2004) Methods for manual pure-tone threshold audiometry (ANSI S3.21-2004) New York: Author.
32. Brown L, Sherbenou RJ, Johnsen SK (1997) Test of nonverbal intelligence: A language free measure of cognitive ability. Austin, TX: Pro-Ed, An International Publisher.
33. Morford JP, Wilkinson E, Villwock A, Piñar P, Kroll JF (2011) When deaf signers read English: Do written words activate their sign translations? Cognition 118: 286–292.
34. Traxler MJ, Corina DO, Morford JP, Hafer S, Hoversten LJ (2014) Deaf readers' response to syntactic complexity: Evidence from self-paced reading. Mem Cognit 42: 97–111.

# Permissions

All chapters in this book were first published in PLOS ONE, by The Public Library of Science; hereby published with permission under the Creative Commons Attribution License or equivalent. Every chapter published in this book has been scrutinized by our experts. Their significance has been extensively debated. The topics covered herein carry significant findings which will fuel the growth of the discipline. They may even be implemented as practical applications or may be referred to as a beginning point for another development.

The contributors of this book come from diverse backgrounds, making this book a truly international effort. This book will bring forth new frontiers with its revolutionizing research information and detailed analysis of the nascent developments around the world.

We would like to thank all the contributing authors for lending their expertise to make the book truly unique. They have played a crucial role in the development of this book. Without their invaluable contributions this book wouldn't have been possible. They have made vital efforts to compile up to date information on the varied aspects of this subject to make this book a valuable addition to the collection of many professionals and students.

This book was conceptualized with the vision of imparting up-to-date information and advanced data in this field. To ensure the same, a matchless editorial board was set up. Every individual on the board went through rigorous rounds of assessment to prove their worth. After which they invested a large part of their time researching and compiling the most relevant data for our readers.

The editorial board has been involved in producing this book since its inception. They have spent rigorous hours researching and exploring the diverse topics which have resulted in the successful publishing of this book. They have passed on their knowledge of decades through this book. To expedite this challenging task, the publisher supported the team at every step. A small team of assistant editors was also appointed to further simplify the editing procedure and attain best results for the readers.

Apart from the editorial board, the designing team has also invested a significant amount of their time in understanding the subject and creating the most relevant covers. They scrutinized every image to scout for the most suitable representation of the subject and create an appropriate cover for the book.

The publishing team has been an ardent support to the editorial, designing and production team. Their endless efforts to recruit the best for this project, has resulted in the accomplishment of this book. They are a veteran in the field of academics and their pool of knowledge is as vast as their experience in printing. Their expertise and guidance has proved useful at every step. Their uncompromising quality standards have made this book an exceptional effort. Their encouragement from time to time has been an inspiration for everyone.

The publisher and the editorial board hope that this book will prove to be a valuable piece of knowledge for researchers, students, practitioners and scholars across the globe.

# List of Contributors

**Yoon-Hyeong Choi**
Department of Preventive Medicine, Gachon University Graduate School of Medicine, Incheon, Korea

**KyooSang Kim**
Occupational Safety and Health Research Institute, Korea Occupational Safety and Health Agency, Incheon, Korea

**Rose Stamp, Jordan Fenlon, Ramas Rentelis, Bencie Woll and Kearsy Cormier**
Deafness, Cognition and Language Research Centre (DCAL), University College London, London, United Kingdom

**Adam Schembri**
Linguistics program and The Centre for Research on Language Diversity, La Trobe University, Melbourne, Australia

**Sobia Shafique, Humaira Ayub, Muhammad Ajmal, Syed Tahir A. Shah, Alamdar Hussain and Maleeha Azam**
COMSATS Institute of Information Technology, Park Road, Islamabad, Pakistan

**Raheel Qamar**
COMSATS Institute of Information Technology, Park Road, Islamabad, Pakistan
Al-Nafees Medical College and Hospital, Isra University, Islamabad, Pakistan

**Saima Siddiqi, Atika Mansoor and Kehkashan Mazhar**
Institute of Biomedical and Genetic Engineering (IBGE), Islamabad, Pakistan

**Margit Schraders, Jaap Oostrik and Celia Zazo Seco**
Department of Otorhinolaryngology, Hearing and Genes, Radboud University Medical Center, Nijmegen, The Netherlands
Nijmegen Centre for Molecular Life Sciences, Radboud University Medical Center, Nijmegen, The Netherlands
Donders Institute for Brain, Cognition and Behaviour, Radboud University Medical Center, Nijmegen, The Netherlands

**Hannie Kremer**
Department of Otorhinolaryngology, Hearing and Genes, Radboud University Medical Center, Nijmegen, The Netherlands
Nijmegen Centre for Molecular Life Sciences, Radboud University Medical Center, Nijmegen, The Netherlands
Donders Institute for Brain, Cognition and Behaviour, Radboud University Medical Center, Nijmegen, The Netherlands
Department of Human Genetics, Radboud university medical center, Nijmegen, The Netherlands

**Ammad Bilal**
Simon Fraser University, Vancouver, British Colombia, Canada

**Tim M. Strom**
Institute of Human Genetics, Helmholtz Zentrum München, German Research Center for Environmental Health, Neuherberg, Germany

**Alejandro Lopez Valdes and Richard B. Reilly**
Trinity Centre for Bioengineering, Trinity College, Dublin, Ireland

**Myles Mc Laughlin**
Trinity Centre for Bioengineering, Trinity College, Dublin, Ireland
Hearing and Speech Laboratory, University of California Irvine, Irvine, California, United States of America

**Fan-Gang Zeng**
Hearing and Speech Laboratory, University of California Irvine, Irvine, California, United States of America

**Laura Viani, Peter Walshe and Jaclyn Smith**
National Cochlear Implant Programme, Beaumont Hospital, Dublin, Ireland

**Hidekane Yoshimura, Shin-ya Nishio and Shin-ichi Usami**
Department of Otorhinolaryngology, Shinshu University School of Medicine, Matsumoto, Nagano, Japan

**Satoshi Iwasaki**
Department of Hearing Implant Sciences, Shinshu University School of Medicine, Matsumoto, Nagano, Japan
Department of Otorhinolaryngology, International University of Health and Welfare, Mita Hospital, Minatoku, Tokyo, Japan

**Kozo Kumakawa**
Department of Otolaryngology, Okinaka Memorial Institute for Medical Research, Toranomon Hospital, Minatoku, Tokyo, Japan

**Tetsuya Tono**
Department of Otorhinolaryngology-Head and Neck Surgery, Miyazaki University School of Medicine, Miyazaki, Miyazaki, Japan

**Yumiko Kobayashi and Hiroaki Sato**
Department of Otolaryngology-Head and Neck Surgery, Iwate Medical University, Morioka, Iwate, Japan

**Kyoko Nagai**
Department of Otolaryngology-Head and Neck Surgery, Gunma University Graduate School of Medicine, Maebashi, Gunma, Japan

**Kotaro Ishikawa**
Department of Otolaryngology, National Rehabilitation Center for Persons with Disabilities, Tokorozawa, Saitama, Japan

**Tetsuo Ikezono**
Department of Otolaryngology, Saitama Medical University, Moroyama, Saitama, Japan

**Yasushi Naito**
Department of Otolaryngology, Kobe City Medical Center General Hospital, Kobe, Hyougo, Japan

**Kunihiro Fukushima**
Department of Otorhinolaryngology, Head and Neck Surgery, Okayama University Postgraduate School of Medicine, Dentistry and Pharmaceutical Science, Okayama, Okayama, Japan

**Chie Oshikawa**
Department of Otorhinolaryngology, Graduate School of Medical Sciences, Kyushu University, Fukuoka, Fukuoka, Japan

**Takashi Kimitsuki**
Department of Otorhinolaryngology, Kyushu Central Hospital, Fukuoka, Fukuoka, Japan

**Hiroshi Nakanishi**
Department of Otorhinolaryngology, Hamamatsu University School of Medicine, Hamamatsu, Shizuoka, Japan

**Weining Rong, Yani Liu, Shaoping Ha, Wenzhou Liu and Xunlun Sheng**
Ningxia Eye Hospital, Ningxia People's Hospital, Ningxia, China

**Xiaoxing Liu**
Department of Ophthalmology, The First Affiliated Hospital of Nanjing Medical University, State Key Laboratory of Reproductive Medicine, Nanjing, China

**Xue Chen**
Department of Ophthalmology, The First Affiliated Hospital of Nanjing Medical University, State Key Laboratory of Reproductive Medicine, Nanjing, China
Department of Ophthalmology and Visual Sciences, The Chinese University of Hong Kong, Hong Kong, China

**Chen Zhao**
Department of Ophthalmology, The First Affiliated Hospital of Nanjing Medical University, State Key Laboratory of Reproductive Medicine, Nanjing, China
State Key Laboratory of Ophthalmology, Zhongshan Ophthalmic Center, Sun Yat Sen University, Guangzhou, China

**Kanxing Zhao**
Tianjin Medical University, Tianjin Eye Hospital, Tianjin Key Laboratory of Ophthalmology and Visual Science, Tianjin, China

**Xiaoli Kang**
Department of Ophthalmology, Xinhua Hospital, Shanghai Jiao Tong University School of Medicine, Shanghai, China

**Melissa A. Calton, Dasom Lee, Srividya Sundaresan, Diana Mendus, Rose Leu, Felix Wangsawihardja and Mirna Mustapha**
Department of Otolaryngology-Head and Neck Surgery, Stanford University, Stanford, California, United States of America

**Kenneth R. Johnson**
The Jackson Laboratory, Bar Harbor, Maine, United States of America

**Julia Campbell**
University of Colorado at Boulder, Department of Speech, Language and Hearing Sciences, Boulder, Colorado, United States of America

**Anu Sharma**
University of Colorado at Boulder, Department of Speech, Language and Hearing Sciences, Boulder, Colorado, United States of America
University of Colorado at Boulder, Institute of Cognitive Science, Boulder, Colorado, United States of America

**Ying-Yee Kong**
Department of Speech Language Pathology and Audiology, Northeastern University, Boston, Massachusetts, United States of America
Bioengineering Program, Northeastern University, Boston, Massachusetts, United States of America

**Ala Mullangi**
Bioengineering Program, Northeastern University, Boston, Massachusetts, United States of America

**Kostas Kokkinakis**
Department of Speech-Language-Hearing, University of Kansas, Lawrence, Kansas, United States of America

**Zhiqiang Hong, Jian Shi and Cheng Du**
Kunshan Municipal Center for Disease Prevention and Control, Kunshan, China

**Huanxi Shen**
Kunshan Municipal Center for Disease Prevention and Control, Kunshan, China
Department of Environmental Genomics, Jiangsu Key Laboratory of Cancer Biomarkers, Prevention and Treatment, Cancer Center, Nanjing Medical University, Nanjing, China

**Jinglian Cao, Lu Ding and Baoli Zhu**
Department of Environmental Genomics, Jiangsu Key Laboratory of Cancer Biomarkers, Prevention and Treatment, Cancer Center, Nanjing Medical University, Nanjing, China
Institute of Occupational Disease Prevention, Jiangsu Provincial Center for Disease Prevention and Control, Nanjing, China

**Zhengdong Zhang**
Department of Environmental Genomics, Jiangsu Key Laboratory of Cancer Biomarkers, Prevention and Treatment, Cancer Center, Nanjing Medical University, Nanjing, China
Department of Genetic Toxicology, the Key Laboratory of Modern Toxicology of Ministry of Education, School of Public Health, Nanjing Medical University, Nanjing, China

**Hengdong Zhang**
Institute of Occupational Disease Prevention, Jiangsu Provincial Center for Disease Prevention and Control, Nanjing, China

**Kai Liu**
Department of Disease Prevention and Control of Yizheng Hospital, Drum Tower Hospital Group of Nanjing, Yizheng, China

**Qian Li**
The First People's Hospital of Kunshan, Kunshan, China

**Jacqueline M. Ogier**
Murdoch Childrens Research Institute, Parkville, Victoria, Australia

**Marina R. Carpinelli**
Murdoch Childrens Research Institute, Parkville, Victoria, Australia
The HEARing Cooperative Research Centre, Parkville, Victoria, Australia
Walter and Eliza Hall Institute of Medical Research, Parkville, Victoria, Australia
Department of Medical Biology, University of Melbourne, Parkville, Victoria, Australia

**Rachel A. Burt**
Murdoch Childrens Research Institute, Parkville, Victoria, Australia
The HEARing Cooperative Research Centre, Parkville, Victoria, Australia
Walter and Eliza Hall Institute of Medical Research, Parkville, Victoria, Australia
Department of Genetics, University of Melbourne, Parkville, Victoria, Australia
Department of Paediatrics, University of Melbourne, Parkville, Victoria, Australia

**Benjamin T. Kile**
Walter and Eliza Hall Institute of Medical Research, Parkville, Victoria, Australia
Department of Medical Biology, University of Melbourne, Parkville, Victoria, Australia
Department of Genetics, University of Melbourne, Parkville, Victoria, Australia

**Benedicta D. Arhatari**
ARC Centre of Excellence for Coherent X-ray Science, Department of Physics, La Trobe University, Bundoora, Victoria, Australia

**R. C. Andrew Symons**
Department of Ophthalmology, Royal Melbourne Hospital, Parkville, Victoria, Australia

**Karl-Heinz Dyballa**
Department of Otolaryngology, Medical University Hannover, Hannover, Germany

**Andreas Buechner and Thomas Lenarz**
Cluster of Excellence hearing4all, Medical University Hannover, Hannover, Germany

**Phillipp Hehrmann and Stefan Fredelake**
Advanced Bionics GmbH, European Research Center, Hannover, Germany

**Enrico Lopriore**
Division of Neonatology, Department of Pediatrics, Leiden University Medical Center, Leiden, The Netherlands

**Martin Offringa**
Child Health Evaluative Sciences, The Hospital for Sick Children Research Institute, University of Toronto, Toronto, Canada

**Selma A. J. Ruiter**
Department of Orthopedagogy, University of Groningen, Groningen, The Netherlands

**Paul F. M. Krabbe and Elise H. Quik**
Department of Epidemiology, University of Groningen, University Medical Center Groningen, Groningen, The Netherlands

**Letty van Toledo-Eppinga, Debbie H. G. M. Nuytemans and Aleid G. van Wassenaer-Leemhuis**
Department of Neonatology, Emma Children's Hospital Academic Medical Center, Amsterdam, The Netherlands

**Manon J. N. Benders and Karen K. M. Korbeeck-van Hof**
Department of Neonatology, Wilhelmina Children's Hospital, University Medical Center Utrecht, Utrecht, The Netherlands

**Richard A. van Lingen and Liesbeth J. M. Groot Jebbink**
Princess Amalia Department of Pediatrics, Department of Neonatology, Isala, Zwolle, The Netherlands

**Djien Liem and Petri Mansvelt**
Division of Neonatology, Department of Pediatrics, UMC St. Radboud Nijmegen, Nijmegen, The Netherlands

**Jan Buijs**
Department of Pediatrics, Máxima Medical Center, Veldhoven, The Netherlands

**Paul Govaert and Ineke van Vliet**
Erasmus MC, Sophia Children's Hospital, Rotterdam, The Netherlands

**Twan L. M. Mulder and Cecile Wolfs**
Department of Pediatrics, Maastricht University Medical Center, GROW-School for Oncology and Developmental Biology, Maastricht, The Netherlands

**Willem P. F. Fetter and Celeste Laarman**
Department of Pediatrics, VU University Medical Center, Amsterdam, The Netherlands

**Simon Maguire, Jeanne Estabel, Neil Ingham, Selina Pearson, Edward Ryder, Damian M. Carragher, James Bussell, Thomas M. Keane, David J. Adams, Christopher J. Lelliott, Ramiro Ramírez-Solis, Natasha A. Karp, Karen P. Steel, Jacqueline K. White and Anna-Karin Gerdin**
Wellcome Trust Sanger Institute, Wellcome Trust Genome Campus, Hinxton, Cambridgeshire, United Kingdom

**Nicolas Walker**
Wellcome Trust Sanger Institute, Wellcome Trust Genome Campus, Hinxton, Cambridgeshire, United Kingdom
Department of Physiology, Development and Neuroscience, University of Cambridge, Cambridge, Cambridgeshire, United Kingdom

**Wai- In Chan**
Department of Haematology, Cambridge Institute for Medical Research, Cambridge, Cambridgeshire, United Kingdom

**Cheryl L. Scudamore**
Department of Pathology and Infectious Diseases, Royal Veterinary College, Hatfield, Hertfordshire, United Kingdom

**Elena Nava, Davide Bottari, Agnes Villwock, Ineke Fengler and Brigitte Röder**
University of Hamburg, Biological Psychology and Neuropsychology, Hamburg, Germany

**Andreas Büchner and Thomas Lenarz**
German Hearing Centre, Medical Clinic Hannover, Hannover, Germany

**Xingchao Wang, Zhenmin Wang, Kai Zhang and Zhixian Gao**
Department of Neurosurgery, Beijing Tiantan Hospital, Capital Medical University, Beijing, China

**Pinan Liu**
Department of Neurosurgery, Beijing Tiantan Hospital, Capital Medical University, Beijing, China
Department of Neural reconstruction, Beijing Neurosurgery Institute, Capital Medical University, Beijing, China

**Yang Fan and Jianqiao Ge and Qihong Zou**
MRI Research Center and Beijing City Key Lab for Medical Physics and Engineering, Peking University, Beijing, China

**Jia-Hong Gao**
MRI Research Center and Beijing City Key Lab for Medical Physics and Engineering, Peking University, Beijing, China
McGovern Institute for Brain Research, Peking University, Beijing, China

**Fu Zhao**
Department of Neural reconstruction, Beijing Neurosurgery Institute, Capital Medical University, Beijing, China

**Yihong Yang**
Neuroimaging Research Branch, National Institute on Drug Abuse, National Institutes of Health, Baltimore, Maryland, United States of America

**Jin Fan**
Department of Psychology, Queens College, The City University of New York, Flushing, New York, United States of America
Department of Psychiatry, Mount Sinai School of Medicine, New York, New York, United States of America
Friedman Brain Institute, Mount Sinai School of Medicine, New York, New York, United States of America
Fishberg Department of Neuroscience, Mount Sinai School of Medicine, New York, New York, United States of America

**Yoshinobu Kidokoro, Keiko Karasawa, Katsuhisa Ikeda and Kazusaku Kamiya**
Juntendo University Faculty of Medicine, Department of Otorhinolaryngology, Tokyo, Japan
Osamu Minowa
BioResource Center, Institute of Physical and Chemical Research (RIKEN), Tsukuba, Japan

**Tetsuo Noda**
BioResource Center, Institute of Physical and Chemical Research (RIKEN), Tsukuba, Japan
Department of Cell Biology, Japanese Foundation for Cancer Research, Cancer Institute, Tokyo, Japan

**Yoshinobu Sugitani**
Department of Cell Biology, Japanese Foundation for Cancer Research, Cancer Institute, Tokyo, Japan

**Douglas E. H. Hartley**
NIHR National Biomedical Research Unit in Hearing, Ropewalk House, Nottingham, United Kingdom
Department of Otolaryngology, School of Clinical Sciences, Nottingham University, Nottingham, United Kingdom
Medical Research Council Institute of Hearing Research, University Park, Nottingham, United Kingdom
Department of Physiology, Anatomy and Genetics, University of Oxford, Oxford, United Kingdom

**Amal Isaiah**
Department of Physiology, Anatomy and Genetics, University of Oxford, Oxford, United Kingdom

**Kimie Matsunaga, Katsuya Tanabe, Hiroshi Inoue, Shigeru Okuya, Yasuharu Ohta, Masaru Akiyama, Akihiko Taguchi, Yukari Kora and Yukio Tanizawa**
Division of Endocrinology, Metabolism, Hematological Science and Therapeutics, Yamaguchi University Graduate School of Medicine, Ube, Yamaguchi, Japan

**Naoko Okayama**
Division of Laboratory Yamaguchi University Hospital, Ube, Yamaguchi, Japan

**Yuichiro Yamada**
Department of Endocrinology, Diabetes, Geriatric Medicine, Akita University Graduate School of Medicine, Akita, Japan

**Yasuhiko Wada**
Department of Health and Nutrition, Kochi University, Kochi, Kochi Japan

**Shin Amemiya**
Department of Pediatrics, Saitama Medical University, Moroyama, Saitama, Japan

**Shigetaka Sugihara**
Department of Pediatrics, Tokyo Women's Medical University Medical Center East, Tokyo, Japan

**Yuzo Nakao**
Division of Ophthalmology, Kinki University Sakai Hospital, Sakai, Osaka, Japan

**Yoshitomo Oka**
Division of Molecular Metabolism and Diabetes, Tohoku University Graduate School of medicine, Sendai, Miyagi, Japan

**Grace Savoy-Burke and Diana Pratt**
Department of Ophthalmology, University of Rochester Medical Center, Rochester, New York, United States of America

**Wei Pan and Amy E. Kiernan**
Department of Ophthalmology, University of Rochester Medical Center, Rochester, New York, United States of America
Department of Biomedical Genetics, University of Rochester Medical Center, Rochester, New York, United States of America

**Lin Gan**
Department of Ophthalmology, University of Rochester Medical Center, Rochester, New York, United States of America
Department of Neurobiology and Anatomy, University of Rochester Medical Center, Rochester, New York, United States of America

**Jianwen Que**
Department of Biomedical Genetics, University of Rochester Medical Center, Rochester, New York, United States of America

**Felicia A. Gilels and Patricia M. White**
Department of Neurobiology and Anatomy, University of Rochester Medical Center, Rochester, New York, United States of America

**Hongyang Wang, Yali Zhao, Yun Gao, Qiong Liu, Dayong Wang, Qian Li, Lan Lan, Na Li, Jing Guan, Zifang Yin, Bing Han, Feifan Zhao, Liang Zong, Wenping Xiong, Lan Yu and Qiuju Wang**
Institute of Otolaryngology, Chinese PLA General Hospital, Medical School of Chinese PLA, Beijing, China

**Yuting Yi, Lijie Song, Xin Yi and Ling Yang**
BGI-Tianjin, Tianjin, China

**Christine Petit**
Unité de Génétique et Physiologie de l'Audition, Institut Pasteur, Paris, France
UMRS 1120, Institut National de la Santé et de la Recherche Me´dicale (INSERM), Paris, France,
Université Pierre et Marie Curie (Paris VI), Paris, France
Collège de France, Paris, France

**Yuan Zhou, Weijing Wu, Zian Xiao, Yuyuan Liu, Jia Liu and Dinghua Xie**
Department of Otolaryngology-Head and Neck Surgery, Institute of Otology, the Second Xiangya Hospital, Central South University, Changsha, Hunan, China

**Jie Qing and Xue Zhong Liu**
Department of Otolaryngology-Head and Neck Surgery, Institute of Otology, the Second Xiangya Hospital, Central South University, Changsha, Hunan, China
Departments of Otolaryngology-Head and Neck Surgery, Leonard M. Miller School of Medicine, University of Miami, Miami, Florida, United States of America

**Denise Yan, Qiong Liu and Lilin Du**
Departments of Otolaryngology-Head and Neck Surgery, Leonard M. Miller School of Medicine, University of Miami, Miami, Florida, United States of America

**Hala Al Taher**
National Institute for Health Research Nottingham Hearing Biomedical Research Unit, Nottingham, United Kingdom

**Derek J. Hoare, Abby McCormack, Magdalena Sereda, Sandra Smith and Deborah A. Hall**
Otology and Hearing group, Division of Clinical Neuroscience, School of Medicine, University of Nottingham, Nottingham, United Kingdom

**Nicolas Van Labeke and Mike Sharples**
Institute of Educational Technology, The Open University, Milton Keynes, United Kingdom

**Victoria L. Kowalkowski**
Medical Research Council Institute of Hearing Research, Nottingham, United Kingdom

**Erin E. Baldwin**
Department of Psychiatry and Biobehavioral Sciences, University of California Los Angeles, Los Angeles, California, United States of America

**Christina G. S. Palmer**
Department of Psychiatry and Biobehavioral Sciences, University of California Los Angeles, Los Angeles, California, United States of America

Department of Human Genetics, University of California Los Angeles, Los Angeles, California, United States of America
Institute for Society and Genetics, University of California Los Angeles, Los Angeles, California, United States of America

**Janet S. Sinsheimer**
Department of Human Genetics, University of California Los Angeles, Los Angeles, California, United States of America
Institute for Society and Genetics, University of California Los Angeles, Los Angeles, California, United States of America
Departments of Biomathematics and Biostatistics, University of California Los Angeles, Los Angeles, California, United States of America

**Patrick Boudreault**
Department of Deaf Studies, California State University Northridge, Northridge, California, United States of America

**Elodie Chiarovano and Pierre-Paul Vidal**
CESEM - CNRS UMR 8194 - Université Paris Descartes, Centre Universitaire des Saints-Pères, Paris, France

**Catherine de Waele**
CESEM - CNRS UMR 8194 - Université Paris Descartes, Centre Universitaire des Saints-Pères, Paris, France
ENT Department - Salpêtrière Hospital, Paris, France

**Cynthia Darlington**
Department of Pharmacology and Toxicology, University of Otago Medical School, Dunedin, New Zealand

**Georges Lamas**
ENT Department - Salpêtrière Hospital, Paris, France

**Brianna O. Flynn**
Bionics Institute, East Melbourne, Victoria, Australia

**Patrick J. Atkinson**
Bionics Institute, East Melbourne, Victoria, Australia
Department of Otolaryngology, University of Melbourne, East Melbourne, Victoria, Australia

**Rachael T. Richardson and Andrew K. Wise**
Bionics Institute, East Melbourne, Victoria, Australia
Department of Otolaryngology, University of Melbourne, East Melbourne, Victoria, Australia
Department of Medical Bionics, University of Melbourne, East Melbourne, Victoria, Australia

**Bryony A. Nayagam**
Bionics Institute, East Melbourne, Victoria, Australia
Department of Otolaryngology, University of Melbourne, East Melbourne, Victoria, Australia
Department of Audiology and Speech Pathology, University of Melbourne, Parkville, Victoria, Australia

**Qian Zhang, Huizhan Liu, Garrett A. Soukup and David Z. Z. He**
Department of Biomedical Sciences, Creighton University School of Medicine, Omaha, Nebraska, United States of America

**Kathy N. Andrew, Jennifer Hoshooley and Marc F. Joanisse**
Department of Psychology and Brain and Mind Institute, The University of Western Ontario, London, Ontario, Canada

# Index